Benson and Pernoll's

Handbook
of *Obstetrics*
& Gynecology

Ninth Edition

Ralph C. Benson, M.D.
Professor Emeritus
Department of Obstetrics and Gynecology
Oregon Health Sciences University
Portland, Oregon

Martin L. Pernoll, M.D.
Chairman
Obstetrics and Gynecology
MacGregor Medical Associates
Houston, Texas

McGraw-Hill, Inc.
Health Professions Division
New York · St. Louis · San Francisco · Auckland · Bogotá · Caracas
Lisbon · London · Madrid · Mexico City · Milan · Montreal · New Delhi
Paris · San Juan · Singapore · Sidney · Tokyo · Toronto

BENSON AND PERNOLL'S HANDBOOK OF OBSTETRICS AND GYNECOLOGY, Ninth Edition

1 2 3 4 5 6 7 8 9 0 DOCDOC 9 9 8 7 6 5 4 3

ISBN 0-07-105405-7

ISSN 1070-731X

The editors were Gail Gavert and Patricia M. Bolger.
The production supervisor was Clara B. Stanley.
The indexer was Irving Condé Tullar.
R.R. Donnelley & Sons was printer and binder.

The following illustrations from Benson, HANDBOOK OF OBSTETRICS AND GYNECOLOGY, Eighth Edition, are reproduced with the kind permission of Appleton & Lange, Norwalk, CT: Figures 2-2, 2-3, 2-6, 20-1, and 29-1.

Special thanks are extended to Laurel V. Schaubert of Biomed Arts Associates, Inc., San Francisco, for her patience and help with the art program.

Contents

Preface

The ninth edition of this text, while still evolving, has been so totally rewritten that it is essentially a new book. The new size, cover, and extraordinary amount of new material suggest the transition of both the book and the field; while the retention of classic and timeless material from previous editions, the use of some of the ageless illustrations, and the title reflect the book's rich heritage.

This edition includes newer aspects of the diagnosis and treatment of genetic abnormalities, hormonal aberrations, obstetric complications, sexually transmitted diseases, and gynecologic neoplasia. Over half of the chapters are new, including The Female Patient, Development and Maldevelopment, Maternal Physiologic Adjustments to Pregnancy, High-Risk Pregnancy, The Infant, Early Pregnancy Complications, Late Pregnancy Complications, Operative Obstetrics, Sexually Transmitted Diseases, Menstrual Abnormalities and Complications, Contraception, The Nonreproductive Years, Endometriosis and Adenomyosis, Infertility and Related Issues, Gynecologic Procedures and Surgery, and Sexual Assault. The remaining chapters have been extensively revised, reorganized, and infused with new material. Uniting the new and previous portions of the book is the overall philosophy of previous editions: Present material that is timely, practical, and clinically useful. While this handbook is not a substitute for a primary textbook, it does contain the essentials of diagnosis and treatment for obstetric and gynecologic disorders. Procedures and medications (with dosages and routes of administration, together with alternatives) are presented, but remember that the choice is rarely inclusive or absolute.

We would like to dedicate this edition to our wives and to our readers.

Jean B. Benson, R.N., wife of Dr. Benson, died of endometrial carcinoma during preparations of this book. She was a warm, compassionate health care provider, a matchless wife, and a loving, devoted mother. For us and so many others, her life and untimely death make the need for correct diagnosis and effective treatment of gynecologic cancer especially poignant and important.

Marcia J.B. Pernoll, M.D., was meticulous in her critique and provided thoughtful as well as painstaking proofreading of the manuscript. Her perspectives as a neonatologist were only slightly less valuable than the woman's perspective she added to all the text.

The readers are truly responsible for the existence of this handbook. Their extraordinary support of its predecessor and their continued demand for another edition led us through three publishers, innumerable editors, and several years of work. We thank you and hope the effort justifies your continued confidence.

Martin L. Pernoll, M.D.
Ralph C. Benson, M.D.

Benson and Pernoll's

Handbook
  of **Obstetrics**
       &
  Gynecology

Chapter 1

The Female Patient

Each female patient presents a unique set of circumstances, beliefs, and expectations. Her sexual and reproductive experiences and organ function are quite individual. She may be fearful of the gynecologic examination or may be uncomfortable confiding things that she considers private or embarrassing. Alternatively, she may be totally matter of fact about her body and its problems. Occasionally, a patient may behave in an overtly sexual manner toward the physician, making him or her uncomfortable. Each patient at every visit is a whole person. She should not be regarded as an assemblage of parts, some of which are more interesting—pregnant or more apt to become cystic or cancerous—than others.

To assist in establishing rapport early in the doctor–patient relationship, ascertain how she prefers to be addressed. Some women prefer the use of their first name, whereas others prefer to be addressed using the formal salutation of Miss, Ms., or Mrs. Make a notation of her preference, since she will recall the inquiry and expect her response to be remembered.

In addition to possessing competence and skill, the care provider must be able to instill confidence about the privacy of all discussions. Above all, the patient must sense that medical personnel truly care about her. A major step toward achieving this goal during the initial visit is to obtain the history in a quiet office with no sense of haste and with the patient fully clothed. Information not readily volunteered early may be disclosed when the patient becomes more comfortable as the interview progresses in a nonjudgmental fashion. Review pertinent episodes in her past medical history, family history, social history, and the review of systems, perhaps using a standardized questionnaire completed by the patient before seeing the care provider. Focusing on details of the patient's concern early in the process may be helpful, since leaving the genitourinary system discussion until last may cause her to believe that you are avoiding her problem. Information about the number of pregnancies, deliveries, abortions, contraception, sexually transmitted diseases, drug usage, sexual practices, and marital status is essential. Current medications and any allergies should be prominent in the review of past history. Ascertain whether or not she has a family doctor, since the physician providing reproductive care may be the only one to examine the patient routinely and must, therefore, provide primary care.

The patient's answers to personal questions may not coincide with the caregiver's personal moral standards, religious beliefs, sexual practices, or experience. However, he or she must not judge but assist with the patient's problems within her frame of reference. Nonetheless, do not neglect to give information about safe sexual practices, proper therapy, and potential consequences of her or her partner's actions. Occasionally, one must stress that certain behaviors may affect not only the patient herself but also her offspring (e.g., drug use, infection). The caregiver must be prepared to consider marital difficulties, sexual dysfunction, or AIDS.

The intitial examination should be a general physical examination, including a breast examination and the gynecologic examination. If the patient is not performing breast self-examination regularly and properly, plans should be made for her to receive instruction in the correct method.

Arrange the examining room to reassure the patient that her privacy is not being invaded via the doors or windows. For example, even the view of a beautiful garden can be distressing to the patient who fears that a gardener may suddenly appear during the examination.

The patient should be undressed completely and draped for examination. Sensitivity to the patient mandates the she not be placed in the dorsal lithotomy position to await the caregiver's arrival. This position may soon become uncomfortable and may leave her feeling vulnerable.

When performing the pelvic examination, have a female nurse or attendant present, if possible, for assistance and to provide a measure of comfort and reassurance to the patient. Explain the procedure before performing any maneuver, and give advance warning of any procedure that may be uncomfortable or even painful. Use instruments deftly. Warn the patient that you will be doing a vaginal or rectal examination before insertion of fingers or instruments. Warming the hands and instruments is a small act that indicates interest in the patient's comfort.

The teenage patient responds to open, honest dialogue. Parent(s), if present, should be asked to wait in the reception room unless the patient (not the parent) insists otherwise. It may be difficult to obtain an accurate history from the teenager because there may be a high degree of misinformation or misunderstanding of the function of sexual organs and the terminology. However, open-ended questions should provide the examiner with a fairly accurate estimate of the patient's knowledge and understanding. Never underestimate the ability of a teenager to deny reality—for example, she may not believe that she is pregnant despite amenorrhea, gross weight gain, and a protuberant abdomen.

Although the elderly patient may no longer be concerned with reproductive function, she may be faced with residual genitourinary problems as a result of pregnancies and aging. Her risk of cancer of the breast and reproductive organs is increased. She is at risk for osteoporosis and fractures. She may still enjoy an active sexual life or may have little or no interest in sexual activity. She may have lost her mate and be lonely and regard the visit to the health care provider as a social event. Alternatively, she may have financial worries that cause her to delay seeking medical help in hope that the problem will go away. Since a higher percentage of the female population is living 20, 30, and even 40 years past menopause, the percentage of gynecologic care required by these patients has increased dramatically. Thus, it is essential to be knowledgeable about the many problems that arise in the geriatric patient.

When the health care provider recommends a particular course of therapy, she or he must be prepared to offer alternatives, to accept a second opinion, and, above all, to allow the patient the opportunity to participate in decision making. There may be instances when financial concerns dictate the best course of action under the circumstances without compromising care. Care providers must recognize, without affront, that what they would choose for themselves may be unacceptable to the patient because of her lifestyle or financial and social situation.

Thus, the patient must be respected as an individual. The expression of that respect must continue through the development of a partnership with the patient to improve her health and well-being.

NORMAL DEVELOPMENT
OF THE UROGENITAL SYSTEM

The female generative and urinary systems develop in close association. However, clarity requires a description of the evolution of each system separately, with mention of important relationships and incorporations during development.

The development of the female urogenital system is well

under way by the *fourth week after implantation,* following the sequence shown in Figures 1-1, 1-2, 1-3, and 1-4. The external female genitalia evolve after about the seventh week.

ORIGIN OF THE OVARIES

During the *fifth to sixth week,* primitive sex cells migrate from the yolk sac into the dorsal mesodermal genital ridge, destined to become the ovary. The sex cells, each likely to develop into a *primordial ovum,* then occupy the outer portion (*cortex*). Soon they are surrounded by smaller, moderately differentiated cells that will develop into *granulosa cells.* Cells just peripheral to the granulosa cells, which appear less differentiated but have otherwise similar stromal elements, will evolve into *theca cells.* Nondescript fibroblasts support a delicate vasculature. Coarse connective tissue and large blood vessels characterize the *medulla.* By the *eighth week,* the ovary is a recognizable organ (Fig. 1-5).

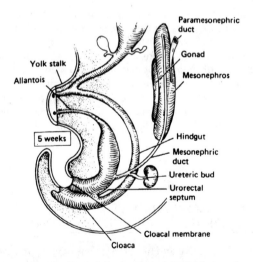

Figure 1-1. Left-side view of urogenital system and cloacal region before subdivision of cloaca by urorectal septum. Position of future paramesonephric duct is shown (begins in the sixth week). Gonad is in the indifferent stage (sexually undifferentiated).

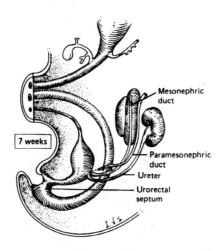

Figure 1-2. Left-side view of urogenital system. Urorectal septum nearly subdivides the cloaca into the urogenital sinus and the anorectal canal. Paramesonephric ducts do not reach the sinus until the ninth week. Gonad is sexually undifferentiated. Note incorporation of caudal segment of mesonephric duct into urogenital sinus (compare with Fig. 2-6).

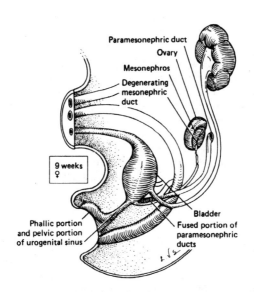

Figure 1-3. Left-side view of urogenital system at an early stage of female sexual differentiation. Paramesonephric (mullerian) ducts have fused caudally (to form uterovaginal primordium) and contacted the pelvic part of the urogenital sinus.

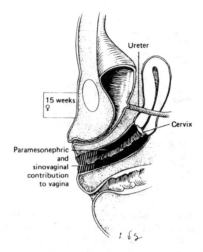

Figure 1-4. Sagittal cutaway view of differentiated urogenital sinus and precanalization stage of vaginal development. The drawing depicts one of several theories about the relative contributions of paramesonephric ducts and sinovaginal bulbs to the vagina (there is little consensus).

Origin of the Female Generative Ducts

The *mullerian ducts* will become the uterine tubes, uterus, cervix, and upper portion of the vagina. The ducts are cordlike structures that begin to differentiate in the embryo at about *6 weeks*. The *upper ducts elongate* and the *lower ducts fuse*. The tract then canalizes to form *patent oviducts, the uterine cavity, the cervical canal,* and *the upper two thirds of the vaginal canal.* The lower *one third of the vagina* is formed from invagination of the cloaca. This duct development requires *4–5 months*.

Origin of the Female External Genitalia

The external genitalia are pericloacal in origin, with the genital tubercle becoming the *mons pubis* and *clitoris*. The *hymen* represents the merge of the upper vaginal (mullerian) portion and the lower vaginal urogenital sinus.

Because of the intricate interdevelopment and the small size of the parts, the sex of the fetus rarely can be determined with

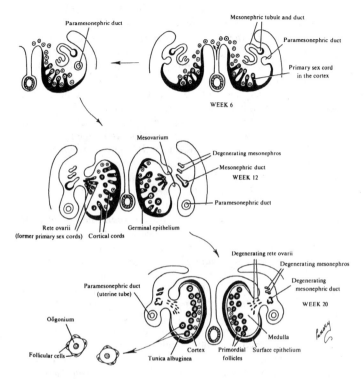

Figure 1-5. Embryology of the ovary. (From B. Pensky, *Review of Medical Embryology.* Macmillan, 1982.)

confidence by ultrasonic scanning or even direct visualization until after the 22nd week.

ORIGIN OF THE KIDNEYS AND URETERS

Three stages mark the development of the human renal excretory apparatus.

1. The *pronephros* (or primordial kidney), a transitional incomplete duct with lateral vestigial tubules, develops in the posterior-lateral mesoderm during the third and fourth weeks. It may transport minimal celomic fluid. The duct alone survives to become the *mesonephric (wolffian) duct.*

2. The *mesonephros* (middle kidney) forms caudal to the pronephros along the mesonephric duct, which finally extends to the cloaca. Along the duct, mesonephric tubules, each with an arteriole and a venule, form primordial glomeruli. The mesonephros, developed by the seventh week, extracts waste products from celomic fluid and blood. By the ninth week, the tubules degenerate. The mesonephric duct is vestigial in the female, but it becomes the epididymis and vas deferens in the male.

3. The *metanephros* (true kidney) begins about the fourth week, as the mesonephric tubules develop and degenerate. The mesonephric diverticulum (ureteric bud) begins to grow out from the mesonephric duct slightly cephalad to the cloaca to become the *ureter* and the metanephros or *permanent kidney.*

During the *fifth through sixth weeks,* the ureter divides within the developing mesonephric mass to form *calices. Collecting and secretory tubules* then appear within the renal mesenchyme to connect the true vascularized *glomeruli* in the renal cortex. There is slight kidney excretion by the tenth week.

During the *second through third months,* the *bladder* develops from the widened lower wolffian ducts that merge with the allantois. The eventual bladder architecture is apparent by the tenth week, when the caudal extension, the *urethra,* finally opens into the urogenital sinus derived from the cloaca.

The *adrenal (suprarenal) glands* begin to form about the *fifth week* from mesenchymal cells, similar to those that produced the nonterminal portion of the ovary, together with nearby cells from the neural folds. A partially organized *adrenal cortex and medulla* are evident by the *ninth through tenth weeks.*

Anomalous female urogenital development, including congenital uterine abnormalities, strange anatomic inclusions, or even pelvic tumors, may represent vestigial male counterparts (Fig. 1-6, Table 1-1).

PEDIATRIC AND ADOLESCENT GYNECOLOGY

The reproductive tract in pediatric and adolescent patients differs from that of the adult, requiring special techniques and equipment for examination. The gynecologic problems addressed in children and adolescents may differ markedly from those of adult women but may be no less serious. Both the anatomy and physiology of

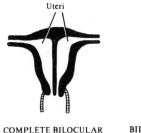

**COMPLETE BILOCULAR
UTERUS**

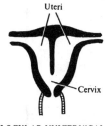

**BILOCULAR UNICERVICAL
UTERUS**

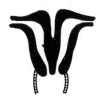

**BICERVICAL UTERUS
BICORNIS**

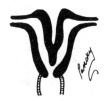

**UNICERVICAL UTERUS
BICORNIS**

UNICORNUATE UTERUS

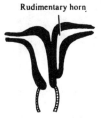

UNILATERAL ATRESIA

Figure 1-6. Congenital uterine abnormalities. (From B. Pensky, *Review
of Medical Embryology.* Macmillan, 1982.)

Table 1-1. Adult Derivatives and Vestigial Remains of Embryonic Urogenital Structures*†

Embryonic structure	Male	Female
Indifferent gonad	*Testis*	*Ovary*
Cortex	Seminiferous tubules	Ovarian follicles
Medulla	Rete testis	Medulla
		Rete ovarii
Gubernaculum	Gubernaculum testis	Ovarian ligament
		Round ligament of uterus
Mesonephric tubules	*Ductuli efferentes*	Epoophoron
	Paradidymis	Paroophoron
Mesonephric duct	Appendix of epididymis	Appendix vesiculosa
	Ductus epididymidis	Duct of epoophoron
	Ductus deferens	Duct of Gartner
	Ureter, pelvis, calyces, and collecting tubules	Ureter, pelvis, calyces, and collecting tubules
	Ejaculatory duct and seminal gland (vesicle)	

Primordium	Male derivative	Female derivative
Paramesonephric duct	Appendix of testis	*Hydatid (of Morgagni)*
		Fallopian tube
		Uterus
Urogenital sinus	*Urinary bladder*	*Urinary bladder*
	Urethra (except glandular portion)	*Urethra*
	Prostatic utricle	*Vagina*
	Prostate gland	*Urethral and paraurethral glands*
	Bulbourethral glands	*Greater vestibular glands*
Mullerian tubercle	Seminal colliculus	*Hymen*
Genital tubercle	*Penis*	*Clitoris*
	Glans penis	*Glans clitoridis*
	Corpora cavernosa penis	*Corpora cavernosa clitoridis*
	Corpus spongiosum	*Bulb of the vestibule*
Urogenital folds	*Ventral (under) aspect of penis*	*Labia minora*
Labioscrotal swellings	*Scrotum*	*Labia majora*

*Modified from K. L. Moore, *The Developing Human: Clinically Oriented Embryology,* 2nd ed. W. B. Saunders Co., 1977.
†Functional derivatives are italicized.

the reproductive tract will change from the hormone-stimulated state of the newborn to the relatively estrogen-free state of the young child to the blossoming of womanhood during adolescence.

ANATOMIC AND PHYSIOLOGIC CONSIDERATIONS

Newborn

The newborn female reproductive tract has experienced *prolonged stimulation by transplacentally acquired maternal hormones.* With transection of the umbilical cord, these hormone levels fall, with slow reversal of their effects over the first month of life. Breast buds are present in most female newborns, and some will produce milk if massaged. Breast massage should be avoided to prevent infection or continued milk production.

At birth, the clitoris is prominent, with a clitoral index of ≤ 0.6 cm^2 (clitoral index = length in centimeters $\times$ width in centimeters). The labia minora are large and may protrude through bulbous labia majora. The hymen is prominent and red, protecting a vagina that averages 4 cm long. A whitish vaginal discharge of mucus and exfoliated cells with an acid pH may be prominent. The uterus may be enlarged (4 cm long), with cervical eversion present. The endometrium may slough and vaginal bleeding may occur within a few days after birth. Parents can be reassured that the *bleeding will stop by 10 days of age.* The ovaries have not descended from the abdomen and cannot be palpated if normal.

Young Child (Under 7 Years)

With little estrogen stimulation, the external genitalia have involuted from birth. The labia majora are flat, and the labia minora are thin, as is the hymen. The clitoris is no longer prominent, but the *clitoral index remains unchanged.* The mucous membranes are pink and only slightly moist. The diameter of the hymenal opening is about 0.4 cm. The vagina is about 5 cm long, and its secretions have an alkaline pH. Vaginal fornices do not develop until puberty. Therefore, the cervix is appositioned against the vaginal vault and is difficult to see or palpate. If seen, the cervical os is a small slit. The regressed uterus does not return to the size of the newborn until 6 years of age. The ovaries have many follicles that decrease in number until menarche, when there are only a few. During this time, the ovaries begin their descent into the true pelvis.

Older Child (7–10 Years)

As *estrogen stimulation returns,* the mons pubis thickens, the labia majora fill out, and the labia minora become more rounded. The hymen thickens, and the opening enlarges to 0.7 cm. The vaginal mucosa thickens, and the vagina elongates to 8 cm. The body of the uterus enlarges primarily by myometrial proliferation. The endometrium gradually thickens. The ovaries enlarge and descend lower into the pelvis. The follicles enlarge, although none will participate in ovulation, then gradually regress in size. *Breast buds may appear.*

Young Adolescent (10–13 Years)

During this phase of development, the *external genitalia continue to approach adult appearance.* Bartholin glands begin to produce mucus immediately before menarche. The hymenal opening enlarges to about 1 cm. The vagina lengthens to adult size (10–12 cm), and vaginal secretions become acidic. The vaginal fornices develop. The body of the uterus becomes twice as long as the cervix. The ovaries descend further into the true pelvis. Breast development continues, with buds progressing to small mounds. Other *secondary sex characteristics develop* (pubic and axillary hair), the body becomes more rounded, and the adolescent growth spurt begins.

GYNECOLOGIC EXAMINATION

Newborn

Since internal examination usually is unnecessary and difficult at this age, *examination is limited to the external genitalia.* Assess the overall appearance, looking for anomalies in addition to ambiguity of sex differentiation. An abnormal or enlarged clitoris may suggest congenital adrenal hyperplasia. Inspect the hymen for patency to rule out imperforate hymen or vaginal agenesis. Rectal examination may palpate the cervix, but normally no other reproductive organs will be felt.

Child

Avoid the use of stirrups, since an adequate view of the genitalia can be obtained with the child in the frog leg position (knees flexed, legs fully abducted) on the examination table or in the mother's lap. Enlisting the child's cooperation is helpful. After a general examination, including inspection and palpation of the breasts, gently palpate the abdomen. Ovarian tumors in this age group usually occur in the low to midabdomen.

Evaluate the external genitalia for evidence of proper hygiene as well as lesions of the skin, inflammation, tumors, excoriations, or vaginal discharge. The labia minora should be separate posteriorly. Ascertain the presence of a vaginal opening. Digital rectal examination must be gentle.

If visualization of the upper one third of the vagina is necessary (e.g., foreign body, abnormal bleeding, screening for in utero DES exposure, penetrating injury), a vaginoscope, cystoscope, or laparoscope may be used. *Examination under anesthesia may be necessary.* In the younger child, a 0.5 cm instrument can be used. In the older child, an 0.8 cm instrument usually can be passed through the hymenal orifice.

Young Adolescent

At this age, the girl may be very sensitive about the changes in her body. She should be an active participant in the history and examination process. She should be asked whether or not she wishes her mother to be present, and *a female assistant should be present if the mother is not.* It is important to reassure her that she may be embarrassed or somewhat uncomfortable but that the examination will not be painful and her hymen will not be damaged. Schedule sufficient time to allow for an unhurried examination and full explanation of each procedure.

Examine the breasts and explain breast self-examination. Stirrups usually are accepted in this age group. After examination of the external genitalia, inspect the cervix and vagina using a long-bladed Huffman-Graves vaginal speculum. If the hymenal opening is of sufficient size, bimanual palpation may be accomplished with a single finger in the vagina. If not, the uterus and ovaries may be palpated using the rectal approach.

After the examination, discuss the findings with the patient and address any concerns. *Patient–doctor confidentiality should be maintained.* If there is some problem of which the parents should be made aware (e.g., pregnancy), advise the patient and convince her that disclosure is necessary for her benefit.

Congenital Anomalies of Reproductive Tract Typically Diagnosed Before Menarche

Abnormalities of the Hymen

There are so many normal variations in the appearance of the hymen (e.g., size and number of orifices, thickness) that essentially the only true anomaly is *imperforate hymen.* The solid membrane of the imperforate hymen is thought to be a persistent portion of the urogenital membrane formed whenever the mesoderm of the primitive streak abnormally invades the urogenital portion of the cloacal membrane.

Obstruction of the vaginal outlet by the imperforate hymen causes a *buildup of vaginal secretions,* initially a *mucocolpos,* and later *hematocolpos* postmenarche. The mucocolpos may be seen as a flat or mildly protruding, thin, shiny membrane. The vagina is distended and may fill the pelvis. Ultrasonography will distinguish between this condition and vaginal agenesis. Hematocolpos is diagnosed in an amenorrheic adolescent with a bulging purplish red hymenal membrane and distended vagina. Blood may fill the uterus (hematometra) and spill from the uterine tubes into the peritoneal cavity.

Imperforate hymen is corrected surgically at the time of diagnosis. In the newborn, the procedure involves simple excision without sutures. In the postmenarchal patient, the membrane must be excised, since simple incision and drainage are likely to result in spontaneous closure and recurrence of hematocolpos.

In some cases, an apparently imperformate hymen has very tiny openings and is termed *microperforate hymen.* Treatment is similar to that for imperforate hymen. A septate vagina may have a single thick median ridge at the hymenal orifice separating the two halves, leaving a double hymenal opening. Surgical correction is necessary if obstruction of vaginal drainage is evident or if it will interfere with intercourse.

Vagina

Vaginal Septum

A vaginal septum may be transverse or longitudinal. The *transverse septum* is the result of faulty canalization of the embryonic vagina and may occur at any level. Septa in the upper portion usually are patent, whereas those in the lower portion of the vagina may be imperforate and result in mucocolpos or hematocolpos. Incomplete septa may be followed until menarche, when complete excision can be performed more easily. A *complete transverse septum should be incised at diagnosis* to allow drainage to occur until menarche, when complete excision of the remaining septum along with the attached dense, subepithelial connective tissue can be performed.

A *longitudinal vaginal septum* results from improper fusion of the distal ends of the mullerian ducts. The septum is fibrous, with an epithelial lining that divides the vagina into two. There may be an accompanying *bicornuate uterus* with one or two cervices. Treatment is necessary only if there is obstruction of drainage from one side of the vagina, if dyspareunia is present, or if it would interfere with vaginal delivery. Rarely, a *double vagina,* complete with two separate muscle layers, occurs and is accompanied by double vulva, bladder, and uterus.

Agenesis

Vaginal agenesis, also known as *Rokitansky sequence,* is believed to be the result of failure of the mullerian ducts to make contact with the posterior portion of the urogenital sinus and often is associated with the absence of uterus and uterine tubes. Defects of the urinary tract (45%) and spine (10%) are common, as is hearing deficiency. On examination, a dimple is noted where the hymenal opening should be, and the rest of the external genitalia appear normal. *Ultrasonography* usually confirms the absent or rudimentary internal genitalia with normal ovaries. Almost all will have a 46,XX karyotype, but male pseudohermaphroditism must be ruled out via *karyotypic documentation.*

The treatment of vaginal agenesis is the creation of a vagina when the patient is contemplating sexual activity. This can be accomplished without surgery by having the patient use a series of progressively larger dilators to exert constant pressure in the dimple where the hymen should be for 20–30 min daily for several months. If this is unsuccessful, a vagina may be created surgically.

Partial vaginal agenesis, usually only of the lower one third, is believed to result from failure of the urogenital sinus epithelium to invade the vagina at 4–5 months gestation. The upper vagina, uterus, and tubes are normal. Visual examination externally is the same as total vaginal agenesis, but ultrasonographic examination confirms the presence of internal genitalia. Rectal examination may reveal a distended upper vagina (especially if postmenarchal), and renal anomalies may be present.

Treatment of partial vaginal agenesis requires drainage of the obstructed upper vagina, usually by creation of a lower vagina.

Uterus

Most uterine anomalies are not diagnosed until after menarche unless other abnormalities of the reproductive tract are present (Chapter 19).

Urethra

Epispadias is the term used to describe the female urethra that opens cephalad to a bifid clitoris as the result of *failure of normal fusion* of the anterior wall of the urogenital sinus. This may be accompanied by exstrophy of the bladder and defects in the abdominal wall and pelvic girdle. Urologic reconstruction is performed in infancy, but gynecologic repair usually is delayed until adolescence.

GYNECOLOGIC DISORDERS IN PREMENARCHAL CHILDREN

Vulvovaginitis

Vulvovaginitis is likely the *most common gynecologic problem in childhood.* The susceptibility of young girls to infection is high because of the thin, atrophic vaginal mucosa (lack of estrogen stimulation), contamination by feces (poor hygiene), and relatively impaired immune mechanisms of the vagina.

Nonspecific vulvovaginitis is a polymicrobial infection associated with disturbed homeostasis, usually secondary to poor hygiene or foreign body. Vulvovaginitis due to secondary inoculation results from bloodborne or contact inoculation of the vagina with pathogens infecting other areas of the body (e.g., urinary tract infection, upper respiratory tract infection). *Specific vulvovaginitis* is primary infection by such organisms as *Neisseria gonorrhoeae, Gardnerella vaginalis, Treponema pallidum,* and herpes simplex.

The *vaginal discharge* (mucopurulent or purulent) from acute vulvovaginitis may be minimal or profuse. If the thin mucous membrane of the vulva or vagina is denuded, there may be a blood-tinged appearance to the discharge. The odor may be very foul. The patient may experience only mild discomfort or severe perineal pruritus and burning, with itching so intense that the child scratches to excoriation with bleeding. The inflamed area may burn when urine passes over it, suggesting urinary tract infection (UTI) when indeed the urinary tract is uninvolved. In these cases, UTI cannot be diagnosed by a clean-catch specimen, since leukocytosis and contamination from the vagina are difficult to eliminate.

Examination of the perineal area reveals erythema or soreness that may be localized or extending to the anus and thighs. A *rectal examination* is essential to evaluate the pelvic organs. *Vaginoscopy* should be performed if the infection is recurrent or refractory to treatment, especially if a foul-smelling bloody discharge (associated with foreign body) is present. The most common foreign body is toilet paper, although various small objects, such as beads and toys, can be found. Radiographs are not reliable for diagnosis, since most objects are not radiopaque. Objects in the lower third of the vagina can be flushed out with warm saline or removed with bayonet forceps, but vaginoscopy is necessary to ensure that no objects remain higher. Recurrent placement of foreign bodies is not unusual.

Vaginal Bleeding

The *source* of vaginal bleeding may be *uterine* (endometrial) in origin or localized to the *vulva/vagina*. If bleeding is *endometrial* in origin, disorders of sexual maturation should be investigated. Otherwise, such lesions as vulvovaginitis, foreign body, vulvar skin lesions, urethral prolapse, trauma, botryoid sarcoma, and adenocarcinoma of the cervix or vagina should be considered.

Urethral Prolapse

When the urethral mucosa protrudes through the meatus, it forms a hemorrhagic, tender vulvar mass. A short course of *estrogen cream* is therapeutic when there is *no urinary retention* and the *mass is small*. If the *mass is large* or *urinary retention is present* or both, *surgical resection* of the prolapsed tissue is required under anesthesia with postoperative urinary catheterization for 24 h.

Trauma

Although most injuries to the genitalia of children are accidental, an *index of suspicion must be maintained* to avoid missing evidence of child abuse or sexual abuse. The description of the accident should fit the injury produced.

Injury to the vulva usually results in hematoma formation that requires no specific therapy other than cold compresses unless the urethra is obstructed or the hematoma is large and continuing to increase in size. If the urethra is obstructed, the bladder must be drained, usually by the suprapubic approach. A large hematoma should be incised and drained, with ligature of the bleeding points. Continued bleeding necessitates packing with gauze for 24 h and prophylactic antibiotics. *Radiographs* of the pelvis may be advisable to rule out fracture.

If the *hymen is lacerated,* bleeding may be minimal, but a penetrating injury must be suspected and vaginoscopy performed even if the patient is asymptomatic. Although most vaginal injuries involve the lateral walls with little bleeding and little pain, a *lesion extending to the vaginal vault requires pelvic exploration* to rule out extension into the broad ligament or peritoneal cavity. Small intravaginal hematomas require no therapy. Large intravaginal hematomas should be incised and drained, with ligature of the bleeding point.

Lichen Sclerosus

Lichen sclerosus (hypotrophic dystrophy) of the vulva is seen most commonly in postmenopausal women but may be seen in young children. Histologic findings are the same in both groups, with no malignant potential in children. Whitish plaques or papules are seen no further than the middle of the labia majora and do not encroach into the vagina. Because this lesion is susceptible to infection and bruises easily, vulvar irritation, pruritus, dysuria, and bleeding from scratching are typical.

Treatment consists of *good hygiene* and short-term use of *hydrocortisone creams* to stop the pruritus and allow healing. About 80% will improve significantly with onset of puberty.

Labial Adhesion

Labial adhesion, which is common in prepubertal children, is believed to be related to the thinness of the skin over the labia minora as the result of *low estrogen levels.* Local irritation can lead to scratching, with injury and adherence in the midline. Most adhesions are asymptomatic and undiagnosed unless interference with urination occurs. Dysuria, pruritus, irritation, and vulvovaginal infections may result. Rarely, total occlusion causes *urinary retention*.

Treatment of symptomatic adhesions consists of 7–10 days of *Premarin cream* twice a day. If medical treatment is unsuccessful, surgical separation may be necessary. Recurrence is common until puberty, when spontaneous resolution can be expected to occur and persist until after menopause.

Genital Tumors

Although uncommon, about 50% of the genital tumors of children are either malignant or premalignant and must be considered whenever such findings as chronic genital ulcer, nontraumatic swelling of the external genitalia, tissue protruding from the vagina, abdominal pain or enlargement, bloody foul discharge, and premature sexual maturation are present.

Benign Tumors

The common benign genital tumors of children are *teratomas, hemangiomas, simple cysts of the hymen, retention cysts of the paraurethral ducts, granulomas,* and *condylomata acuminata.* Small cysts usually require no therapy. Larger cysts require excision and marsupialization of the remaining wall to prevent recurrence. Teratomas require surgical excision. Capillary hemangiomas usually regress spontaneously, but cavernous hemangiomas may bleed extensively if traumatized and must be evaluated for removal or ablation.

Malignant Tumors

Botryoid Sarcoma (Embryonal Carcinoma of the Vagina) Botryoid sarcoma is seen most often in girls under 3 years. It is a rapidly growing tumor arising in the submucosal tissues of the vagina but may involve the cervix as well. The vaginal mucosa protrudes from the vagina in polypoid growths. Biopsy is required for diagnosis. Six months of *chemotherapy* is followed by *surgical removal,* radical hysterectomy, and vaginectomy without oophorectomy. Further chemotherapy for 6–12 months follows. If the tumor cannot be removed, *radiation therapy* is given to shrink the tumor.

Other Malignant Tumors   *Endodermal carcinoma, mesonephric carcinoma,* and *clear cell carcinoma of mullerian origin* (associated with in utero DES exposure) are seen in children or adolescents. Virtually all genital tumors seen in adult women have been reported in children, and the treatment is similar.

Disorders of Sexual Maturation

Before adolescence, the normal pulsatile release of gonadotropin-releasing hormone (GnRH), also called luteinizing hormone-releasing hormone (LHRH), does not occur. With the onset of this hypothalamic activity, the pituitary releases FSH, and the process of ovarian stimulation leads to the production of estrogen. The end-organ response to gradually increasing estrogens and finally progesterone determines the alterations that occur during adolescence and result in puberty. Sexual maturation may progress through *a typical sequence of events over 2–4 years* or may be abnormally accelerated or delayed.

Early in the process leading to puberty, the genital system undergoes marked alterations. The external genitalia gradually assume the adult appearance. The vagina develops progressively thicker mucosa and, while becoming more distinct from the cervix, reaches its adult length (10–12 cm). It also is more distensible and progressively more moist and acidotic with the reappearance of lactobacilli. The uterine corpus enlarges to twice the length of the cervix, and the ovaries descend into the true pelvis.

Late premenarche is marked by accelerated somatic growth and often rapid changes in secondary sexual characteristics. The body habitus begins to assume more feminine characteristics, with breast buds appearing and gradually increasing in size. Thelarche, breast development, is the earliest adolescent change toward puberty, preceding regular ovulation by ~2 years. Pubic hair (pubarche) and axillary hair appear later. The method of *classifying adolescent secondary sexual development* through puberty proposed by Marshall and Tanner (Table 1-2) has become widely accepted. Although puberty is technically defined as the maturation of endocrine and gametogenic function to the point of reproductive capability, it is not uncommon for menarche (the first menses) to be used nearly interchangeably. This is unfortunate, for the first few cycles (generally up to a year) are usually anovulatory. The average age of menarche in the United States is 12.8 years.

Table 1-2. Tanner Classification of Adolescent Development in the Female

Breast development	Pubic hair development	Stage
Papillae elevated (preadolescent), no breast buds	None	I
Breast buds and papillae slightly elevated	Sparse, long, slightly pigmented	II
Breast buds and areolae confluent, elevated	Darker, coarser, curly	III
Areolae and papillae project above breast	Adult-type pubis only	IV
Papillae projected, mature	Lateral distribution	V

Accelerated Sexual Maturation

Sexual precocity is defined as the *onset of sexual maturation ≥2.5 SD earlier than the normal age* (i.e., onset of secondary sexual characteristics < 8 years or menarche < 10 years). Accelerated sexual maturation may be complete or incomplete.

Incomplete Accelerated Sexual Maturation

Premature Thelarche Isolated development of breast tissue (one or both breasts) before age 8 years (excluding the newborn period) is considered premature thelarche and frequently occurs between 1 and 3 years. There is no change in bone growth and no estrogen effect documented in the vagina. Breast biopsy should not be performed, and no specific therapy is indicated.

Premature Pubarche Isolated development of pubic or axillary hair before age 8 years may be idiopathic and of no clinical significance. However, this hair growth may be a sign of excess androgen production from an inborn error of metabolism (congenital adrenal hyperplasia from steroid enzyme deficiency) or tumor. Excess androgen production must be exluded before idiopathic premature pubarche is diagnosed.

Premature Menarche Isolated cyclic vaginal bleeding before age 10 years is considered premature menarche. Estrogen levels are not increased and may be the result of endometrial sensitivity to low level estrogens. *Other causes of vaginal bleeding should be excluded.* There is no adverse effect on growth, future fertility, or menstrual pattern. No therapy is advocated.

Complete Accelerated Sexual Maturation

Immature Hypothalamic-Pituitary-Ovarian Axis Early feminization may result from either ingestion of exogenous estrogens or prolonged use of estrogen-containing creams. Once estrogen product usage is established, immediate discontinuance is advised.

Early endogenous estrogen production is most likely of ovarian origin. *Large follicular cysts, teratomas,* or *cystadenomas* of the ovary may either produce estrogen or stimulate estrogen production. *Granulosa cell tumors, adrenal adenomas,* or *hepatomas* may produce estrogens but are rare.

Mature Hypothalmic-Pituitary-Ovarian Axis These girls experience the orderly process of puberty at an earlier age than normal, typically close to the expected age of puberty but possibly as early as 2–3 years of age. Other than loss of expected adult height from accelerated bone maturation, there is *no adverse effect on fertility or menstrual patterns.* On occasion, CT scan of the brain may reveal a small hamartoma in the hypothalamus.

Precocious puberty may be the result of *CNS lesions* (e.g., tumors, previous fractures, meningitis, or encephalitis). It is believed that irritation of the hypothalamus begins the maturation early, but the overall process may be very prolonged (years). Treatment, if any, is directed toward the CNS lesion.

The *McCune-Albright syndrome,* consisting of polyostotic fibrous dysplasia, irregular cutaneous pigmentation, and precocious puberty, holds an unfavorable prognosis. The precocious puberty usually occurs at a very early age and results in short stature from early epiphyseal closure and pathologic fractures. Many affected girls are *infertile,* with menstrual abnormalities. The cause is unknown, and no specific treatment is available.

Delayed Sexual Maturation

The absence of onset of puberty beyond 2.5 SD of the normal age is considered delayed. Absence of thelarche by 13 years or menarche by 15 years warrants investigation, and evaluation may be initiated earlier if there is concern. Patients with delayed sexual maturation may be classified into one of three categories: *delayed menarche with adequate secondary sexual development, delayed puberty with inadequate or absent secondary sexual development,* or *delayed puberty with virilization.* Obtaining a complete medical, family, and social history is essential, as are plotting growth and performing pubertal developmental staging (Tanner criteria). Complete workup and differential studies are described in Chapter 23.

PREGNANCY IN CHILDREN AND ADOLESCENTS

Precocious or juvenile pregnancy occurs in girls with precocious puberty and has been reported at less than 6 years of age. Most cases involve sexual abuse or incest. There is an increased incidence of premature onset of labor, pregnancy-induced hypertension, and spontaneous abortion. If the patient is under 9 years of age, abnormal labor occurs in > 50% and neonatal loss is 35%.

Adolescent pregnancy is increasing at an alarming rate. The attitudes and expectations of the teenager regarding pregnancy and motherhood usually are far from realistic. Prenatal care and nutrition often are suboptimal. The incidence of cigarette smoking, drug abuse, and sexually transmitted disease is high. Preeclampsia-eclampsia, premature delivery, and intrauterine growth retardation occur more frequently in adolescents than in adult women, making adolescent pregnancy, in general, high risk. Perhaps the best hope for preventing or improving the outcome of adolescent pregnancy lies in *early sex education, conscientious contraceptive counseling,* and *emphasis on prenatal care.*

Chapter 2

Female Reproductive Anatomy and Reproductive Function

FEMALE REPRODUCTIVE ANATOMY

The female reproductive system is composed of the external and internal genitalia. The *external genitalia* (Fig. 2-1) are collectively termed the *pudendum* or *vulva* and are directly visible.

The *internal genitalia* include the *vagina, cervix, uterus, uterine (fallopian) tubes,* and *ovaries* (Figs. 2-2, 2-3). Special instruments are required for inspection of the internal genitalia. Simple specula or other instruments allow direct visualization of the vagina and cervix, but the intraabdominal group can be inspected only by invasive methods (laparotomy, laparoscopy, or culdoscopy) or by sophisticated imaging techniques (ultrasonography, CT scan, magnetic resonance imaging).

EXTERNAL GENITALIA

Mons Pubis (Mons Veneris)

The mons veneris, a rounded pad of fatty tissue overlying the symphysis pubis, develops from the genital tubercle. It is not an organ but a region or a landmark. Coarse, dark hair normally appears over the mons early in puberty. During reproductive life, the pubic hair is abundant, but after the menopause, it becomes sparse. The normal female escutcheon is typically a triangle with the base up, in contrast to the triangle with the base down pattern in males.

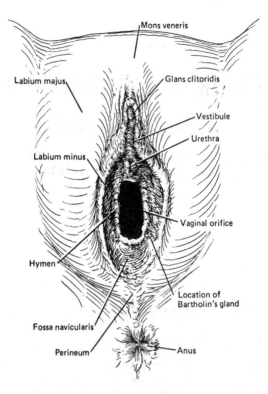

Figure 2-1. External female genitalia.

The skin of the mons contains sudoriferous and sebaceous glands. The amount of subcutaneous fat is determined by heredity, age, nutritional factors, and possibly steroid hormone factors.

Innervation

The sensory nerves of the mons are the *ilioinguinal* and *genitofemoral nerves.*

Blood and Lymph Supply

The mons is supplied by the *external pudendal artery and vein.* The lymphatics merge with those from other parts of the vulva and from the superficial abdomen. The crossed lymphatic circu-

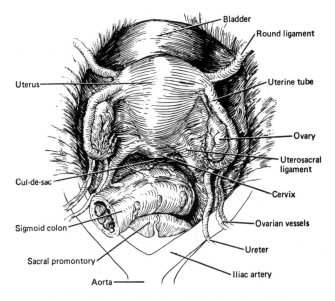

Figure 2-2. Internal female genitalia (superior view).

lation of the labia within the mons is clinically important because it permits metastatic spread of cancer from one side of the vulva to the inguinal glands of the opposite as well as the affected side.

Clinical Importance

Dermatitis is common in the pubic area, and it is important to observe closely if infestation with *Phthirus pubis* (lice, crabs) is suspected. Edema may occur secondary to infections, vulvar varicosities, trauma, or carcinomatous infiltration of the lymphatics. Cancer elsewhere in the vulva also may involve the mons.

Labia Majora

In the adult female, these two raised, rounded, longitudinal folds of skin are the most prominent features of the external genitalia. They are homologous to the male scrotum. They originate from the genital swellings extending posteriorly and dorsally from the

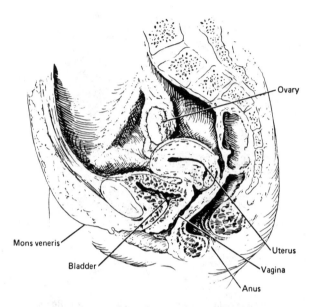

Figure 2-3. Internal female genitalia (midsagittal view).

genital tubercle. From the perineal body, they extend anteriorly around the *labia minora* to merge with the *mons*. The labia normally are closed in nulliparous women but later open progressively with succeeding vaginal deliveries and become thin and atrophic with sparse hair in later life.

The skin of the lateral surfaces of the labia majora is thick and often pigmented. It is covered with coarse hair similar to that of the mons. The skin of the inner labia majora is thin and contains no hairs. The labia majora are made up of connective and areolar tissue, with many sebaceous glands. A thin fascial layer similar to the tunica dartos of the scrotum is present within the labia just below the surface. The round ligament of the uterus passes through the inguinal canal (*canal of Nuck*) to end in a fibrous insertion in the anterior portion of the labia majora.

Small and large coiled subcutaneous sweat glands are situated all over the body except beneath mucocutaneous surfaces, that is, the labia minora or vermilion border of the lips. Normally, the fluid secretion of *small coiled (eccrine) sweat glands,* which have no relationship to hairs, has no odor. *Large coiled (apocrine) sweat glands* that open into hair follicles are found over the mons, the labia majora, and the perineum as well as the axilla. These glands, which begin to secrete an odorous fluid at puberty, are more active during menstruation and pregnancy. The sweat glands are controlled by the sympathetic nervous system.

Sebaceous glands are associated with and open into hair follicles. However, on the labia minora, where hairs are absent, sebaceous glands open on the surface. At puberty, an oily secretion with a slight odor is produced. The fluid lubricates and protects the skin from irritation by vaginal discharge. Gland secretion is mediated by hormonal and psychic stimuli. The activity of the sebaceous glands diminishes in older women.

Innervation

Anteriorly, the labia majora are supplied by the *ilioinguinal and pudendal nerves*. Laterally and posteriorly, they are innervated by the *posterior femoral cutaneous nerve*.

Blood Supply

The labia majora are supplied by the *internal pudendal artery* (derived from the anterior parietal division of the internal iliac or hypogastric artery) and by the *external pudendal artery* (from the femoral artery). Drainage is via the *internal and external pudendal veins*.

Clinical Importance

The labia majora serve no special function. A *cyst of the canal of Nuck* often is mistaken for an indirect inguinal hernia. Adherence of the labia in infants may indicate vulvitis. External force or the complications of labor may cause vulvar hematoma. *Hidradenomas* are tumors that originate in aprocrine sweat glands, but they become malignant only rarely. *Sebaceous cysts,* almost invariably benign but often infected, develop from sebaceous glands.

Labia Minora

The labia minora are small, narrow, elongated folds of skin between the labia majora and the vaginal introitus. They are derived from the skin folds beneath the developing *clitoris*. Normally, the labia minora are in apposition in nulliparas, concealing the *introitus*. Posteriorly, the labia minora merge at the *fourchette*. The labia are separate from the *hymen*, the structure marking the vaginal entrance, or introitus. Anteriorly, each labium merges into a median ridge that fuses with its mate to form the *clitoral frenulum*, an anterior fold that becomes the *prepuce of the clitoris*.

The lateral and anterior surfaces of the labia minora usually are pigmented. Their inner aspect is pink and moist, resembling the vaginal mucosa.

The labia minora have neither hair follicles nor sweat glands but are rich in sebaceous glands.

Innervation and Blood Supply

The innervation of the labia minora is via the *ilioinguinal, pudendal, and hemorrhoidal nerves*. The labia minora are not truly erectile, but a generous vasculature permits marked turgescence with emotional or physical stimulation. They are supplied by the *external and internal pudendal arteries*.

Clinical Importance

The labia minora tend to close the introitus. They increase in size in response to ovarian hormonal stimulation. Indeed, without estrogen stimulation, they all but disappear. *Squamous cell carcinoma* of the vulva often originates in the labia, as do *sebaceous cysts*. The presence of adherent labia minora in the infant is usually due to inflammation. However, *fusion* may indicate sexual maldifferentiation.

Clitoris

This 2–3 cm long homolog of the penis is found in the midline slightly anterior to the urethral meatus. It is composed of two small, erectile corpora, each attached to the periosteum of the symphysis pubis, and a diminutive structure (*glans clitoridis*) that is generously supplied with sensory nerve endings. The glans is partially hooded by the labia minora.

Innervation and Blood Supply

The clitoris is supplied by the *hypogastric and pudendal nerves* and *pelvic sympathetics* and by the *internal pudendal artery and vein.*

Clinical Importance

Cancer of the clitoris is rare, but it is extremely serious because of problems of wide excision and early metastases. The inguinal and femoral nodes usually are involved first.

Vestibule and Urethral Meatus

The triangular area between the labia minora anteriorly onto which the urethra opens, bounded posteriorly by the vaginal orifice, is the *vaginal vestibule.* It is derived from the urogenital sinus and is covered by delicate stratified squamous epithelium.

The *urinary meatus* is visible as an anteroposterior slit or an inverted V. Like the urethra, it is lined by *transitional epithelium.* The vascular mucosa of the meatus often pouts or everts. This makes it appear more red than the neighboring squamous vaginal mucosa.

Innervation and Blood Supply

The vestibule and terminal urethra are supplied by the *pudendal nerve* and by the *internal pudendal artery and vein.*

Clinical Importance

Urethral *caruncles,* as well as *squamous cell or transitional cell carcinoma,* may develop in the urethrovestibular area.

Paraurethral Glands (Skene's Glands)

Immediately within the *urethra,* on its posterolateral aspect, are two small orifices leading to the shallow tubular ducts or glands of Skene, which are wolffian duct remnants. The ducts are lined by transitional cells and are the sparse equivalent of the numerous male prostate glands.

Innervation and Blood Supply

Like the vestibule and urethral meatus, Skene's glands are supplied by the *pudendal nerve* and by the *internal pudendal artery and vein.*

Clinical Importance

Skene's glands, which supply minor amounts of mucus, are especially susceptible to *gonococcal infection*, which may be first evident here. After successful antigonorrheal therapy, nonspecific infection with other purulent organisms is common and results in *recurrent skenitis*. Destruction of the duct using electrocautery or laser may be necessary.

Paravaginal or Vulvovaginal Glands and Ducts (Bartholin's Glands and Ducts) and Hymen

Just external to the hymen are paravaginal, vulvovaginal glands, or Bartholin's glands, the counterpart of Cowper's glands in the male. On either side are two tiny apertures. A narrow duct, 1–2 cm long, connects each of these apertures with a small, flattened, mucus-producing gland that lies between the labia minora and vaginal wall. The *hymen* is a thin, moderately elastic barrier that usually partially but rarely completely occludes the vaginal canal. It is an incomplete double-faced epithelial plate covering a matrix of fibrovascular tissue.

Innervation and Blood Supply

The hymen and area of the Bartholin's glands are supplied by the *pudendal and inferior hemorrhoidal nerves, arteries, and veins.*

Clinical Importance

Bartholinitis may occur with sexually transmitted diseases, especially gonorrhea, and an abscess of Bartholin's duct may require marsupialization.

A tight hymen may result in painful intercourse (*dyspareunia*), in which case hymenotomy or dilatation will be required. The remnants of the lacerated hymen following intercourse or delivery are called *carunculae hymenales (myrtiformes)*. Hymenal or perineal scars also may cause dyspareunia.

Perineal Body, Fourchette, and Fossa Navicularis

The perineal body includes the skin and underlying tissues between the anal orifice and the vaginal entrance. The perineal body is supported by the *transverse perineal muscle* and the lower portions of the *bulbocavernosus muscle.*

The labia minora and majora converge posteriorly to form a low ridge called the *fourchette*. Between this fold and posterior to the hymen is a shallow depression termed the *fossa navicularis*.

Innervation and Blood Supply

These structures are supplied by the *pudendal and inferior hemorrhoidal nerves, arteries, and veins.*

Clinical Importance

The perineal body or fourchette often is *lacerated during childbirth* and may require repair. Because of vascularity, an early or deep episiotomy can result in the loss of several hundred milliliters of blood. Faulty repair may be followed by *dyspareunia* or by reduced sexual satisfaction.

INTERNAL GENITALIA

Vagina

The vagina (Fig. 2-3) is a thin, muscular, partially collapsed rugose canal 8–10 cm long and about 4 cm in diameter. It extends from the hymen at the urogenital cleft to the cervix and curves upward and posteriorly from the vulva. The *cervix* protrudes several centimeters into the upper vagina to form recesses called the *fornices*. Since the posterior lip of the cervix often is longer than its anterior lip, the posterior fornix may be deeper than the anterior fornix. The lateral fornices are similar in size. The vaginal dimensions are reduced during the climacteric, and all fornices, especially the lateral ones, become more shallow.

The vagina lies between the *urinary bladder* and the *rectum* and is supported principally by the *transverse cervical ligaments (cardinal ligaments)* and the *levator ani muscles.*

The peritoneum of the posterior *cul-de-sac (pouch of Douglas)* is closely approximated to the posterior vaginal fornix, a detail of surgical importance.

The vagina is lined by stratified squamous epithelium, which is thick and folded transversely in nulliparas. Many of these *rugae* are lost with repeated vaginal delivery and after the menopause. Normally, no glands are present in the vagina.

Innervation and Blood Supply (Fig. 2-4)

The nerve supply to the vagina is via the *pudendal and hemorrhoidal nerves* and the *pelvic sympathetic system.* The blood supply is from the *vaginal artery* (a descending branch of the uterine artery) and from the *middle hemorrhoidal and internal pudendal arteries.* It is drained by the *pudendal, external hemorrhoidal, and uterine veins.*

The *lymphatic drainage* of the lower vagina is directed toward

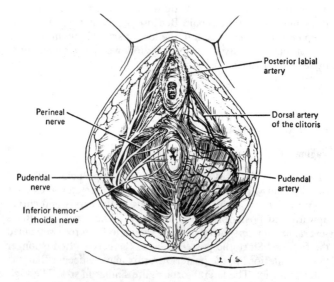

Figure 2-4. Arteries and nerves of female genitalia.

the superficial inguinal nodes; that of the upper vagina is to the presacral, external iliac, and hypogastric nodes. This is important in vulvovaginal infections and cancer spread.

Clinical Importance

Vaginal discharge is common and may be due to local or systemic disorders. Infections of the lower reproductive tract are the most common cause of leukorrhea. Estrogen depletion (senile or atrophic vaginitis) and estrogen or psychic stimulation are other causes. Primary cancer of the vagina is very rare, but secondary spread from cervical cancer is not uncommon.

Cervix

The cervix of the nonpregnant uterus (Fig. 2-3) is a conical, moderately firm organ about 2–4 cm long and some 2.5 cm in outside diameter, with a central, spindle-shaped canal. About half the length of the cervix is supravaginal and close to the bladder anteriorly.

Childbirth lacerations account for most cervical distortions. The external os, which is initially round and only a fraction of a centimeter in diameter, may gape and be much longer as a result of these tears. However, even in the absence of distortions, it is customary to refer to the cervix as having anterior and posterior lips.

The cervix is supported by the *uterosacral ligaments* and *transverse cervical ligaments (cardinal ligaments)*.

The intravaginal portion of the cervix is covered by stratified squamous cells, which usually extend to approximately the external os. The cervical canal is lined by secretory columnar epithelium. The juncture of these two epithelia is variable and is subject to continual revision under the influence of infections, hormones, and trauma. The countless crevices that give the cervical canal a honeycombed appearance on transverse section are infoldings of the mucus-secreting membrane.

Excluding the epithelial covering and the cervical canal, the cervix is composed of *approximately 85% connective tissue* and *15% circular muscle fibers* that join the uterine myometrium above. The anatomic structure of the cervix undergoes marked alteration during pregnancy, labor, and delivery.

Innervation and Blood Supply (Fig. 2-4)

Innervation of the cervix is via the second, third, and fourth *sacral nerves* and the *pelvic sympathetic plexus*. The right and left *cervical artery and vein,* major branches of the uterine circulation, carry most of the blood to and from the cervix.

Clinical Importance

The red appearing, more friable columnar epithelium over the endocervix is responsible for *ectropion* and may contribute to *postcoital bleeding* and *infection.* Additionally, the squamocolumnar junction is the site of >90% of squamous cell carcinomas of the cervix. *Cervical cancer* is the second most common female genital malignant neoplastic disease. (*Endometrial cancer* is the most common.) *Cervical infection* may be a contributor to infertility. Leukorrhea often is due to inflammation of the mucus-secreting membrane.

Uterus

The uterus (Figs. 2-2, 2-3) is an inverted, pear-shaped muscular organ with a narrow central cavity situated deep in the true pelvis between bladder and rectum. The *central cavity,* which is lined by endometrium, is roughly triangular with the base up and is markedly compressed in the anterior-posterior. Each of the upper apices is connected to an *oviduct,* and the lower apex merges with the *cervical canal.*

The uterine tubes join the uterus, one on either side, about two thirds of the distance to the top of the uterus. That portion of the uterus above the tubal insertion is called the *fundus.* Below the insertion is the body (*corpus*) of the uterus, which is continuous with the supravaginal segment of the cervix. In contrast to the cervix, the uterine substance (*myometrium*) is ~85% smooth muscle and only ~15% connective tissue. Except for the anteroinferior portion of the corpus, which is invested by the bladder, the uterus is covered by *peritoneum.*

The adult nonpregnant uterus weighs about 90 g and is about 7–8 cm long and about 4 cm in its widest diameter. However, considerably larger sizes and increased weight occur with hormonal stimulation and after childbirth. During pregnancy, the uterus, which increases to weigh about 1000 g, literally balloons to accommodate the gestation.

The uterus is supported by three paired ligaments. Uppermost are the *round ligaments*, which pass from the uterine fundus anterior to the uterine tube to the internal inguinal canal. Laterally on each side from inferior to the uterine tube extending to the cervix and attached to the pelvic side wall are the *cardinal ligaments*. The *uterosacral ligaments* extend from each sacral attachment to the posterior uterocervical juncture.

In the nulliparous woman, the uterus and cervix usually are directed forward at almost a right angle with the long axis of the vagina. However, 25%–35% of women have retroverted or retroflexed uteri.

Innervation and Blood Supply

The nerves to the uterus include the *superior hypogastric plexus,* the *inferior hypogastric plexus,* the *nervi erigentes,* the *common iliac nerves,* and the *hypogastric ganglion* (Fig. 2-5).

The *uterine artery* (a terminal branch of the hypogastric) is the primary souce of blood to the uterus, and the *ovarian artery* is a minor contributor. The uterine artery passes anterior to the ureter near the uterocervical junction. The veins draining the uterus are primarily the *uterine veins* and secondarily the *ovarian veins*.

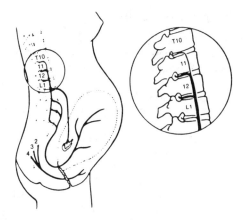

Figure 2-5. Parturition pain pathways. Afferent pain impulses from the cervix and uterus are carried by nerves that accompany sympathetic fibers and enter the neuraxis at T10, T11, T12, and L1. Pain pathways from the perineum travel to S2, S3, and S4 via the pudendal nerve. (From J.J. Bonica, The nature of pain of parturition. *Clin Obstet Gynecol* 1975;2:511.)

Lymphatic drainage may be through the cervix to the *external iliac chain* or via the isthmus to the *lateral sacral nodes*. Lymph drainage within the round ligaments may extend to the superifical inguinal nodes, then to the femoral, and finally to the external iliac chain. Drainage through the suspensory ligament of the ovary proceeds to the lumbar nodes along the aorta, above or below the kidney.

Clinical Importance

The uterus performs its reproductive function with remarkable efficiency. Although menstrual problems are common, they are not usually of uterine origin. Occasionally, *congenital* (e.g., subseptate uterus, uterus unicollis) or *acquired defects* (e.g., Asherman's syndrome) make pregnancy difficult. With the exception of childbirth, the uterus is infrequently subject to infection. The myometrium is rarely the site of malignancy. However, *endometrial cancer* is the most common female genital cancer. The myometrium is very commonly the site of benign uterine *leiomyomas* and, less frequently, is locally honeycombed by endometrium, resulting in *adenomyosis*.

Uterine Tubes (Fallopian Tubes)

Both uterine tubes function to *convey the ova to the uterus from the ovary*. Bilaterally, these tubes lie in the peritonealized superior border of the broad ligament termed the *mesosalpinx*. Each tube is 7–14 cm in length and generally is horizontal near the uterus. On reaching the lower ovarian pole, it courses around the ovary to terminate by contact with the ovarian medial posterior surface.

Each tube is divided into the *isthmus, ampulla,* and *infundibulum*. The most medial segment is the isthmus. It is narrow in diameter, ending its uterine intramural course with an ostium of ~1 mm. More distal to the isthmus is the ampulla, which is more tortuous and wider. The ampulla terminates distally in the funnel-shaped infundibulum, which has as its most distal margin a series of fingerlike diverging processes, the *fimbriae*. The funnel-shaped mouth of the infundibulum, excluding the widely reaching fimbriae, is about 3 mm in diameter and opens into the peritoneal cavity. The infundibulum is loosely supported by the *infundibulopelvic ligament* (suspensory ligament of the ovary).

The tubal wall consists of serous (peritoneal), subserous or adventitial (vascular and fibrous), muscular, and mucous components. The *muscular layer* is composed of outer longitudinal and inner circular smooth muscle layers. The *mucosa* is a ciliated columnar secretory epithelium arranged in longitudinal folds that become more complex in the ampullae. Its ciliary motion is directed toward the uterus.

Innervation and Blood Supply

The oviductal nervous supply is from the *pelvic and ovarian parasympathetic and sympathetic plexuses*. The tubal blood supply is from the *tubal branch of the uterine artery* and from the *ovarian branch of the uterine artery*. The venous drainage is through the tubal veins accompanying the arteries. The lymphatic drainage becomes retroperitoneal to the lumbar aortic nodes.

Clinical Importance

Tubal pregnancy and either intraluminal (usually gonococcal or chlamydial) or peritubal (often streptococcal) *infections* are the most common clinical concerns relative to the uterine tubes. Tubal *distortion* from peritubal scarring by endometriosis or infection, as well as intraluminal problems, may predispose to *infertility*. *Tubal cancer* is very uncommon but serious.

Ovaries

The ovaries are a pair of slightly flattened, ovoid organs that appear mottled pearly white with many surface irregularities. They lie below the pelvic brim and are supported by the *ovarian ligaments* (which extend from the uterus to the medial ovarian pole) and the *infundibulopelvic ligaments*. The ovaries rest in a fossa on the pelvic sidewall lined by peritoneum. They are bounded above by the external iliac vessels, below by the obturator nerve and vessels, posteriorly by the ureter and uterine artery and vein, and anteriorly by the pelvic attachment of the broad ligament. The uterine tubes are draped over the medial surface of the ovaries.

The ovaries weigh 4–8 g each and are usually 2.5–5 × 1.5–3 × 0.7–1.5 cm. They are covered by a cuboidal or low columnar epithelium and are divided into a *medulla* (consisting of numerous blood vessels, lymphatics, nerves, connective tissue, and smooth muscle) and a *cortex* (consisting of fine areolar stroma, many blood vessels, and scattered epithelial cells arranged in follicles).

The *graafian follicles* contain the *oocytes,* which with maturation (i.e., selection for ovulation) enlarge sufficiently to protrude visibly from the ovarian surface. When fully mature, the ovum is released and the follicle is transformed into a *corpus luteum.* This, in turn, is replaced by scar tissue (termed *corpus albicans*).

Innervation and Blood Supply

The ovarian nerve supply is from the *lumbosacral sympathetic chain* and passes to the ovary along the ovarian artery. The *ovarian artery* (usually a branch of the abdominal aorta, although the left not infrequently arises from the left renal artery) is the primary blood supply to the ovary. However, blood is supplied also from the anastomosing *ovarian branch of the uterine artery.* The veins follow the arteries to form the *pampiniform plexus* within the mesovarium. The right ovarian vein empties into the vena cava, whereas the left ovarian vein usually enters the left renal vein. The lymphatics drain retroperitoneally to the aortic lumbar nodes.

Clinical Importance

The principal functions of the ovaries include hormone production and the development of ova for the achievement of pregnancy. These functions may be interrupted by many factors. The ovaries are a frequent site of *benign and malignant ovarian tumors. Torsion* may occur, leading to vascular insufficiency and necrosis.

Ovarian infections also occur, usually in premenopausal women.

THE PELVIC FLOOR

The pelvic floor (Figs. 2-6, 2-7) consists of muscles, ligaments, and fascia arranged in such a manner as to support the pelvic viscera, provide sphincterlike action for the urethra, vagina, and rectum, and permit the passage of a term infant. It is composed of the *upper and lower pelvic diaphragms* and the *vesicovaginal and rectovaginal septa,* which connect the two diaphragms, the *perineal body,* and the *coccyx.* Other structures contributing to the integrity of the pelvic floor include the *transverse cervical (cardinal or Mackerrodt's) ligaments* and the *gluteus maximus muscles.*

The upper pelvic diaphragm is a musculofascial structure made up of *endopelvic fascia, the uterosacral ligaments, and the levator ani muscles* (including the pubococcygeus portion). The lower musculofascial pelvic diaphragm includes the *urogenital diaphragm* and the *sphincter muscles at the vulvar outlet* (ischiocavernosus, bulbocavernosus, and transverse perineal muscles).

All parts of the upper and lower musculofascial diaphragms anchor into the perineal body directly or indirectly, like spokes into the hub of a wheel or shroud lines into the ring of a parachute. For reciprocal support, the layers of the pelvic diaphragms are interwoven and superimposed. They are not fixed but move upon one another. This makes it possible for the birth canal to dilate during passage of the fetus and to close postpartum.

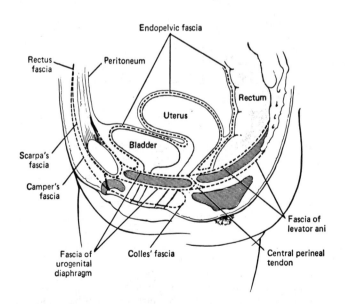

Figure 2-6. Fascial planes of the pelvis. (Modified after Netter.)

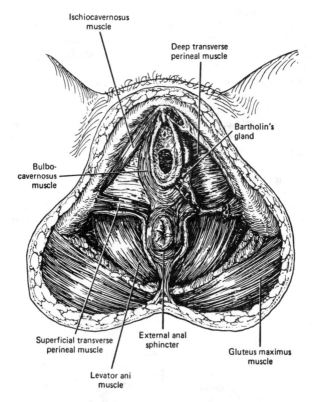

Figure 2-7. Pelvic musculature (inferior view).

The pelvic floor is perforated centrally by three tubular structures: *urethra, vagina,* and *rectum.* Each traverses the pelvic floor at a different angle, which enhances the sphincterlike action of the pelvic muscles.

The different tissues of the musculofascial diaphragm play an important role in providing both support and resilience. The *connective tissue* provides support but no recoil, the *fascia* gives strength but no elasticity, the *elastic tissue* has resilience but little strength, and the *voluntary and smooth muscles* provide stretch and recoil but with limited tolerance.

Weakness or *relaxation* of the pelvic floor may be due to a *neuropathy* or an injury during childbirth, or it may be of congenital or involutional origin.

THE BONY PELVIS

The bony pelvis is composed of four bones, the sacrum and coccyx (posterior) and the two innominate bones laterally and anteriorly. The spinal column articulates (through an arthrodial joint) with the sacrum at L5. Bilaterally, the innominate bones rest on the femurs, articulating by enarthroses (Figs. 2-8, 2-9, 2-10, and 2-11). Within the pelvis itself are two types of joints, a

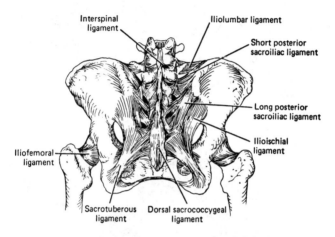

Figure 2-8. The bony pelvis (posterior view).

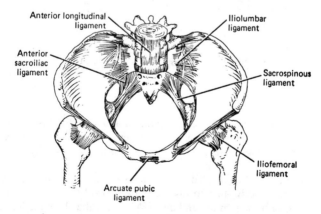

Figure 2-9. The bony pelvis (superior view).

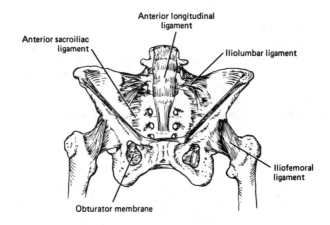

Figure 2-10. The bony pelvis (anterior view).

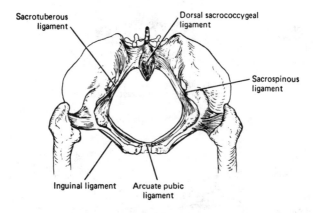

Figure 2-11. The bony pelvis (inferior view).

synchondrosis uniting the two pubic bones and diarthroses between the sacrum and ilium and between the sacrum and coccyx. The innominate bones have three major sections, ilium, ischium, and pubis.

The ilium is composed of the upper part (ala or wing) and a lower part (body) that forms the upper part of the acetabulum, uniting with the ischium and pubis. Medially, the ala of the ilium presents a smooth concave area that anteriorly is the iliac fossa and posteriorly is the iliac tuberosity (superior) and the sacral articulation (inferior). The superior border of the ilium (crest) is bounded by the anterior and posterior superior iliac spines and serves to attach the following muscles: external oblique, internal oblique, transversus (anterior two thirds), latissimus dorsi, quadratus lumborum (posterior), sacrospinalis, tensor fascia latae, and sartorius muscles. The lateral surface of the ilium provides attachments for the gluteal muscles. The posterior border of the iliac is marked by the posterior portion of the greater sciatic notch. Blood supply to the ilium is from the iliolumbar, deep circumflex iliac, obturator, and gluteal arteries.

The ischium has a body, superior and inferior rami, and a tuberosity. The body joins with the ilium and pubis to form the acetabulum. The inner surface is smooth and contiguous with the body of the ilium (above), forming the posterior portion of the lateral wall of the true pelvis. The posterior border forms the anterior portion of the greater sciatic notch. The ischial tuberosity is the most prominent portion of the bone and is the bony portion on which the human sits. The lesser sciatic notch occupies the posterior border of the superior ramus. The inferior ramus joins the inferior ramus of the pubis to form the pubic arch. The ischial spine is an important obstetric landmark, being the narrowest portion of the pelvis, and is located along the inferior ramus. The sacrospinous ligament is found between the ischial spine and the sacrum. The pudendal nerve and vessels pass under the lateral portion of this ligament. Blood comes to the ischium from the obturator, medial, and lateral circumflex arteries.

The pubis has a body and superior and inferior rami. The body contributes to the acetabulum. The rami meet in the midline to form the symphysis pubis, and medially this is marked by the pecten ossis pubis, an irregular ridge. The pubic tubercle is found ~2 cm from the medial edge of the superior ramus. The inferior aspect of the superior ramus is the obturator sulcus. The pubis receives blood from the obturator, medial, and lateral circumflex arteries.

The sacrum is formed by union of 5–6 sacral vertebrae. The fifth lumbar articulates (and occasionally fuses) with the first sacral vertebra. Their anterior portions form the sacral promontory. The posterior surface of the sacrum is convex, the midline forming the median sacral crest (fused spinal processes) and the fused laminae of the sacral vertebrae forming a flattened area laterally. This rough area is marked by absence of the laminae of the fifth and often even the fourth and third sacral vertebrae. This opening of the dorsal wall of the sacral canal is the sacral hiatus. The lateral portions of the sacrum (from fusion of the sacral vertebrae transverse process) articulate with the ileum.

The lower body of the fifth sacral vertebrae articulates with the coccyx. The sacrum receives its blood supply from the middle and lateral (usually 4) sacral arteries.

The coccyx is formed by 4 (occasionally 3 or 5) coccygeal vertebrae, which are most frequently fused into a single bone, and receives its blood supply from the middle sacral artery.

The bony pelvis is divided into two cavities by the iliopectineal line of the innominate bones. The upper cavity, which is larger and shallower, is the false pelvis, and the lower, which is smaller and deeper, is the true pelvis.

THE PELVIC MUSCLES, THEIR NERVES AND BLOOD SUPPLY

Muscles important to the pelvis include those of the abdomen, back, buttock, perineum, and upper extremity. Since many of the muscles have been functionally detailed in preceding portions of this chapter, Table 2-1 summarizes their nerves and blood supply.

MENSTRUATION

Menstruation, or normal periodic uterine bleeding, is a physiologic function occurring only in female primates. It is basically a catabolic process and is under the influence of pituitary and ovarian hormones. Its onset, the *menarche,* usually occurs at age 8–13 years. Its termination, the *menopause,* normally ensues at age 49–50. However, radiologic or surgical intervention may cause *artificial menopause* at an earlier age.

The *interval* between menstrual periods varies according to age, physical and emotional well-being, and environment. The normal menstrual cycle is commonly stated to be 28 days, but intervals of 24 to 32 days are considered normal unless the cycles are grossly irregular. At both the beginning and the end of reproductive life, the cycle is likely to be irregular and unpredictable owing to failure of ovulation. This provides a natural example of the difference between *ovulatory* and *anovulatory menstruation.* On reaching maturity, approximately two thirds of women maintain a reasonably regular periodicity, barring pregnancy, stress, or illness.

The average *duration* of menstrual bleeding is 3–7 days, but this also may vary.

The *average blood loss* in a normal menstrual period is approximately 35–90 ml. About three quarters of this blood is lost during the first 2 days of the period. Women <35 years tend to lose more blood than those >35.

Menstrual discharge contains blood, desquamated endometrial and vaginal epithelial cells, cervical mucus, and bacteria. Prostaglandins have been recovered from menstrual blood, together with enzymes and fibrinolysins from the endometrium. The last prevent clotting of menstrual blood unless bleeding is excessive. Nonetheless, small fragile, fibrin-deficient vaginal clots may form because of the presence of mucoprotein and glucose in an alkaline moiety.

The following factors all may influence menstrual bleeding: (1) fluctuations in ovarian hormones, pituitary hormones, prostaglandin, and enzyme levels, (2) variability of the autonomic nervous system, (4) vascular changes (stasis, spasm-dilatation), and (5) other factors (e.g., unusual nutritional and psychologic states).

The Typical Menstrual Cycle

The menstrual cycle is mediated by complex neuroendocrine mechanisms. A single releasing hormone, *gonadotropin-releasing hormone (GnRH)*, has been identified for the gonadotropins *follicle-stimulating hormone (FSH)* and *luteinizing hormone (LH)*. GnRH is produced in the hypothalamus and transmitted to the anterior pituitary (where the gonadotropins are produced) via the periportal vascular system (Fig. 2-12).

Normal menstrual cycles are carefully regulated by gonadotropin secretion from the anterior pituitary into the systemic circulation. With the onset of each cycle, *follicles* ready for maturation are stimulated to develop by *FSH*. One (rarely more) outstrips the others to form a prominent *graafian follicle*. Regression of the remaining follicles then ensues. Meanwhile, *estrogen* is produced by the *theca lutein cells* of the follicles. The principal ovarian estrogens are estrone (E1), estradiol (E2), and a small amount of estriol (E3). On the eighth and ninth days of the cycle, the estrogen level stops rising, and LH and FSH levels begin to fluctuate. On about the 14th day, a *sudden LH surge triggers rupture* of the follicle and *ovulation* (extrusion of the ovum). Slight bleeding occurs, and the empty

Table 2-1. Motor nerve and blood supply to abdominal and pelvic muscles

Muscle	Motor nerve(s)	Blood supply
ABDOMINAL		
External oblique	T7–L4	Inferior epigastric
Internal oblique	T7–L4	Inferior epigastric, deep circumflex iliac
Transversus abdominus	T7–L1	Deep circumflex iliac
Rectus abdominus	T7–L1	Inferior epigastric
Pyramidalis	T12	Inferior epigastric
PELVIC AND LOWER EXTREMITY		
Cremasteric remnant	Genitofemoral	Inferior epigastric
Psoas minor	L1–L2	Lumbar branch of ileolumbar
Psoas major	L2–L3	Lumbar branch of ileolumbar
Iliacus	Femoral	Iliac branch of ileolumbar
Sartorius	Femoral	Muscular branch of femoral
Rectus femoris	Femoral	Lateral femoral circumflex
Vastus lateralis	Femoral	Lateral femoral circumflex
Vastus medialis	Femoral	Femoral, profunda femoris, popliteal (genicular branch)
Vastus intermedius	Femoral	Lateral femoral circumflex, obturator
Pectineus	Femoral	Medial femoral circumflex, obturator
Gracilis	Obturator	Profunda femoris, obturator, medial femoral circumflex
Abductor longus	Obturator	Medial femoral circumflex, obturator

Muscle	Nerve	Arterial supply
Abductor brevis	Obturator	Medial femoral circumflex, obturator
Abductor magnus	Obturator, sciatic	Medial femoral circumflex, obturator, profunda femoris, popliteal
Biceps femoris	Sciatic	Profunda femoris, popliteal
Tensor fascia latae	Superior gluteal	Lateral femoral circumflex, superior gluteal
Gluteus maximus	Inferior gluteal	Superior and inferior gluteal, profunda femoris
Gluteus medius	Superior gluteal	Superior gluteal
Gluteus minimus	Superior gluteal	Superior gluteal
Obturator internus	Obturator internus gemellus superior	Superior gluteal
Gemellus superior	Obturator internus gemellus superior	Inferior gluteal
Gemellus inferior	Quadratus femoral gemellus inferior	Inferior gluteal
Quadratus femoris	Quadratus femoris gemellus inferior	Medial femoral circumflex
Piriformis	Superior gluteal	Superior and inferior gluteal, pudendal
PERINEAL		
Transverse perinaei	Perineal	Pudendal
Bulbocavernosus	Perineal	Pudendal
Sphincter urethrae	Perineal	Pudendal
Levator ani	S–4, pudendal	Inferior pudendal, inferior hemorrhoidal, inferior gluteal
Sphincter ani externus	Pudendal	Inferior hemorrhoidal, transverse perineal
Coccygeus	Pudendal	Inferior pudendal, inferior gluteal

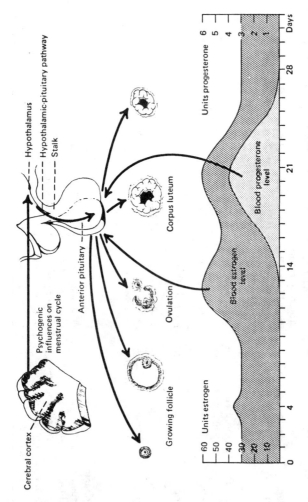

Figure 2-12. Menstrual cycle (hormones, histologic changes, basal body temperature).

follicle soon becomes filled with blood, which clots (*hemor-rhagic follicle*). LH and possibly prolactin stimulate *luteiniza-tion of the granulosa cells,* and a *corpus luteum* is thus formed. The granulosa lutein cells produce *progesterone,* which peaks on about the 23rd or 24th day. If fertilization and nidation of the ovum (pregnancy) have not occured by this time, the *cor-pus luteum regresses.* The levels of *progesterone* and *estrogen decline* thereafter to reach a critical level on about the 28th day, when endometrial bleeding (menstruation) occurs.

Vascular-Hormonal Interaction

Blood is supplied to the endometrium by two types of arterioles: a *tortuous (spiral) type* near or surrounding the endometrial glands that supplies the functionalis layer or outer two thirds of the endometrium, and *short straight vessels* that supply only the basalis layer, the inner third of the endometrium. The *basalis is not shed but remains as a reservoir of tissue for regeneration of the stroma and surface cells of the endometrial glands.* Therefore, only the superficial coiled arteries are involved directly in men-strual bleeding.

For the first week after the onset of menstrual bleeding, the spiral arterioles are short and relatively straight. During the period of thickening of the endometrium, they lengthen. The vessels grow more rapidly than the endometrium, however, and they become coiled, particularly in the midportion of the functionalis. Blood vessels function to support the maturing endometrium under progesterone influence. Four to twenty-four hours before the onset of menstruation, periodic (every 60–90 sec) vasoconstriction alternating with relaxation of the coiled arterioles occurs. By this time, there is considerable de-hydration of the endometrium. The coiled arterioles in the functionalis begin to buckle, stasis occurs in the blood within the arteriovenous channels, necrosis of the terminal arteriolar walls ensues, constriction of these arterioles within the basalis develops, and relaxation and hemorrhage from the peripheral branches begin.

Prostaglandins, largely of the PgF group, are present in con-siderable amounts in endometrium and menstrual blood. They also may participate in the vasoconstriction that precedes men-strual bleeding. Prostaglandins cause intense arterial spasm and smooth muscle contraction. This may explain certain types of *dysmenorrhea.*

Endometrial Cycles (Fig. 2-13)

During reproductive life, the endometrium undergoes continuous cyclic change. Each cycle generally passes through four phases that correspond to ovarian hormone activity and can be identified by endometrial biopsy or multihormone assay (Fig. 2-14).

Proliferative Phase

The proliferative (estrogenic) phase may vary considerably in duration but usually is consistent with each individual. It is usually about 14 days in a 28-day cycle.

The *early proliferative phase* starts on about the fourth or fifth day of the cycle, just before the end of menstruation, and lasts 2–3 days. The end of this phase coincides with about the seventh day of the classic cycle. Surface epithelium is repaired but is thin or defective. Its thickness depends on the loss of tissue during menstrual bleeding. Glands are straight. Nuclei of epithelial cells are pseudostratified, and mitoses are frequent. Stromal cells show relatively large nuclei and little cytoplasm. There are few phagocytes.

The *midproliferative phase* coincides with about the 10th day of the cycle. It differs from the early proliferative phase only in degree. The surface is more regular, the glands are more tortuous, and glandular cells are pseudostratified. The thickness of the endometrium is increased.

The *late proliferative phase* occurs on about the 14th day of the average cycle. The surface is undulating, stromal cells are closely packed, and variable amounts of extracellular fluid are lost. Thickness is about as before, but with greater cellular concentration. The glands are increasingly tortuous and contain minimal secretion. There is no glycogen in the fluid.

Ovulatory Phase

The ovulatory phase occurs with ovulation on about the 14th day of a 28-day cycle. Because there is no appreciable change in the endometrium within the 24–36 h after ovulation, the 14th-day and 15th-day endometrium cannot be distinguished from each other. Distinctive changes appear in gland cells on the 16th day and thereafter, indicating corpus luteum activity and, presumably, ovulation.

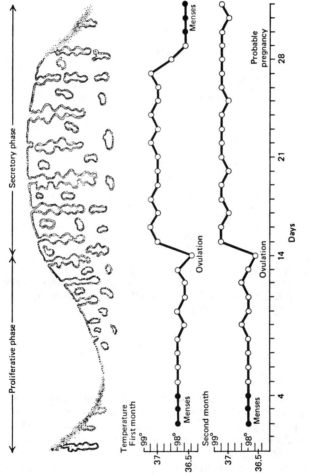

Figure 2-13. Menstrual cycle (hormones, histologic changes, basal body temperature).

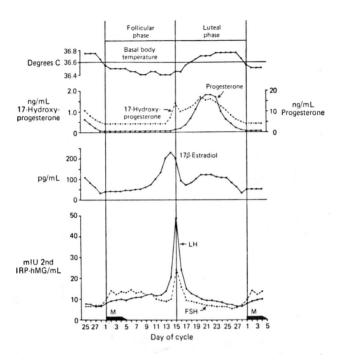

Figure 2-14. Typical basal body temperature and plasma hormone concentration during a normal 28-day human menstrual cycle. M, menstruation; IRP-hMG, international reference standard for gonadotropins. (From A.R. Midgley, in: E.S.E. Hafez, T.N. Evans, eds. *Human Reproduction.* Harper & Row, 1973.)

Secretory Phase

The secretory (progestational) phase technically begins with ovulation. On the 16th day, tortuosity of the glands is increased, there are many mitotic figures, and glycogen-laden basal vacuoles appear. On the 17th day, the most pronounced vacuolization of cells occurs. Almost two thirds of the basal portion of such glands contains glycogen-laden fluid. Slight edema is noted, and mitoses are rare. On the 18th day, secretion of fluid within the glands is apparent. (This corresponds to the time when the ovum is free within the uterine cavity and must derive nourishment from uterine secretions.) On the 22nd day, the glands are more tortuous, but there is less secretory activity, and considerable mucoid secretion is seen in their lumens. Stromal edema is now at a peak. This may facilitate implantation of the ovum. The high points of secretory activity and stromal edema coincide with the period of maximal corpus luteum function. From the 24th to the 27th day, edema regresses, and the stromal cells metamorphose into elements suggestive of decidua cells. The first change is noted in cells around the spiral arterioles, with the appearance of mitotic figures in the perivascular stroma. The glands become more and more tortuous, with serrations of their walls. Secretion of gland cells diminishes. There is infiltration by polymorphonuclear neutrophils and monocytes. Finally, necrosis and slough ensue.

If pregnancy occurs, active secretion and edema persist. The glands become more feathery and serrated. However, the predecidua is not immediately accentuated except around the ovum.

Menstrual Phase

During the menstrual phase, the endometrial edema and degenerative changes that occur at the end of the secretory phase cause tissue necrosis. This is irregularly distributed throughout all endometrial layers except the basalis. The necrosis causes blood vessels to rupture, producing scattered small hemorrhages. These enlarge and coalesce into propagating hematomas, which, in turn, cause endometrial separation and further rupture of small vessels. *Shedding of tissue fragments* usually begins in a patchy fashion about 12 h after bleeding starts in ovulatory cycles. Interestingly, an entire cast of the endometrial cavity is separated in so-called membranous dysmenorrhea. This painful condition results from sudden separation of the entire secretory endometrial lining, presumably because the sequence of events described is abnormally rapid and complete.

About two thirds of the endometrium is presumed to be lost with each ovulatory menstruation. By the time brisk flow ceases, tissue shrinkage and separation have occurred over the greater portion of the surface of the uterine cavity.

After a menstrual period of 4–7 days, bleeding gradually diminishes. Regional ooze is reduced by constriction and thrombosis of the remaining undamaged coiled arterioles, so that spotting finally ceases.

The interval between ovulation and menstruation normally is almost exactly 14 days. In contrast, the preovulatory period, the interval from the first day of menstruation to the day of ovulation, may vary from 7 or 8 days to more than a month. This variability of the preovulatory period accounts for the disparity in the intervals between menstrual periods.

Changes in Cervical Mucus and Vaginal Cytology

The *amount* and *consistency* of cervical mucus vary during the menstrual cycle. If a smear of cervical mucus is allowed to dry in air without fixation and examined under a microscope, characteristic patterns of crystalization can be identified at various stages. At the time of ovulation, the mucus dries to a striking *frondlike pattern (fern test)*. Before and after ovulation and during pregnancy, other characteristic *granular patterns* can be observed.

At about the time of ovulation, the cervical mucus becomes extremely clear and liquid in contrast to the yellowish, viscid mucus normally observed during the extreme preovulatory and postovulatory phases of the cycle. Just before ovulation, a drop of endocervical mucus can be stretched into a thin cobweblike strand 6 cm or longer. This quality (*Spinnerbarkeit*)is related to a high estrogen level and increased saline content.

Vaginal cytology distinctively reflects estrogen and progesterone variations (Fig. 2-15). During reproductive life, the vaginal cytology is characteristic of pregnancy or of the phase of the menstrual cycle. During the late follicular (preovulatory, proliferative) phase (days 12–15 of the menstrual cycle), a cytologic smear of vaginal fluid normally appears estrogenic, with many pyknotic epithelial cells and few white blood cells (WBC). After ovulation, the smear appears progestational, containing curled and clustered epithelial cells and occasional WBC. This is evidence of the luteal phase. A smear during normal pregnancy is marked by smaller, clumped, navicular epithelial cells with a high glycogen content and relatively few WBC.

Systemic Changes

During the preovulatory phase of the menstrual cycle, resting temperatures taken each morning will usually be low (<36.6°C or 98°F). Activity, infection, inadequate sleep, and alcholic beverages before retiring may cause an elevated temperature the following morning. On the day of ovulation, the temperature dips. Then due to the *thermogenic activity of progesterone*, it rises sharply almost 1 degree Fahrenheit (0.5°C) and remains elevated until just before the menstrual period, when it begins to fall toward the low preovulatory levels (Fig. 2-14). This occurs only in ovulating women.

Other systemic changes associated with uterine bleeding after ovulation include (1) extracellular edema, which is the cause of premenstrual weight gain, (2) muscle sensitivity or hypertonicity, producing irritability and agitation (e.g., premenstrual tension

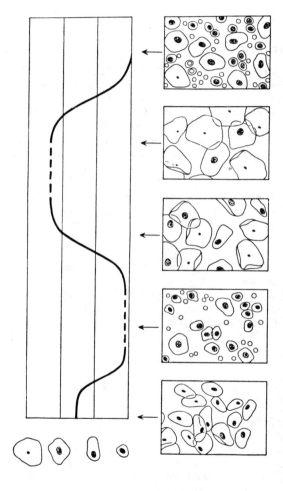

Figure 2-15. Vaginal cytologic picture in various stages of life. *Top.* Graphic representation of the maturation of vaginal epithelium. *Bottom:* Left to right: Epithelial maturation at birth; atrophic cell picture in childhood; beginning of estrogenic influence in puberty; complete maturation in the reproductive period; regression in old age. (From F.K. Beller et al, *Gynecology: A Textbook for Students.* Springer-Verlag, 1974.)

syndrome), (3) vascular alteration, including pelvic hyperemia and increased capillary fragility or a tendency toward bruising, (4) mastalgia due to increased breast size and turgescence, (5) headache (e.g., menstrual migraine), which may be a hormonally mediated vascular headache.

ANOVULATORY CYCLES

In anovulatory cycles, the maturation and differentiation of the endometrium caused by progesterone do not occur. Thus, the sequence of events is greatly altered with variable estrogen alone. Excessive stimulation results in a hypertrophic endometrium, which leads to *irregularly irregular bleeding* (i.e., irregular interval and irregular duration of bleeding). This is usually heavier in amount than normal (ovulatory) menstruation. The period is qualitatively similar to an ovulatory one, but minimal coiling of the spiral arterioles probably can cause only small fissures and no propagating hematomas. Peeling away of the functionalis layer thus takes place only imperfectly in the proliferative or hyperplastic endometrium. Bleeding from terminal arteriolar loops must occur, but tissue loss is minimal. The endometrium continues to proliferate from month to month, with the result that hemorrhage often ensues in subsequent periods from this grossly thickened tissue.

Paucity of estrogen leads to an *atrophic endometrium,* which may also lead to irregularly irregular bleeding but generally is less frequent and much lighter in the amount of blood lost.

OTHER HORMONES IMPORTANT IN FEMALE REPRODUCTION

Under the influence of releasing hormones, other tropic endocrine products are elaborated from the anterior pituitary, including thyrotropin (*TSH*), corticotropin (*ACTH*), growth hormone (*GH*), and melanocyte-stimulating hormone (*MSH*).

In contrast to the anterior lobe of the pituitary, the posterior lobe is linked with the hypothalamus by nerves. The posterior pituitary hormone *vasopressin* (antidiuretic hormone, ADH) controls plasma osmolality and is released by impulses from the supraoptic and paraventricular nuclei to be transported by nerves to the posterior pituitary. *Oxytocin,* which causes uterine muscular and myoepithelial breast ductal cell contraction, to stimulate both labor and lactation, is released and stored in the posterior pituitary by similar complex neuroendocrine mechanisms.

Prolactin may be important in maintenance of the human corpus luteum, but only slight variations in the hormone occur during the menstrual period. Much higher levels are reached during pregnancy, and very high levels of prolactin are the rule during lacatation.

Ovarian stromal cells normally produce small amounts of *androgen,* mainly, *androstenedione.*

Chapter 3

Development and Maldevelopment

GAMETOGENESIS

The *production of ova and sperm* occurs via the process of *meiosis* (whereas somatic cells undergo division via mitosis). *Oogenesis* produces ova, and *spermatogenesis* produces sperm. One spermatogonium results in four sperm, and one oogonium results in one ovum and two polar bodies. Meiosis is a reduction division normally allowing each gamete to contain *23 chromosomes* (*haploid*). Thus, when fertilization occurs and the two haploid gametes unite, the resulting *zygote contains 46 chromosomes* (*diploid*) under normal circumstances.

Two meiotic divisions occur, and each contains several stages.

FIRST MEIOTIC DIVISION

A. Prophase I has five stages.

1. *Leptotene,* wherein the chromatin condenses into individual elongated threadlike structures.

2. *Zygotene,* the migration of single threadlike chromosomes toward the nuclear equatorial plate where homologous chromosomes pair to form bivalents that exchange segments at several points (synapses).

3. *Pachytene,* where chromosomes contract and thicken, then split longitudinally into two chromatids attached at the centromere.

4. *Diplotene* is marked by crossing-over of the nonidentical chromatid constituents of homologous chromosomes at bridges or chiasms. However, the male sex chromatids (X and Y chromatids) do not cross over.

5. *Diakinesis,* the last stage, which occurs when the bivalents

contract, chiasms move toward the ends of the chromosome, homologs pull apart, and the nuclear membrane disappears.

B. During *metaphase I,* the very short and thick bivalents are aligned along the equatorial plate of the cell spindle forms.

C. In *anaphase I,* the centromeres divide so that the homologous chromatids (rather than the identical sister chromatids) are drawn to opposite poles of the spindle.

D. *Telophase I* is marked by spindle breakage, division of cellular cytoplasm, and formation of a nuclear membrane. The cell cytoplasm is equally divided in the male but is unequally distributed in the female. In the latter, most of the cytoplasm goes to the secondary oocyte so that basically only nuclear material becomes the first polar body, which subsequently disintegrates.

SECOND MEIOTIC DIVISION

A. *Metaphase II* reveals new spindle forms, and the chromosomes align along the equatorial plate.

B. In *anaphase II,* the chromatids pull apart to opposite poles of the spindle, with complete division of the centromere.

C. *Telophase II* entails the division of the spindle and cell cytoplasm (again equally in the male and unequally in the female), forming one ovum and the second polar body.

Secondary oocyte development arrests at *metaphase II* until penetration by a sperm. Then meiosis is completed, and the polar body is discarded.

FETAL MALDEVELOPMENT

TERMINOLOGY

A *chromosome is the paired basic structure containing the genes in a linear arrangement.* Humans have 23 pairs of chromosomes (46 total), of which 22 pairs are autosomes and 1 pair (either XX or XY) determine the individual's sex. A *locus is a gene's specific site on a chromosome.* A gene is a sequence of chromosomal nucleotides that forms the production code for specific proteins, i.e., unit of genetic information. Alleles are different genes that occupy the same position on homologous chromosomes and potentially affect a similar function. *Heterozygous refers to dissimilar members of a gene pair,* and *homozygous refers to similar members of a gene pair.* A dominant characteristic is recognized when the phenotypic effect of the gene is the same in the heterozygous state as in the homozygous state. In contrast, a recessive characteristic is one that is only produced in the homozygous state.

The *genotype is the genetic makeup of the individual* and is expressed with the number, then the sex chromosomes, then any specific defects, e.g., 45,XO; 46,XX; 47,XY,21+. The *phenotype is the physical appearance of the individual* with his or her various observed characteristics. The abbreviation p is used for the short arm of chromosomes and q for the long arm (as determined from the chromosome's centromere). Homologous means the same relative position and is often applied to chromosomes and genes.

A *mutagen is an agent* (e.g., physical, chemical) *that induces genetic mutation. Mutations* involve *macromolecular or micromolecular change in germ cell DNA* and are a permanent transmissible alteration. A *teratogen* is an agent (or factor) that *causes defects in the developing organism.* Teratogenic changes may be caused by mutations or by a number of other processes.

In utero development is divided into three phases. The *ovular phase* comprises the first 4 weeks after fertilization. This period is characterized by rapid mitotic divisions, resulting in a blastula. At 5–7 days after fertilization, the products of conception, now characterized by development of the *blastocyst* and separation into microscopically discernible body pole and preplacental zones, implant into the endometrium. Gastrulation begins, and the organ anlagen are relatively positioned. From the 5th through the 8th weeks of pregnancy, the conceptus is termed the *embryo.* This is the *period of organ differentiation.* From the 9th week until delivery, the conceptus is termed a *fetus.* Only a few new structures develop after the 8th week. Thus the fetal period is principally concerned with differentiation, growth, and maturation (Table 3-1).

Developmental age (fetal age) is the age of the offspring calculated from the date of conception. This may be important to embryologists but is rarely used by obstetricians or pediatricians, who are especially concerned with *gestational age,* i.e., the calculated age of the fetus from the first day of the LMP (assuming a 28-day cycle). Gestational age is expressed in *completed weeks.*

CONGENITAL DEFECTS

Congenital anomalies (birth defects, malformations) are significant, usually deleterious, deviations from normal standards of

Table 3-1. Time of insult and potential malformation

Developmental age (weeks)	Malformation
3	Ectromelia
	Ectopia cordis
	Omphalocele
	Sympodia
4	Ectromelia
	Hemivertebra
	Omphalocele
	Tracheoesophageal fistula
5	Carpal or pedal ablation
	Cataract (nuclear)
	Facial clefts
	Hemivertebra
	Microphthalmia
	Tracheoesophageal fistula
6	Agnathia
	Carpal or pedal ablation
	Cataract (lenticular)
	Cleft lip
	Congenital heart disease
	Aortic anomalies
	Gross septal defects
	Microphthalmia
7	Brachycephaly
	Cleft palate
	Congenital heart disease
	Ventricular septal defects
	Pulmonary stenosis
	Digital ablation
	Epicanthus
	Micrognathia
8	Brachycephaly
	Congenital heart disease
	Digital stunting
	Epicanthus
	Nasal bone ablation
	Persistent ostium primum

structure and function. In the United States, the *incidence of congenital anomalies recognizable at birth is 3%–7%*. However, with careful longitudinal follow-up, the incidence may reach 10%. The impact of congenital defects on human life is immense. *Abnormalities are the single major cause of infant mortality* (>20% of all infant deaths). Added to the impact of these deaths is the lost potential and expense to society involving damaged survivors.

Practitioners are most often questioned about congenital defects arising from the following situations: the gravida exposed to a potentially fetotoxic agent, the family that has had an anomalous infant, parents with a previous abnormal offspring or pregnancy loss, or a couple with a known defect who want to reproduce. Although it is not the purpose of this text to provide all the information in detail or the skills necessary to function as a counselor in these circumstances, it is our purpose to describe certain broad principles that may be of value in caring for these patients.

Creation of a Defect

Criteria for the recognition of a defect-creating agent include the following.

1. An *abruptly increased incidence* of a particular defect or association of defects (syndrome)

2. A known *environmental alteration coincident with the increase* in a particular defect

3. *Evident exposure to the environmental alteration* at a stage of pregnancy (usually early) that yields characteristic defect(s)

4. *Absence of other factors* that might create the same abnormality

Nature of the Insult

Causes of some defects are known (% of total): chromosomal aberrations or recognized genetic transmission (23%–25%), drugs and environmental agents (4%–5%), infections (2%–3%), and maternal metabolic aberration (1%–2%). However, the cause remains unknown for 60%–70% of all anomalies.

Known Genetic Transmissions

Known genetic transmissions (~20%) are the largest single ascertainable contributors to mutagenic and teratogenic defects.

Mendelian Inheritance Disorders Roughly half of these conditions may be described by their mendelian inheritance patterns (i.e., autosomal dominant, autosomal recessive, sex-linked, or sex-limited). The chance of an offspring inheriting a characteristic may be determined by the rules of each inheritance pattern.

With *autosomal dominant inheritance, a mutation in one gene of an allelic pair results in a different phenotypic expression or characteristic.* The phenotypic expression of this characteristic (*penetrance*) may vary with environmental or other genetic influences (e.g., with recombination). Examples of autosomal dominant conditions include achondroplasia, color blindness (yellow–blue), Ehlers-Danlos syndrome, Huntington's chorea, Marfan's syndrome, mitral valve prolapse, neurofibromatosis, adult polycystic renal disease, and Von Willebrand's disease. The *rules of autosomal dominant inheritance* follow.

1. The characteristic appears with equal frequency in both sexes.

2. At least one parent must have the characteristic (unless it is a new mutation).

3. Homozygous-normal mating results in all offspring having the characteristic.

4. Heterozygous-normal matings result in 50% of the offspring having the characteristic.

5. If it is a rare trait, most individuals demonstrating the characteristic will be heterozygous.

With *autosomal recessive inheritance, one affected gene of an allelic pair is insufficient to evoke a phenotypic expression of the characteristic* (i.e., different from the normal). However, *with homozygosity, the characteristic appears.* Environment and genetic influences may affect the expressivity of the defect in the carrier state. Examples of autosomal recessive conditions include albinism, chondrodystrophy, myotonia, color blindness (total), cystic fibrosis, dysautonomia, galactosemia, Gaucher's disease, homocystinuria, mucopolysaccharidosis I-H, I-S, III IV, VI, and VII, phenylketonuria, sickle cell anemia, Tay-Sachs disease, and Wilson's disease. The *rules of autosomal recessive inheritance* follow.

1. The characteristic occurs with equal frequency in both sexes.

2. For the characteristic to be present, both parents must be carriers.

3. If both parents are homozygous, all offspring will have the characteristic.

4. If both parents are heterozygous, offspring will have the characteristic in the following distribution: 25% not affected,

50% carrier (heterozygous), 25% with the characteristic (homozygous).

5. Frequent occurrence of rare recessive characteristics is often related to consanguinity.

When a gene on *the X chromosomes is affected, but it is unable to evoke the characteristic if heterozygous, it is said to be X-linked recessive.* However, *the characteristic is expressed in males because of their single X chromosome.* Examples of X-linked recessive conditions include androgen insensitivity syndromes (both complete and incomplete), color blindness (red–green), G-6-PD deficiency, gonadal dysgenesis, hemophilia A and B, Lesch-Nyhan syndrome, and mucopolysaccharidosis II. The *rules of X-linked recessive inheritance* include the following.

1. The characteristic occurs primarily in males.

2. If both parents are unaffected but produce a male with the characteristic, the mother is a carrier.

3. If the father is affected and there is an affected male offspring, the mother must be at least heterozygous for the characteristic.

4. A female with the abnormal characteristic may acquire it by

a. Inheritance of the recessive gene from both her mother and father (father affected, mother heterozygous).

b. Inheritance of the recessive gene from one of her parents and expression occurs as a result of the Lyon hypothesis (functional selection of one X chromosome for this and subsequent progeny).

If a gene on the *X chromosome is affected and able to produce the characteristic in the heterozygous state, it is said to X-linked dominant.* Examples of X-linked dominant conditions include cervicooculoacoustic syndrome, hyperammonemia, and orofacio-digital syndrome I. The *rules of X-linked dominant inheritance* follow.

1. The characteristic affects males and females with equal frequency.

2. Affected male–normal female mating results in 50% affected offspring.

3. Affected homozygous female–normal male mating results in all offspring being affected.

4. Heterozygous female–normal male mating results in 50% affected offspring.

5. Heterozygous females may not demonstrate the dominant characteristic (see Lyon hypothesis).

Multifactorial Inheritance Multifactorial or polygenic inheritance is the *inheritance of a characteristic as a result of the interaction of numerous genes and the environment.* Such inheritance cannot be classified according to mendelian principles. However, it is extremely important in normal inheritance (e.g., human physical features) as well as many common malformations (e.g., anencephaly, cleft palate, meningomyelocele, and pyloric stenosis). That the defects are inheritable is discerned from incidence. That is, the *defects noted occur with a frequency of 0.5–2/1000* in caucasians but occur in 2%–5% of siblings of affected infants with normal parents. That the abnormalities are not entirely environmental is discerned from *concordance* (a higher frequency of such abnormalities in monozygotic than dizygotic twins (e.g., the defects are 4–8 times more common in monozygotic twins.)

Chromosome Abnormalities in Number and Morphology

Chromosomal aberrations are alterations in both number and morphology. They account for *3%–5% of all human anomalies manifest at birth*. The numerical disorders probably most commonly occur during meiosis as a result of failure of the doubled chromosomal complement to be equally divided between the two daughter cells. When subsequently recombined with a normal gamete, this results in one zygote having an extra chromosome (*trisomy*) and another with a missing chromosome (*monosomy*). *Autosomal monosomy is almost always lethal.* However if the monosomy occures in the sex chromosomes, Turner's syndrome (45,XO) results. Most of these individuals are spontaneously aborted, but some survive. *Autosomal trisomy* may occur with all chromosomes, but most commonly results in trisomy 21 (Down syndrome), trisomy 18, and trisomy 13. Again, most are aborted, but a few survive through advanced pregnancy. Sex chromosomal trisomy results in *hyperploidy*.

Another etiology for chromosomal alteration of number and morphology is a parent who has an abnormal chromosomal constituency (e.g., balanced translocation carriers). Morphologic chromosomal defects may also relate to chromosomal breakage (e.g., Fanconi's anemia). Nondisjunction occurring in the postzygotic interval leads to *mosaicism* (cell lines with different combinations of the same basic chromosomal constituency). Mosaicism, not infrequent, must be differentiated from *chimerism* (cell lines from two different chromosomal constituencies), which rarely, if ever, occurs in humans.

Other defect etiologies (drugs and environmental agents, infections, and maternal metabolic imbalance) are discussed under Specific Teratic Agents.

Timing of the Insult

The *stage of development when the insult occurs largely determines the potential adverse effect or malformation*. For example, the free-floating zygote is probably less influenced by deleterious agents than it might be later. An insult that affects the zygote during this interval is most likely to result in abortion. Injury during the 2nd–7th weeks is marked by fetal wastage, structural malformations with time-related specific defects, carcinogenesis, or severe intrauterine growth retardation (Table 3-1). During weeks 9–40, the fetus is likely to develop central nervous system anomalies, behavioral disorder, functional abnormalities, reproductive system defects, and intrauterine growth retardation.

Intensity of the Insult

Most fetotoxic agents may be reduced to a level that is not harmful, and most relatively innocuous agents may be increased in dose even to a lethal level. Thus, it is crucial to ascertain the dosage and the time over which the exposure occurred. Other considerations of dosage must include the nature of the agent and the available information (generally literature) concerning the agent's mutagenic or teratogenic potential.

Host Resistance Mechanisms

Whether or not exposure to a fetotoxic agent creates a defect in a particular situation is influenced by numerous factors: the *interaction of the agent with the maternal organism* (e.g., absorption, penetration, elimination), *transport to the fetus, interaction with the fetus* (e.g., activation, inactivation, excretion), and *reparative phenomena* (e.g., local host factors influencing outcome and genetic mechanisms potentially influencing outcome).

SPECIFIC TERATIC AGENTS

Perinatal Infections

Pregnancy results in decreased maternal resistance to infection. Thus, the potential exists for both reactivation of latent infections and more severe sepsis should infection occur. The developing embryo and fetus are at greatest risk from infective agents during the first trimester, presumably as a result of limited capability for immunologic response. Table 3-2 summarizes some specific infective agents and their potential perinatal or fetotoxicity. Additionally, the effect of various infective agents on the mother (e.g., fever, respiratory distress) may adversely affect the fetus either directly or indirectly (e.g., initiation of premature labor).

Drugs

Despite recent attempts at reduction, the use of multiple prescription and nonprescription drugs during pregnancy continues. Excluding vitamins and iron, the majority of women will take at least one prescription and several nonprescription drugs at some point in pregnancy. Too frequently, this occurs at a critical time, e.g., before the diagnosis of pregnancy. The FDA has established categories of potential for drugs causing birth defects to guide drug usage during pregnancy (Table 3-3).

Drug teratogenicity has such species specificity that it is difficult to extrapolate data from one species to another. Thus, it may be impossible to fully test human teratogenicity in laboratory animals. Indeed, few of the large number of drugs reported to be teratogenic in laboratory animals have been proven to be human teratogens. Nonetheless, there are so many fetotoxic drugs that it is beyond the purpose of this text to detail them. However, every physician and nurse must become familiar with each drug they administer using more complete sources. Table 3-4 includes examples of fetotoxic drugs in several categories.

Ionizing Radiation

Ionizing radiation has long been known to have *both mutagenic and teratogenic effects*. The National Committee on Radiation Protection has stated the amount of ionizing radiation believed to be relatively safe for the embryo is 10 rads. At >15 rads fetal exposure, there is suggestive evidence of an increased incidence of childhood leukemia by age 10. In contrast to older units, modern radiologic equipment has both vastly safer shielding and much lower exposures for imaging (e.g., a chest x-ray should not exceed 0.03 rad).

Table 3-2. Infections with known perinatal or fetal toxicity

Maternal infection	Fetotoxicity
Viruses	
Coxsackie B virus	Myocarditis
Cytomegalovirus	Microcephaly, hydrocephaly, cerebral palsy, brain calcifications, chorioretinitis, deafness, psychomotor and mental retardation, hepatosplenomegaly
Hepatitis	Hepatitis
Herpes simplex virus	Generalized or localized herpes, hydranencephaly, encephalitis, chorioretinitis, thrombocytopenia, petechiae, hemolytic anemia, death
Human immunodeficiency virus (HIV)	Growth retardation, microcephaly, boxlike forehead, flattened nasal bridge, hypertelorism, triangular philtrum, patulous lips
Human parvovirus B19	Fetal death, degenerative changes, eye defects, and congenital anomalies
Mumps	Fetal death, endocardial fibroelastosis, malformations (?)
Poliomyelitis	Spinal or bulbar poliomyelitis
Rubeola	Increased abortions and stillbirth
Rubella	Growth retardation, malformations (cardiac, great vessel, microcephaly), ocular aberrations (microphthalmos, cataract, glaucoma, pigmented retinopathy), newborn bleeding, hepatosplenomegaly, mental retardation, sensorineural deafness, pneumonitis, hepatitis, encephalitis
Vaccinia	Generalized vaccinia, increased abortions
Varicella zoster	Chickenpox or shingles, increased abortions and stillbirths, hydrocephalus, microcephaly, seizures, cataracts, microphthalmia, Horner's syndrome, optic nerve atrophy,

(continued)

Table 3-2. (continued)

Maternal infection	Fetotoxicity
	nystagmus, chorioretinitis, mental retardation, skeletal hypoplasia, urogenital anomalies
Variola	Smallpox, increased abortions and stillbirths
Venezuelan equine encephalitis virus	Microcephaly, hydrocephaly, microphthalmia, cerebral agenesis, CNS necrosis

Spirochetes

Syphilis	Spontaneous abortion, stillbirth, congential syphilis including hydrocephalus, frontal prominence, saddle nose, high arched palate, short maxilla, mulberry molars, notched incisors, enamel dystrophy, 8th nerve deafness, interstitial keratitis, uveitis, glaucoma, mental retardation, convulsive disorders, paralysis or paresis, cardiovascular defects

Bacteria

Gonorrhea	Ophthalmitis
Streptococcus agalactiae (group B beta-hemolytic streptococcus)	Neonatal acute respiratory distress, septicemia, death, meningitis, infection of other organs Possible (not conclusively proven) abortion and premature birth
Listeriosis	Abortions (including habitual), stillbirths, septicemia, meningoencephalitis
Tuberculosis	Congenital tuberculosis

Protozoan

Malaria	Low birth weight, enhanced perinatal mortality
Toxoplasmosis	Microcephaly, chorioretinitis, jaundice

Table 3-3. FDA Teratogenicity drug labeling

Category	Comment
A	Well-controlled human studies have not disclosed any fetal risk.
B	Animal studies have not disclosed any fetal risk or have suggested some risk not confirmed in controlled studies in women or there are not adequate studies in women.
C	Animal studies have revealed adverse fetal effects; there are no adequate controlled studies in women.
D	Some fetal risk, but benefits may outweigh risk (e.g., life-threatening illness, no safer effective drug); patient should be warned.
X	Fetal abnormalities in animal and human studies; risk not outweighed by benefit. *Contraindicated in pregnancy.*

SPECIFIC MATERNAL DISEASES WITH POTENTIAL FETAL DEFECTS

Many conditions affecting the mother will affect the fetus adversely. Some will affect fetal growth and development. Others may cause malformations or deformations.

Diabetes Mellitus

Embryonic exposure to *hyperglycemia enhances the incidence of abortion and fetal defects* (to a threefold increase). The most commonly associated defect is cardiac (transposition of the great vessels, VSD, or coarctation of the aorta), with a fourfold increase over euglycemics. The caudal regression syndrome is the most specific and *rarely occurs except in diabetics.*

Fetal blood glucose levels are approximately 80% of maternal levels. Because insulin does not cross the placenta, the fetal pancreas produces insulin to attempt to regulate fetal blood glucose levels in the normal range. Thus, the fetus responds to hyperglycemia with hyperinsulinemia. Prolonged elevations in maternal blood glucose may result in a macrosomic infant with excessive glycogen storage and fat stores. This glycogen storage may cause sufficient hypertrophy of the cardiac interventricular septum to cause obstruction of outflow of blood from the ventricle and subsequent ischemia.

Excessive fetal secretion of insulin often results in hypoglycemia soon after the maternal supply of glucose is interrupted by clamping of the umbilical cord. The hypoglycemia is usually most pronounced in the first 1–2 h but may continue for ~48 h. Macrosomia may cause *dystocia, delivery complications,* especially *birth injury.* The neonate born of a noncontrolled diabetic mother also has increased incidence of prematurity, respiratory distress syndrome, polycythemia, hyperbilirubinemia, hypomagnesemia, and hypocalcemia.

Thyroid Disorders

Maternal hyperthyroidism may result in *fetal goiter formation.* The *newborn may even experience fatal thyrotoxicosis* if unrecognized and untreated. Symptoms usually appear 1–2 weeks after birth. Maternal antithyroid therapy may lead to perinatal goiter, tracheal obstruction, or hypothyroidism. *Maternal hypothyroidism may be associated with increased fetal wastage and postterm delivery.*

HELLP Syndrome

The surviving fetus (perinatal mortality is as high as 60%) in this condition is almost always premature, with severe growth retardation. The infant may have pancytopenia at birth that may necessitate transfusions of platelets and packed red blood cells after birth.

Systemic Lupus Erythematosus (SLE)

Maternal SLE increases the rate of *abortion* and may result in a perinate with *cardiac arrhythmia,* most notably complete heart block. There are reported cases of *congenital disseminated lupus* in the newborn of affected mothers. *Thrombocytopenia* may be present in the fetus and newborn of mothers with SLE.

Idiopathic Thrombocytopenic Purpura (ITP)

Maternal ITP affects the fetus by causing *thrombocytopenia* in some that may persist 1–4 months after birth. Treatment includes platelet transfusions if the platelet count is <25,000 or active bleeding occurs.

Table 3-4. Fetotoxic drugs

Drug	Fetotoxicity
Aminoglycosides	8th nerve defects, possible ocular damage
Androgens	Masculinization or pseudohermaphroditism
Anticonvulsant therapy	Congenital heart disease (2–3-fold increase); cleft palate (5–10-fold increase)
Antineoplastic agents	Generally potent teratogens
Antithyroid agents	Neonatal goiter, tracheal obstruction, hypospadias, aortic atresia, developmental retardation
Amphetamines	Transposition of the great vessels, withdrawal syndrome
Benzothiadiazides	Thrombocytopenia, altered carbohydrate metabolism, hyperbilirubinemia (if used in late gestation)
Chloroquine	Retinal and 8th nerve damage
Chlorpropamide	Increased anomalies generally
Cocaine	Decreased head circumference, increased CNS anomalies, increased incidence of sudden infant death syndrome
Coumarin (Warfarin)	Nasal hypoplasia, stippled epiphyses, growth retardation, mental retardation (fetal bleeding)
Diethylstilbestrol	Clear cell carcinoma of the vagina and cervix, vaginal adenosis, cervical and vaginal ridges, cervical hoods, and uterine anomalies (T-shaped uterus, constricting band, hypoplastic uterus)
Ethanol	Fetal alcohol syndrome (mental retardation, growth retardation, typical facial features, congenital heart defects, microcephaly, renal anomalies)
Isoniazid (INH)	Severe encephalopathies (may be prevented by concomitant vitamin B_6)
Isoretinoin (Accutane)	Abortion, craniofacial defects (hypoplastic nasal bridge, abnormal ears, microtia, agenesis of ear

(continued)

Table 3-4. (continued)

Drug	Fetotoxicity
	canal, micrognathia, hard and soft palate clefts, etc.), CNS abnormalities (hydrocephaly, hydranencephaly, microcephaly, etc.), cardiovascular abnormalities (transposition, VSD, ASD, truncus arteriosus, PDA, tetralogy of Fallot, etc.), incomplete lobulation of lung lobes
Lithium	Cardiovascular anomalies, congenital heart disease, increased abortion rate
Narcotics (heroin, morphine, methadone)	Withdrawal syndromes (tremors, poor feeding, irritability, seizures)
Oral hypoglycemics	Increased incidence of defects (especially caudal dysplasia)
Phenothiazines	Sight increase in malformations
Phenytoin (Dilantin)	Facial anomalies, microcephaly, mental retardation, nail hypoplasia, growth retardation
Sulfonamides	Neonatal jaundice if used in third trimester
Tetracycline	Stained teeth, do not use in second or third trimester
Thalidomide	Limb reduction anomalies
Trimethadione	Developmental delay, speech difficulty, dysmorphic facies
Vitamin A	Urinary malformations
Vitamin D	Supravalvular aortic stenosis

SPECIFIC IN UTERO FETAL ANOMALIES

Congenital Heart Disease

It is unusual for congenital heart disease (CHD) to harm the fetus in utero unless other congenital anomalies are present. Fetuses are usually carried to term and are appropriately grown. *Problems are recognized after birth*, when the lungs become the organ of respiration, supplanting the placenta. The resistance in the pulmonary vasculature normally decreases from the high level needed in fetal life to bypass the lung circuit to the low level needed to receive about half of the cardiac output for oxygenation by the lungs. If the blood is insufficiently oxygenated (>5 g unsaturated Hgb), cyanosis occurs. This may be caused by lung disease or a cardiac defect with right to left shunting of blood. A murmur and congestive heart failure may be present.

If a fetal cardiac defect is discovered and is determined to be the type likely to require repair soon after delivery, arrangements should be made to have the infant delivered in a tertiary center with neonatal cardiovascular surgery capability to avoid the delay inherent in transport of the infant after birth.

Arrhythmias

The *most common fetal arrhythmias are premature atrial or ventricular contractions.* These can be noted easily on Doppler or real-time ultrasound examinations during the second half of the gestation. Arrhythmias may be regular or irregular. Question the mother about her caffeine intake, e.g., coffee, tea, chocolate or soft drinks, since excessive intake may affect the fetal heart rhythm. Decreasing the intake of these methylxanthines may improve the fetal rhythm.

Even complete heart block may be relatively benign for the fetus if not excessively slow. However, up to 50% will have associated congenital heart defects. When the slow heartbeat is initially detected, the immediate concern is whether this fetus is in severe distress from asphyxia, requiring immediate delivery, or whether time is available for further evaluation and routine delivery. *Fetal echocardiography* may determine whether or not there are associated cardiac defects or signs of congestive heart failure. If congestive heart failure is present and the fetus is believed to be viable, cesarean section delivery should be accomplished if possible in a center where pediatric cardiology services are available to insert a pacemaker in the infant shortly after birth if necessary.

Supraventricular tachycardia (SVT) is a rhythm that must not be allowed to continue without therapy or close observation. Because the heart rate is more rapid (>220 bpm) than with other causes of fetal tachycardia (e.g., maternal fever with chorioamnionitis), this abnormality should not be confused with other conditions. Short bursts of SVT may eventually become continuous. Prolonged SVT may cause congestive heart failure and death. *Treat the mother with digoxin* in high therapeutic dosage to convert the fetal SVT to normal sinus rhythm and continue this drug until delivery. Occasionally, more than one drug may be required to maintain control of the rhythm. Even external electrocardio-version has been performed successfully. After birth, maintain the infant on digitalis (or other appropriate medications) for several months in an attempt to avoid recurrence.

Hydrocephalus

With the increased use of sonography during pregnancy and maternal determination of AFP, hydrocephalus (frequency ~1/2000 deliveries) is often diagnosed long before delivery. When discovered, careful sonographic evaluation of the fetal spine is indicated for evidence of spina bifida, the most commonly associated anomaly. *Hydrocephalus may be a genetic defect* (X-linked recessive and autosomal dominant forms account for ~2% of cases) *or may be part of a genetically related syndrome. It may be caused by isolated aqueductal stenosis (most often Sylvius), various infections, brain tumors, lack of brain substance development, or intracranial hemorrhage.*

The location and the degree of hydrocephalus and plans for the method of delivery may be altered depending on the cause. On rare occasion, massive hydrocephalus with no chance of survival will require decompression of the fetal ventricles to allow delivery by any route. Cesarean section is required for the majority of cases. However, the fetus may be delivered vaginally if labor is preterm or the hydrocephalus is not marked. Nonetheless, hydrocephalus should not be an indication for preterm delivery without evidence of pulmonary maturity, because surgery is very hazardous in infants with respiratory distress syndrome.

The outlook for the infant born with hydrocephalus varies, but it is usually good with regard to mental development. If spina bifida is present, orthopedic, urologic, and physical therapy as well as neurosurgical follow-up are almost always necessary. The child's ability to walk will depend on the level of the neural tube defect (the higher the lesion, the less likely). An encephalocele has a higher risk for both mental and physical handicap than the lower lesions.

Anencephaly

Anencephaly (incidence <1/2000 deliveries) is the result of *incomplete closure of the cranial portion of the neural tube.* The upper brain never develops, the skull bone is absent, and rudimentary brain tissue is covered only by membrane that may weep CSF. It almost always is associated with polyhydramnios. Moreover, the alpha-fetoprotein in the amniotic fluid and maternal serum is elevated unless there is skin covering the defect. Concomitantly, there is an absence of adrenal cortical development. Some will be stillborn. Others may not tolerate the stress of labor. Since *there is no effective therapy* and these infants do not have prolonged survival, heroic measures are contraindicated. Comfort care should be provided to the liveborn.

Intestinal Atresia

Intestinal atresia may occur anywhere in the gastrointestinal tract from the esophagus to the anus. Atresia proximal to the jejunum is frequently associated with polyhydramnios because swallowed amniotic fluid cannot pass far enough into the intestinal tract to be absorbed. Esophageal atresia is most often associated with a tracheoesophageal fistula, a developmental defect (the embryonic foregut is an outpouching from the trachea). Lower intestinal atresia may be secondary to a local vascular accident eliminating blood supply to an area of gut.

Intestinal atresia is frequently associated with many anomalies. The most common is called the VATERR syndrome (vertebral anomalies, anal atresia, tracheoesophageal fistula, renal anomalies, and radial anomalies).

Esophageal atresia, if not identified in utero, should be diagnosed in the first 24 h after birth, since the *infant cannot swallow fluids or even its own saliva* and will sputter, spit, and gag with feedings. Frothy saliva is commonly noted. If esophageal atresia is not associated with a tracheoesophageal fistula (TEF), the abdomen will show no gas on x-ray. If there is an associated TEF, respiratory distress may be evident. Radiographic evaluation should show that gas has passed into the gut (through the lower fistula into the distal esophagus), and an aspiration pattern may be evident in the chest.

Duodenal atresia may be the result of a true developmental stenosis or from obstruction by Ladd's bands or an annular pancreas. Infants with trisomy 21 (Down syndrome) have an increased incidence of duodenal atresia. One may suspect the diagnosis in utero by ultrasound examination. After birth, expect vomiting, which will be bilious if the obstruction is distal to the ampulla of Vater (where bile empties into the duodenum). Typical x-ray findings show a double bubble appearance to the stomach without gas in the bowel.

Jejunal atresia may be associated with polyhydramnios. In

jejunal atresia, the infant will develop bilious vomiting. Abdominal x-ray will show an obstructive pattern. However, *ileal atresia* may not be diagnosed until after discharge (after a short hospital stay). Symptoms are similar to those of jejunal atresia but may appear later because more bowel length is available for distention.

Atresia of the anus is not uncommon, but *atresia of the colon is rare.* The diagnosis of anal atresia is usually made by initial physical examination. Signs of obstruction may not appear before surgery, since drainage of feces may be through a congenital fistula into the vagina, bladder, or urethra.

Oligohydramnios Tetrad

The oligohydramnios tetrad, initially called Potter's syndrome, includes agenesis of the kidneys resulting in oligohydramnios, pulmonary hypoplasia, spadelike hands and feet, peculiar facies with a beaked nose, and creases under the lower eyelids. The fetus, often SGA, usually is in a breech position, does not tolerate the stress of labor, and may be stillborn. When liveborn, the neonate has *immediate respiratory distress and dies of respiratory failure* long before it could die of renal failure. Oligohydramnios is associated with fetal anuria. However, renal agenesis per se is not the cause of pulmonary hypoplasia, which is the result of lack of amniotic fluid and thoracic constraint.

Oligohydramnios without renal agenesis also may cause pulmonary hypoplasia, e.g., prolonged rupture of membranes with continued leakage. Deformation of the face and extremities plus arthrogryposis is usual in long-standing oligohydramnios.

Chapter 4

Maternal Physiologic Adjustments to Pregnancy

FERTILIZATION AND IMPLANTATION

THE PLACENTA

The extruded *ovum* is directed into a uterine tube by its fimbriae and the peritoneal fluid currents. Normally, a few hours after insemination, *spermatozoa* will have passed through the cervix and uterus into the fallopian tubes. *Capacitation* of the sperm (preparation for fertilization) occurs between its passage into the cervix and its reaching the midportion to outer portion of the tube. *Fertilization* occurs when a spermatozoon penetrates the ovum, usually in the outer portion of the fallopian tube. It is unusual for fertilization to occur more than 24 h after ovulation. Indeed, if this occurs, an ectopic pregnancy may result.

The *fertilized ovum* rapidly develops into an embryonic blastocyst. About 3–4 days are required for this minute, free-floating object to reach the uterus. Until implantation, the zygote is nourished by adherent granulosa cells and tubal fluids. Progress is mainly by tubal ciliary action, but peristalsis probably contributes to tubal transit. *Endometrial implantation* ensues 5–6 days later. The favored sites are the anterior and the posterior fundus. This is summarized as follows.

Last menstrual period (LMP)	Cycle days 1–7
Ovulation	Day 14 after LMP
Fertilization	Day 14–15 after LMP
Ovum transit tube to uterus	Days 15–19
Ovum free in uterus	Days 19–21
Implantation	Day 19–21 after LMP
Expected period	Missed or scanty

The early developing embryo with its tissue layers is shown in Figure 4-1.

The *chorion,* or protective covering of the fertilized developing ovum, has an outer ectodermal layer (*trophoblast*). The inner layer is mesenchyme. The trophoblast, initially a poorly defined syncytium, soon develops into two tissue types: an outer confluent but differentiated plasmotrophoblast (*syncytio-* or *syntrophoblast*) and an inner distinct *cytotrophoblast* (Langhans' striae).

The trophoblast produces proteolytic enzymes capable of rapid destruction of endometrium and even myometrium. This allows the zygote to erode quickly into the functionalis layer of the endometrium but usually not beyond the compacta. Deeper

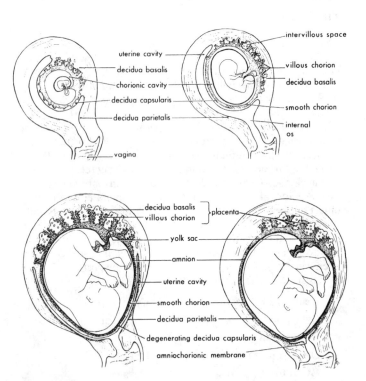

Figure 4-1. Relationships of the fetus, placenta, and membranes to the uterus in early gestation. Top left, 4 weeks. Top right, 6 weeks. Bottom left, 18 weeks. Bottom right, 22 weeks. (From K.L. Moore, *The Developing Human.* W.B. Saunders Co., 1973.)

invasion (placenta accreta) does not occur when there is formation of a layer of hyalinized fibrin (*Nitabuch's striae*).

The total products of conception reach sufficient size to ap-
pose the *decidua parietalis* and obliterate the free space in the
uterine cavity by about the 12th week.

Fetoplacental Circulation

After implantation, small *lacunae* form in the plasmotrophoblast,
and soon they become confluent. These lacunae (future intervillous spaces) fill with blood from tapped veins. An occasional
maternal arteriole is opened also, and, finally, a sluggish circulation becomes established (*hematotrophic phase* of the embryo).

The lacunae soon ramify and enlarge. Concomitantly, vascularized tufts grow down into the blood lakes to form villi for
actual embryonic circulation. The greatest concentration of maternal sinusoids (*intervillous spaces*), as well as most of the villae,
develops in the *chorion frondosum,* the site of the future placenta. As time passes, the vascularity of the decidua capsularis
become obliterated, transforming this structure into a pale translucent membrane (*chorion*) adherent to the *amnionic membrane*
within. Eventually, the fetal villous system that protrudes into
the intervillous blood spaces resemble inverted trees.

The final fetal villus surface, a two-cell layer separating fetal
from maternal blood, is very extensive. It may be as great as 50 m^2
(165 square feet), and the fetal villous capillary system may reach
almost 50 km (~27 miles)—a complex but remarkably workable
system.

Cotyledons (subdivisions of the placenta) can be identified
early in placentation as irregular clefts. At term, one can identify
six or more placental units or cotyledons.

The funis, or *umbilical cord,* usually inserts centrally. Many
variants of placental development are seen (Fig. 4-2), for example, marginal insertion of the cord, bipartite (double) placenta,
or succenturiate lobed placenta (with a small separate accessory
lobe). If even a portion of a cotyledon (or a succenturiate lobe)
is retained after delivery, serious blood loss or infection often
results.

Uteroplacental Circulation

Veins

Many randomly placed venous orifices can be identified over the
entire decidua basalis (basal plate of the placenta). The human

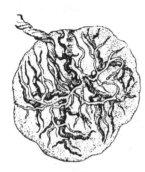

Normal placenta.

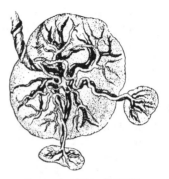

Succenturiate placenta.

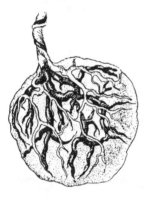

Marginal insertion or battledore placenta.

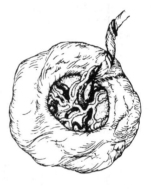

Marked circumvallate or extrachorial placenta.

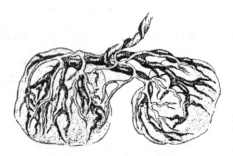

Bipartite placenta.

Figure 4-2. Placental types.

placenta has no peripheral venous collecting system. Collection of venous outflow is a function frequently ascribed to a marginal sinus. However, less than one third of the blood drains from the margin of the placenta. A marginal sinus is not seen even in the early placenta, and subchorionic marginal lakes are not found commonly in the mature placenta. However, dilated maternal vessels are found beneath the periphery of the placenta. These have been described as wreath veins or venous lakes. They may or may not communicate with the intervillous spaces.

Arteries

In contrast to the veins, placental arteries are grouped closer to the decidual attachments of the intercotyledinous septa. As the placenta matures, thrombosis decreases the number of arterial openings into the basal plate. At term, the ratio of veins/arteries is 2:1, approximately that found in other mature organs.

Even in an area beneath a well-formed placenta, some spiral arterioles empty into the intervillous spaces, although many remain coiled and compressed. Arterioles supplying the intervillous spaces appear circuitous and angulated because of fixation of the vessels and growth of the placenta. The tortuosity creates baffles, or points of deflection, that tend to slow the afferent bloodstream.

Near their entry into the intervillous spaces, the terminal maternal arterioles lose their elastic reticulum. Since the distal portions of these vessels are lost with the placenta, bleeding from this source can be controlled only by uterine contraction.

The Mature Placenta

The mature placenta (Fig. 4-3) is a blue-red, rounded, flattened, meaty organ about *15–20 cm in diameter* and *3 cm thick*. It *weighs 400–600 g,* or about one-sixth the normal weight of the term newborn. The umbilical cord (funis) extends from the fetal surface of the placenta to the umbilicus of the fetus. Fetal membranes cover the placental fetal surface and extend from the placental margins to create the space occupied by the fetus, amniotic fluid, and umbilical cord. In multiple pregnancy, one or more placentas may be present depending on the number of ova implanted and the type of segmentation that occurs.

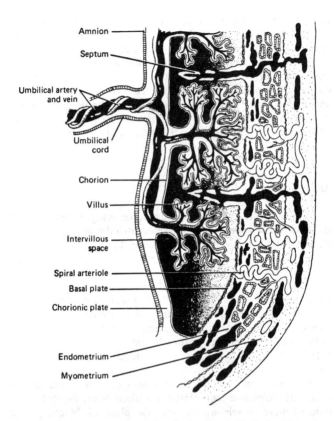

Figure 4-3. Cross section of the placenta. (Modified after Netter.)

Umbilical Cord (Funis)

The umbilical cord is a gray, soft, coiled, easily compressible structure that connects the fetus with its placenta. It *averages 50 cm in length and 2 cm in diameter* (limits of 30–100 cm in length) and is covered by a thin layer of stratified squamous epithelium comparable to fetal skin. The cord contains a framework of loose fibrous connective tissue and is filled with a mucoid material (*Wharton's jelly*). Normally, the cord contains two arteries that carry deoxygenated blood from the fetus and one vein to supply the fetus with oxygenated blood. As a result of aplasia or atrophy, one umbilical artery is absent in about 1% of singletons and 6% of twins. About

17% of these infants with a single umbilical artery have other multisystem structural anomalies. The cause(s) is unknown. Two-vessel cord is more common in African Americans than in others. Age and parity are unrelated factors. *Undergrowth of the fetus* is common with this anomaly, but early delivery cannot be attributed to two-vessel cord.

In the common *marginal insertion* or battledore placenta, the cord inserts at the periphery of the placenta. The battledore placenta poses no special problems.

In the rare *velamentous insertion of the cord,* the cord does not insert on the chorionic plate but inserts on the membranes at a point distant from the chorionic plate. The result poses a hazard. The unsupported umbilical vessels are at grave risk of laceration during labor and delivery, whereupon exsanguination of the fetus may occur.

True knots in the cord, generally in abnormally long cords, are observed in about 1:100 deliveries. Loose or false knots are unimportant, but tight knots may cause cord vessel occlusion, resulting in fetal distress or death.

Fetal Membranes

The *chorion* and *amnion* join the cord, cover the placenta, and extend to envelop the fetus. They strip easily from the fetal surface of the placenta and can be separated by careful dissection.

The amnion is a double-layered translucent membrane. Its outer portion is mesodermal connective tissue, and the inner layer is ectoderm. Eventually, the amnion consists generally of stratified squamous cells with scattered patches of low cuboidal cells. Thickened squamous areas occasionally are observed, especially near the umbilical cord. The chorion is a membrane composed of an outer syncytial layer without cellular divisions and an inner cellular (Langhans') layer.

The placental membranes contain the amniotic fluid and provide a barrier against infection for the fetus. A check for completeness of the membranes at delivery is essential to avoid infection or bleeding usually associated with retained products of conception.

Amniotic Fluid

At term, the fetus is submerged in about 1 liter of clear watery fluid (though *up to 2 liters normally may be present*). The amniotic fluid has a low specific gravity (~1.008) and mild alkalinity (pH ~7.2). The amniotic fluid *protects the fetus* from direct injury, aids in maintaining its temperature, allows free movement of the fetus, minimizes the likelihood of adherence of the fetus to the amniotic membrane, and allows for hormonal, fluid, and electrolyte exchange. It acts as a *repository for fetal secretions and excretions.* It contains fetal squamous debris, flecks of vernix, a few leukocytes, and small quantities of albumin, urates, and other organic and inorganic salts. Hormones and alpha-fetoprotein (AFP), a protein produced by the fetus, also are found in the amniotic fluid. The *electrolyte concentration is equivalent to that of maternal plasma except for calcium,* which is lower (5.5 mg/dl).

Amniotic fluid is variously considered to be a secretion of the amnion, a vascular transudate, or fetal urine. All three sources contribute to its formation in varying amounts at different times in gestation. For example, with lengthening gestations, fetal urine becomes a more important contributor. There is *rapid amniotic fluid turnover* (~350–375 ml/h). Retention of only a few milliliters per hour soon will result in *polyhydramnios* (>2 liters of amniotic fluid), whereas excessive reabsorption or failure of production will cause *oligohydramnios* (<300 ml of amniotic fluid at term).

Placental Physiology

The placenta has two *principal functions:* it acts as a *transfer organ for metabolic products,* and it *produces or metabolizes* the hormones and enzymes necessary for the maintenance of pregnancy. It thus acts as a lung, a gastrointestinal tract, a kidney, and a complex of ductless glands for the conceptus.

The placenta derives most, if not all, of its nourishment from maternal blood. The metabolic activity of the placenta may be measured by its oxygen consumption. Continued growth of the placenta is feasible only to a point, and its functional capacity and oxygen consumption decline in late pregnancy.

Placental Hormones (Figs. 4-4, 4-5)

With the onset of pregnancy, the *pattern* of circulating hormones *changes abruptly* from that of the normal menstrual cycle. Complete sex steroid hormone (estrogen and progesterone) production by the placenta alone is impossible because the necessary enzymes are lacking. However, the fetal and maternal adrenal cortices produce the precursors needed for placental synthesis of

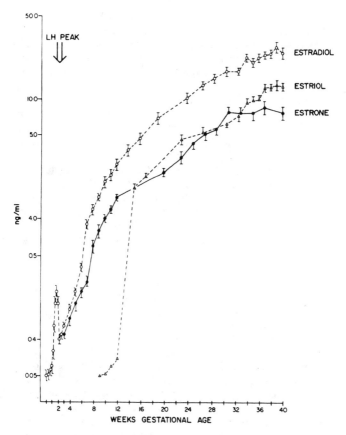

Figure 4-4. The relative concentrations (mean ± standard error) and the incremental patterns patterns of the three major estrogens plotted in the log scale during the course of pregnancy. (Courtesy of J. Marshall.) (From D.N. Danforth and J.R. Scott, eds., *Obstetrics and Gynecology,* 5th ed. J.B. Lippincott Co., 1986.)

the hormones. This is the basis for the concept and term *maternal-fetal-placental unit.*

Estrogens are bound to serum albumin in the maternal circulation and are, therefore, metabolized slowly. *Progesterone,* on the other hand, is not bound and is metabolized rapidly. *Thyroxine* (T$_4$) is bound to alpha-globulin and prealbumin. *Corticosteroids* are held in relatively inactive form in plasma by transcortin.

Thus, the titer of hydroxycorticosteroids is high during pregnancy, although frank Cushing's syndrome is uncommon.

Estrogens Estrogens are produced in ever-increasing amounts by the *syncytiotrophoblast.* The placenta cannot produce the required estrogen precursor but synthesizes estrogens from those supplied by the mother and the fetus. The most potent estrogen, *17β-estradiol,* is derived from dehydroepiandrosterone from both mother and fetus and from testosterone of maternal ovarian origin. This estrogen, like the weakest estrogen, *estriol,* increases approximately 1000-fold from the onset of pregnancy to term. *Estrone,* metabolized principally from androstenedione, synthesized from maternal cholesterol and fetal and maternal dehydroepiandrosterone, increases only 100-fold over the nonpregnant level. Thus, although it seems to be of minor importance, estrone together with estradiol is vital for fetal growth and development.

Estriol, the largest fraction of the total estrogens during pregnancy, is produced largely from fetal 16-hydroxydehydroepiandrosterone. Because the fetal precursors are a vitally important source of estriol, estriol determinations in maternal plasma or urine were used as measures of fetal well-being (e.g., in diabetes mellitus or preeclampsia) before more precise and cost-effective methods were available.

Progestogens *17α-Hydroxyprogesterone* declines to very low levels after an initial (about 2 weeks after the beginning of pregnancy) mild elevation. It probably is produced by the corpus luteum, whose function is almost totally assumed by the placenta after pregnancy is well established (by at least 12 weeks).

In contrast, *progesterone,* which is produced by the placenta, increases daily after the beginning of pregnancy to more than double the prepregnancy value (Fig. 4-5). Progesterone is metabolized about equally by the maternal and the fetal liver and fetal adrenal cortex. The final metabolites are 20α-dihydroprogesterone and pregnanediol.

Progesterone is the principal precursor of the *glucocorticoids* and *mineralocorticoids of the fetus.* Progesterone also can be synthesized in the placenta from acetates or cholesterol (estrogens cannot.) Thus, an assessment of progesterone and its metabolite *pregnanediol* may be an index of placental function, independent of the fetus. This currently is not useful clinically, however.

Chorionic Gonadotropin (hCG) The placental hormone *hCG is produced by the syntrophoblast.* Its concentration rises sharply after implantation of the fertilized ovum and reaches a *peak value of ~100,000 mIU/ml* about the eighth to tenth week. Chorionic gonadotropin then falls sharply to a lower level by

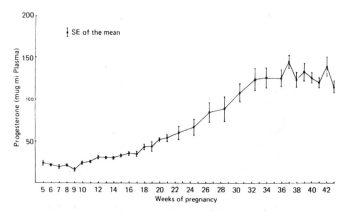

Figure 4-5. Plasma progesterone during pregnancy. (From D.N. Danforth, ed., *Obstetrics and Gynecology,* 4th ed. Harper & Row, 1982.)

about the 120th day and remains at this level to term. It disappears from the circulation at a known rate (Fig. 4-6) of approximately 50% per week. hCG is secreted directly into the maternal blood, with virtually none reaching the fetal circulation.

hCG is *luteotropic* and, like LH, stimulates the production of progesterone, 17-hydroxyprogesterone, and estrogens. The physiologic role of hCG, particularly in later pregnancy, is not known. It apparently is important for maintenance of the corpus luteum in very early pregnancy, but after the first few weeks of gestation, the corpus luteum itself is no longer essential to the maintenance of pregnancy. An immunologic role for hCG (may inhibit lymphocyte response to the "foreign" placenta) has been postulated.

Tests for hCG in the urine have formed the basis for practically all pregnancy tests. This is because of its rapid rise early in pregnancy and continued high output throughout gestation. The alpha subunit of hCG is nearly identical to that of LH, but their beta subunits differ. Thus, radioimmunoassays for the beta subunit of hCG in serum have become the most sensitive tests, ensuring a very early accurate diagnosis of prenancy. hCG is not absolutely specific for pregnancy. Small amounts are secreted by a variety of gastrointestinal and other tumors in both males and females. Thus, it is measured in individuals with suspected tumors as a *tumor marker.*

Plasma Follicle-Stimulating Hormone (FSH) FSH rapidly falls

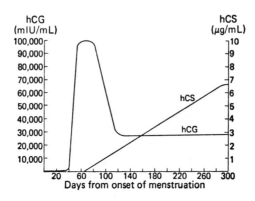

Figure 4-6. hCG and hCS plasma levels during pregnancy. (From W.J. Dignam. In: R.C. Benson, ed., *Current Obstetric & Gynecologic Diagnosis & Treatment,* 4th ed. Lange, 1982.)

to scarcely detectable levels about 10 days after ovulation, never rising again until ovulation occurs following delivery. The activity of the anterior pituitary probably is suppressed by hCG and later by prolactin.

Chorionic Somatomammotropin (hCS) Chorionic somato-mammotropin (hCS), formerly known as placental lactogen (hPL), is a protein hormone produced by the syntrophoblast. It is immunologically and physiologically similar to pituitary growth hormone (hGH). Measurable amounts of hCS are detectable after the eighth week of pregnancy, with a steady increase to term, when normal values of 6–7 Ug/ml are reached (Fig. 4-6).

Other Protein Hormones The placenta also produces *chorionic thyrotropin (CT)* but not corticotropin.

Hemodynamics

There is little short-circuiting of blood from an arterial opening to an adjacent venous outlet. This is because the arterial pressure of the maternal blood (60–70 mm Hg) actually causes it to flow quickly into the low-pressure (20 mm Hg) intervillous space. Maternal arterial blood is directed toward the chorionic plate, whereas venous blood in the placenta tends to flow along and out from the basal plate. Thus, beneficial circulation currents are established.

Maternal blood flow through the placenta at term is about

500 ml/min, whereas the fetus circulates only some 400 ml/min through the placenta. The slow rate of circulation within the placenta is offset by the large capacity of the placenta, which exceeds that of the vessels supplying and draining it, as well as by the excess of maternal over fetal blood. Changes in maternal blood pressure, therefore, have only a gradual effect on the intervillous blood pressure in the placenta. Mechanisms to improve placental transfer are few, however. An increased rate of rhythmic uterine contractions is helpful, but strong, prolonged labor contractions are detrimental to the placental and fetal circulation. An increased fetal heart rate tends to expand the villi during systole. However, this is only a minor aid in circulatory transfer.

The pressure gradient within the fetal circulation changes slowly with the mother's posture, fetal movements, and physical stress. The pressure within the placental intervillous space is about 10 mm Hg when the gravida is lying down. After she stands for a few minutes, this pressure exceeds 30 mm Hg. In comparison, the fetal capillary pressure remains at about 20 mm Hg.

Placental Transfer

Transfer across the placental barrier is accomplished by at least five different processes: simple diffusion, facilitated diffusion, active transport, pinocytosis (engulfment of particles by cells), and leakage through defects.

Simple Diffusion

Substances required for the maintenance of fetal life and the elimination of its waste products are handled largely by diffusion across the placental barrier. Included in this group are oxygen, CO_2, water, electrolytes, and urea. Fetal blood and maternal blood have similar diffusion constants, so that passage of these substances is rapid in either direction. Large quantities of certain substances are involved, and near term, almost 4 liters of water clears the placenta each hour. The principal limiting factors are the relative anatomic inefficiency of the placenta and sluggish blood flow.

Fortunately, fetal oxygen requirements are less than those of the newborn. Oxygen tension in the intervillous space is only about one-half that in the maternal pulmonary veins. The fetus is compensated to a degree because fetal hemoglobin carries slightly more oxygen than adult hemoglobin. Moreover, fetal blood also eliminates CO_2 better than the blood of the newborn.

Facilitated Diffusion

Certain substances important to the fetus (e.g., glucose) are transported across the placenta more rapidly than is possible by simple diffusion. In these instances, a carrier system functions with the chemical gradient, but the system may become saturated at high concentrations. (This mechanism differs from active transport, which operates against the gradient.)

Active Transport

This requires energy, moves against a concentration gradient, and occurs even when the system is saturated. Amino acids, water-soluble vitamins, and large-ion substances, for example, calcium, iron, and iodine, are transported actively. Enzymes probably are involved. Bilirubin is moved from fetus to mother in this manner also. Hence, it is rare for cord blood bilirubin to be >4–5 mg/dl, even with severe fetal hemolytic disease. It also explains why infants are not jaundiced even when their mothers have hepatitis.

Pinocytosis and Leakage Through Defects

The final two mechanisms both accomplish moving substances with such large molecular structures that no other means exist to move them across the placenta.

The Placental Barrier

The human placental barrier is represented initially by two layers of trophoblastic cells that separate the maternal and fetal bloodstreams. The outer layer is the *syntrophoblast,* or *plasmotrophoblast.* The inner layer is the *cytotrophoblast,* or *Langhans' stria.* After the third month, the cytotrophoblast normally loses its continuity, and the cells become less numerous. Therefore, in late pregnancy, the only separation between maternal blood and the fetal vascular endothelium is the syntrophoblast, a single cell layer that is, in essence, a transfer membrane. However, this is a poor barrier, and only a limited number of high molecular weight substances (e.g., insulin, hCG) are blocked completely. Thus, the term *barrier* is something of a misnomer.

Nonetheless, the placenta serves as a time barrier rather than a concentration barrier in most instances. If a drug can be absorbed through the maternal gastrointestinal tract, it can cross the placenta. However, such passage takes time, and the presence of a drug in the cord blood does not necessarily mean that the drug has reached effective levels in the fetal brain.

PLACENTAL DISORDERS

Placental Insufficiency

Placental insufficiency is an obstetric concept to explain *reduced placental function potentially resulting in untoward fetal outcome.* The insufficiency may be *acute* (e.g., after premature partial placental separation leading to fetal distress), or *chronic* (in which there is suboptimal nutritional or gaseous exchange resulting in subnormal fetal growth, oligohydramnios, and possible passage of meconium in utero). The decreased fetal or neonatal growth that occurs with the chronic form is classified as abnormal when the perinate is in the 10th percentile or below. This is a *small for gestational age (SGA)* pregnancy.

Restricted growth potential through diminished placental function may be caused by *abnormal placental anatomy* (e.g., placenta previa, circumvallate placenta, placental hemangioma, twin-to-twin transfusion syndrome). It *is associated more frequently with abnormal placental perfusion* (e.g., cigarette smoking, chronic villitis, infarction, partial separation, premature placental aging). Other *maternal disorders* with decreased placental perfusion include anemia (Hgb <12 g/dl), diabetes mellitus, hypertension, preeclampsia, renal disease (e.g., chronic glomerulonephritis), malnutrition (e.g., inflammatory bowel disease), pancreatitis, lupus erythematosus, and cyanotic heart disease. Finally, it is possible to have restricted growth potential from the enhanced demands imposed by *multiple pregnancy.*

Care must be taken to identify SGA pregnancies with restricted growth potential (exogenous or type II) from those with decreased growth potential (endogenous or type I) because therapy modalities are very different. *Decreased growth potential may be caused by genetic disorders* (e.g., autosomal trisomies, sex chromosome disorders, neural tube defects, dysmorphic syndromes), *congenital infections* (e.g., cytomegalovirus infection, rubella, toxoplasmosis, malaria, listeriosis), *drugs* (e.g., alcohol, tobacco, warfarin, folic acid antagonists), *radiation,* and *small maternal stature.*

Currently, therapy is not possible for the majority of those SGA pregnancies with decreased growth potential (damage), although individualized therapy of the conditions underlying restricted growth potential possibly is of benefit. With serious fetal disorders (acute or chronic), consider delivery by the easiest, least traumatic means. Avoid heavy maternal sedation, anesthesia-induced hypotension, and hypoxia. Ensure proper neonatal support and treatment.

The placenta may be considerably smaller than normal or show premature aging. In addition to the *altered body proportions* (the fetal head is spared at the expense of the body), the SGA perinate has *altered body composition* (including decreased body fat, decreased total protein, decreased total body DNA and RNA, decreased glycogen) and *altered distribution of organ weights.*

The SGA fetus is at risk for *congenital malformations, hypoxia and acidosis,* and *stillbirth.* Neonatally, placental insufficiency may be associated with *hypoglycemia, hypocalcemia, hypothermia, hypoxia and acidosis, meconium aspiration syndrome, polycythemia,* and *congenital malformation.* Unfortunately, there maybe long-term sequelae, including *seizures, cerebral palsy, reduced IQ,* and *learning or behavior disorders.*

Placental and Membranous Tumors

Amnion nodosum (small, pearly irregularities of the amnion) are composed of plaques of benign squamous cells. They may represent localized residui of disease or an incorporation of fetal extradermal derivatives. Amnion nodosum is associated with *oligohydramnios* and major fetal urinary or gastrointestinal tract *anomalies.*

With the exception of *hydatidiform mole,* trophoblastic neoplasms (e.g., *malignant hydatidiform mole, choriocarcinoma*) are rare. *Chorioangiomas* occasionally are associated with fetal maldevelopment of one twin, probably due to shunting of placental blood by the tumor.

Placental Infarcts

Placental infarcts, red to pale brown, firm areas, may be small to massive and located anywhere beneath the chorionic plate.

Infarcts are composed of *degenerating villi and fibrin clot.* They are caused by interference with the maternal blood supply to the intervillous space, for example, thrombosis of a maternal artery to a cotyledon.

Placental infarcts are *rare in early pregnancy.* Occasional small infarcts are common in late normal placentas and may be numerous with preeclampsia. In postdue pregnancy when placental aging becomes evident, scattered small infarcts are common. Gross infarction occurs in partial placental separation. Extensive placental infarction is associated with chronic or acute fetal distress, even fetal death.

Hemorrhagic Endovasculitis

Hemorrhagic endovasculitis (*HEV*) probably is caused by placentitis. In HEV, the blood vessels are injured, and fetal blood is lost into the placenta, causing temporary fetal anemia and hypoxia. Threatened abortion or fever may suggest placentitis. It probably is responsible for growth retardation and early fetal CNS injury (e.g., sensory or motor disability). Whether or not a woman with HEV in one pregnancy will have the abnormality in the next is undetermined.

Placental Infection (Placentitis, Chorioamnionitis)

Bacterial or viral infection of the placenta, particularly the amnion and chorion near the cord insertion, is common after prolonged rupture of the membranes. Maternal chills, fever, uterine tenderness or hypertonicity, and malodorous amniotic fluid are suggestive signs.

Leukocytosis, with a differential shift to the left, increased sedimentation rate, heavy colonization of pathogens on cervical, uterine culture indicates intrauterine sepsis. A steamy or milky appearance of the membranes (due to the presence of polymorphonuclear leukocytes and exudates), together with perivascular leukocytic infiltration of the cord and fetal vessels (omphalitis), is typical. Focal villus inflammation is a late manifestation.

Treat by prompt evacuation of the uterus, oxytocics, and massive parenteral antibiotic therapy against anaerobic and aerobic bacteria. Symptomatic therapy may be the only course in viral infections.

Parametritis, salpingitis, pelvic peritonitis, pelvic thrombophlebitis, or maternal death may ensue, as may perinatal omphalitis, septicemia, septic pneumonia, or death.

PHYSIOLOGIC CHANGES IN PREGNANCY

Maternal Cardiovascular Changes During Pregnancy

Blood

Blood volume, composed of the plasma volume plus the cellular volume, increases 45%–50% during pregnancy. The plasma volume increases more and earlier in gestation than does the cellular volume, although the latter increases about 33% or ~450 ml. This creates a *declining hematocrit* (HCT) until near the 30th week of pregnancy, when the plasma volume plateaus, and is termed the *dilutional* or *physiologic anemia of pregnancy*. With iron supplementation, the erythrocytes increase more rapidly, and the disparity between cellular and plasma volumes is less (Fig 4-7).

Increased plasma volume may be due to augmented plasma renin, secondary to elevated estrogen and progesterone. This encourages sodium retention by stimulating aldosterone secretion. Thus, total *body water is increased,* and *there is a gradual*

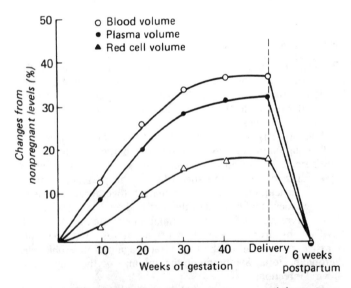

Figure 4-7. Blood volume changes during pregnancy and the postpartum period. (From M.L. Pernoll and R.C. Benson, eds., *Current Obstetric & Gynecologic Diagnosis & Treatment,* 6th ed. Lange, 1987.)

cumulative retention of sodium over the course of an average pregnancy. This results in a total body water increase of 6–8 liters, of which 4–6 liters is extracellular.

The distribution of blood volume varies with changes in body position. Sitting and supine recumbency during the third trimester trap blood in the legs. This also occurs during the *supine hypotensive syndrome* (i.e., bradycardia and hypotension due to reduced blood flow to the heart), when the uterus compresses the inferior vena cava.

The success of pregnancy is correlated with the development and maintenance of a normally expanded maternal blood volume. *Hypovolemia* is associated with *fetal growth retardation and preterm delivery.* Women with multiple pregnancy have more of an increase in blood volume over those with a singleton. However, there is a finite limit, and whereas a significant increase occurs with twins, the amount is much less with each additional fetus.

Leukocytes (primarily polymorphonuclear leukocytes) *increase* from nonpregnant levels (4300–4500/μl) to 5000–12000/μl at term. During labor, leukocytes may rise even higher (to ~25,000/μl).

There is a marked *increase* (~50%) *in fibrinogen* over the course of gestation. This increase is accompanied by a general *enhancement of clotting activity,* which causes a significant rise in the erythrocyte sedimentation rate (ESR). Small decreases in platelet count may occur.

Cardiac Output

Cardiac output (CO), the *product of the heart rate (HR) and stroke volume (SV),* increases ~40% (~1.5 liters/min) during gestation. It reaches the maximum at 20–24 weeks (Fig. 4-8). SV accounts for nearly all of the increase in early pregnancy to reach its peak of 25%–30% at 12–24 weeks. The HR increases by 15 beats/min at term but is influenced by the same variables as in the woman who is not pregnant.

Here, too, *position* of the gravida makes a significant difference—the best being the *left lateral decubitus.* During labor and delivery, contractions express blood from the uterine vascular bed. In the supine position, this increases venous return and transiently augments CO by about 25%, whereas in the lateral recumbent position, there is only a 7%–8% increase. Similarly, SV rises more in the supine vs lateral recumbent (33% vs. 7.7%), and the pulse rate falls less (15% vs 0.7%). The magnitude of

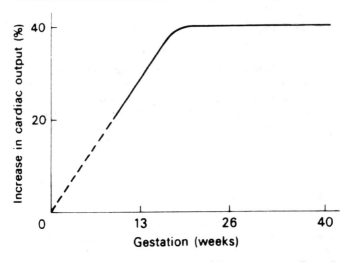

Figure 4-8. Increase in cardiac output during pregnancy. (From F. Hytten and G. Chamberlain, *Clinical Physiology and Obstetrics.* Blackwell Scientific Publications, 1980.)

these changes is modified also by the strength of the uterine contractions.

The enhanced CO is distributed primarily to certain sites. *Uterine blood flow* rises steadily, reaching ~500 ml/min at term. Early in pregnancy, the *renal blood flow* is increased about 30% above the average for nonpregnant women, and the *glomerular filtration rate (GFR)* increases to some 50% above nonpregnant levels. This augmentation persists to term. *Mammary blood flow* increases considerably by term. There is no change in CNS or hepatic blood flow during pregnancy.

Arterial Blood Pressure (BP)

Progesterone causes relaxation of smooth muscle. This is apparent in the venous system and results in dilated pelvic veins, increased vasculature of the uterus, and marked dilatation of the veins in the lower extremities. However, this effect also is noted in the arteries.

BP, the product of CO and peripheral resistance (PR), declines until midpregnancy. This is due to reduced vascular resistance despite the rise in CO. The BP rises under the influence of factors other than progesterone. The latter diminishes peripheral resistance from ~20 weeks gestation to term.

Pulmonary Adjustments to Pregnancy

Capillary dilatation throughout the respiratory tract causes voice changes and makes nose breathing difficult from early pregnancy. Radiologically, *pulmonary vascular markings are enhanced.* Uterine enlargement is accompanied by as much as 4 cm diaphragm elevation, but this altered position does not impede diaphragmatic function. Indeed, the abdominal muscles relax during pregnancy, and, thus, *respiration is more diaphragmatic.* The lower ribcage is flared outward, enhancing the subxiphoid angle and increasing the thoracic circumference by up to 6 cm.

Dead space volume increases because of conducting airway musculature relaxation. Gradual *increase in tidal volume* (35%–50%) occurs with lengthening pregnancy. Diaphragm elevation decreases total lung capacity by 4%–5%. Tidal volume increases 40%. *Functional residual capacity, residual volume,* and *expiratory reserve volume are reduced* by ~20%. *Alveolar ventilation is increased* by ~65% by the combination of larger tidal volume and smaller residual volume. *Inspiratory capacity is increased* 5%–10% by the maximum at 22–24 weeks. There is a *slight increase in respiratory rate, minute ventilation increases* 50%, and by term, *oxygen consumption is increased* 15%–20% above the nonpregnant. *Respiratory minute volume is increased* ~26% (Fig. 4-9).

Hyperventilation of pregnancy (decreased alveolar CO_2 with concomitant lower maternal blood CO_2 while maintaining normal maternal alveolar oxygen tension) occurs as a result of the alterations described. Maternal hyperventilation is due to progesterone action on the respiratory center mediated by peripheral chemoreceptors in the carotid body. This allows the fetus to exchange CO_2 in the most effective manner.

During labor and delivery, many patients hyperventilate. This may lead to respiratory alkalosis with carpopedal spasm. Functional reserve capacity further decreases in the early phase of each contraction (from the redistribution of blood from the uterus), and there may be more efficient gas exchange. Anesthetic administration must be altered accordingly.

Renal Alterations

Dilatation of the renal hila, calices, and *ureters* occurs as early as the late first trimester but usually regresses to normal by the end

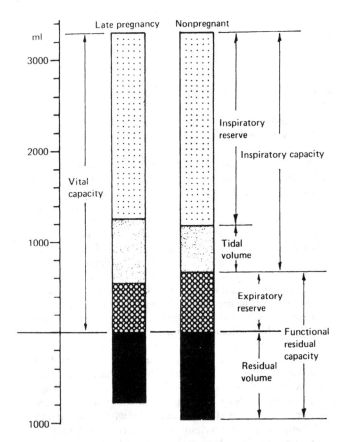

Figure 4-9. Lung volume changes during pregnancy. (From F.E. Hytten and I. Leitch. *The Physiology of Human Pregnancy.* Blackwell Scientific Publications, 1964.)

of the puerperium. The right collecting system exhibits greater dilatation because of compression by the enlarged, dextrorotated uterus. Bilaterial vesicoureteral reflux often occurs during pregnancy. Thus, pregnant women become more susceptible to urinary tract infection.

Renal plasma flow (RPF) increases markedly during pregnancy to attain a maximum of 60%–80% above nonpregnant levels by midgestation. Then, a gradual fall of about 25% occurs by term. The *GFR increases* by ~50% by the second trimester because of increased blood volume and renal blood flow, low-ered oncotic pressure, and endocrine changes. It plateaus in the third trimester to term. The filtration fraction (FF), the ratio of GFR/RPF, decreases during early pregnancy, to rise again in the last trimester. This probably indicates hemodynamic changes within the glomerulus.

Very early in pregnancy, the *creatinine clearance (CC) increases* to ~45% over nonpregnant values. During the second trimester, the CC remains elevated, but in the third trimester, several weeks before term, it gradually falls to nonpregnant levels.

Urea and uric acid are all excreted more effectively during pregnancy, so that the blood concentrations of these substances normally are lower than in the nonpregnant state. More glucose and lactose are excreted during pregnancy. Most amino acids are eliminated more rapidly and in larger amounts during pregnancy. Ascorbic acid and folate losses in the urine occur.

Fluid volume and composition are regulated by renal control of the excretion of sodium and water. Estrogen and cortisol and the renin-angiotensin-aldosterone system contribute to the changes in sodium and water homeostasis during pregnancy. The greatly in-creased GFR during pregnancy causes a considerable increase in sodium filtration, but *tubular reabsorption of sodium is increased.* This results in the positive sodium balance needed to allow for fetal requirements and the increased maternal blood volume. Pro-portionately more water than sodium is retained during the third trimester. This contributes to the commonly observed dependent edema of late pregnancy.

GASTROINTESTINAL ALTERATIONS WITH PREGNANCY

Oral

Salivation often increases and is more acidic. The gums may become hypertrophic and hyperemic, and epulis formation may occur in those without good oral hygiene.

Gastrointestinal

During pregnancy, both *gastrointestinal motility and tone de-crease* (under the influence of increased progesterone). Clini-cally, this leads to delayed gastric emptying, slower transit times, and constipation. There is more gastroesophageal reflux, which leads to *heartburn* and a very real possibility of regurgitation and aspiration if unconscious. The effect of pregnancy on gastric acidity is variable.

The *appendix is displaced superiorly and into the right flank,* and the *bowel is displaced upward and laterally.* This knowledge is most important when appendectomy must be performed in advanced pregnancy.

Liver

No specific gross or microscopic changes in the liver have been noted during pregnancy. Liver function test values in pregnancy are the same as in the nonpregnant state with the following exceptions. (1) Serum albumin decreases slowly during pregnancy from about 4.2 to 3.5 g/dl, with a gradual rise to normal in 6–8 weeks after delivery. (2) Alpha and beta globulin levels increase slightly and gamma-globulin decreases very slightly in pregnancy. (3) Cephalin flocculation is elevated in 25% of pregnancies. (4) Serum alkaline phosphatase increases gradually during pregnancy; at term, average values are 6.3 Bodansky units and 19 King-Armstrong units. Tests unchanged during gestation include those for serum glutamic oxaloacetic transaminase and serum bilirubin levels. The BSP excretion test is unaffected.

Gallbladder

Emptying time is slowed and often is incomplete. The bile's chemical composition is not altered, but bile stasis can lead to gallstones.

MATERNAL WEIGHT GAIN IN PREGNANCY

During the course of pregnancy, the average weight gain will be 22–27 pounds (10–12 kg). At term, the components of weight gain will be distributed as indicated in Figure 4-10. Ideally, only 1.5–3 pounds are gained in the first trimester and 0.8 pounds/week during the second and third trimesters. Inadequate progressive weight gain is often associated with poor fundal growth, reflecting deficient fetal growth. Thus, inadequate progressive weight gain in pregnancy requires investigation for nutritional deficit, maternal illness, malabsorption, or

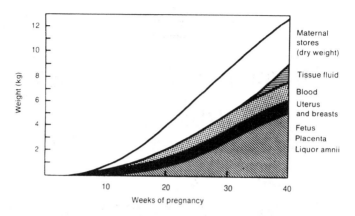

Figure 4-10. The components of weight gain in normal pregnancy. (From F.E. Hytten and A.M. Thomson. Maternal physiological adjustments. In: *Maternal Nutrition and the Course of Pregnancy.* National Academy of Sciences, 1970.)

an abnormal hormonal mileau (e.g., hyperthyroidism). Excessive weight gain in the latter half of pregnancy is worrisome because of the relationship to hypertensive states of pregnancy.

Individualization of maternal weight gain is key to optimal fetal growth. For example, it is recommended that underweight women gain more and obese women less. Women who are heavier at the onset of pregnancy or have excessive weight gain during pregnancy are more prone to have macrosomic babies. By contrast, underweight women and those with inadequate weight gain during pregnancy are more likely to have a fetus with intrauterine growth retardation and a small placenta.

Chapter 5

Diagnosis of Pregnancy and Prenatal Care

The correct early diagnosis of pregnancy is often urgent. For example, a diagnosis is essential to institute studies or treatment of problems that may jeopardize the life or health of mother or offspring or to apprise the infertile couple of the likely success of pregnancy or failure to conceive. Today this is usually accomplished by *early beta-subunit hCG testing* or *ultrasonic scanning* because a definite clinical diagnosis of pregnancy before the second missed period is possible in only about two thirds of patients. However, the practitioner must be familiar with the signs and symptoms of pregnancy to properly test for and treat the early pregnancy.

CLINICAL DIAGNOSIS OF PREGNANCY

Traditionally, the clinical criteria for the diagnosis of pregnancy have been categorized into presumptive, probable, and positive (Table 5-1).

The differential diagnosis of the common signs and symptoms of pregnancy involves other conditions associated with similar complaints or alteration (Table 5-2).

PELVIC FINDINGS OF EARLY PREGNANCY

Critical to the diagnosis of pregnancy by physical examination are the pelvic findings. The presumptive indications of pregnancy include the following.

Table 5-1 Presumptive or probable signs and symptoms of pregnancy*

Symptoms	Signs
Amenorrhea	Leukorrhea
Nausea, vomiting	Changes in color
Breast tingling, mastalgia	consistency, size or
Urinary frequency, urgency	shape of cervix or uterus
Quickening	Temperature elevation (usually by BBT)
	Enlargement of abdomen
	Breasts enlarged, engorged, nipple discharge
	Pelvic souffle (bruit)
	Uterine contractions (with enlarged corpus)

*Although these may be suggestive, even ≥2 are not diagnostic of pregnancy.

1. *Cyanosis of the vagina* (Chadwick's sign, Jacquemier's sign) is present by about 6 weeks.

2. *Softening of the tip of the cervix* (Fig. 5-1) occasionally is noted by the 4th–5th week of pregnancy. However, infection or scarring may prevent softening until late pregnancy.

3. *Softening of the cervicouterine junction* often occurs by 5–6 weeks. A soft spot may be noted anteriorly in the middle of the uterus near its junction with the cervix (Ladin's sign) (Fig. 5-2). A wider zone of softness and compressibility in the lower uterine segment (Hegar's sign) is the most valuable sign of early pregnancy and can usually be noted at ~6 weeks (Fig. 5-3). Ease in flexing the fundus on the cervix (McDonald's sign) generally appears by 7–8 weeks.

4. *Irregular softening and slight enlargement of the fundus* at the site of or on the side of implantation (Von Fernwald's sign) occur by ~5 weeks. Similarly, if implantation is in the region of a uterine cornu, a more pronounced softening and suggestive tumorlike enlargement may occur (Piskacek's sign) (Fig. 5-4).

5. *Generalized enlargement and diffuse softening of the uterine corpus* usually occur ≥ 8 weeks of pregnancy (Fig. 5-5).

ABDOMINAL FINDINGS OF EARLY PREGNANCY

1. *Active movements* usually are palpable ≥ 18 weeks.

Table 5-2 Comparative differential diagnosis of presumptive symptoms and signs of pregnancy

	Cause(s) if pregnant	Differential diagnosis (not pregnant)
Symptoms		
Amenorrhea	hCG, etc.	Pseudocyesis or other psychoneurosis, endocrinopathies (including premature menopause), metabolic disorders (e.g., anemia, malnutrition), obliteration of the uterine cavity, systemic disease (e.g., acute or chronic infection), malignancy
Nausea, vomiting	hCG, etc.	Emotional disorders (e.g., pseudocyesis, anorexia nervosa), GI disorders (gastroenteritis, peptic ulcer, hiatal hernia, appendicitis, intestinal obstruction, food poisoning, acute infections (e.g., influenza, encephalitis)
Mastalgia, breast tingling	Estrogen (duct stimulation), progesterone (alveolar stimulation)	Estrogen with anovulation, chronic cystic mastitis

Urinary urgency, frequency	Estrogen (cystourethral turgescence)	Urinary tract infection (UTI), cystourethritis or cystocele, anxiety, diabetes, pelvic tumors, emotional tension
Quickening	Fetal movements > 14 weeks (approx.)	Increased peristalsis, free adnexal cyst, pseudocyesis, gas, contractions
Constipation	Altered diet; hypoperistalsis	Low fluid, low fiber diet
Fatigue	Progesterone effect	Overwork
Weight gain	Gestational anabolism	Overeating

Signs

Leukorrhea	Estrogen	Vaginitis, cervicitis, genital foreign body, tumor

Pelvic organ alterations

Cyanosis of cervix or Chadwick's sign (>6 weeks)	Hormones of pregnancy	Vascular anomaly or tumor of cervix or uterus
Softening of cervix (>4–5 weeks)	Hormones of pregnancy	Chronic cervicitis
Softening of lower uterine segment (>5–6 weeks), Landin, Hegar's sign	Hormones of pregnancy	Vacular uterine anomaly or tumor
Irregular fundal softening, enlargement (>5 weeks)	Hormones of pregnancy	Myoma
Generalized corpus softening, enlargement (>8 weeks)	Hormones of pregnancy	Adenomyosis or myomata

(continued)

Table 5-2 (*continued*)

	Cause(s) if pregnant	Differential diagnosis (not pregnant)
Temperature elevation basal body temperature (BBT) >2 weeks	Progesterone	Infection, corpus luteum cyst, hCG or progestogen therapy, faulty thermometer
Abdominal enlargement	Uterine size	Obesity, pelvic or abdominal tumor, ascites, obesity, relaxation of abdominal muscles, pelvic and abdominal tumors, ascites, or ventral hernia
Breast changes		
Enlargement, engorgement, secondary areola (>6–8 weeks)	Estrogen and progesterone	Mastitis, malignancy, PMS, pseudocyesis
Colostrum (>16 weeks)	Prolactin, progesterone, etc., excess	Hypothalamic galactorrhea
Pelvic souffle (bruit)	Increased pelvic blood flow	Pelvic tumor or vascular anomaly (aneurysm)
Uterine contractions (with enlarged uterus)	Braxton Hicks contractions	Pseudocyesis, tightening–relaxation of abdominal muscles
Skin pigmentation (chloasma, linea nigra)	Pituitary melanotropin	Ultraviolet exposure (tanning)
Epulis (>12 weeks)	Progesterone	Gingivitis

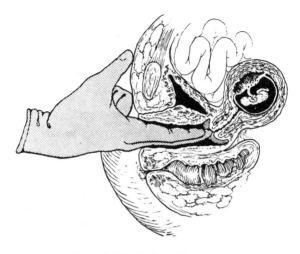

Figure 5-1. Softening of the cervix.

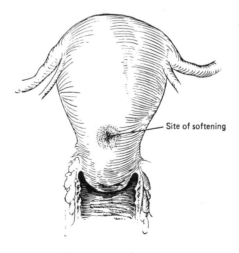

Figure 5-2. Ladin's sign.

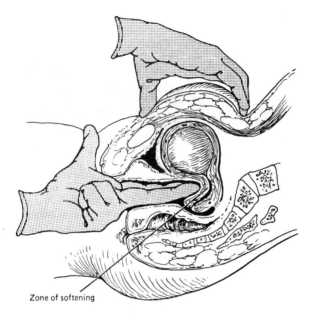

Zone of softening

Figure 5-3. Hegar's sign.

2. By the 16th–18th week, *passive movements* of the fetus may be elucidated by abdominal and vaginal palpation. A firm tap on the uterine wall or vaginal fornix displaces the fetus as a floating body. An impulse then can be felt as a thrust as the fetus moves back to its former position (ballottement). Ascites and tumors must be excluded.

3. After the 24th week, the *fetal outline may be palpated* in many pregnant women.

No subjective evidence of pregnancy is totally diagnostic, however, and laboratory diagnosis is essential.

LABORATORY EVIDENCE OF PREGNANCY

Beta-Subunit hCG

Assays for beta-subunit hCG, commonly used to diagnose pregnancy, have an admitted failure rate (~1%). Moreover, they

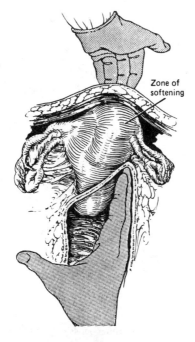

Figure 5-4. Piskacek's sign.

may be positive in nongestational ovarian choriocarcinoma or in uncommon gastrointestinal or testicular tumors. Nevertheless, a positive beta-subunit hCG test may be considered reasonable proof of pregnancy. A true positive followed by a true negative pregnancy test may indicate abortion. The major methods for determining the beta-subunit hCG are as follows.

Immunologic Tests

Immunologic tests for pregnancy (Table 5-3) are based on hCG's *antigenic potential* (direct or indirect agglutination of sensitized RBC or latex particles.) These tests require slides or test tubes for reagents and take from a few minutes to over an hour to complete. Test sensitivities vary widely (250–1400 mIU/ml).

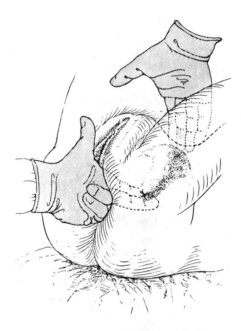

Figure 5-5. Bimanual pelvic examination.

Radioimmunoassay (RIA)

The hCG radioimmunoassay (RIA) requires a gamma counter for the highest sensitivity. The test, reportable in <90 min is extremely accurate (~20 mIU/ml.) Thus, it usually is used when sensitivity is crucial.

Radioreceptor Assay (RRA)

The RRA measures the biologic activity by in vitro binding of hCG to bovine corpus luteum membrane. Unfortunately, hCG and hLH cannot be separated by RRA. A commercially available RRA, Biocept G, has set its negative endpoint high to avoid false positive reports. *The accuracy does not approach that of RIA or ELISA,* however,

Table 5-3 Immunologic tests for pregnancy

Method	Materials	Results
Direct coagulation	Latex particles coated with anti-hCG + serum or urine	Coagulation if hCG is present (pregnant)
Inhibition of coagulation	Anti-hCG + serum or urine *plus* Sensitized red cells *or* Latex particles coated with hCG	Coagulation if hCG is absent (not pregnant); inhibition if hCG is present (pregnant)

Enzyme-Linked Immunoabsorbent Assay (ELISA)

A specified monoclonal antibody produced by hybrid cell technology is used for the ELISA assay. With ELISA, the enzyme induces a color change indicating the hCG level. *ELISA is simple and rapid* (5 min), *no isotopes are used,* and *it can be an office* (serum) *test* (e.g., Prognosis slide test, which measures to 1.5–2.5 mIU/ml). The tube, office or home test (e.g., Preco Rapid Care) measures only to 1.0 mIU/ml. Nevertheless, even ELISA home kits are at least 90% accurate within the range mentioned.

RIA, RRA, or ELISA can be used for the diagnosis of pregnancy as early as 8–12 days after ovulation. *hCH has a doubling time of 1.2–2.5 days during the first 10 weeks of pregnancy,* with a slow decline to about 5000 mIU/ml thereafter.

The latest beta-specific *latex tube or slide tests* that are based on agglutination or agglutination-inhibition are still adequate for the diagnosis of normal pregnancy >1–2 months. However, the ELISA test usually picks up earlier gestations and is more accurate, although after pregnancy, an ELISA test may require weeks to become negative. Therefore, *RIA will continue to be the method employed for serial quantitative studies in problem pregnancies,* particularly trophoblastic disease.

Ultrasonography

Using ultrasonography, *pregnancy can be diagnosed as early as the fourth week* and twins during the sixth week. High resolution real-time ultrasonography can determine gestational age accurately, especially during the first half of pregnancy. During this time, the accuracy of ultrasound for dating a pregnancy is *within 1 week in 95% of cases.* Various parameters, for example, crown-rump, are measured depending on the age of the conceptus.

Gestational Sac Measurements

A *normal gestational sac may be visible at 5 weeks.* It appears as an intrauterine fluid collection surrounded by a rim of echogenic tissue (the choriodecidual layer). Once the mean sac diameter (determined by averaging the AP, transverse, and longitudinal sac dimensions measured from the inner choriodecidual reaction) is >10 mm, a portion of the gestational sac normally should be surrounded by two closely spaced concentric ectogenic lines (the decidua parietalis and decidual capsularis).

In a normal early pregnancy, the *mean gestational sac diame-*

ter increases by ~ 1.2 mm/day. To determine the gestational age (in days), add 30 to the mean gestational sac diameter: a mean sac diameter of 20 mm corresponds to a gestational age of 50 days.

The *secondary yolk sac* can be seen in a gestational sac as early as the sixth week. An *embryonic heartbeat* frequently is identified contiguous with the yolk sac as early as 6 weeks gestational age and should always be present when the mean sac diameter is ≥25 mm (8 weeks).

Fetal Heartbeat

Electronic identification of the fetal heart pulse using *Doppler principle ultrasound* is possible after the eighth week. The early fetal hearbeat is more rapid (160 bpm) and slows with gestation. Near term, the rate is 120–140 bpm.

Mensuration

Mensuration of the fetus (biparietal diameter, abdominal circumference, fetal length, or crown-rump length) or uterine volume may provide accurate estimates of the EDC if taken early and sequentially and compared to known norms.

Tests No Longer Used

Several previously used techniques for pregnancy testing have been abandoned, for example, biologic pregnancy tests because of lower accuracy and extensive preparation time, x-ray demonstration of fetal skeleton because of teratogenic and oncogenic potential, fetal electrocardiography because Doppler ultrasound is more accurate and able to detect an earlier heartbeat, and hormone withdrawal (progesterone) bleeding because it may induce embryologic maldevelopment.

DURATION OF PREGNANCY AND EXPECTED DATE OF CONFINEMENT

ESTIMATED DATE OF CONFINEMENT

After a positive diagnosis, the duration of pregnancy and the *estimated date of confinement (EDC)* must be determined. Since it is uncommon to know the exact onset of pregnancy, these calculations start from the *first day of the last menstrual period (LMP)*. Pregnancy in women lasts about 10 lunar months (9 calendar months). *The average length of pregnancy is 266 days.* The median duration of pregnancy is 269 days. However, only ~6% of patients will deliver spontaneously on their EDC. Most (60%) will deliver within 2 weeks of the EDC. Thus, as in most physiologic events, *term* should be regarded as a season or period of maturity, not a particular day.

A major variable in the calculated duration of pregnancy is recognized because not all women have a 28-day cycle. Hence, the physician also must *consider the length of her cycle.* A patient with a regular 40-day cycle obviously will not ovulate on day 14 but closer to or on day 26. Therefore, her EDC cannot be estimated accurately by Nagele's rule alone. Moreover, some women tend to have long or short gestations as a familial predisposition. Primiparas tend to have slightly longer gestations than multiparas. Thus, the EDC cannot be calculated precisely, although the following clinical approximations have proven useful.

Nagele's Rule

Add 7 days to the first day of the LMP, subtract 3 months, and add 1 year.

$$EDC = (LMP + 7 \text{ days}) - 3 \text{ months} + 1 \text{ year}.$$

For example, if the first day of the LMP was June 4, the EDC will be March 11 of the following year.

Nagele's rule is based on a 28-day menstrual cycle with ovulation occurring on the 14th day. In calculating the EDC, an adjustment should be made if the patient's cycle is shorter of longer than 28 days. The discrepancies caused by 31-day months and the 29-day variation in February of leap year are not correctable by Nagele's rule. Nevertheless, it provides an acceptable estimate of the EDC.

Height of Fundus as Measured Abdominally

The uterus increases from a nonpregnant length ~7 cm to 35 cm at term; it increases 20 times in weight and grows in volume from 500–1000 times. Thus, the *size* of the *uterus should be evaluated at each prenatal visit* to determine the normality of progress. Most examinations involve an estimate of the height of the fundus uteri on the abdomen, not the length of the uterus. The *superior ramus of the pubis, the umbilicus,* and *the xiphoid* are the *fixed reference points* from which the height of the fundus is measured. A rough rule is provided by Table 5-4, and a more precise estimation can be made by the modified McDonald's rule.

Unusually *large measurements suggest an incorrect date of conception, multiple pregnancy, or polyhydramnios.* Unexpectedly *small measurements imply fetal death, fetal undergrowth, developmental abnormality, or oligohydramnios.*

Modified McDonald's Rule

Measure the height of the fundus (over the curve) above the symphysis with a centimeter tape measure. The *distance in centimeters will approximate the gestational age from* 16–38 weeks ± 3 weeks.

The same examiner should measure the fundus whenever possible because variations by personnel may inaccurately suggest pregnancy complications.

Additionally, a rough guide to fetal weight may be calculated from the modified McDonald's uterine measurement (Johnson's rule). However, recall that wide variations in the weights of fetuses in the third trimester may be due to the following.

1. The age–weight patterns of previous infants
2. An expected increase in weight of each successive infant
3. Hereditary traits or acquired disorders affecting infant size, for example, race, nutrition, diabetes mellitus, preeclampsia-eclampsia

Table 5-4. Uterine height and stage of gestation

Week of pregnancy	Approximate height of fundus
12	Just palpable above symphysis
15	Midpoint between umbilicus and symphysis
20	At the umbilicus
28	6 cm above the umbilicus
32	6 cm below the xiphoid
36	2 cm below the xiphoid
40	4 cm below the xiphoid

Johnson's Estimate of Fetal Weight

Fetal weight (in grams) *is equal to the fundal measurements* (in centimeters) *minus* n, *which is 12 if the vertex is at or above the ischial spines or 11 if the vertex is below the spines, multiplied by 155.*

Example: A gravida with a fundal height of 30 cm whose vertex is at −2 station can be represented as 30 − 12 × 155 = 2790 g. If the patient weighs >200 pounds, subtract 1 cm from the fundal measurement. By this calculation, an estimate within 375 g can be expected for about 70% of neonates.

Quickening

A rough estimate of the EDC is possible by adding 22 weeks to the date of quickening in a primigravida or 24 weeks in a multipara.

As in attempting to diagnose pregnancy, the most accurate data for EDC are provided by clinical, laboratory, and ultrasonographic studies.

Early hCG Testing

Determinations of beta-subunit hCG in maternal serum compared with a scale of predetermined quantitative values provide the most accurate estimate of gestational age during the first 8–10 weeks. After this, hCG levels slowly decrease, and the method becomes inaccurate.

Ultrasonography

Early (<20 weeks) *ultrasonographic measurements of the fetal biparietal diameter (BPD), abdominal circumference (AC), crown-rump length, femur length (FL), or total uterine volume* have been correlated accurately with gestational age. However, fetal growth between 20 and 30 weeks is rapid and linear, and there is marked third trimester variability in fetal size (as noted previously). Hence, *initial measurements should be taken and recorded as early as possible with subsequent later determinations.* A comparison of these diameters with standard curves can estimate the gestational age ± 11 days with 95% confidence. When only one measurement is possible or when initial measurements are obtained after the 30th week, the accuracy is much reduced. Nonetheless, during the third trimester, the best estimate of gestational age can be derived from a composite based on BPD, head circumference (HC), AC, and FL measurements. Between 30 and 36 weeks, the gestational age can best be determined by using the BPD-AC-FL measurements (standard deviation 1–2 weeks), whereas between 26 and 42 weeks, the combined use of HC-AC-FL is more accurate (standard deviation 1–2 weeks) (Table 5-5).

PRENATAL CARE

Prenatal care, the management of pregnancy, has numerous purposes.

1. To ensure, as far as possible, an *uncomplicated pregnancy* and the *delivery of a live healthy infant*
2. To *identify and institute care* for any risk state
3. To *individualize the level of care* necessary
4. To *assist the gravida* in her preparation for labor, delivery, and childrearing
5. To *screen for common diseases* that may affect the gravida's or child's life or health
6. To *reinforce good health habits* for the gravida and her family

To achieve these admittedly ideal goals requires an organized and thoughtful approach. Indeed, to be maximally effective, *prenatal care begins before conception*. Although not the only way to provide prenatal care, the following is intended as a guide or functional method that has assisted in fulfilling the stated purposes.

Standard record forms are commercially available. These, completed with explanations when indicated, will amass most of the necessary information. Thus, it is important to identify those data that should be recorded.

HISTORY AND PHYSICAL EXAMINATION

A complete medical history and physical examination early in pregnancy provides the *baseline for diagnosis* and the *treatment* of disorders that may compromise pregnancy.

Table 5-5. Embryonic and fetal growth and development

Fertilization age (weeks)	Crown-rump length*	Crown-heel length*	Weight*	Gross appearance	Internal development
Embryonic stage					
1	0.5 mm	0.5 mm	—	Minute clone free in uterus	Early morula, no organ differentiation
2	2 mm	2 mm	—	Ovoid vesicle superficially buried in endometrium	External trophoblast, flat embryonic disk forming 2 inner vesicles (amnioectomesodermal and endodermal)
3	3 mm	3 mm	—	Early dorsal concavity changes to convexity; head, tail folds form; neural grooves close partially	Optic vesicles appear, double heart recognized, fourteen mesodermal somites present
4	4 mm	4 mm	0.4 g	Head is at right angle to body; limb rudiments obvious, tail prominent	Vitelline duct only communication between umbilical vesicle and intestines, initial stage of most organs has begun
8	1.7 cm	3.5 cm	2 g	Eyes, ears, nose, mouth recognizable, digits formed, tail almost gone	Sensory organ development well along, ossification beginning in occiput, mandible, humerus (diaphysis), and clavicles, small intestines coil within umbilical cord, pleural, pericardial cavities form-

Fetal stage					
12	5.8 cm	11.5 cm	19 g	Skin pink, delicate, resembles a human being, but head is disproportionately large	ing, gonadal development advanced without differentiation. Brain configuration roughly complete, internal sex organs now specific, uterus no longer bicornuate, blood forming in marrow, upper cervical to lower sacral arches and bodies ossify
16	13.5 cm	19 cm	100 g	Scalp hair appears, fetus active, arm-leg ratio now proportionate, sex determination possible	Sex organs grossly formed, myelinization, heart muscle well developed, lobulated kidneys in final situation, meconium in bowel, vagina and anus open, ischium ossified
20	18.5 cm	22 cm	300 g	Legs lengthen appreciably, distance from umbilicus to pubis increases	Sternum ossifies
24	23 cm	32 cm	600 g	Skin reddish and wrinkled, slight subcuticular fat, vernix, primitive respiratory-like movements	Os pubis (horizontal ramus) ossifies, viability possible
28	27 cm	36 cm	1100 g	Skin less wrinkled; more fat, nails appear, if delivered, may survive with optimal care	Testes at internal inguinal ring or below, astragalus ossifies, >50% survive with the best of care

(continued)

Table 5-5. (continued)

Fertilization age (weeks)	Crown-rump length*	Crown-heel length*	Weight*	Gross appearance	Internal development
32	31 cm	41 cm	1800 g	Fetal weight increased proportionately more than length	Middle fourth phalanges ossify, about 90% survive with specialty care
36	35 cm	46 cm	2500 g (for Caucasian)	Skin pale, body rounded, lanugo disappearing, hair fuzzy or wooly, earlobes soft with little cartilage, umbilicus in center of body, scrotum small with few rugae, few sole creases	Distal femoral ossification centers present, >95% survive with individual care
40	40 cm	52 cm	3200+ g	Skin smooth and pink, copious vernix, moderate to profuse silky hair, lanugo hair on shoulders and upper back, earlobes stiffened by thick cartilage, nasal and alar cartilages, nails extend over tips of digits, testes in full, pendulous, rugous scrotum, or labia majora well developed, creases cover sole	Proximal tibial ossification centers present, cuboid, tibia (proximal epiphysis) ossify, over 95% survive with good care

*Approximate.

General Information

Record the patient's correct name, address, birth date, telephone number(s), choice of whom to call in an emergency, and special personal preferences.

History of Present Pregnancy

Obtain the *last menstrual period (LMP)* and *previous menstrual period (PMP)*. Then, calculate the *EDC*. Additionally, note the following.

A. *Current symptoms, signs, and problems*
B. Any *infections, medications, injuries, potential exposure to fetotoxic hazards*, especially those occurring during the present pregnancy
C. Menstrual history
   1. Age at *menarche*
   2. *Interval* between periods
   3. *Duration, amount of flow, intermenstrual spotting*
   4. *Dysmenorrhea*
   5. Leukorrhea
D. *Contraception:* method, duration, acceptance or reason for termination

History of Previous Pregnancies

For *each gestation,* record *duration, type termination, complications, outcome,* and *follow-up.* In those pregnancies resulting in a living child (LC) determine its sex and current well-being and attempt to assess the mother's attitude toward each child. The individual's reproductive history usually is recorded using the following definitions.

Gravidity (G) is the total number of pregnancies, including normal and abnormal intrauterine pregnancies, abortions, ectopic pregnancies, and hydatidiform moles. Multiple pregnancies are counted as a single experience.

Parity (P) is the birth of a >500 g infant or infants, alive or dead. When the weight is not known, use ≥24 weeks gestation. Multiple gestation is again counted as a single occurrence. A nullipara has not delivered an offspring weighing >500 g or of ≥24 weeks gestation.

Abortion (A) is pregnancy that terminates <24th gestational week or in which the fetus weighs <500 g.

Living child or children (LC) expresses the successful outcome of pregnancy.

By convention, this may be written G No., P No., A No., LC No. or further abbreviated to a series of numbers in the order given.

Medical and Surgical History

Record all *allergies* and *drug sensitivities, medications, important illnesses,* and *blood transfusions.*

List (with dates) *all operations* and *serious injuries* and outcomes. Detailed fertility studies should be included. Regarding cesarean deliveries, note the type, indications, trial of labor, and special surgical problems or postoperative complications.

Family History

List *medical, genetic,* and *psychiatric disorders* that may affect the patient or her offspring (e.g., diabetes mellitus, cancer, mental disease). A three-generation pedigree is often revealing.

Patient's Attitudes

Note *reservations* or *preferences as well as fears* manifested by the patient. Is this a wanted pregnancy? Exploring the following areas often will elicit information: her comfort with the pregnancy, prenatal care, early labor care, personal support during labor and delivery, analgesia, anesthesia, delivery, operative intervention, immediate postpartum care for the baby, other hospitalizations, and her response to having a baby.

Estimate the patient's maturity and general emotional stability to assist in *individualizing care.* Is she uncertain or confident?

Physical Examination

Conduct a *complete* general *examination* with special *emphasis* on the *reproductive organs and systems most influenced by pregnancy.* Examination of the head, ears, eyes, nose, and throat should be recorded. Careful *auscultation of the heart and lungs* is mandatory. Serious diseases often are first noted during an obstetric physical examination (e.g., anemia, tuberculosis, breast tumors), thus thoroughness is important. The assessment emphasizes the following.

General Examination

Record the *vital signs* including the blood pressure (BP), pulse, and respiration. Note *weight, height, body build,* and *state of nutrition.* Assess the following.

A. **Skin and hair.** Metabolic disorders (e.g., hypothyroidism) often are first manifested by dermatologic changes.

B. **Mouth.** Evaluate oral hygiene and check for epulis. (Encourage the patient to see her dentist for prophylaxis.)

C. **Neck.** Check for abnormal masses or lymphadenopathy. Expect slight diffuse physiologic enlargement of the thyroid gland in about 60% of pregnant patients.

D. **Breast.** Conduct a careful breast examination. Special attention should be afforded the nipples. This is a good time to initiate a discussion about breastfeeding.

E. **Abdomen.** Especially consider the following.

1. The contour, height (centimeters above the symphysis pubis), and consistency of the uterine fundus and its relationship to other organs or landmarks. Record the location of the fetal heart and its rate.

2. Abdominal organs that are palpable should be identified and abnormalities or extraneous masses identified. These include hernias (umbilical, inguinal, femoral, and lumbar). Hernias often become larger during pregnancy.

F. **Extremities.** Note development, deformity, and restriction of movement of legs, arms, and back. Varicosities and edema must be explained and treated if necessary.

G. **Posture and body mechanics** should be noted.

Pelvic Examination

A stepwise pelvic examination can be performed at any time before term but may be especially meaningful early (e.g., uterine size vs calculated gestational age). Pay particular attention to the following.

A. **Vulvar and vaginal varicosities.** These may bleed at delivery.

B. **Cervix and uterus.** Examine as described in Chapter 16. Near term, it is essential to note cervical consistency, position, and degree of effacement and dilatation. Record the site and extent of previous lacerations of the cervix, since tears may recur at these sites during delivery.

C. **Pelvic masses.** Distinguish between *ovarian* and *other pelvic or retroperitoneal tumors.* In many cases, ultrasonic scan will be useful.

D. **Pelvic measurements.** In most cases, clinical appraisal and recording of the pelvic configuration and major diameters by an experienced physician are adequate. If a pelvis is thought to be contracted, careful note of this should be made for a later evaluation. Clinical measurements necessary for an estimate of the pelvic outlet and inlet diameters are the following.

1. **Biischial diameter (BI)** (normal ≥8 cm) is the distance between the inner margins of the ischial tuberosities, and this constitutes the hypotenuse of the anterior pudendal triangle. The actual distance between the bony margins is usually >11 cm. However, when measured through the soft tissues, a normal value is ≥8 cm. This is known also as the transverse diameter of the outlet or the bituberous, intertuberous (IT), or tuberischial (TI) diameter.

2. **Posterior sagittal diameter of the outlet (PS)** (normal 8–9.5 cm). The PS is the distance from the midpoint of the line between the ischial tuberosities to the external surface of the tip of the sacrum (the tip of the rectal finger). This measurement is taken directly with the rectal finger touching the sacrococcygeal joint while visualizing the ischial intertuberous diameter.

Thoms's or Klein's rule: When the sum of the BI and the PS is more than 15 cm, an infant of normal size usually will pass the outlet safely.

3. **Anteroposterior diameter of the outlet (AP)** (normal ≥11.9 cm). This is the distance from the inferior border of the symphysis to the posterior aspect of the tip of the sacrum.

4. **Interspinous diameter of the midpelvis** (normal ≥10.5). This important measurement has a lower limit of 9.5 cm for passage of an average-sized infant. A reduced interspinous diameter is the most common cause of midpelvic dystocia.

5. **Diagonal conjugate of the inlet (DC)** (normal >11.5 cm) is probably the most important single measurement of the pelvis. It is from the inner inferior border of the symphysis to the midpoint of the sacral promontory (or false promontory, whichever is shorter) (Fig. 5-6). The true conjugate (conjugate vera, CV) is the distance from the anterior midpoint of the sacral or false promontory to the superior margin of the symphysis in the midline. This is calculated to be 1.5 cm shorter than the DC and represents the actual available anteroposterior diameter of the inlet. A DC of ≤11.5 cm or a CV of <10 cm indicates contracture of the pelvic inlet or superior strait. The likelihood of

dystocia, assuming an average-sized infant, in inversely proportional to this measurement. *Significant contracture of pelvic anterior-posterior diameter often is signaled by a term gestation that has failed to engage.*

E. **Palpation**

1. **Pubic arch.** Trace the pubic arch with the examining fingers. The angle formed by the pubic arch (the angle of the rami at the pubis) is usually *110–120 degrees.* In an android pelvis, the angle is narrow (<90 degrees), and the BI is narrow.

2. **Spines of the ischium.** Consider the degree of prominence, sharpness, and extent of encroachment of the spines into the birth canal.

3. **Sacrum.** The contour, depth, and irregularities (e.g., false promontory) are important. Record the curvature as *hollow* (deep), *average* (normally capacious), and *flat* (shallow), and record any irregularity.

4. **Coccyx.** By grasping the coccyx between the fingers of the examining hand, with the other hand placed in the cleft between

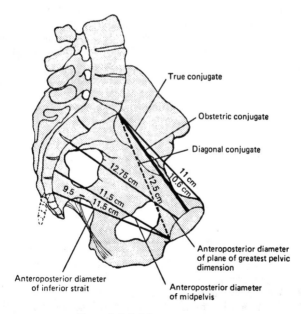

Figure 5-6. Pelvic measurements.

the buttocks, the direction of the coccyx, its degree of movement at the sacrococcygeal articulation, and local tenderness may be determined.

5. **Sacrosciatic notch** (normal >3 cm). The width of this space should be estimated and recorded in centimeters, not imprecise fingerbreadths.

Rectal Examination

Identify hemorrhoids and fissures.

Diagnosis

Record the duration of pregnancy and any anticipated complications.

Prognosis

Record an *initial prediction of the EDC and outcome of the pregnancy* (vaginal or cesarean delivery) together with the likelihood of medical or surgical complications (e.g., diabetes mellitus, inguinal hernia). The prognosis must be altered if obstetric problems develop.

Plan and Treatment

Project the care necessary for this gravida and pregnancy. A model program is noted under Management of Normal Pregnancy.

PROCEDURES AT FIRST OBSTETRIC VISIT

After the history has been taken and the physical examination has been performed
1. Answer questions.
2. Supply written prenatal care instruction, an explanatory

booklet or library references. Ask the patient and her husband to read them carefully before the next visit.

3. Prescribe necessary medications.

4. Arrange an appointment for the first return visit.

5. Request the patient to bring a first voided urine specimen at each subsequent visit.

6. Order laboratory tests.

7. Explain the costs of care.

LABORATORY TESTS

Obviously, laboratory tests must be *individualized for each patient.* Listed below are those commonly ordered for a normal gravida. They should be done *as early as possible,* and certain tests (*) should be repeated at 24–28 and 32–36 weeks gestation.

1. Hemoglobin and hematocrit*, white blood cell count (WBC) with differential count.

2. Serologic test for syphilis (STS or VDRL).

3. Blood group and Rh factor (unsensitized Rh-negative gravidas should have another antibody determination after the 12th and after the 24th week to reveal isoimmunization).

4. Antibody screening test* (a pooled series of about 29 antigens is used to detect the most common sensitizations).

5. Rubella antibody test (need not repeat if immune).

6. Serum alpha-fetoprotein (AFP) determination should be obtained at 16–18 weeks gestation when it is most accurate for detection of neural tube defects.

7. Urinalysis, urine culture (if positive, obtain bacterial sensitivity to antibiotics).

8. Papanicolaou (Pap) smears.

9. Cervical culture for *Neisseria gonorrhoeae* (and proper screening for other suspected sexually transmitted diseases).

10. All African American patients should be screened for sickle cell trait or disease (usually either a blood screening test or hemoglobin electrophoresis).

At this time, the use of certain other tests for screening remains controversial. Thus, in each case, the following should also be considered and discussed as part of the initial assessment. Ultrasonic scan for screening and dating gestation (usually <20 weeks), human immunodeficiency virus (HIV) screening, hepatitis B surface antigen screening, titers for *Toxoplasma gondii,* 1 h blood glucose following 50 g glucose load, tuberculin skin testing, and cervical culture for beta-streptococci (later in gestation).

MANAGEMENT OF NORMAL PREGNANCY

PRENATAL OFFICE VISITS AND EXAMINATIONS

Plan to see the patient once a month until the 32nd week, every 2 weeks until the 36th week, and weekly thereafter until delivery. See her more often if complications arise.

ESSENTIAL PROCEDURES AT EACH VISIT

From the initial office visit until delivery, a *continuing record of the progress of the pregnancy* must be maintained. Include symptoms, signs, habits, contacts or exposures to illnesses, medications, and laboratory test results. Additionally, the following constitute the usual structure of antenatal visits.

1. Ask the patient about her general health and any complaints.

2. Weigh the gravida and record her weight on the prenatal chart. Evaluate weight changes in comparison with the average curve.

3. Record the patient's blood pressure.

4. Examine a urine sample for protein and glucose. If significant glycosuria develops ($\geq 2+$), screen for carbohydrate intolerance. Screening consists of a 50 g oral glucose load and a 1 h blood sugar or fasting blood glucose and a 2 h postprandial blood glucose determination. If these tests are abnormal, order a glucose tolerance test (GTT).

Repeated $> +1$ proteinuria or urinary symptoms will necessitate a clean-catch specimen for culture and microscope study. If the bacterial count is $>100,000$/ml, prescribe appropriate antibiotics. Plan a repeat urine culture 1 week after the conclusion of treatment and again if symptomatology recurs. If the count is $<100,000$ ml, obtain a 24-h urine sample for volume, creatinine clearance, and total protein determination to diagnose possible renal disease.

5. Palpate the abdomen. Measure and note the height of the uterus above the symphysis. Record the fetal heartbeat and any abnormal details. After the 28th week, determine the presentation of the fetus. From the 32nd week on, in addition to these measures, record the position of the fetus, the engagement of the presenting part, and an estimate of the weight of the fetus.

6. Rectal or vaginal examinations may be done at virtually any time (in the absence of bleeding) to confirm the presenting part, establish its station, and determine the status of the cervix.

7. When the EDC, calculated from the LMP, is not supported by the physical findings, employ ultrasonography for abnormal fetal development, gestational age, or growth retardation. Ultrasonography is the obstetrician's major modality in gestational age assessment. Moreover, ultrasonography can be used to evaluate patients with uncertain dates, when the fetus seems too large (due to wrong dates, multiple gestations, hydramnios, macrosomia, associated uterine, or pelvic masses) or too small (wrong dates, oligohydramnios, IUGR). Ultrasonography can aid also in the diagnosis of patients with first trimester bleeding due to ectopic pregnancy, missed abortion, blighted ovum, subchorionic hemorrhage, or hydatidiform mole or third trimester bleeding due to placenta previa, abruptio placentae, or fetal anomalies (e.g., limb defects, neural tube anomalies).

TERM PREGNANCY

Term or fetal maturity at 37–40 weeks is *that period in which the neonate has the maximal likelihood of survival.* Term, a period rather than a day or even a week, is based on the EDC as well as other indices of fetal growth and development.

Full term (ideal maturity) is reached at 40 weeks gestation. The chance for survival then is about 99%. When there are discrepancies in the dates, other observations will be required to diagnose term, or full-term, states.

The fetus at term should weigh >2500 g, with the following approximate measurements: crown-rump 32 cm, crown-heel 47 cm, head circumference 33 cm, thoracic circumference 30 cm, occipital-frontal diameter 11.75 cm, and biparietal diameter 8.25 cm. Numerous determinants other than these measurements are required for a decision regarding age or maturity.

Clinical Findings

Cervical Changes

In early pregnancy, the cervix usually is directed posteriorly in the vagina. As term approaches, the *cervix* becomes soft and *moves anteriorly* into the vaginal axis. Normally, term has been reached when this and *marked effacement and dilatation of 1–2 cm* have occurred. Cervical effacement in primigravidas begins about the

36th week and is almost complete some 2 weeks later. Multiparas rarely achieve total effacement before labor, despite dilatation.

Engagement (Lightening)

When the fetal head descends into the pelvis so that the *biparietal diameter is at or* (more convincingly) *slightly below the brim of the true pelvis* (station 0 to −1), it is termed *engaged*. Engagement in a primigravida precedes delivery by about 2 weeks. Multiparous patients often go into labor before engagement, but if early engagement occurs, term probably has been reached.

NUTRITION IN PREGNANCY

Dietary Requirements

Good maternal nutrition is a major determinant of normal fetal growth and development. The daily dietary allowances recommended by the Food and Nutrition Board of the National Academy of Sciences-National Research Council are listed in Table 5-6. These should be considered approximations because adult patients who are ill or underweight, as well as adolescents who have not completed their growth, will require larger allowances.

Generally it is recommended that the pregnant patient have 36–38 cal/kg/day.

A normal pregnancy diet should include the following daily components (or equivalents): milk, 1 liter (or 1 quart), one average serving of citrus fruit or tomato, a leafy green vegetable, and a yellow vegetable, and two average servings of lean meat, fish, poultry, eggs, bean, or cheese.

Supplemental Mineral and Vitamins

Calcium must be supplemented during pregnancy to meet fetal needs and preserve maternal calcium stores. Milk is relatively inexpensive, and 1 liter (or 1 quart) of cow's milk contains 1 g of calcium, approximately the daily intake recommended during pregnancy (1.2 g) and *33 g of protein.* The milk need not always be in beverage form. It can be used in the preparation of foods, such as soup, custard, or junket. If the patient can not or will not drink whole milk, substitute sources of calcium (e.g., citrus

Table 5-6. Recommended daily dietary allowance for women 18–50 years old, 64 inches tall, and weighing 120 pounds when not pregnant*

Nutrient	Nonpregnant	Increase	
		Pregnant	Lactating
Calories (cal)	2000	+300	+500
Protein (g)	44	+30	+20
Vitamin A (RE)[†]	800	+200	+400
Vitamin D (IU)	200	+200	+200
Vitamin E (mg α-TE)[‡]	8	+2	+3
Vitamin C (mg)	60	+20	+40
Folacin (μg)[§]	400	+400	+100
Niacin (mg NE)[‖]	14	+2	+5
Thiamine (mg)	1.1	+0.4	+0.5
Riboflavin (mg)	1.3	+0.3	+0.5
Vitamin B_6 (mg)	2	+0.6	+0.5
Vitamin B_{12} (μg)	3	+1	+1
Calcium (mg)	800	+400	+400
Phosphorus (mg)	800	+400	+400
Iodine (μg)	150	+25	+50
Iron (mg)	18	+30–60	+30–60
Magnesium (mg)	300	+150	+150
Zinc (mg)	15	+5	+10

*Food and Nutrition Board, National Academy of Science–National Research Council, Revised 1980.
[†]Retinol equivalents. 1 RE = 1 μg retinol or 6 μg β-carotene.
[‡]α-Tocopherol equivalents. 1 α-TE = 1 mg α-tocopherol.
[§]Refers to dietary sources as determined by *Lactobacillus casei* assay after treatment with enzymes to make polyglutamyl forms of the vitamin available to the test organism.
[‖]Niacin equivalents. 1 NE = 1 mg niacin or 60 mg dietary tryptophan.

juice, yogurt, powdered milk) or prescribe a supplement (e.g., calcium carbonate).

Although ample calcium and phosphorus are required by the mother for fetal anabolism, a relative excess of phosphorus may cause leg cramps. Large quantities of milk, meat, cheese, and dicalcium phosphate (taken as a supplement) may impose excessive phosphorus.

Some patients, especially Native Americans, foreign-born African Americans, or certain Orientals, may have a disaccharidase deficiency causing *intolerance to lactose in milk*. For these persons, protein, calcium, and vitamins must be supplied in other forms (e.g., fish, fruits).

Supplemental iron is needed during pregnancy for the fetus and to prevent depletion of the maternal iron stores, especially during the latter part of pregnancy. Iron is the only mineral that usually must be prescribed (i.e., 30–60 mg elemental iron or ferrous sulfate 300 mg bid). Equivalents (ferrous gluconate or fumerate) may be better tolerated.

A pregnant woman who consumes adequate quantities of properly prepared fresh foods needs no other vitamin or mineral supplements, but *many women do not eat enough vitamin-containing foods.* To make certain that the vitamin intake is adequate, the common practice of recommending prenatal vitamin supplements is not harmful in the doses usually prescribed. *Massive doses of any vitamin or vitamin compound should be avoided.* For example, excessive ingestion of vitamins D and A may be fetotoxic.

Patients who do not eat well may benefit from folate supplements. Folic acid (folacin), 0.8 mg/day orally, may be a beneficial dietary supplement for most gravidas. Moreover, routine folate treatment will not harm a pregnant woman with unrecognized pernicious anemia.

Salt Restriction

The requirement for sodium during pregnancy is increased slightly. In any case, overemphasis on salt restriction is unjustified.

Fluids

At least *2–3 quarts of fluid* should be taken daily during pregnancy to accommodate metabolic processes and aid in elimination. Limitation of fluids will neither prevent nor correct fluid retention. *Liquids containing no sodium will not contribute to edema* in the absence of renal failure. Actually, increased intake of water aids slightly in the excretion of sodium and extracellular fluid.

Weight Gain

The *mother's prepregnancy weight and her weight gain during pregnancy are major determinants in the birth weight of the infant.* Women of low weight (e.g., <55 kg) before pregnancy who gain a limited amount of weight (<4500 g) during pregnancy have a higher incidence of low-birth-weight neonates than heavier mothers who gain more weight during pregnancy.

Cumulative energy costs of pregnancy are shown in Figure 5-7. The gravida of average weight requires approximately 2300–2600 cal/day during pregnancy to assure the average weight gain of 11.5–12.5 kg (25–28 pounds) total, whereas the underweight woman, the woman with an SGA fetus, and the woman with a multiple gestation should be encouraged to gain as much weight as possible. In general, younger primigravidas should have more calories than older miltiparas. How much weight should be gained during pregnancy by the obese woman is still debated. In general, there is a great variability of weight gain without apparent harm.

The *gain should be almost linear during the second and third trimesters* with an average of about 0.4 kg/week. Roughly, this should equate to an approximate gain of 0.65 kg by 10 weeks, 4 kg by 20 weeks, 8.5 kg by 30 weeks, and 12.5 kg by 40 weeks. Note that the maternal *weight gain during the first trimester is small and fetal gain is minimal.* During the second trimester, maternal storage of fat, growth of the uterus and breasts, together with an expansion of the blood volume, represent the major components of the gain. During the third trimester, growth of the fetus and placenta and accumulation of amniotic fluid contribute most to the total weight gain but with little maternal weight accumulation.

Extremes are important too (i.e., patients who gain 10 kg in

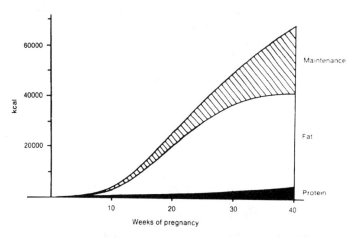

Figure 5-7. The cumulative energy costs of pregnancy. (From F.E. Hytten and I. Leitch. *The Physiology of Human Pregnancy,* 2nd ed. Blackwell Scientific Publications, 1971.)

the first 3 months must not drastically limit future gain to, say, only 2 kg). Similarly, obese women should not attempt to reduce during pregnancy or lactation. This leads to nutritional deficiencies, poor use of protein, and excessive catabolism of fat, causing ketosis and acetonuria. Moreover, an underweight patient who is seen for the first time during the last trimester should not overeat to catch up to her "best weight" at term.

Moderate weight gain is associated with the lowest incidence of low-birth-weight infants and neonatal death. The underweight woman with a small gain in weight during pregnancy should be considered a high-risk patient. Women who gain excessive weight have the usual problems of obesity. Individualization of diet seems the best course of action. *Emphasis should be placed on good nutrition rather than on precise weight control.*

There is no convincing evidence that excessive weight gain causes preeclampsia-eclampsia, but obese gravidas are more likely to have orthopedic problems or postpartum hemorrhage, and their infants are more likely to be macrosomic. The rate of weight gain is important in the diagnosis of preeclampsia-eclampsia. An increase of $\geq$ 1814 g (4 pounds) during any 1–2 week period from 24–35 weeks gestation or $\geq$ 0.9 kg (2 lb) per week from 35 weeks to term will often presage preeclampsia-eclampsia. There has been a marked decline in the incidence of preeclampsia-eclampsia in the United States, and it seems likely that better nutrition may account for at least part of this improvement.

Vegetarians who include dairy products probably will meet their dietary need during pregnancy. However, those with major restrictions (including milk or eggs) probably will need supplements of iron, folic acid, zinc, and vitamin B_{12}.

Teenage gravidas or those with diabetes mellitus or renal disease require special diets. Dietary needs often become apparent during the initial antenatal examination of the skin, nails, hair, mouth, teeth, and musculoskeletal system.

The physician will be more successful as a nutrition counselor if emphasis is placed on what should be eaten rather than what should not be eaten.

MINOR DISCOMFORTS OF NORMAL PREGNANCY

Nausea and Vomiting (Morning Sickness)

About *half of all pregnant women have nausea and vomiting,* often on arising, at some time during pregnancy. This most commonly occurs during the *first 10 weeks, seemingly related to higher levels of hCG*. About 1/1000 gravidas with severe morning sickness develop intractable vomiting (hyperemesis gravidarum, pernicious vomiting of pregnancy). In such cases, a psychiatric consultation may be most useful. Hospitalization may be necessary to correct fluid and electrolyte imbalance or to remove the gravida from a stressful environment or for study. In these severe cases, weight, nitrogen balance, liver enzymes, and fetal growth must be rigorously monitored. The addition of IV vitamins decreases the possibility of hypovitaminosis.

Usually, explanation, reassurance, and symptomatic relief are sufficient. Dietary changes are often helpful. Eating dry toast and jelly immediately on arising, before the nausea begins, helps some patients. Avoidance of disagreeable odors and rich, spicy, or greasy foods is important. Urge the gravida to drink water or other fluids between meals to avoid dehydration and acidosis, which predispose to nausea.

Antinauseants harmless for a nonpregnant woman may have unforeseen or undesirable effects on the fetus. Therefore, during pregnancy, even well-known over-the-counter drugs should be administered only when absolutely indicated and prescribed.

Backache

Virtually all women suffer from at least minor degrees of lumbar backache during pregnancy. Fatigue, muscle spasm, or postural back strain most often is responsible. Relaxation of the pelvic joints from the action of steroid sex hormones or perhaps relaxin also is responsible. Backache often can be relieved by the following measures.

1. *Improvement in posture* is often achieved by the wearing of low heeled shoes. To achieve proper posture, the abdomen should be flattened, the pelvis tilted forward, and the buttocks tucked under to straighten the back.
2. *Prescribe back exercises* under the supervision of a rehabilitation physician, an orthopedist, or a physical therapist.
3. Recommend sleep on a *firm mattress*.
4. *Apply local heat and light massage* to relax tense, taut back muscles.
5. *Give acetaminophen* 0.3–0.6 g orally or equivalent.
6. Obtain *orthopedic consultation* if disability results. Note neurologic signs and symptoms indicative of prolapsed intervertebral disk syndrome, radiculitis.

Heartburn

Heartburn (pyrosis, acid indigestion) results from gastroesophageal regurgitation in almost *10% of all gravidas.* In late pregnancy, this may be aggravated by displacement of the stomach and duodenum by the uterine fundus. Heartburn is most likely to occur when the patient is lying down or bending over. Occasional patients experience severe pyrosis during late pregnancy because of a hiatal hernia. This hernia is reduced spontaneously by parturition. *Symptomatic treatment,* not surgery, is recommended.

Hot tea and change of posture are helpful. Calcium-containing antacids (e.g., Tums) to reduce gastric irritation often are beneficial. Aluminum-based antacids are less desirable.

Syncope and Faintness

Syncope and faintness are common in early pregnancy because of *vasomotor instability* (largely progesterone-related relaxation of vascular smooth muscle). Encourage the patient to eat six small meals a day rather than three large ones. Stimulants (spirits of ammonia, coffee, tea) are indicated for attacks due to postural hypotension.

Leukorrhea

A *gradual increase in the amount of nonirritating vaginal discharge due to estrogen stimulation of cervical mucus is normal* during pregnancy. Such vaginal fluid is milky, thin, and nonirritating unless infection has occurred. Persistent external moisture due to mucus may cause mild pruritus, but itching is rarely severe without infection. Reassure the patient, and suggest protective perineal pads. Excessive leukorrhea accompanied by pruritus or discoloration of the secretion may indicate bleeding or infection, requiring treatment.

Urinary Symptoms

Urinary frequency, urgency, and stress incontinence in multiparas are common, especially in advanced pregnancy. These symptoms usually are due to increased intraabdominal pressure and reduced bladder capacity. Suspect urinary tract disease if dysuria or hematuria is present.

When urgency is particularly troublesome, *limit caffeine,*

spices, and popular beverages. Urised, 1–2 tablets orally every 4 h as necessary, or Levamine, 1 capsule every 2 h, may give relief but rarely is necessary.

Breathlessness

Breathlessness, not actual dyspnea, is a progesterone effect. In nonsmokers and others free of cough or allergic problems, breathlessness occurs as early as the 12th week of pregnancy, and most women have this symptom by the 30th week. There is no effective treatment.

Constipation

Constipation due to sluggish bowel function in pregnancy may be due to progesterone effect and bowel displacement. Emphasize *ample fluids and laxative foods and prescribe a stool softener* (e.g., bran or dactyl sodium sulfosuccinate). Exercise and good bowel habits are helpful. Mild laxatives (e.g., milk of magnesia) are acceptable, but purgatives should be avoided because of the possibility of inducing labor. Mineral oil is contraindicated, since it absorbs fat-soluble vitamins from the bowel and leaks from the anus.

Hemorrhoids

Hemorrhoids, frequent in pregnancy, may cause considerable discomfort. Straining at stool often causes hemorrhoids, especially in women prone to varicosities. *Symptomatic therapy* (hemorrhoidal preparations) is usually sufficient. *Treat constipation early.* At delivery, use elective low forceps with episiotomy when feasible. Surgical treatment rarely is indicated during pregnancy. However, very recently thrombosed, painful hemorrhoids can be incised and evacuated under local anesthesia. Do not suture. Sitz baths, rectal ointments, suppositories, and mild laxatives are indicated postoperatively or postdelivery. Injection treatments to obliterate hemorrhoids during pregnancy are contraindicated. They may cause infection or thrombosis of pelvic veins and are rarely successful because of the great dilatation of many vessels.

Headache

Headache in pregnancy is common and usually due to tension. Refractive errors and ocular imbalance are not caused by normal pregnancy. *Severe, persistent headache in the third trimester must be regarded as symptomatic of preeclampsia-eclampsia until proven otherwise.*

Ankle Swelling

Edema of the lower extremities (not associated with preeclampsia-eclampsia) develops in at least two thirds of women in late pregnancy. Edema is due to water retention and increased venous pressure in the legs. Generalized edema, always serious, must be investigated.

Treatment is largely preventive and symptomatic. The patient should elevate her legs frequently. Restrict excessive salt intake and provide elastic support for varicose veins. Diuretics may reduce edema temporarily but may be harmful to the mother or fetus.

Varicose Veins

Varicosities may develop in the legs or in the vulva. Varices are due to smooth muscle relaxation, weakness of the vascular walls, and incompetent valves. Pressure on the venous return from the legs by the enlarging uterus also is a major factor in the development of varicosities. Large or numerous varicosities are associated with muscle aching, edema, skin ulcers, and emboli.

The patient should *elevate her legs* above the level of her body and control excessive weight gain. *Avoid forceful massage* (especially downward, i.e., against venous return) *and point-pressure over the legs.*

Patients with significant varices should be fitted with elastic stretch stockings. Large vulvar varices cause pudendal discomfort. A vulvar pad snugly held by a menstrual belt may give relief. However, in more severe leg or vulvar varicosities, a Jobst-type leotard garment may be necessary to obtain venous compression. Injection or surgical correction of varicose veins usually is not recommended during pregnancy.

Leg Cramps

Cramping of the muscles of the calf, thigh, or buttocks may occur suddenly after sleep or recumbency in many women after the first trimester of pregnancy. Sudden shortening of the leg muscles by stretching with the toes pointed often precipitates the cramp. Leg cramps may be due to a reduced level of diffusible serum calcium or an increased serum phosphorus level. Symptomatology follows excessive dietary intake of phosphorus in milk, cheese, meat, or calcium phosphate or diminished intake or impaired absorption of calcium. However, fatigue or diminished circulation may be contributing factors.

Treatment should include curtailment of phosphate intake (less milk and nutritional supplements containing calcium phosphate) and increased calcium intake (without phosphorus) as calcium carbonate or calcium lactate. Aluminum hydroxide gel, 8 ml orally tid before meals, absorbs phosphate. Symptomatic treatment consists of leg massage, gentle flexing of the feet, and local heat.

Abdominal Discomfort

Intraabdominal alterations causing distress during pregnancy include the following.

Pressure Pelvic heaviness is caused by the weight of the uterus on the pelvic supports and the abdominal wall. The patient should rest frequently, preferably in the lateral recumbent position.

Round Ligament Tension Tenderness along the course of the round ligament (usually the left) during late pregnancy is due to traction on this structure by the uterus, which is displaced by the large bowel to be rotated slightly to the right. Local heat and change of position are beneficial.

Flatulence, Distention Large meals, gas-forming foods, and chilled beverages are poorly tolerated by pregnant women. Mechanical displacement and compression of the bowel by the enlarged uterus, hypotonia of the intestines, and constipation predispose to gastrointestinal disorders. Dietary modifications often give effective relief. Regular bowel function should be maintained, and exercise is beneficial.

Uterine Contractions So-called *Braxton Hicks contractions* of the uterus may be sharply painful and vexing. The onset of premature labor must always be considered when forceful, regular, extended contractions develop. If contractions remain infrequent and brief in duration, the danger of early delivery is not significant. Sedatives, such as diazepam (Valium) 5–10 mg twice daily, or acetaminophen 0.3–0.6 2–3 times daily, may be of value.

Intraabdominal Disorders Pain may be due to obstruction, inflammation, and other disorders of the gastrointestinal, urinary, neurologic, or vascular system or to pathologic pregnancy or tubal or ovarian disease. These disorders must be diagnosed and treated appropriately.

Fatigue

The pregnant patient is more subject to fatigue during the last trimester of pregnancy because of altered posture and extra weight carried. Anemia and other systemic diseases must be ruled out. *Frequent rest periods are recommended.*

COMMON PREGNANCY CONCERNS

Medications

Discourage the use of drugs in pregnancy because of potential fetal effects. In general, give medication only when urgently required. Avoid new and experimental drugs and all drugs that have been suggested as possible teratogens. Give medicaments, when needed, in the lowest dosage consistent with clinical efficacy. Record all pharmaceuticals taken by the patient during the pregnancy, and caution her about taking any preparation without first discussing it with the physician.

Rest

A daily rest or nap for 1 h, preferably while lying on the side, is desirable. Eight hours of sleep at night is recommended.

Sexual Intercourse

Sexuality continues during pregnancy, and in the normal gravida, *coitus has not been demonstrated to contribute to spontaneous abortion or premature labor.* Thus, coital restraints are neither necessary nor desirable. However, *contraindications to coitus* include premature labor, rupture of the membranes, vaginal bleeding, incompetent cervix, threatened or habitual abortion, multiple pregnancy (after the 28th week), and genital herpesvirus or other sexually transmitted infection.

Douching is seldom necessary and may be harmful. Forceful

douches, especially with a hand bulb syringe, may produce air or fluid embolism.

Physician explanation and questions and answers involving the patient and her spouse are important.

Employment

Most women can continue to work during pregnancy. However, they should not be exposed to hazardous conditions or become seriously fatigued. Exactly how long the pregnant woman can safely remain on the job depends on the type of work, industrial hazards, the policy of the employer, and pregnancy complications. Women with sedentary jobs often work well beyond the 28th week of pregnancy without difficulty. Others whose employment requires more physical exertion may find it advisable to take maternity leave earlier. Rest periods during the day may help to avoid undue fatigue.

The *capacity for work during pregnancy may be affected by weight increase, altered posture, modified physiology* (e.g., cardiovascular, pulmonary, renal), *urinary changes, or complications of pregnancy.* Fatigue may be responsible for increased tension or reduced concentration and alertness. Pregnancy complications rarely are caused by work itself, except when the gravida is exposed to trauma, toxic compounds, or laboratory pathogens. Indeed, the work environment is usually safer than the home or recreational site.

To achieve maximal care during pregnancy, the working gravida should report the pregnancy as soon as the diagnosis is made, and her obstetrician should assess (with the occupational medicine personnel) the potential impact of her employment on the pregnancy (and vice versa). This should be a part of the plan for her pregnancy. The employer should be notified of the plan and any complications or job modifications deemed necessary. The time to cease working must be individualized, but *most current U.S. guidelines recommend return to work 4–6 weeks after delivery.*

Exercise During Pregnancy

Maintaining maternal physical fitness is most desirable during pregnancy. Women who have exercised regularly can withstand the work of labor with less alteration in fetal cord blood.

However, many *variables determine how much exericise can be tolerated without fetal jeopardy* (e.g., reduced uterine blood flow, maternal hyperthermia, or fetal trauma).

During exercise, blood flow is diverted to the muscles and skin and away from the uterus. Unfortunately, the level of exercise associated with a serious decrease in uterine blood flow and how the fetus is affected are yet to be determined. For this reason, women should train for rather than during pregnancy. Nonetheless, the obstetrician cannot (as yet) recommend a specific target maternal heart rate response to exercise because of great individual variation.

Before closure of the neural groove of the embryo, increased maternal core temperature augments the likelihood of neural tube defects (e.g., anencephaly, spina bifida). Later in pregnancy, thermal injuries may cause harm to the fetal thermoregulatory center. However, the critical levels of temperature and time have not been established. Even aerobic exercises during pregnancy can transiently raise the maternal temperature to $\geq 102°F$. Moreover, dehydration increases the temperature rise during exercise. Hence, caution should be advised.

Although abdominal trauma during some exercise (e.g., aerobics) is less likely than with other contact sports, falls or other accidents may jeopardize the placenta or fetus.

In summary, the following recommendations for exercise in pregnancy seem reasonable.

1. *Gravidas accustomed to moderate exercise before pregnancy may continue the program,* but at a slower pace and for a shorter time (i.e., limit exercise by one third, by term, in a linear decrease, in both rate and duration of the accustomed exercise).

2. *Avoid fatigue.*

3. *Do not initiate a new strenuous exercise program* during pregnancy.

4. *Patients who were sedentary before pregnancy should restrict exercise to a moderate program* (e.g., walking or brief swimming).

5. *Hot environments* (e.g., hot tubs or saunas) *should be avoided* during pregnancy.

6. Many *pregnancy complications* (e.g., multiple gestation), *may adversely affect the ability to exercise.*

Alcohol

The safe amount of alcohol intake during pregnancy is still unknown. However, gravidas who consume >6 fluid ounces (180 ml) of whiskey or equivalent daily have at least a 20% likelihood of delivering an infant with features of the *fetal alcohol syndrome.* The patient who never drinks, stops drinking early in pregnancy, or reduces her alcohol intake drastically will have a much better fetal prognosis.

Smoking

Smoking is particularly deleterious during pregnancy. The alterations induced in the mother and fetus are summarized in Table 5-7.

Smoking is especially harmful to women >35 years or those with antepartum bleeding, poor weight gain, anemia, or hypertension. Moreover, *smoking and alcohol intake are synergistically harmful* to the fetus.

Obstetric patients should stop smoking. If this is impossible, restrict tobacco to less than one-half pack of low-nicotine, low-tar cigarettes per day.

Immunizations

Generally, live virus vaccines are contraindicated during pregnancy because of the risk to the fetus. In contrast, killed virus immunization (i.e., poliomyelitis) is permitted. However, the rubella vaccine (a live virus) has, to date, not been incriminated in causing the rubella syndrome. Obviously, *all immunizations must be judged on a risk–benefit basis.*

Table 5-7. Alterations induced by smoking during pregnancy

Gravida	Fetus
Plasma volume reduced	Fetal breathing suppressed
Second trimester abortion, preterm delivery (associated with placenta previa, premature separation of the placenta) increased	Contraction of umbilical arteries diminishes fetal circulation (nicotine effect)
Cardiorespiratory problems augmented	Neonatal birthweight reduced (averages 200 g below normal—directly related to number of cigarettes smoked)
	Perinatal mortality and morbidity increased

Dental Care

"For every child a tooth" is an untrue maxim. Decalcification of the mother's teeth does not occur as a result of pregnancy. Necessary dental fillings or extractions may be performed during pregnancy, preferably under local anesthesia. Routine antibiotic prophylaxis may be necessary in some patients (e.g., with a prolapsed mitral valve). Abortion or premature labor and delivery are not caused even by extensive dental surgery.

Bathing

Bath water does not enter the vagina, and tub baths and swimming are not contraindicated during normal pregnancy. Prolonged exposure to extremely hot or very cold baths should be avoided, however. Showers may be safer than tub baths because with the awkwardness caused by pregnancy, falls in a tub may occur.

Preparation for Breastfeeding

Most women who breastfeed successfully do so naturally without preparation. *The advantages of nursing should be explained carefully to the patient.* If the gravida decides to nurse, institute predelivery breast and nipple care.

The Figure

Pregnancy need not ruin the figure. Avoidance of excessive weight gain, continued daily exercise, and a well-fitted brassiere worn much of the time will help to preserve the figure.

Travel

If a long journey is essential, air travel is best, but pregnant women should not fly at high altitudes in unpressurized aircraft unless oxygen is available. All commercial aircraft are now pressurized to 1525–2130 m (5000–7000 ft), which is safe for pregnant women. To avoid possible delivery en route, most airlines will not permit women to fly during the last month of pregnancy. With all forms of travel, it is advisable for the gravida to walk about approximately once an hour, avoid prolonged extremity dependency, and avoid extreme fatigue.

Travel will not cause abortion or premature labor, but the pregnant woman is jeopardized indirectly by travel, since she may be far from her obstetrician in case of an obstetric emergency. Therefore, with distant travel, she probably should *carry a copy of her antenatal record.*

DIAGNOSIS OF PREVIOUS PREGNANCY

A physician may be required because of medical or legal questions to determine if a woman has had a pregnancy. A reasonably accurate opinion often is possible, based on physical residua of pregnancy or obstetric treatment. The following are suggestive of earlier pregnancy.

Skin	Pigmentation of the nipple areola, evident linear nigra, abdominal, breast, or buttock striae
Breast	Less firm, more pendulous
Abdomen	Relaxation of abdominal wall, diastasis of rectus muscles
Vagina	Widened introitus, cystocele, rectocele
Scars	Lower abdomen (? cesarean section), cervical lacerations, perineal or episiotomy repair

Chapter 6

Course and Conduct of Labor and Delivery

Labor is the normal process of *coordinated, effective involuntary uterine contractions that lead to progressive cervical effacement and dilatation and descent and delivery of the newborn and placenta.* Near its termination, labor may be augmented by voluntary bearing-down efforts to assist in delivery of the conceptus.

False labor is characterized by irregular (both in interval and duration), brief contractions without fundal dominance, cervical change, or a lower station of the fetal vertex or breech.

Dilatation of the cervix is the *diameter of the cervical os expressed in centimenters* (0–10). *Effacement is cervical thinning* that occurs before and especially during first stage labor. Effacement of the cervix is expressed as a percentage of cervical length (normally ~2.5 cm) (Figs. 6-1, 6-2). An uneffaced cervix is 0%; one about 0.25 in length is 100% effaced. Effacement and dilatation are caused by retraction (takeup) of the cervix toward the uterine corpus, not by pressure of the presenting part.

The initiation of labor in the human is poorly understood. Labor may be triggered by one or more significant endocrine or physical changes, for example, abdominal trauma. The onset of labor may occur at any time after well-established pregnancy, but the likelihood increases as term is approached. Labor can be induced or stimulated (augmented) by oxytocic agents (e.g., oxytocin or prostaglandin E_2) (Fig. 6-3).

In ~10% of gravidas, the fetal membranes rupture before the onset of labor. This reduces the capacity of the uterus, thickens the uterine wall, and increases uterine irritability. Labor usually follows. At term, *90% will be in labor within 24 h after membrane rupture.* If labor does not begin in 24 h, the case must be considered complicated by prolonged rupture of the membranes.

Immediately before or early in labor, a small amount of red-tinged mucus may be passed (*bloody show* or mucous plug). This is a collection of thick cervical mucus often mixed with blood and

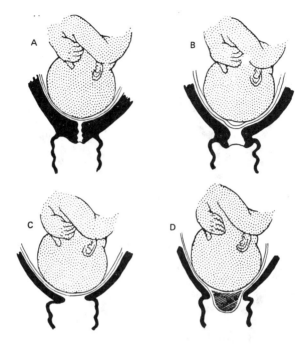

Figure 6-1. Dilatation and effacement of the cervix in a primipara.

is evidence of cervical dilatation and effacement and, frequently, descent of the presenting part.

The beginning of true labor is marked by increasingly frequent, forceful, prolonged, and, finally, regular uterine contractions. Low backache may precede or accompany the uterine contractions (pains). Each contraction starts with a gradual buildup of intensity, and a similar dissipation follows the peak. Normally, the contraction will be at its height before discomfort is felt. Dilatation of the lower birth canal almost always will cause deep pelvic or perineal pain. Nonetheless, occasional nulliparas and some multiparas may have a brief, virtually pain-free labor.

Labor entails the interaction of the so-called 4Ps.

1. The passenger (the fetal size, presentation, position)
2. The pelvis (size and shape)
3. The powers (effective forces of labor, e.g., uterine contractions)
4. The placenta (an obstruction if implanted low in the uterus)

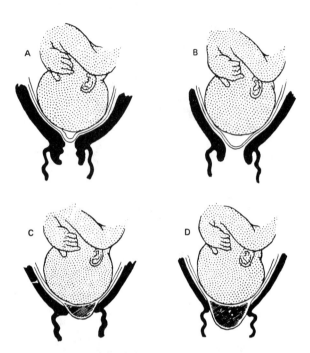

Figure 6-2. Dilatation and effacement of the cervix in a multipara.

Each of these factors, alone or in combination, may make for a normal or a complicated labor and delivery. For example, if the fetus is large and the pelvis is small, labor may be prolonged or progress may be impossible despite strong contractions, even with a placenta normally implanted in the fundus.

NORMAL LABOR

Since, hopefully, the end result of labor is the vaginal delivery of the fetus, membranes, and placenta, the method of judging its progress is based on assessments toward that end. The *first stage of labor begins with the onset of labor and ends with complete (10 cm) dilatation of the cervix.* The first stage is the longest, averaging 8–12 h for primigravidas or 6–8 h for multiparas. However, the first

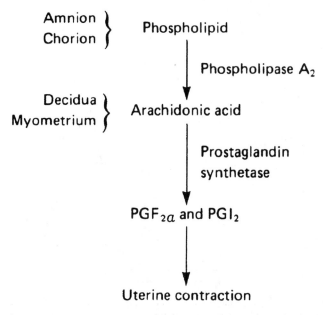

Figure 6-3. Production of prostaglandins in human parturition. (Modified after Liggins.) (From M.L. Pernoll and R.C. Benson, eds. *Current Obstetric & Gynecologic Diagnosis & Treatment,* 6th ed. Lange, 1987.)

stage of labor may be markedly shorter or longer depending on the 4Ps.

Labor is a very dynamic process, and contractions should increase steadily in regularity, intensity, and duration. This is not always the case, and one must set limits concerning the progress of labor (Figs. 6-4, 6-5).

It is useful to divide the first stage of labor into two phases. Thus, the *latent phase of labor* begins with the onset of regular uterine contractions and extends to the start of the *active phase of cervical dilatation* (~3–4 cm).

The *second stage of labor begins when the cervix becomes fully dilated and ends with the complete birth of the infant.* The second stage normally lasts <30 min, and one should be concerned when it extends longer than 1 h (based on fetal morbidity and mortality).

The *third, or placental, stage of labor is the period from birth*

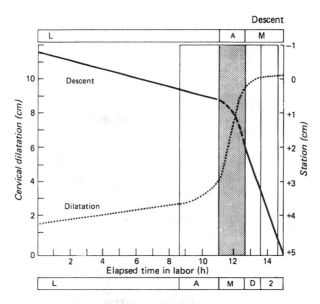

Figure 6-4. Relationship between cervical dilatation and descent of the presenting part in a primipara. L, latent phase. A, acceleration phase. M, phase of maximum slope. D, deceleration phase. 2, second stage. (From M.L. Pernoll and R.C. Benson, eds. *Current Obstetric & Gynecologic Diagnosis & Treatment,* 6th ed. Lange, 1987.)

of the infant to 1 h after delivery of the placenta. The rapidity of separation and means of recovery of the placenta determine the duration of the third stage (Fig. 6-6).

Management of the First Stage of Labor

Initial Examination and Procedures

A. Obtain a *history* of relevant medical details following the last examination.

B. Record the patient's *vital signs* (temperature, pulse, and BP). Examine a clean-catch *urine specimen* for proteinuria and glycosuria.

C. Do a brief *general physical examination.*

D. Palpate the uterus to *determine the fetal presentation, posi-*

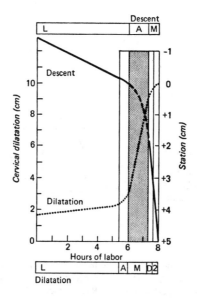

Figure 6-5. Composite mean curves for descent (solid line) and dilatation (broken line) for 389 multiparas. L, latent phase. A, acceleration phase. M, phase of maximum slope. D, deceleration phase. 2, second stage. Relationship is shown between acceleration period of descent and maximum slope of dilatation (shaded area), between latent period of descent and latent plus acceleration phases of dilatation, and between maximum slope of descent and deceleration plase plus second stage. (Redrawn from Friedman and Sachtleben. *Am J Obstet Gynecol* 1965;93:526.)

tion, and engagement (Leopold's maneuvers) (Fig. 6-7). Auscultate the *fetal heartbeat,* and mark the skin where the heartbeat is loudest to note the shift and descent of the point of maximal intensity with progressive labor. This is evidence of internal rotation and descent of the fetus (the mechanism of labor).

E. Note the *frequency, regularity, intensity, and duration* of *uterine contractions* and the *myometrial tone* with and between contractions. Observe the patient's reactions and her tolerance of labor. Restlessness and discomfort often develop as labor progresses.

F. Check for *vaginal bleeding or leakage of amniotic fluid.* Nitrazine indicator paper will turn from green to yellow when moistened with amniotic fluid (pH 7.0). Other tests may be used in doubtful cases.

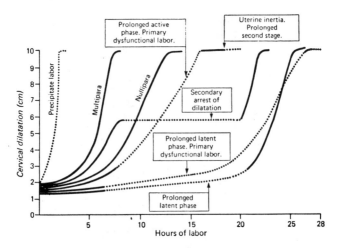

Figure 6-6. Major types of deviation from normal progress of labor may be detected by noting dilatation of the cervix at various intervals after labor begins. (From K.P. Russell. In: R.C. Benson, ed. *Current Obstetric & Gynecologic Diagnosis & Treatment,* 4th ed. Lange, 1982.)

G. *Examine the patient vaginally.* Wear a surgical mask and use a surgically clean glove. Record the time of the following.

1. Identify the *fetal presenting part and its station* in relation to the level of the ischial spines. Station is the level of the head or breech in the pelvis. If the presenting part is at the spines, it is said to be at "zero station." If above the spines, the distance is stated in minus figures (−1 cm, −2 cm, −3 cm, and "floating"). If below the spines, the distance is noted in plus figures (+1 cm, +2 cm, +3 cm, and "on the perineum") (Fig. 6-8). When the most inferior part of the head is at the level of the ischial spines, the station is zero.

Station zero is assumed by projection to be actual engagement, that is, the biparietal diameter at the level of the inlet. However, with considerable moulding, caput succedaneum, or a sincipital presentation of the head, the biparietal diameter may be a significant distance *above* the inlet even though the tip of the vertex is at the spines without true engagement.

2. Dilatation of the cervix by direct palpation is expressed as the diameter of the cervical opening in centimeters. A diameter of 10 cm constitutes full dilatation.

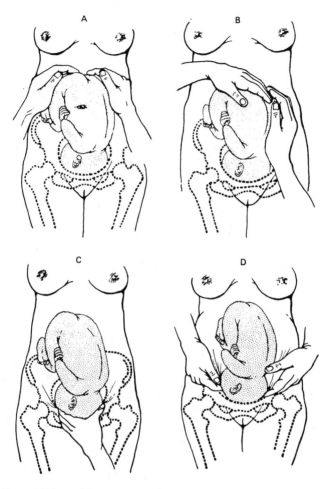

Figure 6-7. Leopold's maneuvers. Determining fetal presentation (A and B), position (C), and engagement (D).

3. Effacement of the cervix (process of thinning out) may occur before labor in the nulligravida but is less likely before the first stage of labor in the multigravida.

4. The position of the presenting part usually can be confirmed by internal examination.

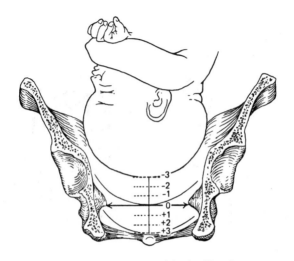

Figure 6-8. Stations of the fetal head.

a. *Vertex presentations* (Fig. 6-9). The fontanelles and the sagittal suture are palpated. The position is determined by the relation of the fetal occiput to the mother's right or left side. This is expressed as OA (occiput directly anterior), LOA (left occiput anterior), LOP (left occiput posterior), and so on.

b. *Breech presentations* are determined by the position of the infant's sacrum in relation to the mother's right or left side. This is expressed as SA (sacrum directly anterior), LSA (left sacrum anterior), LSP (left sacrum posterior), and so on.

c. *Face presentation* is caused by extension of the fetal head on the neck. The chin, a prominent and identifiable facial landmark, is used as the point of reference. As with vertex presentations, the position of the fetal chin is related to the anterior or posterior portion of the left or right side of the mother's pelvis. This is expressed as RMP (right mentum posterior) and so on.

d. *Brow, bregma, and sinciput presentations* are presentations midway between flexion and extension. These usually are temporary attitudes that convert during labor to face or occiput presentation.

e. *Transverse presentations* occur when the long axis of the fetal body is perpendicular to that of the mother. One shoulder

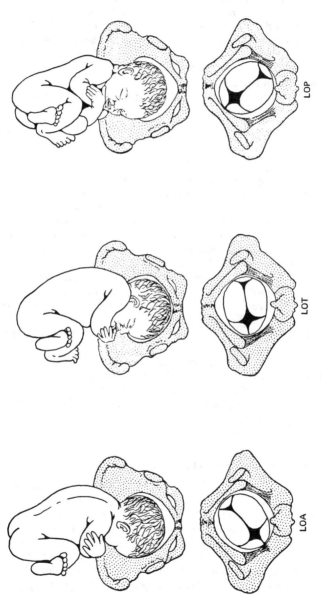

Figure 6-9. Vertex presentation.

(acromion) will occupy the superior strait, but it will be considerably to the right or left of the midline. Transverse presentations are designated by relating the infant's inferior shoulder and back to the mother's back or abdominal wall. Thus, LADP (left acromiodorsoposterior) means that the infant's lower shoulder is to the mother's left, and its back is toward her back.

f. *Compound presentations,* caused by prolapse of a hand, arm, foot, or leg, are complications of one of the other presentations. These unusual presentations generally are recorded descriptively without abbreviations.

Preparation of the Patient for Labor

Following the initial internal examination, do the following.

A. *Prepare and cleanse the pudendum.* Clip the hair short over the entire perineum and the labia, and wash thoroughly with soap or surgical detergent and water. Shaving is unnecessary.

B. If delivery is not imminent, one may *administer a warm* tapwater or mild soapsuds *enema* to evacuate the lower bowel. This should, however, be a shared decision with the patient.

C. *Ambulation,* within reasonable limits, may add to the patient's comfort. However, keep the patient in bed after the membranes have ruptured or until the presenting part has engaged to avoid cord prolapse or compression.

D. Allow only *clear liquids by mouth* during labor to avoid dehydration.

E. Analgesia should not be given until labor is definitely established with the cervix >3 cm dilated. *Analgesics and anesthesia must be ordered on an individual basis,* considering each patient's obstetric problems, the quality of labor, and her desire to be alert or subdued.

Further Examinations and Procedures

A. *Electronic fetal monitoring* (EFM) is simply a prospective means of documenting fetal well-being. The external type is innocuous, and the internal type carries only slight risk. However, although EFM is an excellent diagnostic tool, it is not a substitute for correct clinical judgment. Current retrospective and prospective data support the use of continuous internal EFM for high-risk obstetric patients. Internal EFM is preferable to external EFM because it is more precise and comprehensive in appraising fetal status. Nonetheless, electronic monitoring of low-risk obstetric patients has not demonstrated a beneficial cost/benefit ratio.

B. If continuous EFM is not used, *auscultate and record the fetal heart tones* (FHT) for 1 min following a uterine contraction at least every 30 min during the first stage, at least every 5 min during the second stage, when the membranes rupture and again within 30 min after the rupture, and every 5 min or more often as indicated if complications develop or if meconium passes in vertex presentation.

C. Perform *external and internal examinations* as often as necessary to determine the progress of the labor. Descent and internal rotation of the fetus often can be determined by external palpation alone. Too frequent vaginal or rectal examinations cause the patient discomfort and increase the incidence of intrauterine infection, particularly after rupture of the membranes.

D. *Cleanse the vulvar region* before and after internal examination, after defecation and voiding, or when soiling by vaginal secretions occurs.

E. *Encourage the patient to void frequently.* Palpate the abdomen occasionally for signs of bladder fullness. Catheterize if involuntary distention occurs or if voiding is obviously inadequate.

DELIVERY: MANAGEMENT OF THE NORMAL SECOND STAGE OF LABOR

Vertex Delivery (Tables 6-1, 6-2)

Final preparation for delivery should be completed by the time the presenting part reaches the pelvic floor or sooner if labor is progressing very rapidly.

Spontaneous delivery of the infant presenting by the vertex is divided into three phases: (1) delivery of the head, (2) delivery of the shoulders, and (3) delivery of the body and legs.

Preparation for Delivery

1. Place the patient in a *modified lithotomy position* for delivery. The left lateral decubitus (Sims) or squatting position may be used if a spontaneous uncomplicated birth is anticipated.

2. The physician and assistants must carefully *scrub* their hands and wear *masks, eye protection, and sterile gloves.* Any delivery may become surgically complicated.

3. Administer *anesthesia if necessary* (e.g., pudendal block).

4. *Cleanse the pudendum* with water and surgical detergent.

5. *Drape* the patient with sterile towels or sheets or both.

Table 6-1. Mechanisms of labor: vertex presentation

Engagement	Flexion	Descent	Internal rotation	Extension	External rotation or restitution
Generally occurs in late pregnancy of at onset of labor. Mode of entry into superior strait depends on pelvic configuration	Good flexion is noted in most cases. Flexion aids engagement and descent. (Extension occurs in brow and face presentations)	Depends on pelvic architecture and cephalopelvic relationships. Descent is usually slowly progressive	Takes place during descent. After engagement, vertex usually rotates to the transverse. It must next rotate to the anterior or posterior to pass the ischial spines, whereupon, when the vertex reaches the perineum, rotation from a posterior to an anterior position generally follows	Follows distention of the perineum by the vertex. Head concomitantly stems beneath the symphysis. Extension is complete with delivery of head	Following delivery, head normally rotates to the position it originally occupied at engagement. Next, the shoulders descend in a path similar to that traced by the head. They rotate anteroposteriorly for delivery. Then the head swings back to its position at birth. The body of the infant is delivered next

Table 6-2. Mechanisms of labor: frank breech presentation

Flexion	Descent	Internal rotation	Lateral flexion	External rotation or restitution
Hips: Engagement usually occurs in one of oblique diameters of pelvic inlet	Anterior hip generally descends more rapidly than posterior at both inlet and outlet	Ordinarily takes place when breech reaches levator musculature. Fetal bitrochanteric rotates to AP diameter	Occurs when anterior hip stems beneath symphysis; posterior hip is born first	After birth of breech and legs, infant's body turns toward mother's side to which its back was directed at engagement of shoulders
Shoulders: Bisacromial diameter engages in same diameter as breech	Gradual descent is the rule	Anterior shoulder rotates so as to bring shoulders into AP diameter of outlet	Anterior shoulder at symphysis, and posterior shoulder is delivered first (when body is supported)	
Head: Engages in the same diameter as shoulders. Flexes on entry into superior strait. Biparietal occupies oblique used by shoulders. At outlet, neck or chin arrests beneath symphysis, and head is born by gradual flexion	Follows the shoulders	Occiput (if a posterior) or face (if an occiput anterior) rotates to hollow of sacrum. This brings presenting part to AP diameter of outlet		

6. *Sterile instruments* and necessary supplies previously designated should be arranged conveniently on a table or stand.

7. *Gloves (and gown) must be changed if contamination occurs.*

Delivery of the Head (Figs. 6-10 through 6-14)

1. During the late second stage, the head distends toward the perineum and vulva with each uterine contraction, normally aided by voluntary efforts of the mother. A patch of scalp becomes visible. The presenting part recedes slightly during the intervals of relaxation, but it *crowns* when its widest portion (biparietal diameter) distends the vulva just before emerging.

2. *Do not hasten delivery,* lest serious damage to the mother or child occur. Control the speed of delivery by pressure applied laterally beneath the symphysis as necessary to avoid pudendal laceration or unexpected extrusion of the infant's head. Sudden marked variations in intracranial pressure may cause intracranial hemorrhage. *As the head advances, control its progress and maintain flexion of the head by pressure over the perineum.*

Draw the perineum downward to allow the head to clear the

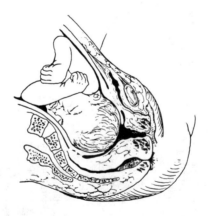

Figure 6-10. Engagement of LOA.

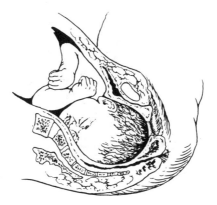

Figure 6-11. LOA position.

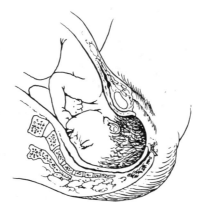

Figure 6-12. Anterior rotation of head.

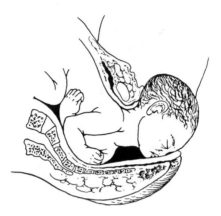

Figure 6-13. Extension of head.

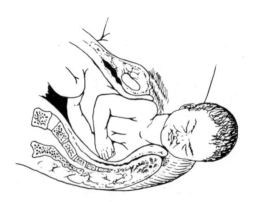

Figure 6-14. External rotation of head.

perineal body. Pressure applied from the coccygeal region upward (*modified Ritgen maneuver*) will extend the head at the proper time and thereby protect the perineum from laceration.

3. If *episiotomy* is elected, it should be performed when the fetal head begins to distend the introitus. In vertex presentations, the forehead soon appears, then the face and chin, and finally the neck.

4. The *cord encircles the neck in about 20% of deliveries.* Note the number of loops. If the nuchal cord is tight, attempt to gently slip the loop(s) of cord over the head. If this cannot be done easily and if this is a singleton, doubly clamp the cord, cut between the forceps, and proceed with the delivery. Wipe fluid from the nose and mouth, then aspirate the nasal and oropharyngeal passages with a soft rubber suction bulb or with a small catheter attached to a deLee-type suction trap.

5. Before *external rotation (restitution),* which occurs next, the head usually is drawn back toward the perineum. This movement precedes engagement of the shoulders, which are now entering the pelvic inlet.

6. From this point on, *support the infant manually* and facilitate the mechanism of labor.

Do not hurry! If strong contractions wane, be patient—labor will resume. Once the airway is clear, the infant can breathe and is not in jeopardy.

Delivery of the Shoulders

Caution: Never exert pressure or strong anterior or posterior traction on the head, neck, or shoulders. Do not hook a finger into the child's axilla to deliver a shoulder. These maneuvers may result in a brachial plexus injury (Erb or Duchenne), a hematoma of the neck, or a shoulder injury.

1. Delivery of the shoulders should be *slow and deliberate.* The shoulders must rotate (or be rotated) to the anteroposterior diameter of the outlet for delivery.

2. Gently *depress the head toward the mother's coccyx until the anterior shoulder impinges against the symphysis. Then lift the head upward.* This aids delivery of the posterior shoulder.

3. The anterior shoulder is next delivered from behind the symphysis by gentle downward traction. The index and third finger should greatly exert pressure on the rami of the mandible while the opposite index and third finger exert equal and gentle pressure on the occiput. (Occasionally, it may be easier to deliver the anterior shoulder first.) Slipping several fingers into the vagina at this

point to assist in delivering the posterior arm is desirable, but *undue pressure must be avoided!*

4. In vertex presentations, a hand may present after the head. Merely sweep the infant's hand and arm over its face, draw the arm out, and deliver the other shoulder as outlined above.

Delivery of the Body and Extremities

The infant's *body and legs should be delivered gradually by easy traction* after the shoulders have been freed.

Immediate Care of the Infant

1. As soon as the infant is delivered, *hold it with the head lowered* (no more than 15 degrees) *to drain fluid and mucus* from the oropharynx. A mucus trap catheter or comparable suction device is useful in clearing the air passages. If the baby is below the level of the placental insertion, blood will drain from the placenta and cord to the newborn. This will amount to 30–90 ml before the cord is clamped or the placenta separates. The excess blood may benefit some neonates (e.g., isoimmunized anemic infants) and harm others (e.g., a plethoric twin).

Placing the newborn on the mother's abdomen before cord pulsations cease has several potential disadvantages: it contaminates the sterile field, the infant is not secure there, and blood drains from the infant to the placenta (usually undesirable).

2. *Evaluate and resuscitate if necessary* (Chapter 8) (Fig. 6-15).

3. *Clamp and cut the cord* when it ceases to pulsate (or sooner if the infant is premature or in distress, or if isoimmunization is probable). Examine the umbilical cord for the normal two arteries and one vein. Apply a sterile cord clamp, cord tie of umbilical tape, or rubber band distal to the skin edge at the cord insertion at the umbilicus. Dress the cord stump with dry gauze.

4. The newborn should be received into warm clean towels or blankets, and *avoid chilling*. Apply means of *identification* (e.g., necklace, bracelet).

5. At this point, the parents may want to hold the newborn and the mother may begin breastfeeding.

6. Next, perform *newborn ocular prophylaxis* (against gonorrhea and *Chlamydia*). Most commonly, erythromycin or tetracy-

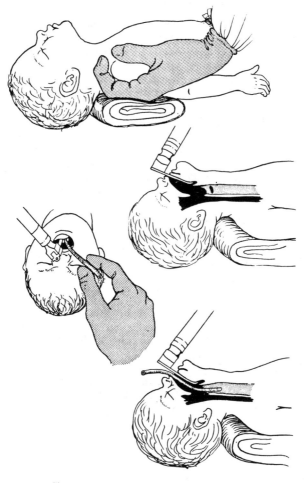

Figure 6-15. Resuscitation of the newborn.

cline ointment is used because they are more protective and provoke less ocular irritation than silver nitrate.

7. *Examine the infant and record Apgar scores,* weight, total length, crown-rump length, shoulder circumference, circumference of the head, and cranial diameters. Note facial, peripheral, genital, or other abnormalities (Chapter 8).

Immediate Care of the Mother Postpartum

1. Carefully *inspect the perineum, vagina, and cervix for lacerations, hematomas, or extension of the episiotomy.* Identify sulcus lacerations, urethral and cervical injury, and other injuries. Lacerations of the birth canal may be described by their extent (expressed as first to fourth degree).

In *first degree lacerations,* only the mucosa or skin or both are damaged. Bleeding usually is minimal.

Second degree lacerations include tears of the mucosa or skin or both plus disruption of the superficial fascia and the transverse perineal muscle. (The anal sphincter is spared.) Bleeding often is brisk.

Third degree lacerations involve the structures indicated in second degree lacerations plus the anal sphincter. Expect moderate blood loss.

Fourth degree lacerations include the structures included in third degree lacerations and entry into the rectal lumen. Bleeding may be profuse, and fecal soiling is inevitable.

2. Control blood loss and repair second to fourth degree lacerations.

MANAGEMENT OF THE THIRD STAGE OF LABOR

Avoid Interference If At All Possible!

Avoid traction on the cord before placental separation and do not knead the fundus to separate the placenta (Credé maneuver). The former may lead to cord laceration and the latter to hemorrhage, uterine inversion, and shock. Maternal morbidity and mortality rates increase with gross blood loss. A uterus that contracts and remains contracted rarely bleeds excessively.

Separation of the Placenta

The placenta is attached to the uterine wall only by anchoring villi and thin-walled blood vessels, all of which eventually tear. In some instances, the placental margin separates first. In others, when the central portion of the placenta is freed initially, bleeding from the retroplacental sinuses may assist placental separation. Incomplete separation, usually due to ineffectual uterine contractions, may allow the retroplacental blood sinuses to remain open, so that severe blood loss may result.

Normal placental separation is manifested first by a firmly con-

tracting, rising fundus. The uterus becomes smaller and changes in shape from discoid to globular. The umbilical cord becomes longer as the placenta descends. There is a palpable and visible prominence above the symphysis (if the bladder is empty) and a slight *gush of blood from the vagina.* These signs normally appear within about 3–4 min after delivery of the infant. The placenta should present at the internal os after four or five firm uterine contractions, whereupon it is expressed into the vagina for delivery.

These signs often are confused with other conditions: uterine anomaly, a second undelivered infant, feces, a tumor, and lacerations of the birth canal.

Recovery of the Placenta

Spontaneous Uterine Expulsion of Placenta

When the uterus is firmly contracted, the mother who has not been anesthetized may be able to *bear down during a contraction to expel the separated placenta.* Although of historic but little clinical significance, a recording of the placenta presenting with the fetal surface to the introitus (*Schultz*) or the maternal surface (*Duncan*) may be made. Spontaneous delivery of the placenta usually is accomplished without difficulty. If it does not occur, however, the following techniques may be used.

Brandt-Andrews Technique (Modified) (Fig. 6-16)

1. Immediately after delivery of the infant, *clamp the umbilical cord close to the vulva.* Palpate the uterus gently without massage to determine whether firm contractions are occurring.

2. After several uterine contractions and a change in size and shape indicate separation of the placenta, hold the clamp at the vulva firmly with one hand, place the fingertips of the other hand on the abdomen, and press between the fundus and symphysis to elevate the fundus. If the placenta has separated, the cord will extrude into the vagina.

3. Further elevate the fundus, apply gentle traction on the cord, and deliver the placenta from the vagina.

Manual Separation and Extraction of Placenta

Manual separation and extraction of the placenta from the fundus of the uterus is an effective direct technique. However,

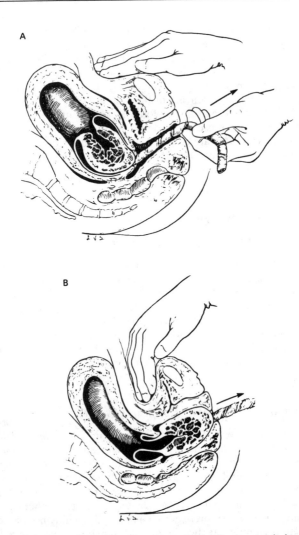

Figure 6-16. Brandt-Andrews maneuver. A. Traction is extended on the cord as the uterus is elevated gently. B. Pressure is exerted between the symphysis and the uterine fundus, forcing the uterus upward and the placenta outward, as traction on the cord is continued. (From R.C. Benson, ed. *Current Obstetric & Gynecologic Diagnosis & Treatment,* 4th ed. Lange, 1982.)

this is invasive and, often, effective anesthesia is required. Manual removal of the placenta should not be undertaken unless it is indicated and the operator is experienced.

1. Prepare the perineum and vulva again with detergent and antiseptic solution.

2. Making the hand as narrow as possible, insert gently into the vagina and palpate for defects in the vagina and cervix. Slowly probe through the cervix with the fingers, taking care not to lacerate the canal. (Brief moderately deep anesthesia may be required if considerable delay has occurred.)

3. Locate and separate the placenta if this can be done easily. Do not attempt to force cleavage against unusual resistance (placenta accreta).

4. Palpate the fundus for defects or tumors.

5. Remove the hand while grasping the completely separated placenta, or leave the placenta if it is firmly adherent (placenta accreta).

Postpartum Oxytocin

After delivery of the placenta, it is common practice (even though not required in the majority of cases) to give *oxytocin 5–10 U IV over 5 min to limit blood loss.*

Postpartum Observation

1. The mother should remain under very *close observation for at least 1 h after delivery of the placenta.* Note her vital signs and reactions. Record the blood pressure, the pulse rate and regularity, and the amount of vaginal blood loss every 15 min, or more often if necessary. Support the uterine fundus. Massage it gently and frequently to maintain firm contraction. Express clots occasionally and *estimate the total blood loss* after 1 h.

2. *Be alert to complaints of severe perineal pain* suggestive of hematoma formation. A rapid pulse and increasing hypotension indicate impending shock, usually due to continued or excessive blood loss. Severe headaches and hyperreflexia may precede eclampsia. A distended bladder (often visible) will lead to enhanced uterine bleeding. Catheterize for retention when necessary. *Do not release any patient to room care until her condition is stable.*

Postpartum Hemorrhage

Postpartum hemorrhage (PPH) is the *rapid or slow loss of >500 ml of blood after delivery.* Early PPH occurs within 24 h of birth. Late PPH may occur 24 h to 4 weeks after birth. *Early PPH may be caused by placental problems* (abruptio placentae, placenta previa, incomplete placental separation), *uterine atony* (anesthesia, marked predelivery uterine distention, abnormal labor, prolonged or excessive oxytocin administration, overdistended urinary bladder), *laceration(s) of the birth canal, rupture of the uterus, blood dyscrasias* (hypofibrogenemia), or *mismanagement* of the third stage of labor. Usually, *late postpartum hemorrhage is due to retained products of conception.* This complication occurs in *5%–10% of term deliveries.* About 2% of these patients must be readmitted to the hospital for transfusion, and some require surgery. *Further complications* of PPH include *shock, anemia, and infection.*

Clinical Assessment The pulse rate should return to normal within the hour after delivery. Hence, *a persistent slight tachycardia may indicate a significant uncompensated blood loss.* Elimination of the placenta and a contracted uterus will restore at least 300 ml of blood to the maternal circulation. This normally causes a systolic elevation of 10–20 mm Hg for several hours after delivery. Therefore, *persistent hypotension suggests excessive blood loss,* which may require replacement. Continued, even moderate postpartum hypertension, especially with associated headache or hyperreflexia, suggests impending pregnancy-induced hypertension (PIH). Magnesium sulfate therapy for the PIH may cause some relaxation of the uterine muscle, but that effect should not deter its indicated usage.

Prevention

A. *Properly manage the placenta*
1. Recover the placenta by spontaneous delivery or Brandt-Andrews maneuver.
2. Avoid the Credé maneuver (kneading of the uterus), and never use the fundus as a piston to push out the placenta.
3. Reserve manual extraction for indicated cases.
B. After placental delivery, *give dilute oxytocin* (5 IU slowly IV).
C. *Anticipate the atonic uterus,* and start dilute oxytocin before delivery of the placenta once it has been ascertained that there is not a second fetus.
D. *Inspect the birth canal* carefully for lacerations.
E. *Explore the uterus* in any patient with possible uterine rupture or retained products of conception. (Some advocate routine exploration in all patients.)

Treatment

A. Obtain a *CBC, coagulation panel, type and crossmatch.*

B. Ensure an open *IV line.*

C. Closely *monitor further blood loss and vital signs.*

D. Initiate appropriate *blood component replacement.*

E. Manually *deliver the partially separated placenta.*

F. Explore the uterus, and carefully *remove any retained products of conception* (this may require uterine curettage).

G. To *reverse uterine atony* after placental recovery

1. Elevate and maintain the fundus out of the pelvis while performing uterine massage.

2. Repeat the prophylactic oxytocin 5 IU slowly IV. If that fails to slow bleeding, consider the addition of prostaglandins or ergonovine (omit the latter if the patient is hypertensive).

H. *Repair the episiotomy and any lacerations* promptly.

I. Perform *hysterectomy for placenta accreta.*

J. *Ligation of uterine arteries or hypogastric arteries* may be lifesaving in certain extreme cases.

K. *Packing the uterus* to control PPH is now done rarely except as a temporary measure (e.g., to stop the flow if blood replacement products are not immediately available). Have available many packs of sterilized gauze about 1 yard wide and 5 yards long (packing takes a considerable amount). A Holmes tubular packing instrument may be helpful but is not essential.

Prognosis The outcome depends on the cause of bleeding, amount of blood lost (in proportion to patient's weight), medical complications, and success of corrective therapy.

AIDS TO NORMAL DELIVERY

THE FATHER

Much has been said of the mother, her needs, and her relationship to the child, but the expectant father has been relatively neglected in the process until recently. Preparation for parenthood begins well before courtship and marriage, but the mother's pregnancy is the beginning of the transition leading to fatherhood. Recognition of the father's concerns leads to discussion and solution of many human problems that surround the expectation of a newborn.

Fathers-to-be experience at least *five emotional stages* (which often overlap): (1) realization or confirmation of pregnancy, (2) awareness of changes in the mother's body and the presence of fetal movements, (3) anticipation of approaching labor, (4) involvement in the delivery process, and (5) new parenthood.

Fears that the father's presence in the delivery room would create a nuisance, add to confusion, or cause infection or legal conflicts have been unjustified. Men who have participated with their spouses in preparation for childbirth have been helpful, supportive, and reassuring. Moreover, properly conducted delivery room experience is almost always a gratifying one for the father, one that assists him in *immediate attachment to the newborn*.

The father may act as a *coach* in addition to the nurse–physician team by assisting with comfort measures. He may be an almost constant *companion* to the patient to offset the loneliness and anxieties of labor. He can be a *messenger,* to report problems or call for help and interpret his wife's needs and wishes to the nurse and doctor. He may serve as an *advocate.* In emergencies, when the mother is sedated or in shock, he can *give informed consent* for treatment that may be life saving. With the father in the delivery room, it is easier for the physician and the parents to welcome a normal newborn or cope with a defective offspring. A well-informed participating father can contribute greatly to the health and well-being of the mother and child, to the benefit of the family relationship and his own self-esteem. All of these factors may prevent or greatly minimize postpartum psychologic problems.

Episiotomy (Perineotomy) and Repair of Episiotomy and Lacerations

An episiotomy is a *pudendal incision* to widen the vulvar orifice to permit easier passage of the infant. The advantages of episiotomy are that *it prevents perineal lacerations, relieves compression of the fetal head, shortens the second stage of labor* by removing the resistance of the pudendal musculature, and *can be repaired more successfully than a jagged tear.* It is used in most primiparas and many multiparas, the most common indications being (1) when a tear is imminent, (2) in most operative deliveries, and (3) to facilitate atraumatic delivery of a premature infant.

Types of Episiotomy (Fig. 6-17)

The tissues incised by an episiotomy are (1) *skin and subcutaneous tissues,* (2) *vaginal mucosa,* (3) *the urogenital septum* (mostly

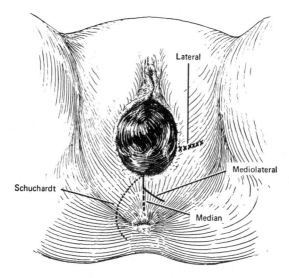

Figure 6-17. Types of episiotomy.

fascia, but also the transverse perineal muscles), (4) *intercolumnar fascia or superior fascia of the pelvic diaphragm,* and (5) the *lowermost fibers of the puborectalis portions of the levator ani muscles* (if the episiotomy is mediolateral and deep). Currently, only two types of episiotomy are used.

Median Episiotomy

This is the easiest episiotomy to accomplish and repair. It is almost bloodless and is less painful postpartum than other types. Incise the median raphe of the perineum almost to the anal sphincter, and extend this separation at least 2–3 cm up to the rectovaginal septum. Occasionally, a third or fourth degree laceration may occur.

Mediolateral Episiotomy

The mediolateral incision is used widely in operative obstetrics because of its safety. Make the incision downward and outward in the direction of the lateral margin of the anal sphincter and at least one-half the distance into the vagina. However, this incision may bleed excessively and may remain painful even after the puerperium.

Timing of Episiotomy

Episiotomy should be done when the head begins to distend the perineum with a mature fetus, before the head encounters the perineal musculature with an immature fetus, immediately preceding application of forceps, and just before breech extraction.

Repair of Episiotomy and Lacerations (Figs. 6-18, 6-19)

Episiotomy Repair

Episiotomy repair is actually a *fascial repair,* not the suture of muscle. *Absorbable suture* (natural or synthetic, usually 000-0000) is preferred. The procedure may employ interrupted or continuous sutures or a combination of both. However, *careful reapproximation of the edges of the divided muscles and surrounding fascia is required.* Avoid mass ligatures and tension on sutures. Do not tie the sutures too tightly, or pain and necrosis may result. In general, *buried sutures* cause less discomfort than through-and-through exposed sutures.

Laceration Repair

In repair of fourth degree lacerations, close the *rectal submucosal layer* with fine interrupted absorbable sutures tied within the lumen of the bowel or a fine continuous suture that everts the mucosal edges. Then approximate the *bowel muscularis* with either a running or interrupted fine absorbable sutures. Close the *rectovaginal septum* as in an episiotomy. Reapproximate the ends of the rectal sphincter by interrupted sutures in the sheath of the sphincter ani. The perimuscular fascia rather than the friable muscle itself affords a much superior closure. Repair the vaginal mucosal and perineal skin defect in the usual running subcuticular fashion; then, suture lacerations.

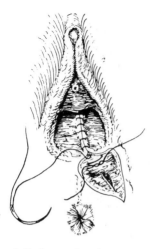

1. Continuous suture of mucosa with inverted suture of perineal body

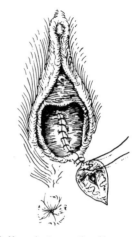

2. Mucosal suture continued in skin and tied with inverted suture

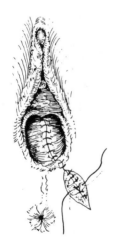

3. Closure of levator ani and perineal musculature

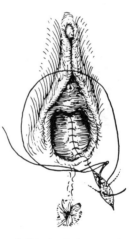

4. Skin closed subcutaneously

Figure 6-18. Episiotomy repair.

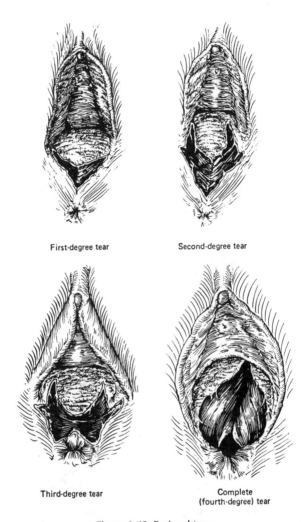

First-degree tear

Second-degree tear

Third-degree tear

Complete
(fourth-degree) tear

Figure 6-19. Perineal tears.

OUTLET FORCEPS

Outlet forceps are used to *extend the head and to guide the infant beneath the symphysis and over the perineum.* Outlet forceps are used only when the vertex is on the perineum (+4 station), with extension beginning. This procedure is indicated (1) when *spontaneous expulsion is inhibited* (e.g., by psychologic circumstances, analgesia, or anesthesia); caudal or spinal anesthesia markedly diminishes the patient's voluntary expulsive efforts, (2) when *uterine inertia* delays or prevents delivery of an infant whose vertex is distending the perineum, (3) when *fetal distress* occurs, and (4) to *prevent laceration* of the introitus.

OBSTETRIC ANALGESIA, AMNESIA, AND REGIONAL ANESTHESIA

Pain in childbirth is normally due to traction on the adnexal, uterine, and cervical supports, *pressure* on the ureters, bladder, urethra, and bowel, *dilatation* of the cervix and lower birth canal, *hypoxia and the accumulation of catabolites* in the myometrium, and *fear, severe tension,* and *anxiety.* In *dystocia,* or abnormal labor, pain often may be due to cephalopelvic disproportion. Tetanic, prolonged, or dysrhythmic uterine contractions may be painful, and intrapartal infection may cause pain.

The *management of any pain requires individualization.* However, with proper preparation, the patient requires much less medication to spare both herself and her infant. Additionally, the gravida's experience is enhanced, she becomes a team member, and she is able to profit from the birth experience, enhancing her love of the newborn.

The following types of pain relief are in use today: positive conditioning of the patient, hypnotics, analgesics, which decrease the patient's pain threshold, amnesics or hypnotics, which obscure the memory of pain and associated disagreeable experiences, regional anesthesia, which interrupts afferent pain pathways, and general anesthesia, which eliminates central perception of discomfort.

Types of Pain Relief

Positive Conditioning

Positive conditioning of the receptive patient during late pregnancy or early labor may reduce tensions and limit the need for pain relief medication. There are a number of successful techniques for accomplishing this, and they should be encouraged even if both patient and physician recognize that other agents may be employed also. Training and the patient's participation are required and, to be successful, are started antenatally.

Analgesics

The commonly employed analgesics are *narcotic drugs,* for example, 50–75 mg IV or IM (low-dose) Demerol. Injectable narcotics in the usual doses elevate the pain threshold by ≥50% to establish a state of relaxation and lethargy. Most of these drugs have a peak action of <90 min and a duration of effect of at least 1–2 h. *Undesirable side effects are* nausea, vomiting, cough suppression, intestinal stasis, and in the early first stage of labor, diminution in the frequency, intensity, and duration of uterine contractions. Frequently, Phenergoin (25 mg) or similar compounds are added because of their antiemetic and potentiating effects. Amnesia is not achieved. Narcotics adversely affect the infant by depressing all CNS functions, especially those of the respiratory center. Early preterm status, growth retardation, trauma, or asphyxia enhances the susceptibility of the infant to narcosis.

Amnestics

Hydroxyzine (Vistaril) and diazepam (Valium) are examples. They are *useful in the first stage of labor* because of a calming effect tranquilizing action. They also *reduce the amount of analgesic drug required.* Both hydroxyzine and diazepam have long half-lives. Their use in the first stage of labor in dosages of 5–15 mg every 4 h does not appear to have a deleterious effect on the newborn.

Nerve Blocks

Consider nerve blocks in two categories: *local anesthetics* and the *true regional blocks.* The former is exemplified by paracervical and pudendal blocks and the latter by epidural and spinal anesthetics. It should be recalled that local anesthetics are generally divided into the *ester-linked* and the *amide-linked.* The ester-linked anesthetics are deactivated locally or in the blood by destruction of the ester linkage. Therefore, they have a shorter action and avoid maternal overdosage. They also have less chance of crossing the placenta in quanties causative of fetal compromise.

Local anesthetics

1. **Paracervical anesthesia.** A *needle guide* (Fig. 6-20) is useful in directing pudendal and paracervical anesthetic blocks. When using a guide $5\frac{1}{2}$ inches long, a $6\frac{1}{2}$-inch 22-gauge spinal needle will protrude only slightly beyond the guide (desirable).

Paracervical anesthesia (Fig. 6-21) is administered when the *cervix is dilated 4 cm or more*. It relieves pain until the presenting

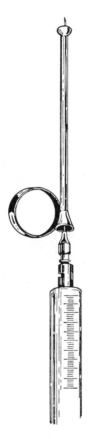

Figure 6-20. Iowa trumpet assembly.

part reaches the lower vagina, when a pudendal and perineal block or other anesthetic may be required. The needle point is inserted just submucosally (0.1–0.2 cm) into the paracervical tissues at the cervicouterine junction at 4 o'clock and 8 o'clock. Inject no more than 10 ml of 1% Procaine on each side.

Exceptional *maternal sensitivity* to the medication or direct vascular injections (manifest by *tachycardia, syncope, seizures*) requires 100% oxygen and supportive measures. Paracervical block may cause *fetal bradycardia* associated with decreased pla-

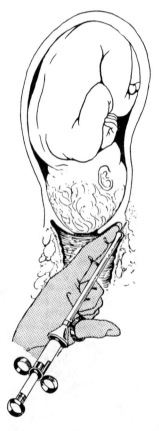

Figure 6-21. Paracervical submucous block.

cental blood flow and, perhaps, a reflex mechanism. However, the majority of serious problems are caused by direct fetal injection. In such cases, it is better to allow the fetus to *recover in utero* than to deliver it in haste.

2. **Pudendal or perineal block** (Fig. 6-22). This permits spontaneous, breech, low forceps, or midforceps delivery with little local pain. It is extremely safe and simple, and the patient maintains her ability to cooperate during labor. The infant rarely is depressed, and blood loss is minimal. Disadvantages

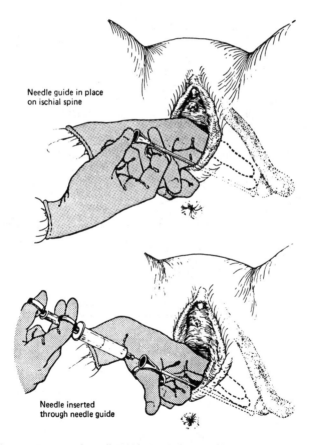

Needle guide in place
on ischial spine

Needle inserted
through needle guide

Figure 6-22. Use of needle guide (Iowa trumpet) in transvaginal anesthetic block.

include discomfort during the injection and a 5-min delay for anesthetic effect.

The two nerves to be blocked on each side of the vagina are the *pudendal and the posterior femoral cutaneous nerves.* The pudendal nerve lies near the inner aspect of the ischial spine and should be blocked there. The posterior femoral cutaneous nerve may be injected beneath the inferior medial border of the ischial tuberosity. The descending branches of the ilioinguinal nerves supply the clitoral region. The perirectal zone is innervated by the hemorrhoidal nerves. The procedure for pudendal and posterior femoral cutaneous block is as follows.

1. Develop a wheal of 0.5%–1% procaine (or equivalent) at the base of each labium majus. Perform all injections through this site.

2. Palpate the ischial spines vaginally or rectally. Slowly guide a 4- or 5-inch, 20- or 21-gauge spinal needle toward each spine while injecting a small amount of procaine ahead of the advancing point. Aspirate, and if the needle is not in a vessel, deposit 5 ml of anesthetic posterior and lateral to the tip of each spine. This blocks the pudendal nerve. Refill the syringe if necessary, leaving the needle in place, and proceed in a similar manner to anesthetize the other areas specified. Keep the needle moving while injecting, and avoid the vaginal mucosa and periosteum.

3. Withdraw the needle about 3 cm and redirect it toward an ischial tuberosity. Inject 3 ml near the center of each tuberosity to anesthetize the inferior hemorrhoidal and lateral femoral cutaneous nerves.

4. Withdraw the needle almost entirely and then slowly advance it toward the symphysis pubica almost to the clitoris, keeping it about 2 cm lateral to the labial fold and about 1–2 cm

Table 6-3. Indications for regional vs general anesthesia

Regional anesthesia	General anesthesia
Recent meal	Need for rapid delivery, fetal
Respiratory infection or asthma	distress
Possible airway problems	Maternal hemorrhage
	Maternal anxiety, hysteria
	Poor uterine relaxation
	Blood coagulopathies
	Neuropathies (epilepsy excluded)
	Bacteremia, viremia

beneath the skin. Inject 5 ml of procaine on each side beneath the symphysis to block the ilioinguinal and genitocrural nerves. Expect prompt flaccid relaxation and good anesthesia for 30–60 min.

Although this procedure is optimal, it is far more common practice today to merely anesthetize the pudendal nerve using the transvaginal technique demonstrated in Figure 6-22. In this technique, the ischial spine is palpated transvaginally and a guide is introduced to facilitate needle placement. The guided needle is placed just inferior and medial to the spine. It is then inserted ~1 cm in the tissue. After aspiration to ascertain that the injection will not be intravascular, the pudendal nerve is blocked by deposition of 5 ml of 0.5%–1% procaine (or equivalent). The procedure is repeated on the contralateral side.

Regional Blocks *Caution:* Special training, skill, and experience are required to administer regional anesthesia. One must become familiar with the techniques and the pitfalls and be knowledgeable in the selection of procedures. Useful generalizations are noted. Table 6-3 details the indications for regional vs general anesthesia, and Table 6-4 shows their relative risks.

Anesthetic administration should never be undertaken without having available analeptic drugs, oxygen, endotracheal equipment, and full resuscitation equipment (to treat complications). To prevent complications, it is *crucial to avoid technical errors* (e.g., intravascular injection of anesthetic drugs or accidental intrathecal injection during epidural anesthesia). The prognosis is best for mother and infant (regardless of the type of anesthesia) when obstetric anesthesiologists, obstetricians, and neonatologists work as a team.

The *major physiologic alterations imposed by gestation must be understood, and necessary alterations in technique must be introduced* (e.g., cardiovascular, respiratory, and gastrointestinal

Table 6-4. Risks of regional vs general anesthesia

Regional anesthesia	General anesthesia
Hypotension	Aspiration of gastric contents
Accidental intravascular or high spinal block	Difficult intubation, e.g., obesity
Postspinal headache	Airway obstruction
Spinal, caudal neuropathy	Prolonged apnea
	Laryngeal pain, edema
	Unfavorable maternal recall

systems and fluid and electrolyte balance). The effective anesthetic dose for epidural or spinal anesthesia is reduced, and maternal uptake and elimination of inhalant anesthetics are increased. In addition, hypoxia is more likely to occur during apnea or airway obstruction. Then, too, the hazard of hypotension and aspiration of gastric contents is increased. All of these problems may affect the fetus secondarily. In cases of marked obesity, endotracheal intubation may be difficult. The fetus may be jeopardized directly by undesirable side effects of drugs or indirectly by reduced uteroplacental circulation.

Prevent aortocaval compression by placing the patient in a supported (wedge or pillow) *oblique or lateral decubitus position* during transport to the delivery room and during delivery. A slight head-down tilt of the bed or table should help also.

Administer *oxygen* by mask to the mother until delivery to improve fetal oxygenation. This is appropriate for both general and regional anesthesia.

Prehydrate the gravida to avoid hypotension and reduced uteroplacental circulation. Rapidly infuse approximately 1 liter of Ringer's lactate solution to increase blood volume and ensure osmotic equilibrium before and after the anesthetic block. (Do not use dextrose solution because delayed neonatal hypoglycemia may develop.) Maintain the patient in slight lateral decubitus position.

For *hypotension,* use a drug with *cardiotonic* (as opposed to vasospastic) *action* (e.g., ephedrine 50 mg IM). Vasopressors with primarily peripheral effects, for example, metaramide (Aramine), phenylephrine (Neo-Synephrine), increase uterine vascular resistance and may be harmful to the fetus.

1. **Epidural anesthesia.** Epidural anesthesia *may be given continuously,* that is, during the latter portion of the first and all of the second stage of labor, or terminally, as a single injection just before delivery. The advantages of properly performed epidural anesthesia are that it causes no fetal asphyxia, the mother remains conscious to witness the birth, blood loss is minimal, vaginal and perineal structures remain relaxed, and headache is unlikely. The technique must be exact, however, and inadvertent massive (high) spinal anesthesia occurs occasionally. Undesirable reactions include rapid absorption syndrome (hypotension, bradycardia, hallucinations, seizures) and postpartal backache and paresthesia.

The *incidence of persistent occiput posterior positions is increased* because the fetal head is not normally rotated on the relaxed pelvic floor. Forceps rotation and delivery, therefore, is more often necessary.

2. **Spinal anesthesia.** Spinal anesthesia (saddleblock) is widely used to alleviate the pain of *delivery.* The advantages of spinal

anesthesia are that fetal hypoxia rarely occurs, blood loss is minimal, the mother remains conscious during delivery, no inhalation anesthetics or analgesic drugs are required, the technique is not difficult, and good relaxation of the pelvic floor and lower birth canal is achieved. Spinal headache occurs in about 5% of patients. Operative delivery is more often required because voluntary expulsive efforts are eliminated. Hypotension may result. Respiratory failure may develop if the anesthetic ascends as a result of rapid injection or straining by the patient.

The procedure for spinal anesthesia is as follows.

1. With the patient lying on her side or sitting, inject 40 mg of procaine (0.8 ml of 5% solution) or comparable drug slowly into the third or fourth lumbar interspace between contractions. Use a 25-gauge needle to pierce the dura. (This avoids leakage of CSF causative of headache.) Elevate the patient's head on a pillow immediately after the injection. Tilt the table up or down to achieve a level of anesthesia at or near the level of the umbilicus. Anesthesia will be maximal in 10–15 min and will last ≥1 h.

2. Record blood pressure and respirations every 5–10 min.

3. Give oxygen for respiratory depression. For hypotension, give vasopressors (e.g., ephedrine 25 mg IV).

4. For cesarean section, tilting the patient about 15–20 degrees to the left by elevating her right hip should avoid vena caval compression by the uterus and possible fetal distress.

General Anesthesia

For occasional deliveries (e.g., instrumented deliveries or cesarean section), general anesthesia may be necessary. This generally is induced by *minimal dose thiopental IV, followed by nitrous oxide-oxygen inhalation and succinylcholine by IV drip.* Considerable experience is required. For general anesthesia of gravid patients, *endotracheal intubation* is essential to prevent aspiration of gastric contents. Table 6-3 details the indications for general and regional anesthesia, and Table 6-4 shows the relative risks of each. Some useful *generalizations* for general anesthesia during pregnancy follow.

1. Prevent hypoxemia by administration of high-flow *oxygen* for 4–5 min before endotracheal intubation when apnea occurs.

2. Avoid aspiration of regurgitated gastric contents by preoperative administration of liquid antacid, *cimetidine,* or equivalent, and insertion of a cuffed endotracheal tube after anesthesia induction. Surgery should await adequate lung aeration.

3. Maintain at least *50% oxygen with anesthetic gas mixtures.*

Avoid hypoventilation, which results in maternal–fetal hypoxemia and acidosis. Prevent hyperventilation, which causes reduced uteroplacental blood flow and decreased fetal oxygenation. Maternal oxygen saturation monitoring is recommended.

Drugs Uncommonly Used Today

Inhalant analgesics (trichlorethylene and nitrous oxide) have been abandoned because of possible overuse and disastrous consequences. Likewise, the use of sedatives has been largely abandoned. They slow mentation, reduce perception of sensory stimuli, and increase suggestion receptivity. In addition, they are poor analgesics, are not amnestics, do not raise the pain threshold appreciably, and they may cause serious fetal depression. Periodic apnea and even abolition of all movements may be prolonged barbiturate effects. The amnesics (e.g., scopolamine) have been retired because their effects are unpredictable and they deprive the patient of her ability to participate. Some patients become somnolent or stuporous, whereas others become restless, hallucinating, and delirious. Phenothiazine drugs (Phenergan) potentiate certain of the desirable (as well as a few of the undesirable) effects of the analgesics, amnesics, and general anesthetics but also have been stopped largely because of their undesirable side effects.

INDUCTION OF LABOR

Induction of labor should be performed *only on specific indications*. There is some risk in any induction, and the *potential benefit must outweigh the risk*.

INDICATIONS

Individual induction of labor, especially in the treatment of *abnormal pregnancy* (preeclampsia-eclampsia, pyelonephritis), reduces maternal and fetal morbidity and mortality. Recall that delivery is either warranted or it is not. *The indication for induction should be so valid that if it fails, delivery is performed by cesarean section.* The following indications for induction of labor are valid in no more than 5%–8% of pregnancies.

1. Maternal infections (e.g., diverticulitis) that fail to resolve and are likely to become more severe unless pregnancy is concluded
2. Partial placental separation with uterine bleeding
3. Preeclampsia-eclampsia (delivery is the treatment for this process)
4. Diabetes mellitus with a mature fetus
5. Renal insufficiency (from any cause)
6. Premature rupture of the membranes when delivery is indicated (Chapter 11)
7. Previous precipitate delivery in a woman who cannot be transported quickly to a hospital
8. Marked polyhydramnios
9. Placental insufficiency
10. Isoimmunization (erythroblastosis)

CONTRAINDICATIONS

1. Cephalopelvic disproportion
2. Unfavorable obstetric circumstances, especially floating or deflected vertex or unfavorable presentation (including breech and multiple pregnancy)
3. Firm, closed, uneffaced posterior cervix (a vaginal examination must be performed before induction so that ripeness of the cervix can be confirmed)
4. Previous uterine or cervical operations (e.g., cesarean section or multiple myomectomy)
5. Maternal cardiac disease (functional class III or IV)
6. Grand multiparity (more than five pregnancies); with oxytocin, the uterus may rupture
7. Fetal distress without induction
8. Placenta previa

DANGERS OF INDUCTION

For the Mother

1. Emotional crisis (fear and anxiety)
2. Failure of induction and subsequent attempts to institute labor or to deliver the fetus

3. Uterine inertia and prolonged labor

4. Tumultuous labor and tetanic uterine contractions with the possiblity of rupture of the uterus, or cervical lacerations

5. Hemorrhagic complications, including abruptio placentae and atonic uterine postpartum hemorrhage

6. Intrauterine infection from examinations, rupture of membranes, or manipulation

7. Hypofibrinogenemia or other clotting abnormality

8. Amniotic fluid embolization

For the Fetus

1. An ill-timed induced delivery exposes the infant to the risks of prematurity.

2. Prolapse of the cord is an early and infection a late complication of amniotomy.

3. Violent labor may result in asphyxia, with subsequent damage.

4. Trauma as a result of the labor or delivery or both

Determining Appropriateness of Induction (the Bishop Score)

Bishop devised a scoring system (Table 6-5) to predict the outcome of induction when no contraindications (e.g., placenta previa) exist. A Bishop score of ≥ 9 indicates that labor may be induced with only a small chance of failure. This has been so

Table 6-5. Bishop score*

Cervical criteria	Score			
	0	1	2	3
Effacement (%)	0–30	40–50	60–70	80
Dilatation (cm)	0	1–2	3–4	5–6
Station of vertex (−3 to +3 scale)	−3	−2	−1, 0	+1, +2
Consistency	Firm	Medium	Soft	
Position	Posterior	Midposition	Anterior	

*From E. H. Bishop. A pelvic scoring for elective induction. *Obstet Gynecol* 1974;24:266.

reliable that it is now applied for many other situations (e.g., premature labor). Induction should not be attempted without determination of the Bishop score.

Preparation for Induction

A. The patient must be in a labor and delivery area with full anesthetic, neonatal, nursing, medical, blood banking, laboratory, and emergency facilities.

B. Vital signs must be obtained, and an IV infusion should be started through a large-bore catheter.

C. Fetal monitoring is always required during induction or stimulation of labor.

D. Prostaglandins (PGE_2 5 mg in a suppository, gel or strip) applied to the cervix the night before induction ripens the cervix (i.e., increases the Bishop score), thus enhancing the likelihood of initiation of labor.

E. Enemas and purges for the preparation or induction of labor (by reflex uterine hyperactivity) are harmful and painful and often are unsuccessful. They are contraindicated.

F. Ergot preparations are contraindicated for induction. They cause sustained contractions and must not be used before delivery for any reason.

Methods of Induction

Surgical Methods

Amniotomy is the safest (as measured by mortality and morbidity), easiest, and surest way to induce labor. Release of amniotic fluid shortens the muscle bundles of the myometrium. The strength and duration of the contractions are thereby increased. Amniotomy is painless and causes few complications.

Rupture of the membranes is accomplished through the partially dilated cervix using a hook or other sharp instrument. *Do not displace the infant's head!* Keep the patient in bed in Fowler's position after amniotomy so that slow drainage of fluid can occur. Anticipate labor <6 h if the patient is at term.

Stripping of the membranes (alone) is not recommended, since the result is unpredictable. This technique involves inserting a finger between the margin of the partially dilated cervix and the membranes and separating the two by a circular motion. It usually is uncomfortable and may be painful. It probably enhances the natural production of cervical prostaglandins. Unfortunately, untimely membrane rupture, damage leading to bleeding from a low-lying placenta, or mild amnionitis may occur.

Medical Methods

Parenteral administration of a very dilute solution of *oxytocin* is a most effective medical means of inducing labor.

The dosage of oxytocin must be individualized. The administration of oxytocin is really a biologic assay: the smallest possible effective dose must be determined for each patient and then used to initiate labor. In most cases, it is sufficient to add 0.1 ml of oxytocin (1 U Pitocin or Syntocinon) to 1 liter of 5% dextrose in water. Thus, each milliliter of solution will contain 1 mU of oxytocin.

Begin induction or augmentation at 1 mU/min. Increase oxytocin arithmetically by 2 mU increments (e.g., $1,3,5...n$ mU/min at 15-min intervals).

Doses greater than 15 mU/min are of concern. Those above 40 mU/min cause renal alterations and should not be necessary except in rare circumstances. Administration is controlled by the use of a constant infusion pump.

Constant observation by qualified attendants (preferably a physician) is required.

When contractions of 40–60 mm Hg (internal monitor pressure) or 40–60 sec (on the external monitor) occur at intervals of 1–4 min, the oxytocin dose should not be increased further. If contractions cease or become weak and ineffectual after a satisfactory start, the infusion may be resumed. *The infusion should be slowed or terminated if contractions exceed 60 mm Hg, exceed 60-sec duration, or have an interval of <2 min or if the fetus shows any signs of fetal distress (Chapter 5).*

It is not uncommon for the first induction attempt to fail; thus *repeated (serial) induction* must be considered. The criteria for a failed induction include inability to establish a consistent labor pattern (meeting the cited standards) and failure to affect cervical dilatation, effacement, or descent. Prospective discussion with the gravida and her family concerning the possibility of serial induction is very useful.

Should labor fail to start in one 6-h interval of induction *with intact membranes* (e.g., diabetes, preeclampsia) and both mother and fetus remain stable, efforts should cease for 6–18 h. This will allow the mother and myometrium to recover. Prostaglandin E_2

cervical application should be considered. Another 6-h attempt should follow. If this too fails, another 6–18 h rest interval is undertaken (again, if all is stable). At the start of the next 6-h induction, the membranes should be ruptured. If induction should fail cesarean section is warranted and should be done as soon as it is ascertained that induction is a failure.

Induction *with ruptured membranes* must proceed more rapidly and should not exceed 24 h from the time of rupture. However, it is still preferable to proceed in approximate 6-h increments.

Chapter 7

High-Risk Pregnancy

Although pregnancy may be classified as a normal physiologic condition, it is fraught with considerable risk to both mother and offspring. Fortunately, *most of the risk occurs to a minority of patients.* Thus, it is prudent to *identify those at risk and attempt to prevent the morbidity and mortality.* Some factors contributing to risk are quite obvious, but others are very subtle. Thus, care must be taken in definitions, screening programs, and application of the tools available for diagnosis and treatment. The following is but one of the ways to approach this multifaceted set of circumstances.

DEFINITION, INCIDENCE, AND IMPORTANCE

A high-risk pregnancy is one in which the mother or perinate is or will be in jeopardy (death or serious complications) *during gestation or in the puerperium/neonatal interval.* Estimates of the incidence of high-risk pregnancy vary widely depending mainly on the criteria used for definition and the accuracy of the data collection. Nevertheless, by most standards, ~20% of established pregnancies in the United States are at some risk and ~5% are at very high risk. About half can be identified antenatally and another quarter during labor (Table 7-1). For example, at least the *majority of perinatal deaths are associated with prematurity or congenital anomalies.* If these two conditions are excluded, 60% of fetal and >50% of neonatal deaths are associated with only five obstetric complications: *breech presentation, premature separation of the placenta, preeclampsia-eclampsia, multiple pregnancy, and urinary tract infection.* Certain less common complications (e.g., cord prolapse) also cause an inordinately high proportion or perinatal losses. Of course, a low-risk pregnancy (not endangered by present or forseeable complications) can become high risk at any time.

Table 7-1. Identification of specific obstetric risk factors

INITIAL EVALUATION
Biologic factors

High risk	Some risk
Maternal age <15 or ≥35 years	Maternal age 15–19 years
Morbid obesity	>20% of standard height for weight
Poor nutrition	
Maternal malignancy	<20% of standard height for weight
Ovarian neoplasms	
Genetic or familial disorder	Short stature (≤60 inches)
Incompetent cervix	Uterine leiomyomata
Cervical malformation	Pelvic or spinal deformity
Uterine malformation	
Congenital anomaly	
Genital tract anomalies	

Obstetric history

High risk	Some risk
Parity of ≥8	Parity of >5
Three or more abortions	Prolonged labor or dystocia
Stillborn or neonatal loss	Infertility
Previous pregnancy with	Prior ABO incompatibility
Premature labor	Prior fetal malpresentation
Birth weight <2500 g	Previous PIH
Birth weight >4000 g	Genital tract infections
Genetic disorder	Human papillomavirus (HPV)
Congenital anomaly	Herpes
Isoimmunization	Gonorrhea
Eclampsia	Chlamydia
Birth damaged infant	Group B *Streptococcus*
Special neonatal care	
Medically indicated pregnancy termination	
Molar gestation	

Medical and surgical history

High risk	Some risk
Hypertension (moderate to severe)	Mild hypertension
	Class I heart disease
Severe renal disease	Gestational diabetes
Class II–IV heart disease	Recurrent urinary infections
Insulin-regulated diabetes	Positive serology
Endocrine ablation (thyroid)	Sickle cell trait
Abnormal cervical cytology	Epilepsy
Sickle cell disease	Emotional disorders
Pulmonary disease	Smoking

(continued)

Table 7-1. (continued)

INITIAL EVALUATION
Medical and surgical history

High risk	Some risk
Liver disease	Pelvic inflammatory disease
Recurrent pyelonephritis	Previous ectopic pregnancy
Collagen vascular disease	Physical abuse
Malignancy	
Gastrointestinal disease	
Substance abuse	
Heavy smoking (>10 day)	

EVALUATION ON EACH PRENATAL VISIT, EARLY PREGNANCY (≤20 WEEKS)

High risk	Some risk
Teratic exposure	Unresponsive urinary tract infection
Failure of uterine growth	Possible ectopic gestation
Antenatal diagnosis indicated	Missed abortion
Isoimmunization	Severe hyperemesis gravidarum
Severe anemia (≤9 g Hgb)	Positive serology
Multiple gestation	Sexually transmitted disease
Fetal anomalies	Unresponsive anemia
Cervical incompetence	Vaginal bleeding
Insulin-regulated diabetes	Diet-regulated diabetes
Fetal anomalies	
Nonimmune hydrops	
Renal agenesis (Potter's)	

EVALUATION ON EACH PRENATAL VISIT, LATER PREGNANCY (>20 WEEKS)

High risk	Some risk
IUGR	Pregnancy ≥42 1/2 weeks
Anemia (≤9 g Hgb)	Preeclampsia
Severe preeclampsia	Breech (for vaginal delivery)
Eclampsia	Placenta previa
Isoimmunization	Premature onset of labor (<36 weeks)
Oligohydramnios	Premature rupture (<38 weeks)
Hydramnios	Chronic or acute pyelonephritis
Thromboembolic disease	Abnormal fetal position
Abruptio placentae	
Abnormal antepartum test (NST, CST, BPP)	
Prolonged membrane rupture	
Fetal infections	

(continued)

Table 7-1. (continued)

INTRAPARTUM EVALUATION High risk	Some risk
High-risk factors above	Mild PIH
Severe PIH or eclampsia	Rupture of membranes >12 h
Hydraminos or oligohydramnios	Primary dysfunctional labor
Amnionitis	Secondary arrest of dilatation
Prolonged rupture (>24 h)	Labor >20 h
Uterine rupture	Second stage >2.5 h
Abruptio placentae	Precipitous labor
Placenta previa	Prolonged latent phase
Meconium in amniotic fluid	Uterine tetany
Abnormal presentation	Induction of labor
Multiple gestation	Operative forceps
Fetal weight <1500 g	Vacuum extraction
Fetal weight >4000 g	General anesthesia
Abnormal FHR patterns	Abnormal maternal vital signs
Breech delivery	Fetal presentation not descending with labor
Prolapsed cord	
Fetal acidosis	
Shoulder dystocia	
Maternal distress	

The *early identification of risk factors is vital* for both avoidance of serious problems and proper treatment of complications responsible for increased maternal and perinatal mortality and morbidity. Despite steady improvement, at least three quarters of obstetric deaths (9/100,000 births) and at least one half of newborn deaths (10/1000 births) in the United States are preventable.

PRENATAL CARE, A DIAGNOSTIC AND THERAPEUTIC PROGRAM

Good prenatal care is preventive medicine of a high order. It provides an opportunity to identify the individual's risk status and appropriately individualize care for each patient. Moreover, it has been amply demonstrated that those *gravidas who receive good prenatal care materially improve both their own and their offspring's chance* of successfully negotiating this most hazardous interval of life.

Maternal, fetal, or neonatal hazard often can be foretold by critical assessment of the gravida's history, physical examination, and antenatal course (Table 7-2). Dozens of factors during pregnancy, labor, delivery, and the early puerperium suggest added risk; for example, unwanted pregnancy, ignorance, exposure to toxic products, and unwillingness or inability to obtain good early obstetric care relate to high-risk pregnancy. Whatever the problem, prevention, early diagnosis, and proper treatment will greatly reduce the perinatal mortality and morbidity rates. Thus, most clinicians include these factors in their plan for prenatal care (Chapter 5) and actively search for and treat them as the pregnancy progresses.

Additionally, several risk scoring systems to predict jeopardy have been suggested. Although risk scoring systems are not as sensitive or as specific as originally thought, they may provide a useful method to ensure that most of the risk-producing states are screened in each gestation.

HISTORICAL SCREENING

Poverty, ignorance, substance abuse, and unwanted pregnancy are sociologic conditions *associated with high-risk pregnancy.* These may take years to alleviate, and their solutions have little to do with medicine. For example, low socioeconomic and single marital status (in an adolescent) are two important obstetric high-risk factors. Although physicians cannot do much to remedy the underlying problem, proper diet, rest, social support, proper antenatal care, and good patient cooperation can improve the prognosis of such an adolescent to approximate that of most middle-income gravidas. Thus, *our purpose is to deal primarily with factors that can be influenced by medical management* and the currently available diagnostic and therapeutic modalities.

A *uniform perinatal record* is very useful to assist the physician in evaluating high-risk pregnancy. Some commercially available forms may use risk lists, whereas others rate factors according to their importance. Whatever system is used, it must be applied assiduously.

Maternal Age

The lowest rates of maternal and perinatal morbidity and mortality occur at maternal age 20–29. Thus, younger and older women are at greater risk.

Adolescent pregnancy has a higher frequency of low birth weight infants, and in those younger than 16 years there is increased risk of pregnancy-induced hypertension. Mothers age 35 or older are at high risk, and those over 40 years are at extraordinary risk. The most common problems are *increased chromosomal abnormalities, chronic hypertension, pregnancy-induced hypertension, obesity, uterine myomas, increased incidence of age-related medical problems* (e.g., diabetes), *and an increased risk of being delivered by cesarean section.* The risk of *trisomy* is directly related to age, rising from 0.9% at age 35–36 to 7.8% at age 43–44 years. Prenatal diagnosis screening questions (Table 7-2) should be asked of each older gravida and the follow-up documented. Starting the screening as early as maternal age 32 has merit. Women with a low level of serum alpha-fetoprotein (AFP), regardless of age, should be considered for amniocentesis, since they have an increased risk of trisomic offspring.

In summary, it is important to ascertain the following. Does the patient, her husband, or their family have heritable disorders? What is the health of first-degree relatives (siblings, parents, offspring), second-degree relatives (uncles, aunts, nephews, nieces, and grandparents), and third-degree relatives (first cousins)? What are the probable reproductive outcomes? Is there drug exposure (both husband and wife)? What are the parental ages (paternal risk $\geq$ 55)? What is the ethnic origin (because of enhanced risk of several disease states, e.g., Tay-Sachs disease in Ashkenazi Jews, beta-thalassemia in Italians and Greeks, sickle cell anemia in African Americans, and alpha-thalassemia in Southeast Asians)?

Obstetric History

The *number of previous pregnancies* is important. To para 5, there is increased chance of successful pregnancy. However, after 5, the risk from uterine inertia, postpartum hemorrhage, placenta previa, and abruptio placentae begins an almost exponential increase. A *history of infertility* places a patient at increased risk because of a greater incidence of fetal wastage. There is a correlation between the *outcome of previous pregnancies* and what may happen to the current pregnancy.

Thus, the following obstetric historical findings signal risk:

Table 7-2. Prenatal diagnosis screening questions

	Circle Appropriate Answer	
1. Will you be age 35 or older when the baby is due?	Yes	No
2. Have you or the baby's father or anyone in either of your families ever had		
a. Down syndrome?	Yes	No
b. Spina bifida or meningomyelocele (open spine)?	Yes	No
c. Hemophilia (blood will not clot)?	Yes	No
d. Muscular dystrophy?	Yes	No
3. Have you or the baby's father had a child born dead or alive with a birth defect not listed in Question 2?	Yes	No
If yes, describe:_____		
4. Do you or the baby's father have any close relatives who are mentally retarded?	Yes	No
If Yes, list cause if known:_____		
5. Do you or the baby's father or close relative in either of your families have any inherited genetic or chromosomal disease or disorder not listed above?	Yes	No
6. Have you or the spouse of this baby's father in a previous marriage had three or more *spontaneous* pregnancy losses?	Yes	No
7. Do you or the baby's father have any close relatives descended from Jewish people who lived in Eastern Europe (Ashkenazi Jews)?	Yes	No
If Yes, have either you or the baby's father been screened for Tay-Sachs disease?	Yes	No
If Yes, indicate results and who screened:_____		

(*continued on next page*)

Table 7-2. (continued)

	Circle Appropriate Answer	
8. If patient or spouse is African American: Have you or the baby's father or any close relative been screened for sickle cell trait and found to be positive?	Yes	No

I have discussed with my doctor the above questions which are answered Yes and understand that I am at increased risk for:

_____

and that it is usually possible to diagnose an affected fetus by testing amniotic fluid at about 16 weeks of pregnancy or placental tissue at an earlier time in pregnancy and I DO NOT want the test. _____

       (Patient Signature)   (Date)

Patient wants amniocentesis and fetal diagnoses for:_____

_____

Patient referred for further testing or counseling concerning:

_____
_____

*Modified from Antenatal Diagnosis, NIH Publication No. 79-193, April 1979.

habitual abortion, pregnancy terminated for a medical indication, stillbirth, neonatal death, preterm or SGA birth, birth of a baby >4000 g, isoimmunization, pregnancy-induced hypertension, baby with known or suspected genetic disorder or congenital anomaly, and birth-damaged infant or infant requiring special neonatal care. Other historical risk factors include operative deliveries (cesarean section, midforceps or breech extraction), prolonged labor or dystocia, severe psychiatric disturbances associated with pregnancy, and closely spaced pregnancies (<3 months).

Reproductive Tract Disorders

Abnormalities of the reproductive tract cause at least 25% of recidive reproductive losses. Thus, a history of *incompetent cervix, septate uterus, bicornuate uterus, or uterine leiomyomas* may warn of pregnancy risk. Other reproductive tract aberrations that may place the pregnancy at risk because they can require therapy during pregnancy include *cervical dysplasia and ovarian tumors*. Should intervention be necessary, the safest time to perform surgery is during the second trimester, when both post-surgical abortion and preterm labor have the lowest incidence.

Exposure to Fetotoxic Agent

For discussion of the topic, see Chapter 5.

Medical Complications of Pregnancy

Some of the systemic diseases creating risk in pregnancy include *blood disorders* (e.g., coagulopathy, sickle cell disease), *cancer, cerebral aneurysms or tumors, chronic hypertension, connective tissue disease* (e.g., systemic lupus erythematosus), *diabetes mellitus, endocrine ablation, epilepsy, gastrointestinal and liver disease, heart disease, pulmonary disease, renal disease* (e.g., glomerulonephritis), and *thyroid disorders*.

Family History

A detailed family history keyed to mental retardation, multiple gestation, and heritable diseases is mandatory. Risk assessment is aided by a three-generation pedigree.

Physical Examination

Stature

Women less than 5 feet (150 cm) tall have increased fetopelvic disproportion. Thus, short stature is an indication for careful bony pelvis assessment.

Weight

Ideal weight is necessarily predicated on height and body habitus, and abnormalities of weight must be individualized. Both *underweight and overweight signal risk* for the perinate. Moreover, the maternal prepregnancy weight and gain during pregnancy are related directly to birthweight. The woman who weighs <100 pounds (45 kg) when not pregnant has an increased chance of having an SGA infant. Women who are obese for height have a greater chance of pregnancy complicated by LGA birth, dysfunctional labor, and shoulder dystocia. The morbidly obese increase their risk even further.

Blood Pressure

Hypertension poses great risk to pregnancy and should be evaluated immediately (Chapter 13). Although occasional hypotension from orthostasis or from the supine hypotensive syndrome is of concern, it is easily managed symptomatically.

Breasts

When a mass is found, the usual breast *cancer workup cannot be delayed by the pregnancy.*

Heart

Diastolic murmurs, systolic murmurs ≥grade 3, and arrhythmias always require a medical evaluation.

Vascular System

Severe varicosities tend to thrombose during pregnancy (p. 395).

Pelvic Evaluation

Pelvic problems relating to risk include *genital prolapse, fixation of a retroflexed and retroverted uterus, uterine anomalies, cervical tumors, cervical laceration, cervical incompetence, genital condylomata accuminata* (which may cause neonatal laryngeal papillomas), *genital herpes, group B streptococcal infections, abnormalities of the ovaries, abnormalities of the uterine tubes, and abnormalities of the bony pelvis* or pelvic capacity.

 A diagnosis and a plan of management for each of the conditions placing the patient at risk must be proposed.

COURSE OF PREGNANCY

ANTENATAL VISITS

Antenatal visits must be more frequent for high-risk than for normal obstetric patients to accurately appraise the pregnancy and identify and correct problems. Antenatal visits also provide an opportunity for education about problems, their solution, and counseling.

The etiologies of many serious problems that develop during pregnancy are reviewed elsewhere. Thus, only the major categories are summarized here.

Abnormal Vital Signs

The most frequent aberrations of vital signs signaling risk during pregnancy are *abnormal weight or blood pressure.* As noted previously, failure to gain weight during pregnancy often is associated with an SGA perinate, and excessive weight gain is associated with an LGA perinate. *Fever* may trigger preterm labor and may injure the fetal CNS. *Pregnancy-induced hypertension* (PIH) is most often indicated by a $\geq$ 140/90 blood pressure or a $\geq$ 30 mm Hg systolic or a $\geq$ 15 mm Hg diastolic rise. Other symptoms of PIH include proteinuria and significant edema (Chapter 13).

Common Laboratory Abnormalities

The most common abnormal laboratory values during pregnancy are *urinary* (bacteria, protein, or glucose) *or hematologic. Significant bacteriuria* ($>$100,000 bacteria/ml) places the patient at risk for pyelonephritis, premature rupture of membranes, and premature onset of labor. *Diabetes mellitus* (even if only gestational) is related to a number of pregnancy risks (p. 416). Moreover, gestational diabetic mothers require follow-up after delivery because they are at increased risk of developing chemical diabetes. Hematologic risks, the most common being *anemia and isoimmunization,* are detailed in Chapter 14.

Problematic Symptoms or Signs

Symptoms or signs of greatest concern during the course of pregnancy include *vaginal bleeding, uterine growth out of proportion to dates,* and *the untimely termination of pregnancy.* Uterine bleeding in early or late pregnancy warns of jeopardy to the pregnancy

(Chapter 10 and 11). A discrepancy of uterine size for dates requires ultrasonic scanning for explanation. If the size is less than reasonable for dates, it is due most frequently to an error in dates, an SGA fetus, a congenital anomaly, or oligohydraminos. If the uterus is larger than expected for dates, it most commonly indicates polyhydramnios, multiple gestation, fetal anomaly, an LGA fetus, or an error in dates. Preterm termination of pregnancy, with or without rupture of membranes is second only to congenital anomalies as a cause of morbidity and mortality. Postterm pregnancy termination poses risks of uteroplacental insufficiency, meconium-containing amniotic fluid, and complicated labor or trauma during labor and delivery (from excessive size).

Surgery During Pregnancy

Although not increased by pregnancy, *acute appendicitis* is the most common surgical emergency during gestation. The major pregnancy complications of acute appendicitis (similar to all abdominal surgery) include premature delivery and peritonitis.

If all physical trauma (e.g., assault, motor vehicle accidents, and falls) were categorized as surgical emergencies, trauma would head the list. The patient with significant physical trauma during pregnancy has a marked risk of abruptio placentae.

Immunizations During Pregnancy

Current recommendations concerning immunizations during pregnancy are summarized in Table 7-3.

COURSE OF LABOR

Common problems during the course of labor include dystocia, fetal distress, and meconium-stained amniotic fluid.

DYSTOCIA

Dystocia is abnormal or difficult labor. It occurs in <10% of nulliparas and is less common in multiparas. The etiology of

Table 7-3. Recommendations for immunizations during pregnancy

Cholera	Comply only to meet international travel requirements
Hepatitis A	Immunize gravida after exposure
	Newborns of mothers who are incubating or ill should receive 1 dose after birth
Hepatitis B	Newborn should receive hyperimmune globulin soon after delivery, followed by vaccination
Influenza	Immunize gravida following criteria recommended for general population
Measles	Live virus vaccine during pregnancy contraindicated on theoretical grounds
	Pooled immune globulins for postexposure prophylaxis
Mumps	Theoretically contraindicated during pregnancy
Plague	Immunize only if there is substantial infection risk
Poliomyelitis	Not routinely recommended but mandatory in epidemics or when traveling to epidemic areas
Rabies	Same as nonpregnant
Rubella	Contraindicated (although teratogenicity negligible in follow-up of those inadvertently given the vaccine)
Tetanus and diphtheria	Give toxoid if no primary series or no booster in 10 years
	Postexposure prophylaxis in unvaccinated with tetanus immune globulin plus toxoid
Typhoid	Recommended if traveling to endemic area
Varicella	Varicella-zoster immune globulin for exposure
	Indicated for newborns whose mothers developed varicella within 4 days before or 2 days after delivery
Yellow fever	Postpone travel if possible but immunize before travel to high-risk areas

dystocia is typically ascribed to one or a combination of the 4 Ps (pelvis, passenger, powers, and placenta).

The most common pelvic abnormalities associated with dystocia include *bony size or configuration, birth canal soft tissue aberration* (e.g., congenital anomalies, scarring of the birth canal, conglutination of the external cervix os, massive condylomata accuminata), and *other reproductive organ neoplasia* (e.g., cervical carcinoma, ovarian cyst, uterine leiomyoma), including a *distended bladder or bowel.*

Abnormalities of the passenger (*fetal dystocia*) include *excessive fetal size* (>4000 g), *malpositions* (e.g., breech, transverse lie), *congenital anomalies* (e.g., hydrocephalus, sacrococcygeal teratoma), and *multiple gestations* (e.g., malpresentation, locking twins—twin A breech, twin B vertex).

Uterine dystocia (i.e., uterine activity that does not elicit the normal progress of labor) is referred to as an abnormality of the powers. Commonly, uterine dystocia includes *hypertonic, hypotonic,* or *discoordinate uterine activity,* although lack of voluntary expulsive effort during the second stage of labor also may delay delivery.

Abnormal placental location (e.g., placenta previa or low-lying posterior implantation) decreases pelvic capacity by lying over the sacral promontory.

Pelvic Types

As noted in Chapter 1, the female pelvis is classified into four major types, although various combinations may occur (Fig. 7-1, Table 7-4).

The *gynecoid pelvis* is the most favorable for vaginal delivery and is seen in ~50% of women in the United States. It is characterized by oval inlet (transverse diameter slightly exceeds the anteroposterior diameter), straight sidewalls, nonprominent ischial spines, a wide subpubic arch, and a concave sacrum.

The *android* (male-like) *pelvis* is found in ~33% of Caucasian and 15% of African American women. The android inlet is wedge-shaped, the pelvic sidewalls are convergent, the ischial spines are prominent, the subpubic arch is narrow, and the sacrum is inclined anteriorly in its lower one third. It is likely to be associated with persistent occiput posterior position and deep transverse arrest dystocia.

The *anthropoid pelvis* is found in ~20% of Caucasian women and ~85% of African American women. It is marked by an oval inlet (but the anteroposterior diameter exceeds the transverse),

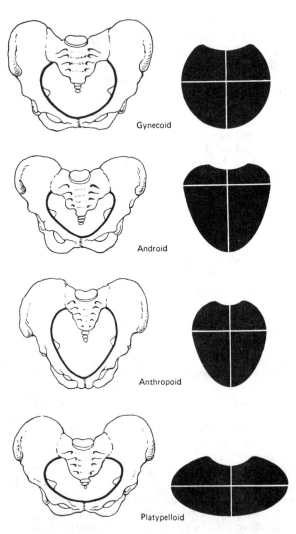

Gynecoid

Android

Anthropoid

Platypelloid

Figure 7-1. Pelvic types. White lines in the diagrams at right show the greatest diameters of the pelves at left.

Table 7-4. Pelvic types*

	Gynecoid	Android	Anthropoid	Platypelloid
Inlet	Rounded or slightly heart-shaped. Ample anterior and posterior segments	Wedge-shaped or rounded triangle. Posterior segment wide, flat; anterior narrow, pointed	Anteroposterior ovoid with length of anterior and posterior segments increased. Transverse diameter reduced	Transverse ovoid; increased transverse AP diameter of both segments
Sacrum	Curved, average length	Straight with forward inclination	Normally curved but long and narrow	Curved, short
Sacrosciatic notch	Medium width	Narrow	Wide, shallow	Slightly narrowed
Side walls (AP view)	Straight, divergent, or convergent	Usually convergent	Straight	Straight or slightly divergent
Side walls (lateral view; "lateral bore")	Straight, divergent, or convergent	Usually convergent	Often straight	Straight or divergent
Interspinous diameter	Wide	Shortened	Shortened	Increased
Pubic arch	Curved	Straight	Slightly curved	Curved
Subpubic angle	Wide	Very narrow	Narrow	Wide
Biischial diameter	Wide	Shortened	Often shortened	Wide

*After Caldwell and Moloy.

the pelvic side walls diverge, and the sacrum is inclined posteriorly. This type pelvis is most likely to be associated with occiput posterior dystocia.

The *platypelloid pelvis* is rare (<3% of all women) and is characterized by a wide transverse diameter of the inlet. Inlet dystocia is common because the fetal head cannot enter the true pelvis. Transverse arrest may occur in the midpelvis because internal rotation is compromised by unfavorable pelvic diameters.

Critical Pelvic Measurements

Critical pelvic dimensions (for average-sized fetuses) include a *diagonal conjugate ≥12.5 cm, an obstetric conjugate (anteroposterior of the inlet) ≥10 cm, and a transverse of the midpelvis of ≥9.5 cm* (Table 7-5).

Inlet Contracture

Inlet contracture can be expected if the *anteroposterior is <10 cm or the transverse is <12 cm (or both)*. This is suggested clinically by one or more of the following: a floating vertex presentation at term or in early labor, an inability to perform the Muller-Hillis maneuver (manually pushing the fetal head into the pelvis with gentle fundal pressure), presenting part not well applied to the cervix in labor, an abnormal presentation (e.g., breech, trans-

Table 7-5. Measurements in clinical pelvimetry

Measurement	Normal value	Abnormal value (possibly inadequate)
Biischial diameter (BI)	≥ 8 cm	<8 cm
Posterior sagittal diameter of outlet (PS)	8–9.5 cm (direct)	<8 cm
Anteroposterior diameter of outlet (AP)	≥ 11.9 cm	<11.9 cm
Interspinous diameter of midpelvis	≥ 10.5 cm	<9.5 cm
Diagonal conjugate (DC)	>11.5 cm	<11.5 cm
True conjugate (CV)	>10 cm	<10 cm
Angle of pubic arch	110–120°	<90°

verse lie), cord prolapse, poor progress in labor, uterine dysto-cia, excessive molding of the fetal head, or caput succedaneum formation. *Complications* include prolonged labor, prolonged rupture of the membranes, and pathologic retraction ring at the junction of the lower uterine segment and fundus (Bandl's retrac-tion ring, signifying impending uterine rupture). Cesarean sec-tion usually is necessary for the true inlet contracture.

Midpelvic Contracture

Midpelvic contracture nearly always occurs as a result of an *in-terspinous diameter of <9.5 cm*. This may be suspected if the pelvic sidewalls are convergent, and a narrow pelvic arch is pres-ent. Other clinical suggestions include prolonged second stage of labor, persistent occiput posterior, deep transverse arrest, uter-ine dystocia, or excessive molding of the fetal head. As with inlet dystocia, neglected midpelvic dystocia may result in uterine rup-ture or fistulae due to pressure necrosis. Cesarean section is the treatment of choice because instrumental delivery may lead to fetal or maternal injuries.

Outlet Contracture

Isolated outlet dystocia is very rare, but this occurs if the *in-tertuberous diameter is not >8 cm or the sum of the intertuberous and the posterior sagittal diameter of the outlet is ≤ 15 cm.*

Fetal Abnormalities Causing Dystocia

Abnormalities of Presentation and Position

Abnormalities of fetal (passenger) *presentation and attitude* (*lie*) *complicate* ~5% of all labors. The most common of all fetal abnormalities causing dystocia is *breech presentation.* The most common of the *vertex* positions are *occiput posterior* and *occiput transverse* malpositions. Whereas these positions may occur nor-mally, their persistence is abnormal. Occiput posterior is associ-ated with partial deflection of the fetal head and presentation of the larger posterior portion of the head (as opposed to the smaller anterior portion) to the transverse of the midpelvis. The diagnosis is made by vaginal examination (confirmed by palpat-ing the fetal ear). Persistent occiput transverse is associated with pelvic dystocia, platypelloid or android pelves, or uterine dystocia. *Deep transverse arrest* occurs in the midpelvis and usually is due to an inadequate midpelvic diameter, as in an android pelvis.

Selection of proper treatment that will be the least traumatic to mother and perinate requires clinical acumen.

Sinciput or brow presentations usually are transient fetal presentations with various degrees of deflection of the fetal head, which hopefully convert to face or vertex as labor proceeds. Thus, *expectant management* is the first recommendation. Of course, fetopelvic disproportion, uterine inertia and arrested progress, prematurity, and grand multiparity may mandate intervention.

Face presentation occurs in ~0.2% of deliveries and is most commonly associated with *congenital malformations* (e.g., anencephaly), *fetopelvic disproportion, prematurity,* or *grand multiparity. Mentum posterior position,* in all but very small prematures, is not safely deliverable vaginally. Delivery of some mentum anterior presentations is possible, but most require cesarean section.

Abnormal fetal lie is most commonly *transverse or oblique* and occurs in ~0.33% of deliveries (six times more frequent in *premature births*). Other causative associations include grand multiparity, pelvic contracture, and abnormal placental implantation. *External cephalic version* during the third trimester is most useful in conversion to a vertex. One of the major risks is a 20 times increase in cord prolapse with rupture of the membranes. A *compound presentation* occurs when the presenting part is accompanied by a prolapsed extremity. Gentle pinching of the digits may cause the fetus to retract the extremity. Should this and spontaneous restitution fail to occur or if dystocia is also a problem, consider cesarean section.

Macrosomia

Macrosomia is defined as fetal size >4000 g and occurs in ~5% of deliveries. Macrosomia may be associated with shoulder dystocia. The large-for-dates fetus may be related to maternal diabetes mellitus or marked obesity. The differential diagnosis must also include inaccurate calculation of the duration of gestation, multiple pregnancy, hydramnios, or uterine tumor.

Abnormal Labor (Powers)

Consider two components in evaluating labor: the *contractions per se* and the *cumulative effect of the contractions* as determined by the progress of labor.

Evaluation of Uterine Contractions (Fig. 7-2)

The evaluation of contractions requires an affirmative answer to the following five questions.

1. *Is there fundal dominance?* The relative intensity of contraction normally is greater in the fundus than in the midportion or lower uterine segment. Absence of fundal dominance may indicate lack of a uterine synchrony (as occurs with false labor).

2. *Does the uterus relax between contractions?* Normal resting tone is 12–15 mm Hg. When it is increased without oxytocin stimulation, suspect abruptio placentae.

3. *Is the average value of the intensity of contractions >24 mm Hg?* In the active phase of labor, intrauterine pressure often increases to 40–60 mm Hg.

4. *Is the frequency of contractions about 3–5 min?* With normal labor, the frequency of contractions progresses from one every 3–5 min to one every 2–3 min during the active phase.

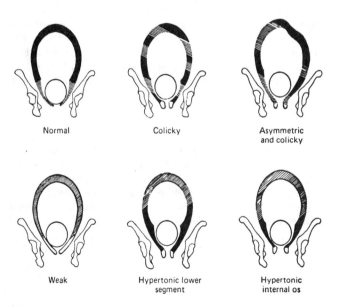

Figure 7-2. Normal and dysfunctional uterine contraction types. (After Jeffcoate.) Black, strong contraction; shaded, slight contraction; white, atonic areas.

5. *Do the contractions last longer than 30 sec?* The duration of effective contractions is abnormal if they exceed 60 sec.

Abnormal Contractions

Hypotonic dysfunction Hypotonic dysfunction is character-ized by contractions with *insufficient force* (<25 mm Hg) *or an irregular or infrequent rhythm or both.* Hypotonic dysfunction is more common in nulligravidas during the active phase of labor but may be associated with excessive sedation, early administration of conduction anesthesia, and uterine overdistention (e.g., multiple gestation, polyhydramnios). If there is no contraindication (e.g., fetopelvic disproportion, multiple gestation, malpresentation, al-lergy), hypotonic dysfunction responds well to oxytocin.

Hypertonic dysfunction. Hypertonic and uncoordinated dys-function often occur together and may be accompanied by eleva-tion of uterine resting tone, lack of fundal dominance, and increased uterine pain. Hypertonic dysfunction generally is asso-ciated with overzealous oxytocin use, abruptio placentae, or fetopelvic disproportion. Fetal distress is a common association. Hypertonic dysfunction may result in precipitate delivery. Treat-ment is problematic but often includes tocolysis, amyl nitrate, cessation of oxytocin, or cesarean section (if indicated for mal-presentation, fetopelvic disproportion, or fetal distress). The fetus subjected to hypertonic dysfunction is at increased risk of fetal distress, intracranial hemorrhage, or perinatal injury. Lac-erations of the birth canal also may result from rapid delivery.

Evaluation of Labor

Usually, dystocia is heralded by an *abnormal labor pattern.* Fig-ures 6-4 and 6-5 detail one method of assessment and describe the normal course of labor. *Decreasing perinatal risk requires the recognition of aberrations* of labor and *proper intervention.*

Abnormal patterns of labor (Fig. 6-6) include a prolonged latent phase, a protracted active phase (dilatation), protracted descent, a prolonged deceleration phase, the secondary arrest of dilatation, or the arrest of descent. In contrast, precipitate labor may also occur.

Abnormal Labor Patterns

Prolonged latent phase The *latent phase begins with the onset of regular contractions and ends at the beginning of the active phase of* *labor* (3–4 cm cervical dilatation). The average latent phase is ~6 h for nulliparas and ~5 h for multiparas, with the upper limit of normal at 20 h for nulliparas and 14 h for multiparas. The usual *causes* of a prolonged latent phase *include excessive analgesics or analgesics administered too early in labor, conduction anesthesia performed before the active phase, an unfavorable cervix* (e.g., a low Bishop score or scarring), *uterine dysfunction* (e.g., weak, irregular, uncoordinated, or ineffective uterine contractions), and *fetopelvic disproportion.* False labor may be the correct diagnosis in 10% of cases in this category. The recommended treatment of prolonged latent stage is the discontinuation of medications or anesthesia, correction of fluid or electrolyte deficiencies, and morphine 8–12 mg (determined on a weight basis) to rest the gravida for 6–12 h. Then, about 5% of patients will require an oxytocin infusion, but nearly all with a prolonged latent phase will proceed to vaginal delivery without fetal complications.

Protraction disorders The *active phase of labor starts at 3–4 cm and ends with complete (10 cm) cervical dilatation.* Dilatation is protracted if labor is proceeding at <1.2 cm/h in a nullipara and <1.5 cm/h in a multipara. Descent is protracted if there is <1 cm/h descent in a nullipara and <2 cm/h descent in a multipara. The causes of protraction disorders include *fetopelvic disproportion* (33%), *malpositions* (e.g., occiput posterior), *ineffectual contractions* (e.g., excessive sedation, conduction anesthesia above the T10 dermatome), and *soft tissue dystocia.*

Protraction disorders require an assessment of the quality of labor and the diagnosis (or elimination) of fetopelvic dystocia. The quality of labor usually is investigated using *electronic fetal monitoring* with an intrauterine catheter to determine pressure changes. In the past, x-ray pelvimetry was used commonly to diagnose fetopelvic disproportion, but today diagnosis is by physical determination of pelvic contours and diameters, often confirmed by ultrasonography.

Cesarean section is indicated for the patient with *fetopelvic disproportion.* If disproportion can be excluded and if the fetal status remains satisfactory and labor is adequate, avoid oxytocin and inhibitory factors (e.g., analgesia). Ensure support (hydration and close observation) in anticipation of vaginal delivery. If contractions are inadequate but with a satisfactory fetal status, oxytocin stimulation (with close maternal and fetal monitoring) is indicated. Nonetheless, labor may still be prolonged. *Expect about two thirds of these patients to have vaginal delivery.*

Arrest disorders The *deceleration phase starts at nearly 10 cm dilatation and continues to complete dilatation.* The deceleration phase is arrested or prolonged if it continues for >3 h in nulliparas or >1 h in multiparas. A secondary arrest of dilatation occurs when there is no progress in dilatation for ≥2 h during the active phase. An arrest of descent occurs with failure to progress for ≥1 h during the active phase of labor. A later failure of descent may occur when there is no descent during the deceleration phase or second stage of labor.

Causes of arrest disorders include *fetopelvic disproportion* (~50%), *fetal malpositions* (e.g., occiput posterior, face, brow), *conduction anesthesia labor impairment,* and *excessive sedation.* As with the protraction disorders, each patient must have careful evaluation for fetopelvic disproportion and fetal well-being. If disproportion is present, cesarean section is indicated. In the absence of disproportion or contraindication to its use, oxytocin stimulation is generally effective therapy. This is likely if a postarrest rate of dilatation or descent is greater than or equal to the prearrest rate. Hydration, allowing excessive analgesia or conduction anesthesia to dissipate, and other supportive measure also may be helpful. Arrest disorders generally carry a *poor prognosis for vaginal delivery and have increased perinatal morbidity and mortality.*

Precipitate labor Precipitate labor and delivery may occur as a result of either very rapid dilatation or descent. Precipitate dilatation is defined as *active phase dilatation of ≥5 cm/h in a primipara or ≥10 cm/h in a multipara.* Precipitate descent is active phase descent of ≥5 cm/h in a primipara or ≥10 cm/h in a multipara. Precipitate labor usually results from very forceful contractions (e.g., oxytocin-induced or as a result of abruptio placentae) or low birth canal resistance (e.g., multiparity). Discontinue oxytocin if it is in use. However, there is no current effective treatment, and physical attempts to retard delivery are absolutely contraindicated.

Precipitate labor may cause *maternal amniotic fluid embolism, uterine rupture, cervical lacerations, or lacerations of the birth canal.* There is associated postpartum uterine hypotonicity, with resulting risk of hemorrhage. The perinate is at extraordinary risk from hypoxia (impeded uteroplacental exchange because of the contractions) and perinatal intracranial hemorrhage (direct or indirect trauma). Unattended delivery (direct injury, no resuscitation, chilling) further jeopardizes the newborn.

FETAL DISTRESS

Fetal distress is the infant's critical response to stress, most usually deprivation. It implies that physiologic reserve mechanisms have been exceeded or exhausted and that pathologic changes are occurring or are about to occur that affect vital organ function to the point of temporary or permanent injury or death. The most immediate of fetal needs are (as in the adult) the acquisition of oxygen and the elimination of carbon dioxide. Thus, the metabolic derangements signaling acute fetal distress are hypoxia, hypercarbia, and acidosis.

Usually, asphyxia, or hypoxia, is induced by only three mechanisms: decreased maternal uteroplacental blood flow, decreased maternal oxygenation, and decreased umbilical blood flow. During a moderate asphyxic episode, the fetus can compensate by the diversion of blood flow to the most vital organs, by limiting oxygen consumption over a prolonged interval (e.g., postmaturity), or by shifting to anaerobic metabolism. If the asphyxic stress is severe, prolonged, or becomes more pronounced, these compensatory mechanisms ultimately fail, and fetal distress becomes evident.

Fetal distress also may be chronic, that is, a longer interval of sublethal fetal deprivation that affects growth and development. This may be associated with a reduction of placental perfusion by placental abnormality or by deficient fetal metabolism. Some degree of either acute or chronic fetal distress may exist in up to 20% of all patients.

Chronic Fetal Distress

Reduced placental perfusion results from *maternal conditions,* including *vascular spasm* or *inability to adjust to pregnancy* (e.g., chronic hypertension, pregnancy-induced hypertension, diabetes with pelvic vascular calcification), *inadequate systemic circulation* (e.g., severe maternal heart disease, severe anemia), or *insufficient oxygenation of the blood* (e.g., cyanotic heart disease, long-term pulmonary shunting, residence at high altitude).

Placental causes of chronic fetal distress include *premature placental aging and diabetes mellitus. Fetal causes* of chronic fetal distress include the *postmaturity syndrome, multiple gestation, twin-to-twin transfusion, congenital anomalies, maternal–fetal transfusion,* and *erythroblastosis fetalis.*

Chronic fetal distress is most commonly diagnosed by serial ultrasonic examinations or by testing for fetal well-being. Once diagnosed, chronic fetal distress or deprivation requires very close follow-up.

Treatment is supportive but nonspecific. This consists of correcting the underlying condition(s) if possible, maximizing the fetal opportunity to acquire metabolic substrate (oxygen and glu- cose) by maternal therapy with bedrest, enhanced nutrition and oxygen, elimination of maternal limitations complicating the underlying condition (e.g., infection), and special surveillance during delivery and in the immediate newborn interval (Chapter 8).

Acute Fetal Distress

Acute fetal distress usually is caused by *compromise of the fetal respiratory lifeline* (Table 7-6) and is a *true medical emergency.* If steps are not taken, the fetus will likely die or be severely compromised. Thus, the health care provider must have a clear and orderly plan of treatment.

Most acute fetal distress is detected during labor. Often, EFM

Table 7-6. Representative causes of acute fetal distress

Maternal	Hypotension (e.g., supine hypotensive syndrome)
	Hypoxia or hypercarbia (e.g., maternal aspiration syndrome)
	Impaired respiration (shock-lung, bronchospasm)
	Pregnancy-induced hypertension
	Shock (hemorrhagic, cardiac, septic)
	Sickle cell crisis
Uterine	Hypertonia or polysystole
	Excessive oxytocin
	Uterine rupture
Placental	Abruptio placentae
	Placenta previa
	Premature placental aging
Cord	Prolapse
	Ruptured vasa previa
	Tight or short cord
	True knot
Fetus	Cardiac failure (hydrops fetalis, tachyarrhythmia, myocarditis)
	Congenital anomaly
	Hemorrhage
	Isoimmunization

will reveal decreased placental perfusion with contractions. Most of the criteria for fetal distress are based on EFM information (p. 228).

The treatment of fetal distress (rescue) seeks to restore or maintain uteroplacental–fetal blood flow and acid-base balance. The treatment of fetal distress is straightforward. However, prognosis depends largely on the underlying cause of the fetal distress and current fetal status.

1. *Change maternal position* to relieve pressure on the umbilical cord and improve uterine blood flow, especially from the lateral recumbent position when the uterus impedes blood return via the inferior vena cava.

2. *Correct hypotension.* If change of position fails to correct hypotension, shift the uterus off the great vessels by manual pressure, elevate the legs, apply elastic leg bandages, and administer fluids rapidly IV. Cardiotonics (e.g., ephedrine) may be necessary to restore abdominal pressure.

3. *Decrease uterine activity.* Discontinue oxytocin if in use. Tocolytics, now being tested, have not yet been approved for general use in acute situations.

4. *Hyperoxygenate.* Give 6–7 liters/min of oxygen by mask and guarantee complete maternal oxygenation to enhance maternal–fetal oxygen transfer.

5. *Correct metabolic imbalances.* If the mother is acidotic, administer sodium bicarbonate to correct the imbalance. However, the fetus may respond slowly. Maternal hypoglycemia should respond to hypertonic glucose (50 g IV).

6. *Confirm the diagnosis.* Fetal scalp blood pH sampling should confirm a presumptive diagnosis of acidosis and hypoxia in life-threatening situations.

7. *Alert necessary personnel of the emergency.* Rarely can the obstetrician alone provide the total care necessary for the compromised perinate and mother. Thus, obstetric nursing service, anesthesiology, and the neonatologist or neonatal resuscitation team should be alerted.

8. *Deliver the perinate.* If these steps fail, delivery must be effected to save the perinate. The mode of delivery must be individualized based on the status of labor, imminence of vaginal delivery, and maternal factors.

MECONIUM STAINING OF AMNIOTIC FLUID

See discussion on page 265.

METHODS OF FETAL ASSESSMENT

ULTRASONOGRAPHY

Clinical ultrasound involves high-frequency sound waves produced by applying alternating current to a piezoelectric substance. The transducer is coupled to the patient by a transmitting medium (e.g., mineral oil), and the generated sound waves pass through the soft tissue (ultrasound will not pass through well-mineralized bone) until an interface of different tissue densities is encountered. Part of the sound is then reflected. The transducer broadcasts only a short part of a duty cycle. Most of the time is spent receiving. Thus, the *returning sound is collected and subsequently analyzed.* One or many transducers may be used, and they may be movable or fixed. A number of such devices are available, and a variety of information may be gathered.

The ability to visualize the fetus probably has contributed more than any other advance in the diagnosis and treatment of the fetus as a patient. Examples of useful ultrasonic scannings include very early identification of normal and abnormal gestation (e.g., blighted ovum, ectopic), measurement of fetal growth, estimation of fetal weight, observation of fetal organs (e.g., the heart) and the determination of fetal well-being, identification of multiple gestation, detailing of fetal anomalies, differential comparison of various fetal parts, demonstration of hydramnios or oligohydramnios, visualization of the cord and measurement of cord blood flows, visualization of the placenta (e.g., maturity, placement, size, blood clot, tumors), demonstration of placental aberrations (e.g., hydatidiform mole, molar degeneration, chorioangiomas), visualization of uterine tumors or anomalies, and revelation of cervical abnormalities (e.g., incompetent cervix).

Ultrasound measurements, biparietal diameter (BPD) and fetal length (FL), *are most accurate <20 weeks.* Unfortunately, because of biologic variations, each measurement is less accurate during the latter half of pregnancy. During the third trimester, gestational age can best be derived from a composite of BPD, head circumference (HC), abdominal circumference (AC), and femur length (FL) measurements. Additionally, for the purpose of obtaining accurate fetal data, it is best to obtain serial measurements.

AMNIOCENTESIS

Amniocentesis is the *aspiration of amniotic fluid.* Amniocentesis is useful for antenatal diagnosis, physiologic maturity testing, and the investigation of disorders (e.g., isoimmunization). Amniocentesis is almost always performed transabdominally because of the greater infection risk if performed transvaginally. Occasionally, amniocentesis is used in treatment (e.g., hydramnios).

Perform an ultrasonic scan immediately before amniocentesis for neeedle guidance. The minimal information recorded from the ultrasonic examination should include the number of fetuses, the fetal cardiac activity, the fetal biparietal (and often femur length or abdominal circumference), placental site, and location of the best position for needle placement.

Procedure

Prepare the abdomen with a bactericidal agent and inject a local anesthetic (elective). Use the smallest needle that will adequately remove the sample (usually a 22 gauge), and enter the amniotic cavity for only a short distance. Remove ~15 ml of fluid for diagnostic purposes. Document fetal well-being by ultrasonic scan at the termination of the procedure. Administer *Rh-immune globulin* to the Rh-negative unsensitized patient receiving amniocentesis.

Amniotic fluid normally is clear to slightly yellow-tinged. It may contain flecks of vernix or lanugo hair in later pregnancy. If bloody, maternal blood probably was aspirated. However, RBC do not interfere with fetal cell growth or other analyses. Examine green to greenish brown fluid under the microscope. If particulate matter (meconium) and not old blood (fetal bleeding) is seen, ~50% fetal mortality is likely. *Tobacco brown* amniotic fluid usually is associated with *fetal death,* whereas *light brown, dark red, or wine-colored fluid* is indicative of *intraamniotic hemorrhage* (the color depends on the Hgb content). This is associated with pregnancy loss in ~one third of cases. An *elevation of AFP* in the discolored fluid portends *fetal death, spontaneous abortion,* or *fetal anomaly* (e.g., anencephaly).

With experience, transabdominal amniocentesis under ultrasonographic guidance results in <0.5% complications, using a needle ≤ 20 gauge and only one needle insertion. Complications include maternal bleeding, bruising or hematoma formation, fetal bleeding, possible fetal penetration injury, and infection.

Fetal Heart Rate Monitoring

Observation of the fetal heart rate is the most directly available means of assessing fetal status. Reliable changes in the fetal heart rate are caused by fetal hypoxia and acidosis. Nonetheless, disastrous results have been reported in the presence of a normal fetal heart rate. Thus, to enhance accuracy, the heart rate of the fetus or adult is only one detail that must be evaluated with other available information.

Basal Fetal Heart Rate

Baseline The fetal heart rate (FHR) in early gestation is higher than at term, when it is 120–160 bpm. Gradual slowing amounts to ~20 bpm and occurs linearly throughout the pregnancy. The *baseline or basal FHR is the average rate prevailing apart from beat-to-beat variability and periodic changes.*

Tachycardia Tachycardia occurs when the baseline *FHR >160 bpm lasting for >10 min.* It is further quantified as moderate (160–180 bpm) or severe (>180 bpm) (Table 7-7). Tachycardia may

Table 7-7. Summary of mature fetal heart rate parameters

Feature	Parameters	Interpretation
Baseline heart rate	120–160 bpm	Normal
Tachycardia		
Moderate	161–180 bpm	Nonreassuring
Marked	>180 bpm	Abnormal
Bradycardia		
Moderate	100–119 bpm	Nonreassuring
Marked	>100 bpm	Abnormal
Short-term variability	5–15 bpm	Reassuring
Long-term variability	Present	Reassuring
Periodic changes		
Accelerations	>15 bpm for >15 sec	Well-being
Decelerations		
Early	10–40 bpm	Head compression
Late	5–60 bpm	Hypoxia/acidosis
Variable	10–60 bpm	Cord compression
Combinations		Nonreassuring

result from maternal fever, maternal hyperthroidism, fetal infection, or fetal distress.

Bradycardia Bradycardia is defined as an *FHR <120 bpm*. Moderate bradycardia (100–119 bpm) may be associated with severe fetal distress, whereas severe bradycardia (FHR <100 bpm) is likely to be agonal or due to heart block.

Beat-to-beat variation (short-term variability) There is a beat-to-beat variation of the fetal heart in the mature fetus; that is, the time interval between heartbeats varies slightly. The internal EFM normally records small, rapid, rhythmic fluctuations with an amplitude of 5–15 bpm. This variation is referred to as *beat-to-beat variability* or as *short-term variability*. This is a normal finding in the mature fetus but may not be present in the premature (but normal) fetus, the sleeping fetus, and medicated fetuses (e.g., alphaprodine, atropine, barbiturates, conduction anesthesia, diazepam, general anesthesia, meperidine, morphine, phenothiazines, and magnesium sulfate in large doses). Good FHR short-term variability in the absence of such mitigating factors indicates adequate CNS oxygenation. If normal FHR variability is apparent 5 min before birth, a good Apgar rating is likely irrespective of earlier periodic changes, assuming no congenital anomalies.

When FHR beat-to-beat variability is significantly decreased and cannot be explained by the above factors, *shift the mother to a different position, give her oxygen by mask, and maintain normal blood pressure*. With failure of these measures to improve beat-to-beat variability, fetal assessment by scalp sampling or stimulation tests should be undertaken to further test fetal well-being.

Long-term variability There may be a periodicity to these beat-to-beat alterations (i.e., the short-term variability appears to have a rhythmic reproducible pattern). This is termed *long-term variability*. If present, long-term variability is a sign of well-being but is altered by the same factors affecting short-term variability.

Periodic Changes

The periodic changes are deviations from the baseline in response to fetal stimulation, movements, or uterine contractions. Periodic changes may be of two types, accelerations or decelerations.

Accelerations To be classified as an acceleration, the FHR must increase >15 bpm, and this must last for >15 sec. An acceleration usually evokes a rather smooth pattern when viewed on EFM and is believed to be *a solid indication of fetal well-being*. Moreover, accelerations may be triggered in the normal

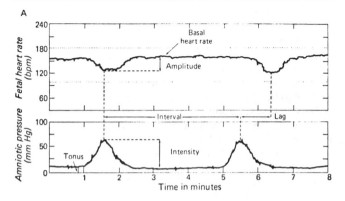

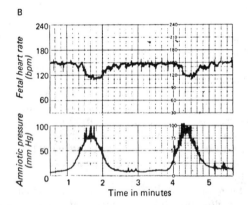

Figure 7-3. Fetal heart rate tracings. A. Schematic tracing. B. Early deceleration. (From S.G. Babson et al., *Management of High-Risk Pregnancy and Intensive Care of the Neonate,* 3rd ed. Mosby, 1975.)

mature fetus by body motion, acoustic stimulation, stimulation of the fetal scalp, and other stimuli.

Decelerations Decelerations (Fig. 7-3) are periodic declines in heart rate (from the baseline), usually in response to uterine contractions. Indeed, on antepartum monitoring, spontaneous deceleration is a very ominous finding and should be viewed with concern. Early and late deceleration patterns are uniform, occurring as exact mirror images (on EFM) of the uterine contractions.

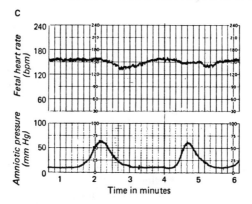

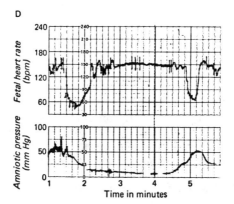

Figure 7-3 (cont.). Fetal heart rate tracings. C. Late deceleration. D. Variable deceleration. (From S.G. Babson et al., *Management of High-Risk Pregnancy and Intensive Care of the Neonate,* 3rd ed. Mosby, 1975.)

With *early decelerations,* the onset of the deceleration occurs with the onset of the contraction, the nadir of the heart rate occurs with the apex of the contraction, and the heart rate increases back to baseline as the contraction ebbs. Early deceleration is caused by compression of the fetal head and is much more common with ruptured membranes. It is a *benign finding,* and no therapy is required. However, if early deceleration patterns are severe, prolonged, persistent, or accompanied by thick meconium staining, the problem may be serious. Therapy includes changing of maternal position (lateral recumbent is best) and ruling out umbilical cord compression (sterile vaginal examination). In some cases, with administration of atropine to the mother the fetus receives enough to block the cause (i.e., vagal stimulation).

Late decelerations appear like early decelerations except with late decelerations, *the pattern occurs later than the contraction;* that is, the onset of FHR deceleration occurs *after* the contraction onset, the nadir of FHR occurs *after* the apex of the contraction, and the FHR deceleration continues *after* the contraction has abated. Late deceleration is most commonly associated with uteroplacental insufficiency and is a consequence of hypoxia and metabolic disorders. *Thus, this is the most ominous fetal heart rate pattern.* In less severe cases, the FHR may transiently exceed the baseline after termination of the deceleration. With severely affected fetuses, the FHR takes longer to return to baseline from the deceleration and does not transiently accelerate. However, in some with severe compromise, the fetus will have a baseline tachycardia.

Significant changes during contractions may be subtle, and the FHR may be within the normal range. Thus, careful interpretation is necessary. This is particularly true for the postdate fetus because the findings of late decelerations are less obvious than at an earlier stage of gestation. Treatment involves decreasing uterine activity (e.g., terminate oxytocin), correcting maternal hypotension, hyperoxygenating, and expanding maternal blood volume. *Should these steps not be immediately effective, deliver the infant.*

Variable decelerations are not uniform and vary widely in configuration. They may begin at any time in relation to the contraction, and often both onset and cessation are marked by sudden changes in the FHR. Variable decelerations may be nonrepetitive and are caused by umbilical cord compression. Decelerations are classified as *severe if they last* >60 sec or lead to an FHR of ≤ 90 bpm. If vaginal examination reveals no palpable cord, maternal positional changes do not resolve the pattern, or the decelerations are severe, do fetal scalp blood sampling if feasible to determine the degree of fetal compromise. In the absence of fetal scalp sampling availability, a high presenting part, or other compromising factors, deliver the infant without delay.

The *most common combined deceleration pattern* is that of *variable and late decelerations.* This is a most ominous pattern and usually consists of variable onset of the pattern, with a late pattern then developing. Nearly all fetuses with this pattern are severely compromised, and *immediate delivery should be consid-*

ered if the simple steps outlined for late decelerations do not cause the pattern to improve.

Methods of Fetal Monitoring

The fetal heart rate may be obtained by manual stethoscope, Doppler ultrasound, direct ultrasonic visualization, phonocardiography, and direct electrocardiography. Direct ultrasonic visualization is not practical for prolonged observation (e.g., during labor), and phonocardiography is much more difficult to achieve than Doppler ultrasonic heart monitoring. Availability of equipment, the physician's experience with the various techniques, and the patient's risk state must determine the method for monitoring.

Stethoscopic Monitoring

Stethoscopic monitoring of fetal heart tones to assess fetal well-being currently is adequate for screening low-risk patients. Ascertain the baseline FHR by careful auscultation between contractions and listen for 30 sec after contractions to determine if there are decelerations from the baseline. This should be performed every 30 min during the first stage of labor. In the second stage auscultation should be accomplished every 15 min and in the delivery room every 10 min. Stethoscopic monitoring is convincingly inadequate in the high-risk cases.

Electronic Fetal Monitoring

Fetal monitors currently available provide either external or internal sensing of the FHR and the associated contraction sequence while creating a permanent record of the data.

External Fetal Monitoring Most external fetal monitors use a *Doppler ultrasound transducer* applied to the mother's abdomen. The transducer detects fetal heart activity and triggers the rate-computing circuitry. A disadvantage of this method is imprecision in detection of beat-to-beat variability. What appears to be normal or increased variability may be artifact because of merging of the ultrasound pickup. However, if the baseline appears smooth when an ultrasound transducer is used, the beat-to-beat variability may be decreased. Direct ECG internal monitoring is the only reliable method of achieving recognition of the beat-to-beat variability (Fig. 7-4).

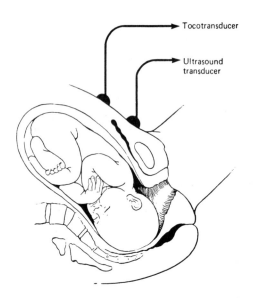

Figure 7-4. External fetal heart rate monitoring. (Redrawn from E.H.G. Hon, *Hospital Practice* 5:91, 1970.)

A *tocotransducer* that responds to changes in pressure transmitted from the uterus to the abdominal wall is used to *monitor uterine activity* externally. Unfortunately, the external monitor does not provide quantitative data regarding the intensity of uterine contractions—only their frequency and duration. Additionally, the input signals often are distorted when the patient moves or if the belt is loosened. Obesity may further reduce the quality of the external FHR recording. Therefore, the abdominal transducer must be readjusted often to ensure good recording. Nonetheless, because external fetal monitoring is noninvasive, it is almost devoid of clinical complications.

Internal Fetal Monitoring Internal fetal heart monitoring (Fig. 7-5) during labor yields data relatively free of artifacts caused by patient movement. However, internal monitoring cannot be used before the cervix is dilated >1 cm and the membranes are ruptured to permit placement of the scalp electrode. The fetal R wave is used by the rate-computing circuit of the internal fetal monitor

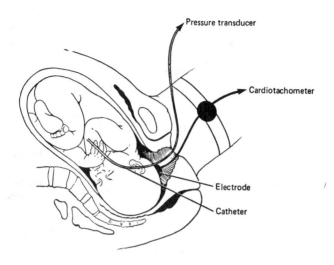

Figure 7-5. Internal fetal heart rate monitoring. (Redrawn from E.H.G. Hon, *Hospital Practice* 5:91, 1970.)

to develop a beat-to-beat recording that accurately depicts baseline irregularity and the widest ranges of the FHR.

When an intrauterine catheter attached to a pressure transducer can be inserted, an accurate record of intrauterine pressure usually can be obtained. Thus, the *intensity of contractions can be determined,* and an abnormal elevation of uterine tone between contractions can be recognized. This information is useful clinically, especially when oxytocin induction or augmentation of labor is considered or when premature separation of the placenta occurs.

There are few clinical problems attributable to internal FHR monitoring. Minor infections can be anticipated in ~1% of cases, but serious fetal scalp infection is rare. Perforation of the uterus or slight placental bleeding with the introduction of the pressure catheter may occur. Amnionitis may develop with prolonged monitoring using an indwelling catheter (>6 h).

It may be difficult to obtain proper pressure readings and ensure subsequent recordings: calibration may not be proper, air bubbles may be present in the line or transducer, pressure leaks or kinks in the catheter system may develop, a valve may be loose, a stopcock may be defective, or a damaged cable or coupling may be the problem. There are few technical problems with the electrode. However, if the internal electrode is applied to the cervix accidentally, the mother's heart rate will be recorded instead of the fetal heart rate.

Retain the entire monitoring strip or representative portions, including abnormal strip recordings, as part of the patient's record.

Most obstetric patients accept fetal monitoring as a part of better perinatal care and insurance against fetal damage or death despite the technology involved.

The *indications for internal fetal monitoring include* advanced maternal age, previous cesarean section, diabetes mellitus, significant cardiac or hypertensive disease, moderate or severe isoimmunization, medical complications of pregnancy, multiple gestation, pregnancy-induced hypertension, moderate or severe anemia, pyelonephritis, uterine bleeding, polyhydramnios, fetal growth retardation or compromise (abnormal clinical or laboratory tests), premature labor, meconium-stained amniotic fluid, postdatism (≥ 42 weeks), abnormal fetal heart rates or patterns obtained by other methods, augmentation of labor, dysfunctional labor, uterine bleeding, and prolonged first or second stage or labor.

Electronic Monitoring Diagnosis of Fetal Distress

During labor, severe FHR variable decelerations, late decelerations, fetal bradycardia, and decreased FHR variability should be viewed as indicative of fetal compromise. Loss of beat-to-beat variability, together with bradycardia, indicate probable asphyxia. The addition of severe variable or late FHR decelerations is further evidence of asphyxia.

FETAL SCALP BLOOD pH DETERMINATIONS

The fetal blood pH is mediated in the short term by respiratory exchange of O_2 and CO_2 (via the placenta). In the long term, pH depends on the concentrations of lactic and pyruvic acids that accumulate because of anaerobic metabolism. Interruption of placental blood flow (e.g., by cord compression) will produce respiratory acidosis. If the interruption is brief, rapid recovery is likely. However, prolonged hypoxia induces anaerobic metabolism, which leads to metabolic acidosis. Then, recovery takes much longer.

Fetal scalp blood pH determinations can be attempted after the cervix is >3 cm dilated, after the membranes are ruptured and the vertex is engaging or engaged in the pelvis. Proper instrumentation must be available, and laboratory capability must be assured. A sterile drape is applied. The fetal scalp is exposed using a conical endoscope. An antiseptic is applied, then silicone gel is spread over the incision site, and a 2 mm puncture is made. *Capillary blood* that beads up on the silicone film *is collected in several* heparinized capillary tubes. The time of collection is recorded, and the specimens are immediately sent to the laboratory for pH determination. Pressure against the puncture site during 1–2 uterine contractions should ensure clotting and prevent fetal bleeding from the incision site. Poor technique or excessive scalp hair may lead to an inadequate blood sample.

Fetal scalp blood sampling should be considered for persistent late decelerations, for persistent severe variable decelerations, when meconium staining of the amniotic fluid is associated with abnormal FHR patterns, for unexplained fetal tachycardia, or with decreased baseline variability.

Interpretation of results:

Normal pH	7.25–7.35
Borderline pH	7.20–7.25
Abnormal (low) pH	<7.20

For decisive action, obtain more than one sample report. A correlation must exist between the FHR monitor pattern and the pH report. Only a fair agreement between the scalp blood pH and the Apgar score can be expected because of other factors, for example, materal hyperventilation, drug effect, slow collection, or amniotic fluid contamination. Nonetheless, *fetal scalp blood pH monitoring will aid in the confirmation or refutation of otherwise difficult to diagnose cases of fetal distress.*

SPECIFIC TESTING FOR FETAL WELL-BEING

EVALUATION OF ABNORMAL ALPHA-FETOPROTEIN (AFP) DETERMINATION

Nearly all AFP is of fetal origin. It is initially produced in the yolk sac, but, by the 13th week, when AFP peaks in both fetal serum and amniotic fluid (AF), it is of hepatic origin. The AFP concentration in the fetal serum is 150 times that in AF. However, some of this protein is excreted in fetal urine, and AFP eventually passes from the amniotic fluid into the maternal serum (levels ~0.1%–1% of that in the fetal serum).

Over 5% of women screened at 16–18 weeks gestation *will have an elevated maternal serum AFP.* Normal levels are highly dependent on length of gestation. Thus, exact knowledge of gestational age is critical. The test is used to screen for open neural tube defects. Nonetheless, *the vast majority of elevations will be false positives* caused by inaccurate gestational dating, multiple gestation, fetal demise, a dying fetus, congenital nephrosis (an autosomal recessive trait), bladder neck obstruction, esophageal or duodenal atresia, exomphalos, sacrococcygeal teratoma, pilonidal sinus, Turner syndrome (45,XO), Potter's syndrome (renal agenesis), fetal blood in amniotic fluid, fetomaternal hemorrhage, abdominal pregnancy, some low-birth-weight fetuses, or many noncentral nervous system structural abnormalities. Therefore, even the false positives may represent serious problems; hence, an evaluation will be necessary to identify the cause of the elevation. However, only 1 in 25 with a single elevated AFP screening study will actually have a neural tube defect. Stated another way, *24 of 25 women with a single elevated AFP value will eventually prove to have a normal fetus.*

The secondary screen generally consists of repeating the maternal AFP determination and performing a detailed ultrasonography (searching for fetal defects and carefully determining the ultrasonic gestational age). This generally will reveal the cause of the initial AFP elevation. However, if the AFP is ≥2.5 times the mean for the gestational age and ultrasonography does not yield a specific diagnosis, further studies will be necessary.

Perform amniocentesis for amniotic fluid AFP, AF acetylcholinesterase, and possibly *for a karyotype.* AF acetylcholinesterase levels (if available) are significantly elevated in open neural tube defects, and it is more specific than AFP.

False negative tests are uncommon, but *low maternal serum AFP* levels require investigation because they may be associated with *genetic abnormalities, especially trisomies.*

ANTENATAL GENETIC DIAGNOSIS

Eliciting genetic information is discussed earlier in this chapter. A complete evaluation of those potentially affected with genetic disorders is beyond the purpose of this text. Nonetheless, we summarize the conditions amenable to prenatal diagnosis and the techniques available for obtaining tissue for analysis.

Conditions Amenable to Antenatal Diagnosis

About 90% of antenatal diagnostic tests are done *to diagnose or rule out chromosomal disorders.* The most common indication for study is advanced maternal age (≥35 years, although ≥32 seems more logical). It is known that with aging, women have a greater chance of having a chromosomally abnormal baby. Although mothers ≥35 have ~6% of all pregnancies, they account for >25% of all neonates with Down syndrome.

Other indications for antenatal diagnosis include a previous offspring with a chromosomal defect, three or more spontaneous abortions, patient or husband with chromosome anomaly (e.g., a parent who is a known translocation carrier), possible X-linked disease (e.g., hemophilia—usually only able to tell sex of offspring), risk of an inborn error of metabolism (e.g., Tay-Sachs), and risk of a neural tube defect. Many other disorders will soon be detectable. Thus, when a specific case is encountered, the *practitioner should consult a center doing antenatal genetic diagnosis* to ascertain testing available for the specific condition, the techniques usually applied, and at what stage of gestation the testing is best accomplished.

Requirements to Provide Antenatal Diagnosis

Antenatal diagnosis is complex and requires experienced personnel: an obstetrician experienced in the techniques, a medical genetics group with biochemical and cytogenetic expertise, a genetic counseling service, and professional referral services.

Antenatal Diagnosis Techniques

The tissue for analysis may be acquired by several routes.

Amniocentesis Amniocentesis is ideally performed at 14–16 weeks, when there is approximately 200 ml of amniotic fluid and many viable cells in the fluid. Although diagnosis of many genetic diseases can be made using chorionic villus sampling, others will require amniocentesis (e.g., anomalies associated with marked elevation of AFP).

Chorionic Villi Sampling Chorionic villi sampling (CVS) offers a newer, earlier approach to the prenatal diagnosis of many genetic disorders. Between 8 and 12 weeks, the fetus is enclosed by the amniotic sac with a space between the thin inner amniotic membrane and the thicker outer chorionic membrane. On the external surface of the chorion are delicate, fernlike villous projections, the *chorion frondosum*. During the late first trimester, these villi are evenly distributed. Later, some of the villi develop into a dense, shaggy concentration that finally attaches to the uterine wall to form the placenta.

To accomplish CVS, insert a thin, soft plaster catheter transcervically into the chorion frondosum under high-resolution linear array ultrasonography, and gently suction portions of the villi for study. The timing is important because, much earlier or later, the risk of complications increases. The recovered 5–8 g of tissue is useful for preliminary direct evaluation, but many chromosomal, DNA, or enzyme studies require fetal cell culture.

The advantages of CVS are that it is feasible at 8–12 weeks gestation, same-day determination of fetal sex and chromosome number is possible, and it avoids membrane puncture. The main disadvantages are that some chromosome morphology is less precise on direct tissue preparation, great care must be taken in preparation or an artificially high incidence of mosaicism may result (i.e., the syncytiotrophoblast must be removed), spontaneous abortion may be more frequent than with amniocentesis, an enhanced number of limb-reduction defects may occur, and serious infections may result.

Direct fetal blood sampling   Some disease states are so problematic and the diagnosis is so important that cordocentesis may be required to sample fetal blood directly. This complicated procedure, although quite safe in experienced hands, is best performed in a limited number of centers.

Tests of Physiologic Maturity

The physiologic maturity of the fetus can be determined by the amniotic fluid lecithin/sphingomyelin ratio (LS ratio), phosphotidylglycerol (Pg) determinations, and other tests for pulmonary surfactant. Creatinine content, bilirubin concentration, and fluid osmolality tests have largely been abandoned.

Rapid Surfactant Test (RST, Bubble Test)   This is a simple, rapid, and reliable technique for predicting fetal lung maturity. Amniotic fluid is centrifuged at 2000 rpm for 15 min, and the supernatant is then drawn off. Two dilutions of supernatant and 95% ethanol are made (1:1 and 1:2). The tubes are capped and

Table 7-8. Correlation of rapid surfactant test (RST) with lecithin/sphingomyelin (LS) ratio

Predicted Fetal Pulmonary Maturity	LS Ratio	RST
Mature	>2	Complete ring of bubbles persists 15 min at 1:1 and 1:2 dilutions
Intermediate	1.5–2	Complete ring of bubbles persists 15 min at 1:1 dilution only
Immature	<1.5	No complete ring of bubbles at either dilution

shaken vigorously for 30 sec and observed for the appearance of bubbles at the surface. The predicted fetal pulmonary maturity has been correlated with the LS ratio as shown in Table 7-8.

Phosphatidylglycerol Test Phosphatidylglycerol (Pg) constitutes about 10% of surfactant phospholipids, and its presence appears to improve the functioning of lung surfactant. Unfortunately double thin-layer chromatography is required for the Pg determination.

NONSTRESS TESTING

The nonstress test is an appraisal of fetal well-being based on the observation that the normal fetus will have characteristic periodic accelerations in the FHR patterns, and the unhealthy fetus will not. Average baseline variability and acceleration of the FHR in response to fetal movement indicate that the fetus is not in jeopardy and has a good reserve. This is assessed by external fetal monitoring without stimuli (stress) to the fetus.

If the fetal CNS is depressed because of hypoxia, acidosis, or drugs, the baseline variability may be reduced and FHR acceleration with fetal movement absent. These patterns may be noted also during fetal sleep. If sleep is likely, the fetus should be stimulated by abdominal palpation.

Major *indications* for nonstress testing *are a history of stillbirth or serious anomaly, drug abuse, possible asphyxia or other circulatory problem* (e.g., meconium-stained amniotic fluid before labor, hemoglobinopathy, Rh isoimmunization), *suspected intrauterine growth retardation, medical complications of pregnancy* (e.g., diabetes mellitus of classes B–H, chronic renal disease, systemic lupus erythematosus), *hypertensive disorders complicating pregnancy, and prolonged pregnancy.*

The first nonstress test is rarely required before the 28th week of pregnancy. The maternal history or status generally indicates the time for the initial test (e.g., about the 32nd week in mild diabetics).

Procedure

1. Place the patient in bed in the semi-Fowler position at ~30 degrees elevation.

2. Record maternal blood pressure on the FHR record every 10 min.

3. Continue the test for 20 min.

a. If the test is reactive (see below), end the test and repeat in 7 days.

b. If nonreactive, continue the test for 20 min more.

c. If the test remains nonreactive, proceed to manual stimulation, acoustic stimulation, administration of food or glucose to the mother or, in the very high risk patient, to the contraction stress test.

Interpretation

The test is reactive if there are ≥2 accelerations of FHR that reach >15 bpm above the baseline and are at least ≥15 sec in duration in a 20 min interval. A nonreactive test does not meet the criteria for the reactive test. If there is no fetal movement, the test is unsatisfactory.

CONTRACTION STRESS TEST

The contraction stress test (CST) is a useful method for determining fetal well-being. It is a stress test based on the fact that uterine contractions decrease uteroplacental blood flow. This transient decrease may be enough to evoke a significant response in the compromised fetus.

Before the onset of labor, *mothers with obstetric problems associated with uteroplacental compromise* (e.g., small-for-dates fetus) are candidates for the CST fetal evaluation. *Contra-indications* include placenta previa and women at high risk for premature labor (e.g., those with incompetent cervix, multiple pregnancy, or ruptured membranes with a premature offspring).

Although prognostication may be difficult, the incidence of perinatal mortality and morbidity is much higher in high-risk patients with a positive CST than in those with a negative CST.

There are two methods of evoking contractions: the nipple (or breast) stimulation and the oxytocin contraction test.

Nipple Stimulation Test

Nipple stimulation, which releases oxytocin in late pregnancy, is used to accomplish the uterine contraction test. Nipple stimulation is effective in about 90% of cases, is noninvasive, and over-dosage is unlikely.

The test is conducted like the oxytocin challenge test with the same end points. There is no standardized nipple stimulation procedure as yet. However, an effective plan requires the gravida to roll one nipple between her fingers for 1 min. (Longer stimulation may evoke exaggerated uterine activity.) After 3 min, if moderate uterine contractions have not ensued, she may manipulate both nipples for 5–10 min. If this is not effective, proceed to an oxytocin challenge test.

The Oxytocin Challenge Test (OCT)

Procedure

The gravida is placed in the semi-Fowler position and slightly on one side. An external FHR monitor (usually Doppler ultrasound) and a uterine activity (toco) monitor are placed on the mother's abdomen. FHR and uterine activity are observed for 10–30 min (baseline). Oxytocin is then administered by controlled IV infusion (IVAC, Harvard pump, or comparable device) at 0.5 mU/min. Oxytocin dosage is increased slowly until at least three contractions develop in a 10 min period. Slow (every 20 min) stepup may be required, but hyperstimulation—contractions at intervals of 2 min or less or contractions over 90 sec in duration—must be avoided, or fetal distress and emergency cesarean section may be necessary. The CST requires 60–90 min to perform. Interpretation depends on strict adherence to the protocol to avoid false positive CSTs.

Interpretation

A positive CST is one in which persistent late deceleration occurs (i.e., a drop in FHR with onset at or beyond the peak of uterine contraction). The minimal degree of deceleration in FHR (bpm) has not been acceptably defined. Some specialists have agreed on 5, and others regard any perceptible deceleration as significant. Nonetheless, decelerations must occur and persist with most contractions.

When the CST is positive, about 10% of fetuses will die within 1 week if undelivered. When the state of the cervix is favorable, a closely monitored labor may be chosen. Before vaginal delivery of any high-risk patient is attempted, place an internal electrode and monitor the patient by direct means during labor.

In most cases, a convincingly positive CST is an indication for prompt cesarean section because 50%–75% of these patients who are allowed to go into labor have late decelerations.

A suspicious or equivocal CST hyperstimulation or an unsatisfactory test cannot be interpreted and must be repeated in 24 h.

A negative CST is temporarily reassuring, but the outcome of any high-risk pregnancy must be guarded. Intrauterine death is unlikely to occur within 7 days with a negative CST. The CST should be repeated in 1 week or less. If labor, unfavorable symptomatology, or serious laboratory indices develop, the need for cesarean section must be assessed.

DAILY FETAL MOVEMENT COUNTING

Frequent movements of the fetus (as perceived by the mother) have been a reassuring sign for centuries. Investigators have reported a marked decrease in fetal movements during fetal distress or just before fetal death. Comparisons of daily fetal movement counts (DFMC) with movement recorded electronically for a 12 h period have revealed that almost 90% of all fetal movements can be identified by the mother. Thus, this simple, cost-effective test can be used as a first screening in complicated pregnancies, as a routine test in normal gestation, or as a supplement to other testing.

Normally, the number of fetal movements decreases late in pregnancy. However, in uteroplacental insufficiency (fetal distress), the frequency of fetal movement decreases markedly, to cease at fetal death. Although the test has not yet been standardized, fewer than 10 fetal movements in a 12 h period probably mandates additional evaluation.

BIOPHYSICAL PROFILE

In high-risk patients, high-resolution dynamic ultrasonography may be used to obtain a fetal biophysical profile (BPP). This is derived from assessment of the following variables: fetal movement, tone, breathing, nonstress test, and approximate amniotic fluid volume. Chronic asphyxia, a common cause of perinatal death with associated diminished fetal movements and oligohydramnios, results in depressed fetal CNS activity. During ultrasound examination (10–30 min), fetal movements are observed and are assigned a score of 2 when normal and 1 when abnormal. When the results of this screening test are markedly abnormal, a 50–100-fold increase in perinatal mortality is likely.

Ideally, this type of testing should be begun in high-risk patients at about 30 weeks gestation and repeated at weekly intervals.

OTHER TESTS OF FETAL WELL-BEING

Estriol determinations have been largely abandoned for fetal assessment.

APPRAISAL OF FETAL HEALTH IN LABOR

1. *Consider pertinent details* in the history, the general physical and obstetric examination, pelvimetry, and fetal heart tones (monitored externally or internally).
2. *Evaluate the character and progress of labor* (e.g., Friedman's curve) and the passage of blood or meconium-stained amniotic fluid.
3. *Identify fetal distress* (i.e., abnormal FHR patterns either direct or indirect), with special concern for bradycardia or late severe variable deceleration, and acidosis in samples of fetal scalp blood.

Chapter 8

The Infant

NEWBORN

The *neonatal,* or newborn, *period* is defined (e.g., for mortality data) as *the first 28 days of life.* Thus, it is a portion of the infant interval that extends from birth through the first year of life. However, there is a greater mortality during the tumultuous neonatal period than in all ensuing life until the eighth decade.

Obviously, the infant's status at birth is affected by its status in utero, especially during stressful labor and delivery. The condition at the moment of birth varies from an active, crying normal newborn, to one who is totally unresponsive and likely to die without immediate resuscitation. Thus, providers of obstetric and newborn care must be prepared (with trained personnel, proper equipment, and necessary medications) to render comprehensive emergency support and care for the newborn.

IMMEDIATE EVALUATION AND CARE AT DELIVERY

Apgar Score

A *rapid evaluation* is mandatory during the first few seconds after birth as the cord is being clamped. *Muscle tone and activity* can be assessed even before delivery of the body is complete. Most infants are slightly blue (color) at birth, but they rapidly turn pink with effective *respiration* save for the distal extremities. Palpating the cord pulsations or auscultating the chest for 15 sec affords a contemporary *heart rate.*

These parameters are combined into a screening assessment of the newborn's immediate adjustment, the Apgar score, recorded at 1 and 5 min after birth. This scoring system provides points between 0 and 2 for each of five categories, including *color, tone, respiratory effort, reflex activity, and heart rate* (Table 8-1). The best possible Apgar score is 10; the lowest score is 0.

Table 8-1. Apgar score of newborn infant

	Score		
	0	1	2
A	Appearance (color)	Blue or pale	Body pink, extremities blue	Completely pink
P	Pulse (heart rate)	Absent	<100	>100
G	Grimace (reflex irritability in response to stimulation of sole of foot)	No response	Grimace	Cry
A	Activity (muscle tone)	Limp	Some flexion of extremities	Active motion
R	Respiration (respiratory effort)	Absent	Slow, irregular	Good, crying

Interpretation of the score often guides immediate therapy: *≥7 is considered normal, 4–6 is compromised, and 0–3 is a medical emergency.* The scores may be recorded every 5 min until a score of 7 or above is reached. Thus, an Apgar score recorded as 1,3,5,8 would be interpreted as 1 at 1 min, 3 at 5 min, 5 at 10 min, and 8 at 15 min.

The Apgar scores are not a good measure of asphyxia or of long-term outcome. Moreover, *certain groups of neonates will not score well,* including the *premature* (when the neonate lacks sufficient neuromuscular development), the *narcotized fetus,* and the *traumatized fetus.* A variety of problems apply to the fetus, including maternal general anesthesia sufficient to anesthetize the fetus. The narcotized newborn may have no tone, no respiratory effort, no reflex activity, and blue color. Nevertheless, he may have a good heartbeat for an Apgar score of 2 with a normal cord pH and no asphyxia. Of course, asphyxia will rapidly ensue if respiratory support is not provided until recovery is sufficient for spontaneous respiration.

Arterial Cord pH

The arterial cord pH is another indicator of status at birth. Normally, arterial cord pH is ≥7.21. A pH <7.00 indicates significant acidosis, although an isolated sample cannot determine if the fetal condition is improving or deteriorating. Nonetheless, an arterial cord blood gas is useful in the high-risk patient, in cases of unexpectedly low Apgar score, in prematures, in the narcotized newborn, in the traumatized newborn, and in uncertain or unexplained situations. Scandinavians use a scoring system at birth that combines the Apgar score and the cord pH for a better indicator of overall status.

Drying, Warming, Positioning, Suctioning, Identification, and Prophylaxis

The wet newborn rapidly chills due to evaporative heat loss. *Rapid gentle drying* with warm towels or blankets under a radiant warmer or a warming surface *minimizes cold stress.* Cold stress can result in hypothermia, hypoglycemia, and respiratory distress. While drying, continue to evaluate responsiveness. If the infant is not breathing (apneic), this tactile stimulation may be sufficient to initiate respiratory effort. Because the infant may be draining fluid from the lungs or gastric contents (vomiting), the *head should be keep flat or somewhat lower than the feet,* and oropharyngeal suction should be applied (gently) as necessary to prevent aspiration. Routinely aspirating gastric contents by oro-gastric or nasogastric tube is contraindicated because the fluid is an important source of glucose immediately after birth.

When the newborn has stabilized, place *identity bands* and administer *prophylactic ophthalmic treatment* against gonorrhea and chlamydia using 1% silver nitrate, erythromycin (0.5%), or tetracycline (1%) ointment. The last two are preferred therapy against chlamydia. The newborn should be kept warm while *bonding with the parents.*

Initial Physical and Laboratory Observations

Next, record the *vital signs* (temperature, respiratory rate, and heart rate), *weigh,* and *measure* (head circumference and length). Do a gestational assessment using either a complete Dubowitz evaluation of neurologic and physical characteristics or a modified Dubowitz (Ballard) examination (Table 8-2).

Evaluate the *appropriateness of growth for gestation* in every newborn by plotting weight, length, and head circumference against norms for gestational age. Morbidity varies significantly within a single weight group depending on maturity. Infants below the 10th percentile in weight for gestation are classified small for gestational age (SGA). SGA is associated with many causative factors, including intrauterine infection, genetic abnormalities, maternal drug ingestion, maternal small stature, multiple gestation, placental insufficiency, and maternal hypertension.

Infants weighing above the 10th percentile for gestation are large for gestational age (LGA). LGA is associated with infants of diabetic mothers, maternal obesity, hydrops fetalis, post-datism, multiparity, advanced maternal age, large maternal stature, and congenital disorders (e.g., Beckwith-Weidemann).

A *physical examination* should be performed by the nursing staff as well as the baby's physician. Administer vitamin K to prevent hemorrhagic disease of the newborn, because vitamin K stores are low at birth and vitamin K in breast milk is minimal. Do a *blood glucose screening for hypoglycemia* (Chemstrips BG are preferable to Dextrostix because they are more accurate in the higher hematocrit range found in newborns), and obtain a *hematocrit* level to determine anemia or polycythemia. If the blood glucose level is low (<45 mg/dl) on the initial screening test, obtain a true blood glucose level and initiate therapy. If the hematocrit is abnormal, undertake appropriate studies.

Vital signs should be continued even if stable and monitored every 4–8 h. A *bath* using mild soap and water is usually given during this period to wash off blood and meconium.

NEWBORN EXAMINATION

Many physical and neurologic findings are recorded as part of the gestational assessment examination and summarized in Table 8-2.

General Appearance

Note the infant's activity, proportions, obvious defects, cry, and respiratory effort.

Skin

Look for skin tags, moles, discolorations, and other defects of skin. The skin will vary in thickness depending on the length of gestation, ranging from very thin and red in the preterm infant to pale and leathery in the postterm infant. Vernix (a whitish fatty coating most evident from 36 to 39 weeks) may be present (before a bath). Perfusion can be assessed by capillary refill (normally <3 sec) after blanching the skin of the extremity or chest by finger pressure. Bruising is not uncommon. Localized petechiae are not unusual (especially on the head and back), but generalized petechiae warrant further investigation. Jaundice is abnormal. Meconium staining may be present, especially around the nails or umbilical cord, but should not be confused with jaundice. Acrocyanosis (blueness of the hands and feet) is normal because of the high hemoglobin levels present. Plethora (ruddy color) may be noted with crying if the baby is polycythemic.

Head

Note the shape of the head (round, elongated, asymmetric), separation or fusion of sutures, presence and size of the anterior and posterior fontanelles, and edema of the scalp (caput succedaneum), which was the presenting part.

Eyes

Check pupil size and shape and look for conjunctival hemorrhage.

Ears

Note auricular size, shape, and placement and determine the presence of an open auditory canal.

Nose

Ascertain that both nares are patent by gently occluding one nostril at a time, and observe for air flow while holding the mouth closed. Note abnormalities in size, shape, septum, philtrum, and nasal bridge.

Mouth and Pharynx

A cleft lip will be obvious if present. Inspect the gums for cysts or neonatal teeth. Check the palate for clefts. A submucous cleft of the palate may not be seen but can be palpated with a finger in the mouth. Note the presence of the uvula and whether it is bifid. A frenulum below the tip of the tongue is not uncommon. Look for symmetric movement of the lips with crying.

Neck

Assess the neck length and check for webbing, cysts, masses, or torticollis.

Chest

Note intercostal or subcostal retractions. Check the spacing of the nipples. Asymmetry of the chest may indicate pneumothorax.

Lungs

Auscultate to evaluate the presence of rales or rhonchi. *Are breath sounds equal?* Diaphragmatic hernia and pneumothorax must be excluded.

Table 8-2. Newborn mature rating and classification: Estimation of gestational age by maturity rating

NEUROMUSCULAR MATURITY

	0	1	2	3	4	5
Posture						
Square Window (Wrist)	90°	60°	45°	30°	0°	
Arm Recoil	180°		100°-180°	90°-100°	< 90°	
Popliteal Angle	180°	160°	130°	110°	90°	< 90°
Scarf Sign						
Heel to Ear						

PHYSICAL MATURITY

	0	1	2	3	4	5
SKIN	gelatinous red, transparent	smooth pink, visible veins	superficial peeling &/or rash, few veins	cracking pale area, rare veins	parchment, deep cracking, no vessels	leathery, cracked, wrinkled
LANUGO	none	abundant	thinning	bald areas	mostly bald	
PLANTAR CREASES	no crease	faint red marks	anterior transverse crease only	creases ant. 2/3	creases cover entire sole	
BREAST	barely percept.	flat areola, no bud	stippled areola, 1–2 mm bud	raised areola, 3–4 mm bud	full areola, 5–10 mm bud	
EAR	pinna flat, stays folded	sl. curved pinna, soft with slow recoil	well-curv. pinna, soft but ready recoil	formed & firm with instant recoil	thick cartilage, ear stiff	
GENITALS Male	scrotum empty, no rugae		testes descending, few rugae	testes down, good rugae	testes pendulous, deep rugae	
GENITALS Female	prominent clitoris & labia minora		majora & minora equally prominent	majora large, minora small	clitoris & minora completely covered	

Table 8-2 (cont.)

Gestation by Dates _____ wks

Birth Date _____ Hour _____ am
                                          pm

APGAR _____ 1 min _____ 5 min

MATURITY RATING

Score	Wks
5	26
10	28
15	30
20	32
25	34
30	36
35	38
40	40
45	42
50	44

SCORING SECTION

	1st Exam=X	2nd Exam=O
Estimating Gest Age by Maturity Rating	_____Weeks	_____Weeks
Time of Exam	Date _____ am Hour _____pm	Date _____ am Hour _____pm
Age at Exam	_____ Hours	_____ Hours
Signature of Examiner	_____ M.D.	_____ M.D.

Scoring system from J.L. Ballard et al., A simplified assessment of gestational age. *Pediatr Res* 11:374, 1977. Adapted from A.Y. Sweet. In: M.H. Klaus and A.A. Fanaroff, eds., *Care of the High-Risk Infant,* 2nd ed. W.B. Saunders Co., 1979.

Heart

Record rate and rhythm as well as presence, timing, and location of murmurs (fully one third of all newborns will have a murmur detected in this transition period). Muffled heart tones suggest pneumomediastinum. Displaced heart tones suggest pneumothorax or diaphragmatic hernia. Palpate brachial and radial pulses for presence and strength. Absent or diminished femoral pulses suggest coarctation of the aorta.

Abdomen

Observe movement with each breath, protuberance, or scaphoid appearance. Palpate for masses or enlargement of the liver, spleen, kidneys, or bladder. Check the umbilical cord for evidence of herniation or infection and the number of vessels, normally three. Anomalies in an infant with a two-vessel cord are increased.

Genitalia

The male penis should be evaluated for length, torsion, hypospadias, or epispadias. The scrotum should contain two testicles of similar size. Asymmetry may indicate a unilateral hydrocele. Bilateral hydrocele is not uncommon, especially with breech position. If the testis is not felt in the scrotum, feel along the inguinal canal for incomplete descent before diagnosing cryptorchidism.

In the female, the relative size of the labia majora and minora should be noted, and vaginal patency should be assessed. Vaginal tags are not unusual, nor is a whitish discharge. Look for introital cysts.

Anus

Check for anal location, patency, and tone.

Hips

Gently assess for range of motion and signs of dislocation.

Clavicles

Palpate the clavicles to ascertain presence, crepitus (fracture), and symmetry.

Extremities

Count the numbers of fingers and toes. Exclude syndactyly (webbing of fingers or toes). Assess the shape, symmetry, and length of each extremity or digit and check range of motion.

Spine

Observe for curvature and evidence of spina bifida or masses.

Central Nervous System (CNS)

Evaluate tone and general activity levels. Is the cry normal? Do all extremities move equally? Birth injury to the brachial plexus may be present in an upper extremity that does not move or has limited movement. Test the Moro reflex. Assess the tonic neck reflex and Babinski reflex. The normal infant makes a stepping motion if the foot is placed on a hard surface. Check the grasp reflex. Test cranial nerve II by observing the newborn fix and follow a bright object 10–12 inches in front of the face for about a 60-degree arc. Suck and swallow tests cranial nerves V,VII,X, XI, and XII. The ocular movement with the doll's eyes maneuver (rotating the infant upright at arm's length in both directions) will evaluate cranial nerves III, IV, VI, and VIII (vestibular only). Testing the auditory portion of VIII requires observation of the infant's response to sound (awakens if asleep, quiets if awake).

Cord Care

The cord may be painted once with triple dye to speed drying and minimize bacterial infection. To help keep the cord dry, apply isopropyl alcohol several times a day until the cord separates (<2 weeks). Erythema or purulence should be evaluated for the possibility of omphalitis.

FEEDING

The initial feeding may occur shortly after delivery. Sterile water or glucose/water has no advantage over milk with regard to chemical pneumonitis if aspiration occurs. If the baby is formula-fed, low-calorie formula or dilute formula often is ordered for the first day because relatively small amounts of colostrum and breast milk are produced for the first 24–48 h. Formula feeding should be offered at least every 3–4 h, but breastfeeding may be more frequent.

VOIDING AND DEFECATION

The newborn will *void within the first 24 h unless an abnormality is present*. The first voiding frequently occurs in the delivery room. Hence, accurate recording then and later should be used to avoid undue concern. The normal newborn will *pass meconium in the first 48 h of life* (~10% before birth). Meconium is the accumulation of bile salts, swallowed lanugo, shed intestinal cells, and intestinal secretions. It is sticky and dark green to black in appearance. With the initiation of feeding, the stool undergoes a transition phase that is partly meconium and partly food residue. Eventually, the stool becomes yellow to green and seedy in appearance. Stool passage may be as infrequent as every other day to as frequent as a small stool with each feeding.

CIRCUMCISION

Circumcision (surgical removal of the penile foreskin) usually is performed by either the pediatrician or the obstetrician. Although circumcision has been practiced for many centuries (for religious reasons), *there is controversy as to the medical value of routine circumcision.* Circumcision should not be performed on infants with bleeding disorders or when penile anomalies are present (e.g., hypospadias), since the foreskin may be needed for reconstructive surgery. Recent reports have suggested that the incidence of urinary tract infection in uncircumcised males is higher than in the circumcised population. The major risks of circumcision are bleeding, infection, and scar formation. The advantages and disadvantages must be discussed with the parents to obtain informed consent for the procedure. Consider the pain involved and offer local anesthesia.

Screening for Metabolic Disorders

All states have screening programs for certain metabolic disorders causing mental retardation that are preventable by diet or medication if begun early enough in life. The most common of these disorders are phenylketonuria and hypothyroidism. However, galactosemia, Tay-Sachs disease, and others are increasing in frequency. Testing for sickle cell disease or trait in the African American population should be routine.

Discharge

On the day of discharge, the *physical examination should be repeated* because some findings not evident on the day of birth (e.g., heart murmurs, cephalhematoma, jaundice) may have appeared. *Routine baby care should be discussed and arrangements made for follow-up care.* Follow-up is especially important with early discharge (often <36 h after delivery). Hypoplastic left heart may only manifest itself after closure of the ductus arteriosus and is rapidly fatal without therapy. Signs of sepsis may not appear before discharge. Thus, *parents must be made aware of the need to seek assistance at the earliest sign of trouble.* The experienced nursery staff will not be present in the home to recognize the danger signals. The *proper use of an infant car seat* must be impressed on the family because a babe in arms is at high risk in a moving vehicle.

Resuscitation

Anticipation is the key to the best possible outcome. A low-risk pregnancy can suddenly change into high risk (e.g., predelivery cord prolapse or postdelivery diaphragmatic hernia). Resuscitative equipment and personnel trained in resuscitation should be present. Ideally there should be three people, one to manage the airway, another to assess the cardiac function, and another to provide necessary drugs and equipment and record the time and the procedures performed. Rapid drying and a radiant heat source are essential to minimize hypothermia during resuscitation.

  Newborn resuscitation follows the same ABCs applied to resuscitation of the adult.

Airway

A patent airway is essential. Because the newborn frequently has mucus or meconium in the oropharynx, use suction devices to aspirate mucus or meconium from the oropharynx. Bulb suction can clear the oropharynx, but a suction catheter or endotracheal tube connected to suction will be required to clear the trachea. Because of the risk of AIDS, avoid mouth-to-mouth and mouth-to-endotracheal tube suction unless there is no other option available (e.g., home delivery). *Provide a source of oxygen* (FIO_2 1.0) *once the airway is clear if the infant is cyanotic.* When spontaneous breathing is well established with good color, maintain oxygen therapy until the infant is stable. The risk of oxygen toxicity in a term infant after a brief period is negligible. However, it is better to give too much rather than too little oxygen because the infant may be acidotic and at high risk for persistent pulmonary hypertension. A preterm infant often requires an oxygen saturation monitor. This is easily applied to an extremity, with adjustment of the oxygen level saturation between 90% and 95%.

Breathing

Mask and Bag

If the infant is not breathing spontaneously but has an Apgar score of ≥4, gentle stimulation with drying and warmth may initiate respirations. Without response, begin assisted ventilation by bag and mask using 100% oxygen (FIO_2 1.0). A self-inflating bag should have a reservoir or rebreathing device, or only about 40% oxygen ($FIO_2 \sim 0.40$) will be available to the infant. Check the FIO_2 setting if the gas source is attached to a blender and adjust to 1.0.

The *mask should be the proper size for the baby* (preterm and term sizes are available). Adjust the mask so that it is snug to avoid air leaks. Be careful not to inadvertently press the top of the mask against the eyes. The newborn tongue is relatively large, so *lift the mandible toward the mask by fingers at the angle of the jaw rather than pressing the mask down on the face.*

A few breaths may be necessary to inflate the lungs and initiate spontaneous respiration. Watch the infant closely, and auscultate the chest to ensure adequate air exchange whether respiration is spontaneous or assisted. Continue bag and mask resuscitation at ~40 breaths/min. If the infant is not receiving adequate ventilation via bag and mask, use endotracheal intubation.

Endotracheal Tube

If the infant has an Apgar score of ≥3 without spontaneous respiratory effort, or if respiration is insufficient with bag and mask resuscitation, accomplish endotracheal intubation. Multiple attempts at intubation by the unskilled can do more harm than good (e.g., perforation of the hypopharynx, trachea or esophagus, prolonged hypoxemia as attempts are made, intubation of the esophagus). *This is a skill that any provider delivering babies must have acquired.*

The endotracheal tube size should be determined by the infant's size and weight. A 3.5-mm internal diameter tube is sufficient for most term infants to allow adequate clearing. A 2.5-mm tube is the smallest that should be used and should be able to accommodate infants up to 1250 g. Between 1250 and 2500 g, a 3.0-mm tube should be adequate. If a tube is too small, the work of breathing will be increased and air can leak around it (cuffed endotracheal tubes are never to be used in newborns). If the endotracheal tube is too large and is forced into the trachea, damage and stenosis may follow.

Do not insert the endotracheal tube too far into the airway. To prevent this, estimate the depth of insertion based on the infant's weight. Use only endotracheal tubes with markings in centimeters. The tip of the tube to the lip edge should be remembered as the rule of 1-2-3-4 and 7-8-9-10. For a 1 kg infant, the tip to lip distance should be 7 cm. For 2 kg, the tip to lip distance should be 8 cm. For 3 kg, it should be 9 cm, and for 4 kg, 10 cm. For weights in between, estimate the distance (e.g., 7.5 cm for 1500 g). Always auscultate for equal air exchange and air leaks after insertion before taping the tube in place. Another method of endotracheal tube location can be applied by feeling in the suprasternal notch as the tube is inserted. Stop advancement of the tube just after the tip passes the examining finger. *X-ray confirmation of tube location will be necessary later if the endotracheal tube remains in place.*

Frequently, the infant will become vigorous, with good respiratory effort, after several minutes of assisted ventilation, and the endotracheal tube can be removed. Observe for recurrence of respiratory distress or cyanosis. Insert an *orogastric* or *nasogastric tube* to allow decompression of the stomach from insufflated gas.

Cardiac

Assessment of heart rate should be performed by both *auscultation of the chest and palpation of brachial pulse.* Feeling the cord for pulsations immediately after birth may be helpful in determining heart rate. Bradycardia (<90 bpm) usually responds rapidly to the administration of oxygen and assisted ventilation. If heart rate persists at 60 bpm or less despite respiratory support, cardiac resuscitation should be initiated. The sternum should be depressed using finger pressure over the middle of the sternum (not the lower one third) 1–1.5 cm. The overlapping thumbs may be used with the hands encircling the chest or the index and third fingers pressing simultaneously at a rate of 100–120 bpm. Assisted ventilation should be continued with periodic auscultation to ensure adequate air exchange and heart rate.

If the infant does not respond, administer IV glucose and alkali (do not mix together because of hyperosmolality). Glucose is a necessary energy source for the cardiac muscle and brain. Glucose levels may fall precipitously if anaerobic glycolysis is occurring. With this process, lactic acid levels build rapidly in the blood, and cardiac response is decreased. *Give 2 ml/kg of 10% glucose solution if Chemstrip BG is low or glucose screening is not readily available.* Sodium bicarbonate is the preferred alkali source in this situation, but its osmolality (~1400) requires dilution of the standard stock solution (1 mEq/ml) with water to minimize rapid shifts in blood osmolarity. Avoid overcorrection of the acidosis. Rapid calculation of the dose to be administered pending blood gas analysis is 1–2 mEq/kg administered no faster than 1 mEq/kg/min. Because sodium bicarbonate is caustic if extravasated, administration into a large peripheral vein, the umbilical artery, or an umbilical venous catheter positioned above the diaphragm (to avoid hepatic necrosis) is recommended.

While intravascular access is being attempted, *epinephrine can be absorbed via the trachea using the endotracheal tube* in a dose of 0.1 ml/kg of a 1:10,000 solution. Since epinephrine is less effective in an acidotic environment, repeat the dose intravascularly after the bicarbonate has been administered if bradycardia persists.

Once an adequate heart rate has been established, discontinue cardiac massage and observe for adequate pulses and assess blood pressure. If the infant is hypotensive, expand the blood volume with Plasmanate or normal saline 10 ml/kg over 30–60 min. Blood products may be necessary if the cause of the infant's distress is blood loss. Pressor agents, such as dopamine (1–4 μg/kg/min to promote renal blood flow) and dobutamine (5–20 μg/kg/min) may be necessary as a continuous IV drip once in the nursery to maintain adequate blood pressure.

PROBLEMS ASSOCIATED WITH PREMATURITY

RESPIRATORY DISTRESS SYNDROME (RDS)

Respiratory distress syndrome (also called hyaline membrane disease) *is the most common cause of mortality and morbidity in the nonanomalous preterm infant.* The incidence is directly related to gestational age—the more preterm the infant, the greater the risk ($\sim 60\%$ at 30 weeks, 20% at 34 weeks). Term infants can develop RDS, but this is uncommon, except perhaps in infants of diabetic mothers (IDM), where the overall incidence of RDS is two to three times higher than in infants of nondiabetic mothers.

The pathophysiology of RDS is a vicious cycle of *decreased alveolar surfactant leading to increased alveolar surface tension, resulting in generalized atelectasis.* This atelectasis causes both hypoventilation and uneven ventilation–perfusion, which in turn cause CO_2 retention and hypoxemia. These in turn cause acidosis and subsequent capillary endothelial damage. Capillary damage results in leakage of plasma proteins and fibrin, which produce a diffusion gradient, further increasing CO_2 retention, hypoxemia, and acidosis, which in turn reduce surfactant synthesis, storage, and release. If this cycle cannot be broken, the patient dies. If hypoxemia and acidosis can be brought under control, the alveolar cells have the opportunity to recover sufficiently to produce and release surfactant, thereby reducing atelectasis and allowing better ventilation and perfusion.

RDS is exacerbated by predelivery or postdelivery asphyxia, acidosis, or hypothermia. Assess pulmonary maturity antenatally by determining the lecithin/sphingomyelin (LS) ratio of amniotic fluid or the presence or absence of phosphatidyl glycerol (Pg). *The incidence of RDS is decreased in infants experiencing certain types of stress* (e.g., IUGR, prolonged rupture of the membranes, maternal hypertension). RDS (both amount and severity) may also be decreased by administration of glucocorticoid to the mother at least 24–48 h before delivery at 28–32 weeks gestation when preterm delivery is anticipated. RDS is now being *prevented or treated postdelivery by synthetic or bovine surfactant administered into the trachea.*

RDS may be present at birth or within the first 4–6 h of life. Consider other causes if respiratory distress begins thereafter. The infant will have any combination of tachypnea (RR >60), retractions (substernal, intercostal), nasal flaring, grunting respirations, or cyanosis. The chest x-ray shows intermediate expansion of the chest with a reticulogranular (ground glass) appearance and air bronchograms. The blood gases show progressive acidosis (predominantly respiratory) with hypoxemia and hypercarbia.

Assisted ventilation frequently is necessary to assure adequate oxygenation and gas exchange. Reduce the $Paco_2$ to a normal or near normal range to correct acidosis, maintain a neutral thermal environment, and provide appropriate IV glucose to maintain adequate blood sugar levels and to provide some caloric intake. Avoid fluid overload, which may contribute to significant PDA.

PULMONARY AIR LEAK

Microscopic tears in the airway/alveolar lining allow air to pass along the vascular sheath, into the interstitium or the pleural space. The location of the free air determines its designation as *pneumothorax, pneumomediastinum, pulmonary interstitial emphysema, pneumopericardium, or pneumoperitoneum.* The incidence is ~1% of all live births. Air leak is not limited to preterm infants. Not all infants with pulmonary air leak will be symptomatic. About 25% of infants with RDS develop an air leak syndrome, and up to 50% of infants with meconium aspiration syndrome will suffer an air leak.

Suspect air leak in any newborn with respiratory distress, especially after resuscitation, and in infants on ventilators with deterioration or with muffled heart tones.

The *diagnosis of air leak is made by chest x-ray,* and both anteroposterior (AP) and lateral views are necessary initially to determine location and size. Thereafter, an AP view will be sufficient in most cases for follow-up.

Transillumination of the chest also can be used to diagnose pulmonary air leak, but it requires a dark room. The area of free air shows greater transmission of light around the light source than does the unaffected side. If air leak is diagnosed, request neonatal consultation.

PATENT DUCTUS ARTERIOSUS (PDA)

The ductus arteriosus (between the aorta and pulmonary artery) is necessarily patent in utero to allow circulatory bypass of the lungs, but the ductus closes rapidly after the first breath in a vasoconstrictive response to increased Pao_2. This response is mediated by prostaglandin. *Final closure may take 1–8 days in the term infant,* but in the preterm, this process may take weeks. As many as 75% of preterm infants <1000 g have a clinically evident PDA.

PDA may cause a range of problems from an asymptomatic intermittent murmur at the left upper sternal border to florid congestive heart failure. Obtain pediatric cardiology consultation.

INTRACRANIAL HEMORRHAGE

Four relatively common types of intracranial hemorrhage are recognized: *subarachnoid, subependymal germinal matrix/intraventricular (SEH/IVH), subdural, and cerebellar.*

Fetal intracranial hemorrhage occurs, but most significant hemorrhages occur after birth in the preterm infant, although term infants are not immune.

Subarachnoid Hemorrhage

Subarachnoid hemorrhage is the *most common hemorrhage in newborns* (presumably either due to trauma involving molding of the head for delivery or related to asphyxia). Most do not result in significant bleeding, and the infant is asymptomatic. A lumbar puncture may reveal RBCs. Cranial ultrasonography or CT scan will eliminate or elucidate other origins of the bleeding.

Subependymal Germinal Matrix/Intraventricular (SEH/IVH)

Because the germinal matrix (a highly vascularized area adjacent to the ventricular area of the brain) is present until ~35 weeks gestation, intraventricular and periventricular hemorrhage are common (20%–40%) in preterm infants. Ultrasonography or CT scan should provide the diagnosis.

Because the germinal matrix is most prominent at the head of the caudate nucleus at the level of the foramen of Monro, this is the site of most hemorrhages. Bleeding limited to the subependymal area of the germinal matrix is termed subependymal hemorrhage (SEH). When the bleeding ruptures through the germinal matrix and into the ventricular system, it is called intraventricular hemorrhage (IVH). IVH is mild when there is no ventricular dilation. It becomes moderate when the ventricle(s) dilate and severe when the hemorrhage extends into the parenchyma of the brain. The latter two gradations are associated with increased incidence of morbidity and mortality. *Many will develop post-hemorrhagic hydrocephalus within 2–3 weeks of the original hemorrhage.* Some cases of hydrocephalus will resolve spontaneously, whereas others will require drainage procedure(s). Developmental delay or neurologic deficits or both will be present in as many as two thirds of the infants with moderate to severe IVH.

Subdural Hemorrhage

Subdural hemorrhage occurs with trauma when there is excessive molding of the head and sudden tearing of the superficial veins over the cerebral cortex or the venous sinuses of the posterior fossa during delivery of the head. The usual circumstances are *precipitous labor and delivery in a primigravida, high or mid-forceps delivery, or an LGA baby. If hemorrhage occurs in the cerebellar fossa, death occurs rapidly* due to compression of brainstem. When the hemorrhage occurs over the cerebral hemispheres, the early symptomatology may be anemia, unexplained jaundice, seizures, or other signs of increasing intracranial pressure (bulging fontanel, altered states of consciousness). Later signs (4–6 weeks) may include increasing head circumference, failure to thrive, or vomiting. CT scan is better than ultrasonography in defining the exact location, quantity of blood, and extent of hemorrhage.

Cerebellar Hemorrhage

Cerebellar hemorrhage *most commonly occurs in the preterm infant concomitant with asphyxia or trauma.* Such hemorrhage frequently results in a progressive downhill course to death. Symptoms in those with nonlethal hemorrhage are apnea, high-pitched cry, hypotonia, vomiting, absent Moro reflex, and rapidly increasing head circumference. Although cerebellar hemorrhage can be diagnosed by cranial ultrasonography, CT scan may give better delineation.

RETINOPATHY OF PREMATURITY (ROP)

Formerly known as retrolental fibroplasia, ROP is a *disorder of the immature retinal vascular system.* The retinal vessels are incompletely developed until about 34–36 weeks gestation, with the temporal area the last site to mature. *The more preterm the infant, the greater the risk of developing ROP.*

Vasoconstriction of the retinal arteries occurs in response to increased arterial oxygen tension (Pao_2), similar to the vasoconstriction of the ductus arteriosus after birth in response to the sudden increase in Pao_2. This vasoconstriction may be a protective response and cause no harm to fully developed retinas, but localized hypoperfusion and hypoxemia in the incompletely vascularized retina stimulate proliferation of new vessel formation (neovascularization) in an attempt to supply the underperfused areas. The subsequent hemorrhage(s) into the vitreous and retina causes fibrous proliferation, scar retraction, and in the worst case, retinal detachment and blindness.

Hyperoxemia can occur in infants breathing room air. Thus ROP has been reported in preterm infants who have never received supplemental oxygen. Likewise Fio_2 1.0 is not necessarily harmful to the retina if normoxemia is maintained. Because of fluctuating Pao_2 despite constant Fio_2 delivery, *continuous monitoring of blood oxygen is a necessity in small preterm infants.*

APNEA

Apnea in the newborn is *cessation of respiration for 15 sec, frequently accompanied by cyanosis or bradycardia.* Respiratory irregularity is common in preterm infants due to immaturity. Practically all preterm infants <34 weeks will have apnea at some point. Before deciding that apnea is secondary to immaturity of the neonatal respiratory control centers, other causes must be investigated and treated if present. These include drugs, both maternal (e.g., magnesium, narcotics) and neonatal (e.g., narcotics, Prostin), infections (e.g., sepsis, meningitis, NEC), metabolic disturbances (e.g., hypoglycemia, hyponatremia, hypocalcemia), CNS abnormalities (e.g., seizures, intracranial hemorrhage), temperature abnormalities (e.g., hypothermia or hyperthermia), decreased oxygenation (e.g., hypoxemia, anemia, left to right shunt from PDA). *Apnea may be obstructive* (chest wall moves with respiratory effort but no nasal air flow occurs), *central* (CNS) in origin, or *mixed* (a combination of the two).

Treatment of apnea of prematurity consists of multiple modalities ranging from stimulation for infrequent episodes, changing position (may be helpful in obstructive apnea), methylxanthines (theophylline, caffeine) for recurrent apnea, to nasal CPAP or assisted ventilation for intractable apnea.

BONDING/SEPARATION ANXIETY

Parents are frequently and legitimately concerned about bonding with their sick or preterm infant. With more liberal visiting and handling policies of current NICUs, visiting is more often a problem when the mother and baby are in different locations (hospital, city, or state) or have transportation problems. This is one advantage of maternal transport for delivery rather than neonatal transport after birth.

Nursing personnel can be a tremendous asset in helping parents cope with the stresses associated with prematurity. Recording the *frequency and length of parental visits* (or lack thereof) and *parental response* (e.g., talking to the baby, making eye contact) is the first step in recognizing a problem and finding resources to solve it. Weekly letters and Polaroid pictures sent to the parents can help. *Parent support groups* can also relieve some anxiety. *NICU social workers* are available in most centers and can be invaluable in helping parents deal with financial worries and so on. Since the typical weight at discharge has decreased to the 4 to $4\frac{1}{2}$ pound range, more and more NICUs are providing facilities for the *parents to room in with the baby* 1 or 2 nights before discharge to allow a better transition from hospital to home and assure competence and confidence in handling the preterm infant, giving medication, and similar activities.

INFECTION

Because the immune system is incompletely developed in the newborn, *infection is one of the more common causes of morbidity and mortality.* Mortality is higher in the preterm than in the term infant. Sepsis and pneumonitis predominate in the first few days of life. Meningitis and urinary tract infection become more frequent after the first week.

Many infants are born prematurely because of chorioamnionitis and are infected before or at birth. *Determining the offending organism* in the neonate *can be difficult* for several reasons: only a small blood sample is available for culture (1 ml or less), the organism may be bacterial (aerobic or anaerobic), fungal, or viral, and skin contaminants are relatively common because of difficulty in obtaining free-flowing blood.

Laboratory findings associated with neonatal infection include leukocytosis (WBC >30,000), leukopenia (WBC <5000), increased immature neutrophils (left shift, immature: total neutrophils >0.2), thrombocytopenia (platelets <100,000), metabolic acidosis, and increased WBC in CSF (>30). *Chest radiographs* may show pneumonitis, and *gram stain* of the tracheal aspirate may reveal organisms. Culture and gram stain of the gastric contents immediately after birth may indicate the presence of amnionitis but not necessarily neonatal infection. Since group B beta-hemolytic streptococcus is the most common neonatal bacterium causing infection, *latex agglutination testing* of blood, urine, and CSF can be helpful, especially if cultures are negative.

Treatment consists of broad-spectrum antibiotics until the offending organism can be isolated and antibiotic sensitivity can be determined.

PROBLEMS ASSOCIATED WITH THE TERM INFANT

TRANSIENT TACHYPNEA OF THE NEWBORN (TTN)

TTN may result from delayed clearing of pulmonary fluid. It is not an aspiration syndrome. Pulmonary fluid is produced by the lungs and has a different protein and electrolyte content from amniotic fluid. TTN occurs more frequently after cesarean delivery without labor, presumably because the onset of labor terminates production of pulmonary fluid, and fluid is more effectively squeezed out of the lungs when the chest is compressed passing through the birth canal. The respirations usually are 80–120 per min, usually without grunting. The tachypnea is present shortly after birth. Cyanosis will be present if the spontaneous hyperventilation is inadequate to maintain oxygenation. Blood gases in room air usually show normal pH and $Paco_2$ (CO_2 diffuses 20 times faster than O_2), with low to normal Pao_2. The chest x-ray shows good chest expansion with some haziness and, frequently, fluid in the interlobar fissures (seen best between RUL and RML).

TTN is usually self-limiting and generally resolves in <36 h. *Maintain adequate oxygenation,* usually by oxyhood until the fluid can resorb spontaneously. Assisted ventilation is rarely necessary, and mortality is unusual.

HYPERBILIRUBINEMIA

Jaundice (icterus, yellow skin) *is present in ~50% of all newborns.* Unconjugated hyperbilirubinemia (level >1.0–1.5 mg/dl) is present in almost all. It is important to distinguish between physiologic and pathologic hyperbilirubinemia to provide appropriate therapy.

Bilirubin is produced primarily as the breakdown product of heme from RBCs. Free bilirubin rapidly binds with albumin and is transported to the liver, where it is conjugated with glucuronic acid to form a water-soluble product for excretion in bile. Once in the intestine, the bilirubin becomes unconjugated and may be reabsorbed via the portal system, converted to urobilinogen, and excreted via the kidneys or excreted in stool.

The *two forms of bilirubin* that are of clinical significance in the newborn are the *unconjugated fraction* (indirect reaction, fat-soluble, commonly elevated) and the *conjugated fraction* (direct reaction, water-soluble, less commonly elevated). Physiologic elevation of unconjugated bilirubin is a combination of increased production (e.g., naturally shorter life span of fetal RBCs, bruising) and decreased excretion (e.g., increased enteric resorption of bilirubin, decreased activity of hepatic glucuronyl transferase).

Physiologic hyperbilirubinemia may be as high as *12 mg/dl in term infants* (mean peak at 3 days) and *14 mg/dl in preterm infants,* with a later mean peak (5 days). Note that a physiologic level does not exclude the risk of harmful effects (especially in the premature). *Elevated conjugated bilirubin* (level >1.5–2 mg/dl) is *never physiologic.* Causes include primary hepatitis (e.g., viral, bacterial, protozoal, idiopathic), toxic hepatitis (e.g., drugs, necrosis, sepsis, parenteral alimentation), metabolic disorders (e.g., galactosemia, alpha$_1$-antitrypsin deficiency, cystic fibrosis, Gaucher's disease), and ductal disturbances (e.g., biliary atresia, choledochal cyst).

Pathologic causes of unconjugated hyperbilirubinemia secondary to increased production include *isoimmunization* (Rh, ABO, and other blood group incompatibilities), *RBC biochemical defects* (e.g., G6PD deficiency, pyruvate kinase deficiency), *infection* (bacterial, viral, fungal), and *blood sequestration* (e.g., cephalhematoma, IVH, bruising, abdominal hemorrhage). *Pathologic causes of decreased excretion* include *conjugation defects* (e.g., Crigler-Najjar, type II glucuronyl transferase deficiency, breast milk jaundice) and *increased reabsorption* (e.g., intestinal obstruction, gastrointestinal hemorrhage). Unconjugated hyperbilirubinemia of *undetermined etiology* may be seen in infants of diabetic mothers and hypothyroidism.

Bilirubin encephalopathy results from cytotoxic effects of unconjugated bilirubin on neurons (especially basal ganglia, hippocampal cortex, and subthalamic nuclei). Severe disease progresses from lethargy and hypotonia to rigidity, opisthotonos, high-pitched cry, fever, and seizures ending in death in 50%. The survivors have residual choreoathetoid cerebral palsy, hearing deficits, paralysis of downward gaze, and occasionally mental retardation. Infants having sequelae of subclinical disease are categorized as having minimal brain dysfunction. Conditions that increase the risk of bilirubin encephalopathy are prematurity, hypoxia, sepsis, acidosis, hypoglycemia, rapid hemolysis, drugs that compete for bilirubin binding sites (e.g., sulfonamides), and low albumin states.

Appropriate initial *laboratory studies* include both *total and direct bilirubin levels, CBC with platelet count, blood type, and Coombs' test*. Further studies are indicated depending on results and clinical findings.

Treatment is intended to decrease the unconjugated bilirubin level before damage can occur and to eliminate the cause if possible. The recommended maximum tolerance of total bilirubin levels ranges from 10 to 20 mg/dl depending on birth weight, gestational age, associated risk factors, and etiology of hyperbilirubinemia. There is some suggestion that breast milk jaundice is better tolerated, and higher levels may not be harmful.

Double volume exchange transfusion is the most rapid and effective method to decrease bilirubin levels (usually ~50%) but carries the risk inherent in simple blood transfusion as well as hypoglycemia, sepsis, acidosis, platelet washout, arrhythmia, and death. The most frequent treatment is phototherapy, which uses wavelengths in the blue spectrum to photoisomerize bilirubin to allow excretion without conjugation. The eyes must be shielded, and increased water loss from the skin and gastrointestinal tract (diarrhea is a common side effect) necessitates adequate fluid intake. Phototherapy is contraindicated in direct hyperbilirubinemia. Phenobarbital stimulates protein synthesis and hepatic enzyme production and can decrease both direct and indirect bilirubin levels over a period of 24–48 h and may be helpful when phototherapy is not indicated.

PROBLEMS ASSOCIATED WITH THE POSTTERM INFANT

MECONIUM ASPIRATION SYNDROME WITH PERSISTENT PULMONARY HYPERTENSION

Postterm infants have the *highest incidence of meconium passage in utero*. They also are at greater risk of asphyxia during labor and delivery as a result of progressive uteroplacental insufficiency.

Pathophysiology

When asphyxia occurs, the postterm fetus may gasp and swallow meconium (often very thick from the large volume passed and lower amniotic fluid available for mixture), filling both the airway and stomach. With the first breath after birth, the meconium is inhaled further into the small airways and subsequent breaths (spontaneous or with resuscitative efforts) may cause pulmonary air leak (from the ballvalve effect of the meconium obstructing the airway on exhalation), further compromising ventilation, perfusion, and oxygenation. The meconium causes a chemical pneumonitis. *The resultant respiratory distress may persist for 7–10 days.*

Because these infants are frequently acidotic and hypoxemic, vasodilation of the pulmonary arteries is inhibited, resulting in *persistent pulmonary hypertension of the newborn (PPHN)*, formerly called persistent fetal circulation (PFC). PPHN is responsible for a vicious cycle in which the lungs receive insufficient cardiac output to properly oxygenate the systemic circuit. High pulmonary artery pressure causes right to left shunting of blood across the patent foramen ovale or PDA where pressures are lower. Continued hypoxemia or acidosis results in further vasoconstriction of the pulmonary circuit and even less pulmonary blood flow. PPHN may also be associated with RDS, hypoglycemia, sepsis, or hyperviscosity or may be idiopathic in origin.

Chest x-ray may reveal coarse infiltrates more on the right than left due to the takeoff position of the left mainstem bronchus. Pulmonary air leak should be evaluated and treated if present.

Treatment

The best treatment of meconium aspiration is prevention. Suctioning the nasopharynx and oropharynx (trachea in skilled hands) before delivery of the body can be extremely helpful. Tracheal suctioning need not be performed in every meconium-stained baby but should be performed in cases of thick (pea soup) meconium, depression, or respiratory distress at birth. A 14 F suction catheter has the same external diameter as a 3.5 mm endotracheal tube and is large enough to remove most particulate meconium.

Meconium regurgitated into the oropharynx from a stomach overdistended by bag and mask ventilation often is aspirated.

Thus, this is one instance where emptying the gastric contents can be beneficial.

Antibiotic therapy is indicated in the patient with residual respiratory distress or infiltrate on chest x-ray for two reasons. Sepsis may have been the precipitating factor in meconium passage in utero, and meconium is a good culture medium.

PERINATAL ASPHYXIA

Although asphyxia may occur without regard to gestational age, the *incidence is higher in preterm and postterm infants than in term infants.* Factors associated with increased risk for asphyxia include

1. Sudden disruption of fetoplacental exchange (e.g., cord prolapse, placental abruption, bleeding placenta previa, nuchal cord)

2. Chronic decreased fetoplacental exchange (e.g., postmaturity, IUGR)

3. Decreased maternal/placental blood flow (e.g., hypotension, hypertension, uterine tetany)

4. Decreased maternal oxygenation (e.g., cardiopulmonary disease, hypoventilation, hypoxia)

5. Delayed or improper resuscitation

Physical damage varies with gestational age. The periventricular area and subependymal germinal matrix are more susceptible in the preterm infant. In the term newborn, the typically affected areas are the cortical and CNS subcortical gray matter. Damage to the latter results in hypoxic ischemic encephalopathy (HIE). The most severe degree of asphyxia results in brain necrosis (if survival is more than 24 h postinsult) and death. During the asphyxial episode, all organs of the body are exposed (some more than others due to redistribution of blood flow to the vital organs). Renal failure or cardiac failure, or both, postasphyxia indicate significant insult and of themselves may cause further CNS damage, impede recovery, or cause death.

Signs of CNS dysfunction include an altered state of consciousness, poor sucking, poor feeding, respiratory pattern abnormalities (including apnea), seizure activity, abnormal pupillary response, decreased oculovestibular response, and a tight or bulging fontanel. When it occurs, *seizure activity usually begins 12–24 h after birth, but it can occur as early as 2–6 h.* When status epilepticus or serial seizures persist for over 24 h, the risk of death or sequelae is highest, but not without exception. Seizures should be treated promptly, and efforts should be made to maintain adequate glucose levels and oxygenation, since apnea frequently accompanies seizure activity. The two signs most predictive of long-term sequelae are duration of seizure activity and altered states of consciousness.

Chapter 9

The Puerperium

The puerperium, arbitrarily designated as the *6 weeks following childbirth,* is the period of adjustment after pregnancy, when lactation is possible and the mother's body returns to the non-pregnant state.

PHYSIOLOGIC EVENTS OF THE PUERPERIUM

CARDIOVASCULAR AND BLOOD

Cardiac output peaks immediately after delivery, at which time it is 80% above the prelabor value in most normal patients. This is accompanied by *elevated venous pressure and increased stroke volume.* Rapid changes toward normal nonpregnant values occur thereafter, particularly during the first week, with a gradual decline during the next 3–4 weeks to prepregnancy values.

The *HCT rises ~5% above the predelivery value* in patients having an uncomplicated vaginal delivery. This occurs, despite the average blood loss of ~500 ml, as a result of renal elimination of both intravascular and extravascular fluids that have accumulated during pregnancy. Indeed, *blood volume decreases by ~20% by the fifth postpartum day.* Following cesarean delivery, there is an ~5% drop in hematocrit by the fifth day postpartum as a result of the average blood loss of 1000 ml. The average puerperal fluid loss is ~4 kg (9 pounds). Gradual weight loss follows.

Most women with normal blood values during pregnancy and an average blood loss at delivery show a *relative polycythemia* during the second week postpartum. Iron supplementation is not necessary for normal nonlactating postpartum women if the HCT or hemoglobin concentration 5 days after delivery is about the same as the normal predelivery value.

The normal slightly hypercoagulable state found during pregnancy is further enhanced during the puerperium, thus predisposing to thrombosis. By 3–5 days after delivery, platelet adhesiveness will have increased considerably, with lesser increases in platelet count and factor V and VIII values. However, fibrinolytic activity also increases. These values all diminish after the first week, returning to normal by about the fourth week.

LUNGS, RENAL, AND REPRODUCTIVE TRACT

Postpartum lung volume and capacity changes are at nonpregnant levels by 6 weeks. The hypotonic and slightly elongated and *dilated ureters and renal pelvis revert to normal* by the third month. Nearly 50% of patients have mild proteinuria during the first week, but renal function returns to prepregnant levels during the early puerperium.

The *uterus involutes* most rapidly after delivery and is complete by the sixth week postpartum. This is chiefly a result of contraction and decrease in the size of individual myometrial cells (Fig. 9-1). However, following a term gestation, the uterus remains slightly larger than before pregnancy because of some added connective tissue and a persistent slightly augmented vasculature. Endometrial regeneration is complete by the third week postpartum, except for the placental site, which requries 5–6 weeks. Microscopic evidence of placental implantation (primarily fibrous tissue) remains permanently.

Lochia rubra, the bloody discharge that follows delivery, normally becomes more serous and lighter in color (*lochia serosa*) after 2–3 days. In another week, the lochia becomes mucoid and yellowish due to the inclusion of leukocytes and disintegrating decidual elements. Discharge usually ceases about the fourth week after delivery.

The *cervix gradually closes* during the puerperium. The external os is converted to a transverse slit ~2 weeks after delivery. The distended *vagina* gradually *returns to its prepartum state* by the third week after vaginal delivery. The rugae remain flattened and the torn hymen heals irregularly.

The *voluntary muscles of the pelvic floor* gradually regain their tone, although trauma during vaginal delivery may weaken the musculature and predispose to genital hernias. Overdistention of the abdominal wall during pregnancy may cause rectus diastasis (separation).

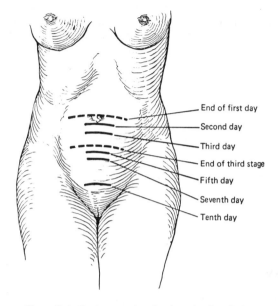

Figure 9-1. Postpartum levels of uterine involution.

RETURN OF OVULATION AND MENSTRUATION

Hormone changes immediately after delivery are abrupt. *Estrogen, progesterone, and hCG levels fall to the nonpregnant range within 1 week.* The *prolactin level increases* considerably during the first week, especially in patients who are nursing, and remains high during lactation. A state of relative estrogen deficiency occurs during the puerperium, especially in women who nurse their babies. This may lead to a menopausal appearing vagina and dyspareunia. Vaginal cytologic studies will reveal near-atrophic smears.

Nursing mothers rarely menstruate in <6 weeks postpartum. However, ~50% will ovulate on or before that time. *After abortion ≤ 15th week,* the average time required for return of ovulation is 2–3 weeks, and menstruation should occur within 4–5 weeks. If pregnancy was >15 weeks duration, ovulation should occur within 4–6 weeks, and menses should resume within 6–7 weeks. However, the time of the first ovulatory cycle after delivery is variable. In nonlactating women, ovulation may occur as early as the 25th–35th day postpartum. Menstruation resumes in about 40% of nonlactating women by the sixth week. By 12 weeks after delivery, 70%–80% of nonlactating women will have begun to menstruate again.

CARE DURING THE FIRST WEEK OF THE PUERPERIUM

Length of Hospitalization and Vital Signs

Most patients can return home safely 1–2 days after delivery. However, to effectively screen for puerperal problems (especially sepsis) the *temperature, pulse, and respiration rate should be ascertained every 4 h for 2–3 days.* Give $Rh_o(D)$ immune globulin (300 μg IM within 72 h of delivery) to unsensitized Rh-negative women who deliver Rh-positive offspring.

Exercise and Early Ambulation

Early ambulation is encouraged. It provides a sense of well-being, hastens involution of the uterus, and may reduce the incidence of thrombosis. Nonetheless, the patient should avoid lifting, straining, or pushing. Rest periods are essential.

Diet

A regular diet is permissible as soon as the patient is hungry and is free from the effects of analgesics, amnesics, or anesthetics. High-protein foods, fruits, and vegetables are recommended. A high fluid intake is advised, especially for nursing mothers. Even lactating women probably require no more than 2600–2800 kcal/day, and caloric excess has the usual consequences.

BLADDER CARE

Avoid overdistention of the bladder, which is normally hypotonic immediately after delivery. *Postpartum polyuria* for several days after delivery causes the bladder to fill in a relatively short time, and *frequent voiding is necessary.* The gravida may be unaware of the distending bladder, and thus timed voiding (every 1–2 h) may be necessary. If overdistention occurs, decompression by catheter may be required. If catheterization yields >1000 ml or is required ≥3 times/day during the first several days after delivery, a retention catheter for 12–24 h may assist in regaining bladder tone.

BOWEL FUNCTION

Normally, bowel function continues without serious problems. A mild ileus may follow anesthetics or some analgesics. This can generally be reversed by a mild laxative (e.g., Milk of Magnesia). A rectal suppository, such as bisacodyl (Dulcolax), or a small tapwater enema may be required.

ANALGESICS AND SEDATIVES

Acetaminophen (325–550 mg every 4 h) is usually sufficient for pain, but in more severe cases, codeine 30–60 mg every 4 h may be added. If the latter is insufficient for pain relief, seek a more serious problem (e.g., hematoma) as the cause of the pain.

Hospital procedures, noise, and strange surroundings are not conducive to sleep. *Mild sedatives at bedtime may be necessary* to ensure a good night's rest. The medication selected should allow the gravida to awaken easily and be alert to care for the baby without a later hangover effect.

CARE OF EPISIOTOMY AND LACERATIONS

Gently cleanse the perineum with soap or detergent and water at least once or twice each day and after defecation. Keep the pudendum clean and dry. However, Sitz baths bid or tid may be very beneficial, especially if hemorrhoidal discomfort is a problem. Healing should occur rapidly. Dry heat applied to the perineum with an infrared lamp for 20–30 min tid often relieves discomfort and promotes healing. Greasy ointments or salves to the perineum cause skin maceration and may foster infection.

Inspect the episiotomy or repaired lacerations daily. Perform vaginal or rectal examination if a hematoma or infection seems likely. Drain the sutured area if suppuration develops.

BATHS

As soon as the patient is able, she may take a shower, sitz bath, or tub bath. Water does not ascend into the vagina with the patient sitting in a bathtub.

CARE DURING CONVALESCENCE

Hygiene, diet, and other care are essentially the same as noted. Discuss with the gravida the normally decreasing amounts of sanguineous *vaginal discharge,* which lasts about 3 weeks. Mention the possibility of a "small period" during the 4–5 weeks after delivery. This should allay later concerns. The seriousness of *infection* should be stressed and its signs (local heat, pain, redness, fever) reiterated. Instruct the patient as to what to do should any of these signs develop. A *brassiere,* worn constantly, especially if she is nursing, may assist with breast discomfort. A girdle is rarely necessary. Vaginal douches should be used only on specific indication. *Coitus should not be resumed until an episiotomy or lacerations have healed* (generally 4 weeks). The postpartum dialogue is an opportunity for the patient to voice her *desire for future reproduction* and for the physician to assist (if necessary) with contraception.

Activity and responsibility should increase gradually. During the first 3–4 weeks postpartum, a limited regimen is recommended (light duty), but *full activity should be anticipated by* about 6 weeks postpartum.

Active exercise involving the pubococcygeus muscles (*Kegel exercises*) may enhance resolution of pelvic floor relaxation and urinary stress incontinence even if significant anatomic defects (e.g., cystocele) are present. Repeated contraction of the pubococcygeus muscle (as with attempts to stop voiding or a bowel movement in progress) for 5–10 min 3–4 times daily may restore muscle tone and function.

POSTPARTUM EXAMINATIONS

FIRST POSTPARTUM EXAMINATION

Examine the patient about *4 weeks after delivery.* By this time, *healing of the perineum should be complete, the lochia should have ceased, the cervix should be closed, and the uterus should have nearly returned to its prepartum size.* Hopefully, the examination will occur before intercourse so that any minor abnormalities can be corrected and, again, the type of contraception can be discussed. General inquiry and examination should estimate the time for return to full activity and employment. Specifically the first postpartum examination should include

Weight Ideally, the patient will have returned to her *approximate prepregnancy weight.* The abdominal muscle tone will be improving, but this is largely exercise-dependent.

Breasts *Note abnormalities* of the nipples, lactation, the adequacy of support, and the presence of redness, tenderness, or masses.

Uterine Bleeding *Heavy or persistent uterine bleeding* requires definitive investigation and treatment. A course of an oxytocic (e.g., ergonovine) may be beneficial. However, dilatation and curettage may be required.

Vaginal Discharge *Leukorrhea ceases* in about two thirds of the patients by 4–5 weeks. Infections require diagnosis and specific treatment.

Pelvic Do a *complete pelvic examination:* speculum, bimanual, and rectovaginal evaluation. The postpartum examination should afford the best opportunity for bimanual examination of the intraabdominal organs because some abdominal relaxation will have persisted. Examine the episiotomy and repaired lacerations. Perineovaginal support should be ascertained.

Uterine subinvolution may be the result of infection, retroposition, or retained products of conception. Treatment must be directed toward correction of the specific problem. If *uterine prolapse* (descensus) is present, its degree should be noted and related to symptoms. If prolapse is marked and persists for >4 months, consider surgical correction.

Repeat specific laboratory tests that were abnormal during pregnancy. Treat problems identified (e.g., anemia).

Contraception *Discuss family planning.* Prescribe the contraceptive method most suitable and acceptable to the couple.

FURTHER EXAMINATIONS

If further therapy is necessary other visits should be scheduled. A gynecologic examination and cervical cytologic study should be performed ~6 months after delivery. At that time, menstrual or other problems should be evaluated.

LACTATION

Lactation begins about 48–72 h after delivery, with sudden engorgement of the breasts. However, the infant can begin nursing almost immediately after birth, since colostrum will be available.

PHYSIOLOGY AND PATHOPHYSIOLOGY OF LACTATION

Estrogen and progesterone, present in large amounts during pregnancy, *stimulate the ductal and alveolar systems of the breast,* respectively. This causes proliferation and differentiation of the mammary glands and the production of clear, thin, serumlike colostrum as early as the third month of pregnancy. Colostrum continues to be secreted to term. Nonetheless, the high level of estrogen during pregnancy inhibits the binding of prolactin (hPL) in breast tissue, so milk is not produced. *After delivery, estrogen, progesterone, and hCS levels fall sharply, and hPL stimulates the mammary alveoli to produce milk.* Interestingly, the hPL level needed to maintain lactation is lower than that achieved during pregnancy. Optimal levels of insulin and thyroid and adrenal hormones play a secondary roles in lactation.

Suckling is not required for the initiation of lactation. However, nursing is necessary for continued milk production (suckling stimulates periodic hPL secretion). Suckling also stimulates release of oxytocin from the posterior pituitary via a breast-to-pituitary neural reflex. In addition to its effect on uterine smooth muscle, oxytocin contracts the periacinar muscle fibers of the breast, causing ejection of milk into the major collecting sinuses that converge on the nipple. This is called the *milk ejection or milk letdown reflex.* Tension and fatigue inhibit the letdown reflex, but the infant's cry and nursing stimulate it.

The infant does not nurse by developing intermittent negative pressure but by a rhythmic grasping of the areola. Thus, milk is worked into the mouth. Very little force is required in nursing because the breast reservoirs can be emptied and refilled independent of suction. Nursing mothers develop a sensation of drawing and tightening—a draught or concentration—within the breast at the beginning of suckling after the initial breast engorgement disappears. Mothers are thus conscious of the milk ejection reflex, which may even cause milk to spurt or run out. The milk letdown phenomenon is inhibited by drugs, pain, breast engorgement, or adverse psychic conditioning, such as embarrassment.

For several days after initial milk production (breast filling), the milk ejection reflex may be deficient. Then, the breasts become so distended that the nipples appear retracted, the areolas are unyielding to the nursling's efforts, and the infant obtains little or no milk. Manual expression of milk or the administration of oxytocin (or both) will usually start the flow and relieve the engorgement, whereupon nursing may be more successful.

The mother should nurse her infant at *both breasts at each feeding* because overfilling of the breasts is the main cause of decreased milk production. Nursing at only one breast at a feeding leaves the other breast full, and the distention of the full breast inhibits the letdown reflex. This causes a reduction in milk output in both breasts. Thus, alternating breasts from one feeding to the next may increase engorgement distress and reduce milk output. It is also advisable to move the infant from one breast to the other every 5–10 min to minimize nipple maceration.

ADVANTAGES AND DISADVANTAGES OF BREASTFEEDING

For the Mother

Breastfeeding is convenient, costs nothing, is emotionally satisfying for most women, and speeds uterine involution. Suckling promotes favorable maternal–infant interaction. Moreover, mothers who breastfeed may derive some protection against breast cancer.

The disadvantages are that regular nursing may restrict activities, and nipple tenderness or mastitis may develop.

For the Infant

Breast milk is digestible, readily available, at the proper temperature, and free from bacterial contamination. The composition is ideal. As a result, breastfed infants have fewer digestive or allergy problems. The child receives passive antibodies, infant–maternal bonding is enhanced, and the child is less likely to become obese (compared to formula-fed babies). There are no known disadvantages to the breastfeeding of an infant if the mother is healthy and willing and the supply of milk is adequate.

CONTRAINDICATIONS TO BREASTFEEDING

Absolute contraindications to breastfeeding are *epidemic mastitis, breast cancer, active pulmonary tuberculosis, and maternal intake of antithyroid medications, cancer chemotherapeutic agents, or certain other toxic drugs.* Indeed, when prescribing medications for the nursing mother, it is essential to consider their potential impact on the infant. Breastfeeding may be impossible for weak, ill, or very premature infants, or those with cleft palate, choanal atresia, or phenylketonuria (PKU). However, expressed breast milk may be saved and given at a later date except in the case of PKU.

DRUGS IN BREAST MILK

Innumerable drugs may be detected in a parturient's blood and milk. Numerous drugs harmful to the nursing infant pass into breast milk, including chloramphenicol, metronidazole, nitrofurantoin, sulfonamides, and antithyroid drugs.

TEACHING BREASTFEEDING

Success or failure of breastfeeding is related to the amount of factual information and emotional support available to the mother. Although this may be useful at the time of delivery, it may be much more effective if included as part of the prenatal educational program. Organizations, such as the La Leche League, the Nursing Mothers of Australia, and the Plunkett Society in New Zealand, have been very effective in promoting breastfeeding.

Demonstrations of infant care and formula preparation are also generally a part of nursing service programs. Several important points bear emphasis.

1. The patient should wash the nipples daily with unscented mild soap and water, using a washcloth (beginning in the last trimester). After drying, she may apply hydrated lanolin. Perfumed soaps and skin or hand creams should not be used because they may contain irritants. The application of alcohol is inadvisable, since it dries and hardens the skin.

2. Inverted or short nipples should be drawn gently outward each day to increase their length temporarily.

3. The nipples should be protected with plastic film or nipple shields.

4. A well-fitted brassiere (worn even at night) supports the breasts, improves circulation, and avoids trauma.

5. Expressing colostrum gently several times each day during the last 4–6 weeks of pregnancy stimulates the flow of the fluid.

6. Beginning on the first postpartum day, if not contraindicated, the normal newborn should nurse at each breast on demand or approximately every 3–4 h for 3 min total nursing time per breast per feeding. Increase the time by 1 min each day, not exceeding 7 min per breast per feeding. The average infant obtains 60%–90% of the milk in 4 min of nursing. Suckling for longer than 7 min often causes maceration and cracking of the nipples (with subsequent risk of mastitis).

7. A glass of cool water 5 min before nursing or another method of psychologic preparation (especially fluids) strengthens the reflex of milk ejection. Ample fluids are especially important, but beer, wine, and spirits will not increase milk production more than water.

8. Avoid engorgement and trapping of milk by gentle expression of excess milk before nursing or by use of oxytocin, 10 units in 0.25 ml of normal saline as a nasal spray, just before infant feeding.

MILK PRODUCTION

Normally, the mother's yield of breast milk is directly proportionate to the infant's demand, assuming that free secretion of milk has been established and feedings are given every 3–4 h. With nursing, the average milk production on the second postpartum day is about 120 ml, on the third postpartum day at least 180 ml, and by the fourth day about 240 ml. A rule of thumb for calculation of milk production for a given day during the first week after delivery is *multiply the number of the postpartum day by 60*. This gives the approximate milliliters of milk/24 h. Sustained milk production should be achieved by most mothers after 10–14 days. A yield of 120–180 ml of milk per feeding is common by the end of the second week.

Oral contraceptives and estrogens adversely affect the amount of milk produced, but few other commonly used drugs have this capability.

Nipple Fissures

Fissured nipples have painful cracks that may lead to mastitis. Apply dry heat and nonmedicated, nonperfumed hydrous lanolin for benefit. Prefeeding manual expression of milk will reduce breast engorgement and make nursing easier. A nipple shield may also be used. Finally, the nursing infant should alternate from breast to breast after no more than 5 min to promote healing.

Suppression of Lactation

If the patient does not choose to nurse her infant, *estrogen or androgen administration* (or a combination of both) decreases hPL, or *mechanical inhibition of lactation* (breast binding) may be effective. All are most effective only if started immediately after delivery, and all have a high failure rate. Moreover, concerns about the undesirable side effects of estrogen particularly (e.g., thromboembolism) have led to decreasing use of sex steroids.

A dopamine-agonist, *bromocriptine* (Parlodel) 2.5 mg orally for 14 days, *inhibits prolactin secretion* and will suppress lactation. However, prolonged treatment with this drug may be necessary, and side effects (e.g., nasal congestion, headache, or nausea) occasionally develop.

Mechanical Suppression

The patient should not nurse and should not express milk or pump her breasts. A tight compression uplift binder for 72 h and a snug brassiere thereafter are necessary. Ice packs and analgesics (e.g., acetaminophen or aspirin and codeine) may be used if necessary. Fluid restriction and laxatives are not helpful in suppression of lactation.

At first, the breast will become distended, firm, and tender. After 48–72 h, lactation usually ceases and pain subisdes. Involution will be complete in about 1 month.

PUERPERAL PATHOLOGY

Puerperal pathology is so highly weighted to infectious disease that even the definition of postpartum morbidity remains a definition implying infection (i.e., a temperature of >101.8°F on two consecutive occasions 6 h apart more than 24 h after delivery). The *three major problems are urinary tract infection, puerperal mastitis, and puerperal sepsis.* Nevertheless, other noninfectious problems may complicate the puerperium.

PUERPERAL MASTITIS

Puerperal mastitis is breast infection during the 6 weeks following childbirth. Generally, it is unilateral. The usual cause is *Staphylococcus aureus.* About 0.5%–1.0% of parturients are affected, and most of these are primiparas. There are two types of puerperal mastitis.

1. The *sporadic form* is an acute cellulitis involving interlobular connective and adipose tissues. A nipple fissure is the usual avenue of infection. Localized pain, tenderness, segmental erythema, and fever result. The milk is not infected.

2. *Epidemic mastitis* is a fulminating infection of the breast glandular system, with symptoms and signs similar to but more acute than those of sporadic mastitis. A nursery *Staphylococcus* carrier is most often incriminated, where an infant acquires the infection, which is then spread into its mother's ductal system after the regurgitation of a small amount of infected milk.

Diagnostically, it is crucial to culture the milk and to culture the neonate. Perform serial CBCs, blood cultures, and other laboratory tests as indicated.

Treat both types of acute mastitis *with antibiotics capable of destruction of penicillinase-resistant pathogens* (e.g., oxacillin, cephalothin, or equivalent). In the sporadic form, continued suckling is advisable because nursing prevents engorgement and decreases the likelihood of abscess formation. Often, a nipple shield will decrease maternal discomfort. In the epidemic form, the infant harbors the pathogenic organism. Hence, antibiotic therapy, prompt weaning, suppression of lactation, cold packs, and a snug breast binder are recommended.

Usually, if proper antibiotic therapy is initiated before the onset of suppuration, the signs and symptoms of infection should begin to resolve within 24 h. Puerperal mastitis that has not subsided in 2–3 days has most likely progressed to an abscess. Then, surgical drainage of all infected loculations is necessary to resolve the abscess.

Prevention is obviously more effective in the sporadic type and involves good hygiene (i.e., cleansing the nipples with plain soap and water, avoiding topical alcohol, and prevention of nipple fissures). Helpful methods to prevent the latter are (1) to place a finger in the corner of the infant's mouth to break its sucking force at the end of feeding and (2) to not allow lengthy feeding at one breast or maceration may occur.

Therapy for the infant is not usually necessary, even in the epidemic form.

PUERPERAL SEPSIS
(SEE ALSO SEPTIC SHOCK, P. 334)

Any infection of the genital tract occurring as a complication of abortion, labor, or delivery is termed puerperal sepsis. Streptococci, staphylococci, clostridia, coliform bacteria, or *Bacteroides* are the pathogens most often identified. Cellulitis resulting from vaginal or cervical lacerations may be the initial site of infection, as may the endometrium, particularly in the zone of placental attachment (the equivalent of a large surface wound). Debility (anemia, undernutrition), serious systemic disorders, prolonged rupture of the membranes, protracted labor, and traumatic delivery predispose to puerperal infection.

The *incidence* of puerperal sepsis in U.S. hospitals is *<3% in low-risk, vaginally delivered patients.* The incidence rises (nearly exponentially) with increasing obstetric risk and operative delivery. Puerperal sepsis is exceeded only by hemorrhage and preeclampsia-eclampsia as a major cause of maternal death in this country.

Clinical Findings

Many genital tract infections are mild and cause few or slight symptoms. Others are fulminating and may be fatal within a short time.

Symptoms and Signs Malaise, headache, anorexia, and remittent slight elevations in temperature and a rise in pulse rate generally begin 3–4 days after delivery. Vague discomfort in the perineum or lower abdomen and nausea and vomiting may follow. Often, the lochia becomes foul or profuse. High fever (childbed fever), rapid pulse, ileus, localization of pain, and tenderness in the pelvis may be observed during the next 1–2 days. Bacteremic shock may develop.

Physical Examination At the first suspicion of puerperal infection, conduct a careful aseptic pelvic examination. The repair of any laceration or episiotomy must be scrutinized for signs of sepsis. A sterile ring forceps should be used to open the cervix to guarantee free flow of lochia. Perform a careful bimanual examination (including rectovaginal) to identify potential sites of infection. Culture the cervical canal, and obtain a urine culture for predominant organisms and their sensitivity to major antibiotics. If improvement does not follow after 48–72 h of intensive multiple antibiotic therapy, careful reexamination for an abscess should be conducted.

Laboratory Findings *Polymorphonuclear leukocytosis* and an *increased sedimentation rate* indicate infection. Identification of pathogens from cervical and uterine lochia by culture and sensitivity tests will require 24–48 h, but stained smears should be obtained immediately for a preliminary diagnosis.

Ultrasonography and X-Ray Findings X-ray studies are not helpful except to exclude gastrointestinal, urinary, or pulmonary problems. Ultrasonography may be useful for the localization of an abscess or to diagnose or rule out retained products of conception or pelvic thrombophlebitis.

Complications and Sequelae

Genital tract infections commonly progress from endometritis to endomyometritis to pelvic cellulitis and peritonitis or septic pelvic thrombophlebitis. Abscess formation, septicemia, pulmonary embolism, septic shock, and death may result.

Differential Diagnosis

Febrile complications of the puerperium unrelated to genital tract infection include *mastitis, urinary and respiratory infection, and enteritis,* in that order of frequency.

Prevention

Avoidance of puerperal sepsis requires strict aseptic technique during pelvic examination and delivery. Minimize obstetric trauma because injured tissues are susceptible to infection.

Treatment

Emergency Measures

Treat septic shock (see p. 334).

General Measures

1. Place the patient in the semi-Fowler position.
2. Order a clear liquid diet for at least several days if ileus is not present.
3. Administer IV fluids to maintain proper electrolyte and fluid balance. Dilute oxytocin in the infusion should maintain a contracted uterus.
4. Administer analgesics, sedative-hypnotic drugs, or laxatives as required.

Specific Measures

1. Initially, give antibiotics in large doses (e.g., penicillin G 5 million units IV plus kanamycin 1 g IM, immediately follow with penicillin 1.2 million units with kanamycin 0.5 g IM 4 times daily). In infections likely to be anaerobic, particularly if *Bacteroides* is thought to be present, substitute clindomycin 600 mg IM for kanamycin. When the results of culture and sensitivity studies are reported, continue therapy with the antibiotic of choice in large and repeated doses.
2. For the serious infection, it is often necessary to admit the patient to an intensive care unit and to perform hemodynamic monitoring.
3. For treatment of disseminated intravascular coagulation, see p. 500.

Surgical Measures

1. Surgical drainage of abscesses usually is necessary, and the pelvic approach is preferred.

2. Percutaneous insertion of an inferior vena caval umbrella may be necessary in cases of septic pulmonary thromboembolism.

3. Hysterectomy is indicated for serious uterine infections unresponsive to antibiotics (e.g., a postabortal uterine abscess or an infected hydatidiform mole). In such cases, it may be possible to spare the ovaries using continued high-dose antibiotics. However, the outcome may still be uncertain.

4. Ligation of the ovarian veins may be life saving in repeated septic pulmonary embolization from septic pelvic thrombophlebitis.

Prognosis

The maternal mortality due to puerperal sepsis in the United States is about 0.2%, but it is vastly greater in some developing countries. Puerperal infections have the potential to cause abscesses in the remaining pelvic organs (e.g., ovaries), impair subsequent fertility, and require subsequent surgery.

PUERPERAL INVERSION OF UTERUS

An inverted uterus is one partially or completely turned inside-out. Inversion of the uterus may be *partial* (herniation of the fundus into the uterine cavity) or *complete* (extrusion of the corpus through the cervix into or beyond the vagina). Either type may be spontaneous or induced and acute or chronic. Acute spontaneous puerperal inversion is due to straining by the patient soon after delivery. *Acute induced puerperal inversion* may be due to

1. Traction of the cord before placental separation

2. Severe kneading of the fundus to induce placental separation or expulsion

3. Improperly executed manual separation or extraction of an adherent placenta

Chronic induced puerperal inversion is due to the same causes as the acute variety that are unrecognized after delivery. The incidence of uterine inversion is about 1:15,000 deliveries (lowest where obstetric care is of the highest quality).

Clinical Findings

1. Acute complete inversion causes sudden agonizing pain and an explosive sensation of fullness extending downward into the

vagina. Hemorrhage and profound shock occur in >50% of patients. If inversion is partial, pain and bleeding will be less severe.

2. In complete inversion, a large bleeding mass will be obvious outside the introitus, often with the placenta still attached.

3. In partial inversion, bimanual examination will reveal a cup-shaped depression at the fundus with a mass palpable above or bulging through the cervix.

4. Chronic partial uterine inversion is characterized by persistent, otherwise unexplained bleeding and discomfort. Bimanual examination or an instrument passed through the partially closed cervix may reveal the abnormality.

Differential Diagnosis

A *large submucous myoma* at the external cervical os may cause the same signs as inversion, but the fundus will be large and rounded without a craterlike depression.

Complications

Shock, hemorrhage, or death may ensue in acute complete inversion, especially when mismanaged. Anemia, infection, or embolization may develop in partial or chronic cases.

Prevention

Avoid traction on the cord until definite separation of the placenta has occurred. Do not knead the fundus. Supervise the patient until the uterus is rounded and firmly contracted.

Treatment

1. Control shock with IV fluids, plasma, whole blood, and oxytocin before attempting definitive treatment. *Caution:* do not give ergotrate, or cervical contraction may block fundal replacement.

2. Attempt to replace the uterus by abdominovaginal means. If the placenta is still attached, *leave it attached* (this limits additional bleeding). Deep brief general anesthesia may be required. Cervical constriction may be relaxed by whiffs of amyl nitrite vapor or epinephrine 0.3–0.6 ml of a 1:1000 solution IM.

Countertraction on the cervix while directing the inverted portion of the uterus upward facilitates replacement.

Another method of correcting acute or subacute puerperal uterine inversion is as follows. Under general anesthesia, lift the uterus out of the pelvis by grasping the inverted fundus with the vaginal gloved hand, then apply steady pressure toward the umbilicus. Retain the fist within the uterus until the corpus is well contracted (prostaglandins or ergot may be desirable) to prevent recurrence of inversion. Packs are not effective and maintain distention.

3. If correction cannot be accomplished quickly by manipulation, surgical replacement may be mandatory. This must be accomplished by abdominal laparotomy. Visualization generally reveals that the ovaries are close together in the midline, and the uterus is not visible. The ovarian ligaments, tubes, and round ligaments disappear into a tightly closed hole. A linear incision in the posterior wall of the cervix at the level of the uterocervical junction (usually between the uterosacral ligaments) relaxes the stricture, and with gentle manipulation from above and below, the uterine fundus is replaced. The incision may then be repaired in at least two layers with an absorbable synthetic suture. Oxytocics are administered after the fundus is delivered.

Prognosis

Manual replacement is effective in >85% of cases. Prophylactic administration of antibiotics may be warranted, for there is a high rate of infection after uterine inversion. Recurrence of inversion or in a subsequent pregnancy may occur.

Chapter 10

Early Pregnancy Complications

SPONTANEOUS ABORTION

Spontaneous abortion (miscarriage) is the *termination of pregnancy before completion of the 20th gestational week*. The term applies to both live and stillborn fetuses weighing ≤500 g. However, a fetus need not be identified if other products of conception are present (e.g., placenta or membranes). Familiarity with the local legal definition is mandatory because there is considerable state to state variation.

Spontaneous abortion is the unintended result of 15%–40% of all known pregnancies. The earlier the gestation, the more likely is abortion. About 75% occur before 16 weeks, and approximately 60% occur before 12 weeks. A major difficulty in detailing exact numbers is the variability of methods for pregnancy diagnosis. For example, a serum beta-subunit hCG determination will detect very early pregnancies (and thus more losses) than the standard available urine pregnancy tests. At least 80% of all pregnancies terminate spontaneously before the woman or physician is aware of the pregnancy (*subclinical or undiagnosed spontaneous abortion*). Table 10-1 estimates the losses with in vitro fertilization (which would be included in the subclinical category).

ABORTION DEFINITIONS

Many different variables apply to abortion, and a number of definitions are required. It is assumed that all definitions refer to spontaneous abortion, if not otherwise specified.

Early abortion occurs <12th gestational week.

Late abortion occurs between 12 and 20 weeks gestation.

Table 10-1. In vitro fertilization losses

16% of fertilized ova do not divide
15% of fertilized ova are lost before implantation (first gestational week)
27% are lost during implantation (second gestational week)
10.5% are lost following the first missed menses
Total loss is 68.5%

Threatened abortion refers to intrauterine bleeding <20th week of completed gestation, with or without uterine contraction, without cervical dilatation, and without expulsion of the products of conception (POC). Moreover, ultrasound must reveal the fetus to show signs of life (e.g., heartbeat or motion). In threatened abortion, the previable gestation is in jeopardy, but the pregnancy continues.

Inevitable abortion is intrauterine bleeding before the 20th completed gestational week, with continued cervical dilatation but without expulsion of the POC. In inevitable abortion, momentary evacuation of part or all of the conceptus is likely. Abortion is considered inevitable with two or more of the following.

1. Moderate effacement of the cervix
2. Cervical dilatation >3 cm
3. Rupture of the membranes
4. Bleeding for >7 days
5. Persistence of cramps despite narcotic analgesics
6. Signs of termination of pregnancy (e.g., absent mastalgia)

Incomplete abortion is the expulsion of some but not all of the POC >20th completed gestational week.

Complete abortion is expulsion of all the POC >20th completed gestational week. When the entire conceptus has been expelled, pain ceases, but slight spotting persists for a few days.

Missed abortion is death of the embryo or fetus <20th completed gestational week, but the POC are retained in utero for ≥8 weeks. Symptoms of pregnancy disappear, and there may be a brownish vaginal discharge but no free bleeding. Pain and tenderness are absent, the cervix is semifirm and closed or only slightly patulous, the uterus becomes smaller and irregularly softened, and the adnexa are normal. Fetal death at 18–26 weeks followed by missed labor and retention for >6 weeks may be associated with maternal fibrinogen depletion (*dead fetus syndrome*). Consider administration of cryoprecipitate to prevent hemorrhage from hypofibrinogenemia before evacuation of the uterus (Fig. 10-1).

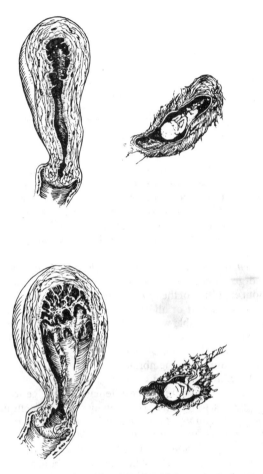

Figure 10·1. Top. Complete abortion. At right, product of complete abortion. Bottom. Incomplete abortion. At right, product of incomplete abortion.

Infected abortion is that associated with infection of the internal genitalia.

Septic abortion is infected abortion with dissemination of bacteria via the maternal circulation.

Habitual abortion is the spontaneous, consecutive loss of 3 or more nonviable pregnancies.

Induced abortion is the purposeful interruption of pregnancy by medical or surgical techniques.

ETIOLOGY OF SPONTANEOUS ABORTION

Early Abortion

Abnormal products of conception are the overwhelming cause of spontaneous abortion. At least 10% of human conceptuses have chromosomal abnormalities, and most of these are aborted. Indeed, 50%–60% of first trimester spontaneous abortions have an abnormal karyotype (vs ~7% in elective induced abortion). The most common karyotypic abnormalities are trisomy (52%), polyploidy (26%), and X monosomy (15%). Major interruptions of embryogenesis (e.g., failure of the fetus to develop or neural tube defects) account for some of the rest. These are largely multifactorial in etiology (an admixture of genetic and environmental). Additional factors include infections (e.g., cytomegalovirus), endocrine abnormalities (e.g., failure of the corpus luteum), and genital tract abnormalities (e.g., subseptate uterus). The cause of a significant number of early abortions remains unknown.

Late Abortion

Worldwide, the major causes of abortion during the second trimester are *infections* (e.g., syphilis, malaria), *circumvallate placenta, maternal metabolic imbalances* (e.g., diabetes mellitus, severe hypothyroidism), *maternal physiologic impairment* (e.g., cardiac disorders, hypertension), *maternal dietary insufficiency* (e.g., bulimia, avitaminosis B or C), *isoimmunizations, exposure to fetotoxic factors* (e.g., lead poisoning, substance abuse), *trauma* (e.g., direct or indirect abdominal injury), and *uterine or cervical defects* (e.g., cervical incompetency). A wide variety of other etiologies may induce abortion, including severe electric shock, although there is no convincing evidence that abortion may be induced by psychic stimuli (e.g., severe fright, grief, anger, or anxiety).

DIAGNOSIS OF ABORTION

Clinical

Obtain a complete history and perform a general physical (including pelvic) examination on every patient to determine if special laboratory or other studies are necessary to detect diseases or deficiency states.

Classically, the *symptoms of abortion are uterine cramping* (with or without suprapubic pain) *and vaginal bleeding* in the presence of previable pregnancy. The integration of the physical examination with these symptoms allows a tentative diagnosis.

Laboratory Studies

In many cases, a serum pregnancy test is useful. Minimal laboratory studies should include culture and sensitivity of cervical mucus or blood (to identify pathogens in infection) and a complete blood count. In some cases, determination of progesterone levels may be useful to detect corpus luteum failure. When hemorrhage is present, blood typing and crossmatching as well as a coagulation panel are necessary.

Genetic analysis of aborted material may determine chromosomal abnormality as the etiology. This often provides invaluable information for counseling.

Diagnosis of Fetal Death

The immunoassay (IA) and radioimmunoassay (RIA) pregnancy tests identify hormones produced by the trophoblast. However, even with death of the embryo or early fetus, groups of trophoblastic cells may remain attached and temporarily viable. Therefore, these pregnancy tests may remain positive for a time. In any event, when a negative RIA test is reported, the pregnancy is over, although gestational debris may be retained.

With a clinical diagnosis of inevitable abortion, ultrasonography is less useful than it is in threatened abortion, when ultrasonography may distinguish a living from a nonliving gestation. Using real-time ultrasonography, the absence of gross motion and especially heartbeat is indicative of fetal death. In some cases, absence of a fetus or fetal disorganization also may be detected. Rarely, gas in the great vessels will be observed.

If cardiac motion is present, as is normally noted <8 gestational weeks (mean sac diameter 2.5 cm), the prognosis is more favorable.

DIFFERENTIAL DIAGNOSIS

Ectopic gestation is differentiated from spontaneous abortion by the additional symptoms and signs of unilateral pelvic pain or tender adnexal mass. *Membranous dysmenorrhea* may closely mimic spontaneous abortion, but decidua and villi are absent in the endometrial cast and pregnancy tests (even RIA) are negative. *Hyperestrogenism* may lead to marked proliferative endometrium with symptoms of cramping and bleeding. *Hydatidiform mole* usually ends in abortion (<5 months) but is marked by a very high hCG titer and fetal absence. *Pedunculated myoma* or *cervical neoplasia* may also be confused with spontaneous abortion.

COMPLICATIONS

Hemorrhage and infection are major causes of maternal mortality or morbidity. Although very rare, about three fourths of cases of choriocarcinoma follow abortion. Infertility may result from inflammatory tubal occlusion after infected abortion. Rh sensitization may be avoided by administration of Rh immune globulin (see p. 311).

PREVENTION

Some abortions may be prevented by treatment of maternal deficiencies or disorders before or during pregnancy (e.g., diabetes mellitus, hypertension). Closure of an incompetent cervix will prevent certain abortion.

The usual technique for correction of cervical incompetency, *cervical cerclage,* involves placement of a suture or a nonabsorbable Mersilene or comparable strand, ribbon, or band beneath the mucosa and pericervical fascia at the cervicouterine junction. It may be done during the pregnant state for correction of cervical incompetence (Fig. 10-2) or accomplished between pregnancies. The physician must then decide whether to release the ligature during labor for vaginal delivery or to perform cesarean section near term.

TREATMENT

Rapid assessment of the patient's hemodynamic status should be performed (e.g., blood pressure, pulse rate). A rare critical case

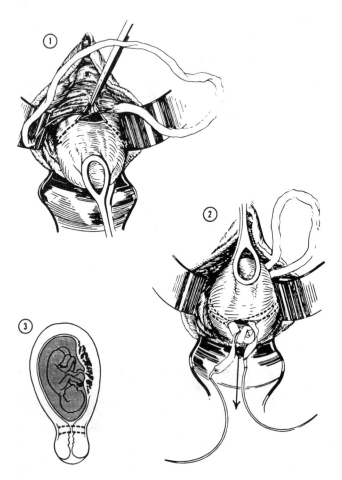

Figure 10-2. Cerclage of the cervix (Shirodkar) with incompetent os in pregnant patient.

will require hemodynamic monitoring. In all except those with minimal bleeding (e.g., a stable complete abortion or an early threatened abortion), establishing an intravenous line is necessary. Administer antishock therapy, including fluid and blood replacement when indicated.

Complete Abortion

Observation (at least 1 h) for further bleeding may be sufficient. If the products of conception are available, they should be studied for completeness and may be submitted for genetic analysis or other pathologic assessment. In questionable cases, *ultrasonic uterine scanning* may detail remaining products of conception. After observation, the patient suffering complete abortion may return home with instructions to note signs of infection (fever, chills, pain), observe for vaginal hemorrhage, and refrain from intercourse or douching until reexamined in about 2 weeks to determine lack of cervical closure or other abnormalities.

Threatened Abortion

Place the patient at *bedrest* after immediate danger from hemorrhage and infection has passed. Clinical judgment dictates whether bedrest may be accomplished at home (generally only in a nontroubling situation) or in the hospital. *Coitus and douches are contraindicated.*

Ultrasonic scanning is useful to determine fetal well-being. Obviously, a major determinant of prognosis is the recognition of fetal life and normality of fetal structures. Abortions without signs of fetal life should be managed as inevitable or incomplete abortions after appropriate discussion with the patient and family.

Progesterone therapy has theoretical value in <5% of abortions (those due to documented deficiency). In such cases, one may administer progesterone parenterally or by vaginal suppository. However, progesterone treatment remains controversial. The main points of contention include proper case selection, questionable efficacy, the potential to continue the retention of an abnormal pregnancy (i.e., missed abortion), and possible teratogenesis. Other therapy (e.g., tocolytics) is even more questionable.

In case of questionable fetal viability, the prognosis is best when bleeding and cramping quickly subside, with evidence of cervical closure. *The longer the symptoms persist, the more ominous the situation.*

The prognosis for the patient is good if all products of conception are evacuated or removed and if hydatidiform mole and choriocarcinoma can be ruled out.

Correction of maternal disorders may make future successful pregnancies possible. However, if an aborted fetus is found to have an abnormal karyotype, it may be desirable for the parents to obtain a genetic workup. In such cases, genetic investigation involving chorionic villus sampling or amniocentesis may be prudent during the next pregnancy. However, in certain severe transmissible genetic disorders, a determination of the exact defect in one or both parents will assist them and the practitioner to select artificial insemination (AID) or in vitro fertilization of donor egg or in vitro fertilization with donor egg and donor sperm or adoption or sterilization.

Inevitable and Incomplete Abortion

Once the patient's hemodynamic status has been assessed and treatment started, *retained tissue must be removed* or bleeding will continue. *Oxytocics* (e.g., oxytocin 10 IU/500 ml of 5% dextrose in Ringer's lactate solution IV at ~125 ml/h) should contract the uterus, limit blood loss, aid in the expulsion of clots or tissue, and decrease the possibility of uterine perforation during dilatation and curettage. Ergonovine should be given only *after* the diagnosis of complete abortion is certain.

In some cases, tissue at the external os may simply be removed with sponge forceps. In others, it will be necessary to perform a suction D & C. Although it is rarely required, a sharp curettage may be lightly performed after the suction D & C to ascertain completeness. A heavy or extensive sharp curettage is potentially hazardous because it may lead to uterine synechia.

The removal of products of conception usually may be performed safely under paracervical block in an outpatient facility. However, a limiting factor is the ability to adequately observe the patient after the procedure. In cases of heavy bleeding or if the abortion has occurred in the second trimester, hospitalization is usually necessary.

The majority of patients receiving outpatient care may be released after observation (1–6 h) confirms the return of physiologic function and absence of early complications. Discharge instructions for the uncomplicated case are as noted for complete abortion.

The *major complication of D & C is uterine perforation*. If this is suspected, the patient must be observed in the hospital for signs of intraperitoneal bleeding, rupture of the bowel or bladder, or peritonitis. Exploratory laparotomy and broad-spectrum antibiotic therapy may be necessary.

OTHER ABORTION PROBLEMS

Missed Abortion

Ultrasonic scanning is usually definitive in the *diagnosis* of fetal death. It also assists in the differential diagnosis of a normal pregnancy with inaccurate dates, pelvic tumor, or the loss of a multiple gestation.

Current *treatment* of missed abortion is induction of labor using prostaglandin E_2 suppositories, enhanced if necessary with dilute IV oxytocin.

The major risk of missed abortion is the possibility of hypofibrinogenemia. Thus, if the products of conception are contained longer than 4 weeks after fetal death, close monitoring of the serum fibrinogen is mandatory.

Infected or Septic Abortion

With infected abortion, expect *pelvic and abdominal pain and fever* (100–105°F). On physical examination there is often *suprapubic tenderness* and *signs of peritonitis*. The pelvic examination will likely, but may not necessarily, reveal a malodorous cervical discharge, pain on motion of the cervix, or uterine tenderness. Hypothermia may precede endotoxic shock, and jaundice may be due to hemolysis. Oliguria or renal failure is a serious complication.

The necessary *laboratory* information includes a complete blood count, urinalysis, culture of cervix or uterus or both, serum electrolytes, and a coagulation profile. Chest and abdominal x-ray films are necessary to diagnose or rule out septic emboli, gas beneath the diaphragm (uterine perforation), foreign body in the uterus (possible criminal abortion), and gas in the pelvic tissues from gas-forming organisms.

Treatment consists of hospitalization, high-dose IV antibiotic therapy (individualized to the suspected organisms), fluid and electrolyte support, and careful monitoring of vital signs and urinary output. These patients must be considered serious, even potentially critical. Hemodynamic monitoring may be necessary in the more severe cases (for determination of cardiac output, blood volume, blood gases).

The uterus must be emptied, and this should be accomplished by D & C as soon as the patient is stable. All products of conception must be removed, even though a thorough curettage of infected uterus greatly enhances the risk of uterine synechia (Asherman's syndrome). Abdominal hysterectomy may be necessary when clostridia or bacteroides are the causative organisms, when there is necrosis of the uterus, with complete uterine perforations (e.g., bowel injury), or when the patient responds poorly to septic shock treatment.

Pelvic thrombophlebitis and septic emboli may be grave sequelae of septic abortion. Consider additional, more specific antibiotic and also anticoagulant therapy. If repeated septic emboli occur, anticoagulants are contraindicated. Pelvic vein ligation or percutaneous umbrella occlusion of the vena cava may be necessary for septic embolization.

Habitual Abortion

Based on very conservative data (a 15%–40% chance of loss of any given pregnancy), three consecutive losses are required to approach statistical significance (<1%). The risk of first trimester abortion after one loss is 24%, after two losses 26%, and after three losses 32%. Thus, data from a series of cases with only two consecutive losses may not be valid.

The most likely *causes* of habitual abortion are genetic abnormality, reproductive tract anatomic abnormalities, hormonal abnormalities, infections, abnormal immunologic factors, or systemic disease. However, the cause remains unknown at least in one third of all habitual abortions.

Thus, the *incidence* of habitual abortion varies with parental genetic abnormalities (e.g., balanced translocation carrier parent, hyperploidy), maternal systemic diseases (e.g., hypertension, diabetes mellitus, SLE), maternal hormonal abnormalities (e.g., hypothyroidism), maternal genital tract abnormalities, and parental sharing of similar HLA-A and HLA-B (and possibly abortion, stillbirth, or infant with malformations).

Possible *etiologies for genetic errors* include parental chromosome translocation, recombination defects, other genetic factors (e.g., homozygous dominant inheritance), environmental agents (i.e., radiation, chemicals, medications), or delayed fertilization. In an abortion with an abnormal karyotype, there is an ~80% chance of the next abortus having an abnormal karyotype (vs ~50%–60% if the first has a normal karyotype).

Even after three spontaneous abortions, the probability of a fourth is <1 in 3. However, even this chance justifies investigation to determine a demonstrable cause. In addition to routine history and physical examination, the following are useful.

1. Prepare a three-generation pedigree for both partners and complete a thorough reproductive history (including pathologic and karyotypic information from previous abortions).

2. Obtain a karyotypic study of both parents.

3. Perform a hysterosalpingogram, hysteroscopy, or laparoscopy to rule out anatomic abnormalities of the reproductive tract.

4. Order laboratory studies for T_3, T_4, TSH, glucose abnormality screening (1 or 2 h postprandial), SMA, and antinuclear antibodies or antibodies to double-stranded DNA.

5. Arrange for immunologic screening for both parents. Currently, this includes HLA-A and HLA-B and transferrin C typing. An immunologic consultation also may be useful.

6. Biopsy the endometrium during the luteal phase, or obtain serum progesterone to assess the corpus luteum, or do both.

7. Perform infectious screening of cervical or endometrial tissue by culture for *Listeria monocytogenes, Chlamydia, Mycoplasma, U. urealyticum, Neisseria gonorrhoeae,* cytomegalovirus, and herpes simplex and serum titers for *Treponema pallidum, Brucella abortus,* and *Toxoplasma gondii.*

Therapy must be guided by the diagnostic workup.

1. *Genetic error.* Consider artificial insemination by donor or in vitro fertilization with donor ova or sperm.

2. *Anatomic abnormalities of the reproductive tract.* Employ uterine operations (e.g., Jones, Tompkins, Strassman procedure, myomectomy), cervical cerclage (abdominal or vaginal), or cervical reconstruction.

3. *Hormonal abnormalities.* When deficient, administer thyroid, progesterone, clomiphene citrate.

4. *Infection.* Give appropriate antibiotics.

5. *Immunologic factors.* Assess the need for administration of purified paternal lymphocytes to counter blocking antibodies (should be performed only in a center regularly using this therapy).

6. Treat *systemic disorders* appropriately using disease-specific therapy.

ECTOPIC PREGNANCY

A *fertilized ovum implanted outside the uterine cavity* is an ectopic pregnancy. Ectopic pregnancy usually results from conditions that delay or prevent the transit of a fertilized ovum through the fallopian tube. Over 50% are associated with tubal inflammatory changes (previous or chronic salpingitis). Other important etiologic factors include zygote abnormalities, transmigration of the ovum, postmidcycle ovulation–fertilization, or exogenous hormones.

The *incidence* of ectopic pregnancy has risen dramatically during the past two decades in the United States to >1:100 pregnancies (from ~1:500). The increase, most notable among nonwhite women, is attributable to tubal infection, endometriosis, and an enhanced chance of ectopic gestation after failed laparoscopic tubal ligation. Unknown factors also are likely.

Ectopic pregnancy is a *major cause of maternal mortality* mainly because of uncontrolled hemorrhage and shock (0.1%–0.2% in the United States, but the rate is higher in developing countries). Fetal mortality in ectopic pregnancy is nearly universal.

CLASSIFICATIONS

Ectopic pregnancy is classified according to the site of implantation (the following is in decreasing order of occurrence).

1. *Tubal* (>99%) ectopic pregnancies are further subdivided into the anatomic section involved: ampullary (55%), isthmic (25%), fimbrial (17%), interstitial (angular, cornual) (2%), and bilateral (very rare) (Fig. 10-3).

2. *Ovarian* pregnancy (0.5%) may follow fertilization of an unextruded ovum.

3. *Abdominal* (~1/15,000 pregnancies) pregnancy may be primary, with the initial implantation of the zygote outside the tube (e.g., on the liver), or secondary to expulsion or rupture of a tubal pregnancy.

4. *Cervical* implantation (rare) is suggested by a greatly enlarged cervix (often as large as the nonpregnant uterus, known as the "hourglass sign"). This is an enlarged, highly vascularized, bleeding cervix, with tight internal os and a gaping external os.

5. *Uterine* ectopic gestations (rare) may occur with implantation in the cornua, a uterine diverticulum, uterine sacculation, rudimentary horn, or the muscular wall (intramural).

6. *Combined* intrauterine pregnancy (heterotopic). This occurs in 1/17,000–30,000 pregnancies.

7. Other rare possibilities include *intraligamentous*. Pregnancy even follows hysterectomy.

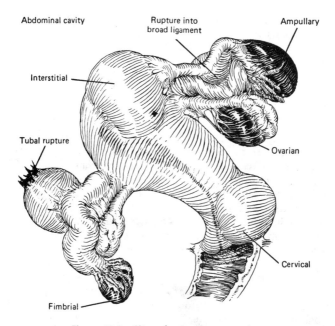

Figure 10-3. Sites of ectopic pregnancies.

Findings at Diagnosis

Unruptured ectopic gestation is characterized by brief amenorrhea, unilateral adnexal tenderness, and fullness. Before the advent of high-resolution ultrasound, <2% of ectopic pregnancies were unruptured when discovered. However, almost 50% are now diagnosed at this stage.

Sharp unilateral lower abdominal or pelvic pain or both (and possible backache) after brief amenorrhea and irregular bleeding are the usual complaints with an *acute* (rupturing or recently ruptured) *ectopic gestation*. Some 70% will have a tender pelvic mass. Scant, persistent uterine bleeding will be noted in about 80%. Collapse and shock (from bleeding), often precipitated by a vaginal examination, occur in at least 10%. A history of abnormal menses or infertility will be recorded in about 60% of these patients.

Chronic ectopic gestation (now unusual). Pelvic discomfort is variable. Expect an adnexal or cul-de-sac mass. This eventually may become crepitant. A bluish discoloration in or about the umbilicus (Cullen's sign of hematoperitoneum) may appear in neglected cases. By this time, the pregnancy usually is over, but pain persists and infection may intervene.

PATHOLOGIC PHYSIOLOGY

Whereas the usual early signs of pregnancy are noted in the cervix, the uterus becomes minimally enlarged and slightly softened with an ectopic gestation. The endometrium contains decidua (but no trophoblast) and has a characteristic microscopic appearance termed the "Arias-Stella reaction."

In ectopic gestation, the corpus luteum of pregnancy functions as long as the trophoblast remains viable. Amenorrhea results from trophoblast production of hCG and corpus luteum secretion of progesterone. Slight endometrial bleeding generally occurs, presumably with abnormal hormonal patterns, following a variable interval of amenorrhea. Endometrial separation and bleeding occur when the trophoblast is withdrawn (e.g., with rupture). Only in uncommon interstitial pregnancy does blood from the tube drain via the uterus into the vagina.

Lower abdominal, pelvic, or low back pain may be secondary to tubal distention or rupture. Isthmic pregnancy usually ruptures in about 6 weeks, and hemorrhage due to ampullary pregnancy occurs at 8–12 weeks. Cornual pregnancies are most commonly carried to the second trimester before rupture. Intraabdominal pregnancy may terminate anytime with bleeding. A pelvic mass is caused by enlargement of the conceptus, hematoma formation, bowel distortion by adhesions, or infection. If the fetus dies without extensive bleeding, it may become infected, mummified, calcified (lithopedian), or an adipocere (fatty replacement).

CLINICAL FINDINGS

No specific symptoms are diagnostic of ectopic pregnancy. However, as indicated in the percentages of findings in a proven series, the symptomatology is strongly suggestive: secondary amenorrhea of <2 week duration (68%), abnormal uterine bleeding (75%), and unilateral lower abdominal or pelvic pain (99%). The most consistent sign is adnexal tenderness (96%), and unilateral tenderness on turning the patient (positive Adler sign) is inconsistent but important if present.

Culdocentesis (transvaginal passage of a needle into the cul-de-sac) is useful for the determination of free blood in the abdominal cavity. Grasp the posterior lip of the cervix with an Allis clamp or tenaculum and cleanse the vagina (e.g., with povidone-iodine). Infiltrate local anesthetic into the vaginal wall between the uterosacral ligaments. Pass an 18-gauge spinal needle (attached to a 10 ml syringe) 1–4 mm into the cul-de-sac while exerting gentle countertraction on the cervix.

Blood recovered by culdocentesis is evidence of hematoperitoneum if the blood does not clot (having already clotted and partially liquefied in 95% of ruptured ectopic gestations), RBC rouleaux are absent, and the RBCs are crenated.

Laparoscopy usually is diagnostic in early and unruptured ectopic pregnancy. However, if culdocentesis reveals free intraperitoneal blood and the patient is a surgical emergency, laparoscopy will unduly delay therapy. Proceed to laparotomy.

LABORATORY FINDINGS

An indirect but very accurate diagnosis of ectopic pregnancy may be achieved by using a *correlation of high-resolution ultrasonography and quantitative RIA of serum hCG*. Specifically, if the hCG is >6500 IU/ml and no uterine gestational sac is evident, the patient must be presumed to have an ectopic pregnancy, and laparoscopy is indicated. If the hCG level is <6000 IU/ml, abdominal ultrasonography usually will not (<15%) reveal the ectopic gestational sac.

The enhanced resolution afforded by higher-frequency transvaginal ultrasonography (especially if repeated in ~3 days when the first is not diagnostic) offers a sensitivity approaching 100% and a specificity of ~98%. The positive predictive value approaches 98%, and the negative predictive value is ~100%.

The serum hCG increases less rapidly in most ectopic pregnancies than in normal pregnancies (when it should double every 2–4 days). However, if the hCG level rises 70%–100% in 48 h and no intrauterine sac can be seen, ectopic pregnancy is probable.

DIFFERENTIAL DIAGNOSIS

Conditions clinically similar to ectopic pregnancy include appendicitis, salpingitis, ruptured corpus luteum cyst, ruptured ovarian follicle, abortion, ovarian torsion, and urinary tract infection (Table 10-2, pp. 306–307).

COMPLICATIONS

Without surgical intervention, a ruptured ectopic pregnancy may cause *life-threatening hemorrhage* ($\geq 0.1\%$ results in maternal death). *Infection* often follows neglected ruptured ectopic pregnancy. *Sterility or other reproductive failure* may occur after or as a result of ectopic pregnancy (in 30%–50% of patients who have had surgical removal of a tube for an ectopic gestation). Obstruction and fistulas may develop after hematoperitoneum, peritonitis, or lithopedian formation. Rh immune globulin administration prevents Rh isoimmunization (see p. 311).

PREVENTION

1. Properly treat salpingitis.
2. Completely remove products of conception (D & C) in incomplete abortion.
3. Peritonealize all areas at surgery (to avoid adhesions).

TREATMENT

Nearly 20% of ectopic gestations occur as surgical emergencies. Operate immediately on diagnosis. Delay is justified only to correct shock.

A. *Emergency treatment*

1. Hospitalize the patient.
2. Insert a large-bore IV into a large vein.
3. Obtain hemogram, clotting panel, and blood for type and crossmatch.
4. Administer antishock measures as indicated: IV crystalloids, blood component transfusion, keep the patient comfortably warm, give oxygen, and apply MAST compression trousers or moderately snug tourniquets around the upper legs.

B. *Surgical treatment* (either laparoscopy or laparotomy)

1. Choice of procedure depends on surgical judgment. Laparotomy is the best procedure for the patient with a surgical

emergency. Currently, laparoscopy with antimesenteric linear salpingostomy (preferably by laser) is being used increasingly for unruptured ectopic pregnancies and nonemergency situations. As the diagnostic capability of ultrasound increases, laparoscopy is less necessary for diagnosis but is assuming greater importance in therapy.

2. Control hemorrhage (blood and clots need not be completely removed; they will be absorbed and limit anemia, or the filtered citrated blood may be used for autotransfusion).

3. Remove the products of conception (secondary implantation may occur with incomplete removal).

4. Preserve normal or minimally damaged tubes or other organs. If the pregnancy is early or if tubal missed abortion has occurred, perform salpingostomy to enucleate the pregnancy and preserve the tube. Ligate bleeding points. Suture closure is not necessary.

5. Indications for organ removal include

a. Uncontrollable hemorrhage.

b. Severely damaged tube (requires cornual excision—not resection—to prevent repeat ectopic pregnancy and endosalpingosis of the stump).

c. Hysterectomy is usually required in ruptured interstitial or cervical pregnancy.

d. Oophorectomy is necessary in ovarian pregnancy but is not recommended in cases where tubal removal is required.

C. *Supportive treatment*

1. Give broad-spectrum antibiotics for infection.

2. Prescribe oral or IM iron therapy or both to replenish iron stores.

D. *Medical therapy*

Currently, methotrexate (intraamniotic or systemic with leucovorin) for the treatment of certain unruptured ectopic gestations is being investigated. This is not yet recommended for general use, but it may be useful in certain circumstances (e.g., cervical pregnancy). Injection inactivation of the corpus luteum also is being studied.

PROGNOSIS

Ectopic pregnancy is a life-threatening disorder in >10% of cases, and >1% of these patients die of internal hemorrhage and shock or of later complications. Survival of the fetus in extrauterine pregnancy is exceptional.

Table 10-2 Differential diagnosis of ectopic pregnancy

	Ectopic pregnancy	Appendicitis	Salpingitis	Ruptured corpus luteum cyst	Uterine abortion
Pain	Unilateral cramps and tenderness before rupture	Epigastric, periumbilical, then right lower quadrant pain; tenderness localizing at McBurney's point; rebound tenderness	Usually in both lower quadrants, with or without rebound	Unilateral, becoming general with progressive bleeding	Midline cramps
Nausea and vomiting	Occasionally before, frequently after rupture	Usual, precedes shift of pain to right lower quadrant	Infrequent	Rare	Almost never
Menstruation	Some aberration: missed period, spotting	Unrelated to menses	Hypermenorrhea or metrorrhagia, or both	Period delayed, then bleeding, often with pain	Amenorrhea, then spotting, then brisk bleeding

Temperature and pulse	37.2–37.8°C (99–100°F); pulse variable: normal before, rapid after rupture	37.2–37.8°C (99–100°F); pulse rapid: 99–100	37.2–40°C (99–104°F); pulse elevated in proportion to fever	Not over 37.2°C (99°F); pulse normal unless blood loss marked, then rapid	To 37.2°C (99°F) if spontaneous; to 40°C (104°F) if infected
Pelvic examination	Unilateral tenderness, especially on movement of cervix; crepitant mass on one side or in cul-de-sac	No masses	Bilateral tenderness on movement of cervix; masses only when pyosalpinx or hydrosalpinx is present	Tenderness over affected ovary; no masses	Cervix slightly patulous; uterus slightly enlarged, irregularly softened; tender with infection
Laboratory findings	White cell count to 15,000/µl; red cell count strikingly low if blood loss large; sedimentation rate slightly elevated	White cell count 10,000–18,000/µl (rarely normal); red cell count normal; sedimentation rate slightly elevated	White cell count 15,000–30,000/µl; red cell count normal; sedimentation rate markedly elevated	White cell count normal to 10,000/µl; red cell count normal; sedimentation rate normal	White cell count 15,000/µl if spontaneous; to 30,000/µl if induced (infection); red cell count normal; sedimentation rate slightly to moderately elevated

Ectopic pregnancy *recurs in about 15%* of cases, but most patients who have had one ectopic pregnancy later have normal pregnancies.

In combined extrauterine and intrauterine pregnancy, one or the other usually is diagnosed—rarely both. Generally, the extrauterine pregnancy succumbs, and 60% of the intrauterine pregnancies go on to viability.

ISOIMMUNIZATION

Isoimmunization is the *development of antibodies against the antigens of a genetically dissimilar individual.* Antigens may be transferred by exposure to blood products or by mingling of fetal blood with the maternal blood. The latter occurs throughout pregnancy but usually reaches levels sufficient to provoke a response in late gestation or during delivery. Once the mother is immunized, even minute amounts of subsequent antigen act as a stimulus, causing a rise in maternal antibody production.

When the mother becomes sensitized, a variety of antigens are produced. The gamma globulin antibodies (IgG) can cross the placenta and destroy fetal RBCs. If the fetal hematopoietic system is not able to compensate for the RBC destruction, hemolytic anemia occurs. The increased destruction of RBC results in heme as well as increased levels of unconjugated bilirubin. Both heme and unconjugated bilirubin are neurotoxic. In utero these are efficiently transferred across the placenta. However, when the cord is severed, the immature liver cannot conjugate bilirubin efficiently (due to low levels of glucuronyltransferase), and hyperbilirubinemia develops. Jaundice ensues, and as bilirubin and heme accumulate in the plasma, bilirubin may cross the blood–brain barrier to be deposited in the nuclear zones of the midbrain and brainstem, causing kernicterus.

The *Rh antigen* (Rh factor) *is the most common cause of maternal isoimmunization.* Individuals who carry the Rh factor are described as Rh positive; those who lack the factor are termed Rh negative. Rh isoimmunization occurs only in the Rh-negative individual. If an Rh-negative woman is carrying an Rh-positive fetus, the stage is set for fetal isoimmune hemolytic disease.

Other blood groups causing isoimmunization with an IgG response and thus the potential for fetal hemolytic disease include (in descending order of occurrence) *Kell, Duffy, Kidd, MNS,*

Diego, and P factors. Although Lutheran and Xg groups may cause fetal hemolysis, it is usually less severe.

RH ISOIMMUNIZATION

Severe isoimmune hemolytic disease has the potential to occur in ~1/200 pregnancies in the United States. The vast majority of these are due to Rh isoimmunization. The *incidence of Rh negativity differs markedly among races:* Basques (30%–35%), other Caucasians (10%–12%), African Americans (8%), Native American (1%). The risk of isoimmunization for an Rh-positive ABO-compatible infant with an Rh-negative mother is ~16%. Of these, ~2% will occur antepartum, 7% within 6 months of delivery, and 7% early in the subsequent pregnancy. ABO incompatibility affords some protection from isoimmunization, but not enough for reliance. It is imperative that every pregnant woman be screened for her Rh status, since with the administration of immune globulin (RhIgG), kernicterus can be virtually eliminated.

Diagnosis

1. Screen all pregnant women (including those who have aborted or have ectopic pregnancy) for ABO type, Rh, and other pertinent antibodies (e.g., Hemantigen screen).
2. If the woman is Rh-negative and unsensitized
a. Test the husband for ABO and Rh.
b. Repeat the antibody screen at 28 and 35 weeks.
c. Administer prophylactic RhIgG.
3. If the mother is sensitized
a. Serial dilutions of the indirect Coombs' test are a guide to the maternal response but do not correlate well with the fetal status. Any dilution of ≥1:8 must be investigated by amniotic fluid analysis. Positive tests of lesser dilutions warrant a repeat study in ~2 weeks.
b. Spectrophotometric analysis of the amniotic fluid will determine the relative degree of fetal jeopardy (Fig. 10-4). This should start at 16–18 weeks.
c. Serial fetal ultrasonography (start at 14–16 weeks) is used to determine normal growth as well as presence of ascites or hydramnios.
4. Investigate for fetomaternal hemorrhage

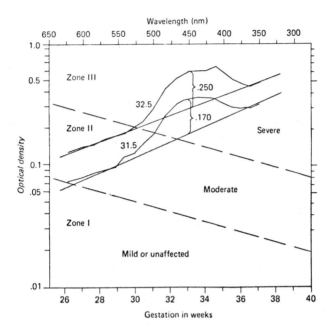

Figure 10-4. Transabdominal amniocentesis: spectrophotometric analysis of amniotic fluid surrounding an erythroblastotic fetus. Amniocentesis was performed at $31\frac{1}{2}$ and $32\frac{1}{2}$ weeks. The spectral absorption curve was obtained by plotting the optical densities at various wavelengths on 2-cycle semilogarithmic graph paper. A tangential line joining the lowest portions of this curve approximates the values for unstained amniotic fluid and is the baseline for calculations. The difference between the involved and uninvolved curves is measured at 450 nm (the wavelength at which maximum absorption by bilirubin or bilirubin-like products occurs) and plotted at the appropriate number of weeks of gestation (dotted line). The case illustrated shows rapid progression from moderate to severe disease. Under such conditions, fetal death often is imminent. Immediate delivery usually is necessary if the gestational age will permit. Otherwise, intrauterine fetal transfusion may be considered. (From S.G. Babson and R.C. Benson, *Clinical Perinatology.* Mosby, 1971.)

a. Determine significant blood loss by newborn hematocrit or hemoglobin determination or both.

b. Ascertain the presence of fetal hemoglobin in the maternal circulation (e.g., Kleihauer-Betke, hemoglobin electrophoresis).

Prevention

All of the *following information pertains to Rh-negative pregnancies* because immune globulins are not available for the other blood group isoimmune hemolytic disorders.

1. *Abortion.* Approximately 2% of spontaneous abortions and 4%–5% of induced abortions will undergo isoimmunization. Spontaneous early first trimester abortions may be treated adequately with 50 μg RhIgG, However, later abortions and induced abortions require the usual dose (300 μg).

2. *Amniocentesis.* There is an 11% chance of sensitization if the needle enters the placenta. Administer 300 μg of RhIgG after amniocentesis in the unsensitized patient.

3. *Routine prophylaxis.* In the unsensitized, Rh-negative woman with a negative antibody screen, 300 μg of RhIgG should be administered at 28 weeks. This confers relative protection for ~12 weeks and substantially reduces the chance of becoming sensitized before delivery. The 28 week prophylaxis does not alter the delivery plan. However, if the pregnancy goes beyond 40 weeks, it may be prudent to administer antepartum prophylactic RhIgG again.

4. *Antepartum hemorrhage.* Patients with placenta previa or abruptio placentae who do not deliver immediately should receive 300 μg of RhIgG. If the pregnancy is carried 12 weeks from the time of the first administration, another prophylactic dose is recommended.

5. *Abdominal trauma.* Auto accidents, physical assault involving the abdomen, or external version may result in the release of fetal RBC into the maternal circulation. Hence, to prevent isoimmunization, 300 μg of RhIgG is recommended after the incident.

6. *Fetal death.* In cases of fetal death, there is often loss of fetal RBCs into the maternal circulation and occasionally fetomaternal exsanguination. Thus, investigation for fetal hemorrhage and dose-specific RhIgG (minimally 300 μg) are both necessary.

7. *Delivery.* If the infant of an Rh-negative woman is Rh-positive or Du-positive, administer 300 μg of RhIgG within 72 h.

8. *Fetomaternal hemorrhage.* Fetomaternal hemorrhage may result with multiple gestation, manual removal of the placenta,

cesarean section with placental incision, precipitous delivery, tetanic labor, abruptio placentae, and placenta previa. When the approximate amount of fetal blood has been ascertained, the amount of RhIgG to be administered is based on 25 μg/ml of fetal blood.

Treatment and Prognosis

1. *Mildly affected fetus* (Liley zone 1). Continue ultrasonic monitoring every 2 weeks, repeat amniocentesis in 2–3 weeks, and plan for delivery at term or with fetal pulmonary maturity. Testing for fetal well-being may be desirable. In summary, intervention is usually not necessary, and only minimal neonatal treatment leads to a good prognosis.

2. *Moderately affected fetus* (lower Liley zone 2). Continue ultrasonic monitoring and add weekly biophysical profile testing. Repeat amniocentesis every 1–2 weeks. Deliver before term as soon as pulmonary maturity is compatible with survival. If delivery is necessary before pulmonary maturity, administer betamethasone within 48 h before delivery. In summary, careful monitoring is necessary to determine that the fetus is not worsening. If the fetus remains in lower zone 2, usually only early delivery and neonatal therapy are necessary for a satisfactory prognosis.

3. *Severely affected fetus* (upper Liley zone 2 and zone 3). Intervention generally is necessary for the fetus to reach a gestational age when delivery and extrauterine risks are less than risks of in utero therapy. Weekly or more frequent ultrasonic scans and tests of fetal well-being are necessary. Amniocentesis is done approximately weekly to determine fetal status and pulmonary maturity. Intrauterine transfusion, using O-negative, low-titer, glycerolized RBC may be required to save the immature, severely anemic fetus. Although this procedure is beyond the scope of this text, it may be accomplished safely by ultrasonically guided intravascular transfusion. Once started, repeated in utero transfusion is necessary because fetal hematopoiesis decreases or ceases. In summary, with this poor prognostic situation, direct intervention is usually necessary to save the perinate's life.

ABO Hemolytic Disease

Potential maternal–infant ABO incompatibility occurs in 20%–25% of pregnancies but *causes a recognizable neonatal problem in only 10% of those at risk.* Moreover, the problem nearly always affects A (especially A1) or B infants of group O mothers, and 40%–50% of cases occur in the firstborn (vs 1%–2% of Rh problems). The maternal antibodies are variable, and the neonatal direct Coombs' test may be either positive or negative. Although ABO isoimmunization produces an IgG response, for unknown reasons, it generally causes a much milder hemolytic disease. Serious fetal anemia is rare, and such sequelae as stillbirth or hydrops almost never occur.

Characteristically, during the first day after birth, the neonate with ABO hemolytic disease shows the onset of indirect hyperbilirubinemia. The neonate may have hepatosplenomegaly. Usually, management requires only bilirubin surveillance and phototherapy (~10% of cases), although occasionally (~1%), exchange transfusion is necessary. Serious sequelae are rare.

Chapter 11

Late Pregnancy Complications

THIRD TRIMESTER HEMORRHAGE

DEFINITION AND ETIOLOGY

The only bleeding that normally occurs during late pregnancy is a very small amount (<15 ml) with loss of the mucous plug prior to delivery. All other bleeding is abnormal and merits investigation. A useful list of the causes of third trimester bleeding is demonstrated in Table 11-1.

One must *distinguish between obstetric and nonobstetric bleeding* (the two major classifications). Nonobstetric causes are much less common in pregnancy and generally are less hazardous.

Of the obstetric causes, various forms of *placental bleeding* account for the vast majority. The most frequent are *placenta previa* or *premature separation* of a normally implanted placenta. *Rupture of the uterus,* rare without previous uterine surgery, occurs in about 1% of patients previously delivered by cesarean section. Uterine rupture may cause vaginal bleeding, but most of the loss will be concealed. *Nonplacental bleeding,* rare during pregnancy, may be due to *blood dyscrasia* or *lower genital tract disorders* (e.g., cervical or vaginal infections, neoplasms, or varices). Generally, the bleeding is slight, even with carcinoma of the cervix.

INCIDENCE AND IMPORTANCE

Significant vaginal bleeding occurs in 5%–10% of late pregnancies and must be carefully evaluated because *obstetric hemorrhage is the largest cause of maternal morbidity* and mortality.

Table 11-1. Etiologic classification of third trimester bleeding

Risk	Causes	
	Obstetric	Nonobstetric
High	Placenta previa	Coagulopathies
	Abruptio placentae	Cervicouterine neoplasms
	Uterine rupture	Lower genital malignancies
	Vasa previa with fetal bleeding	
Moderate	Circumvallate placenta	Vaginal varices
	Marginal sinus rupture	Vaginal lacerations
Low	Cervical mucous extru-sion (bloody show)	Cervicitis, eversion, erosion, polyps

Additionally, *it is a significant factor in perinatal morbidity and mortality.* Most patients have <500 ml bleeding, but serious hemorrhage >500 ml will occur in 2%–3% of pregnancies. Overall, multiparas are more commonly affected.

DIAGNOSIS OF THE CAUSE OF BLEEDING

Initial Examination

There are three principles of investigation of third trimester hemorrhage.

1. Because of the extreme hazard of uncontrollable bleeding with placenta previa, vaginal or rectal examination must be avoided until that diagnosis can be excluded.

2. All third trimester vaginal bleeding must be investigated in a hospital with the capability of dealing with maternal hemorrhage and perinatal compromise.

3. Immediate assessment of blood loss and hemodynamic status guides the earliest stage of therapy. Recall that the signs and symptoms of hypovolemic shock include pallor with clammy skin, orthostatic hypotension, syncope, thirst, dyspnea, restlessness, agitation, anxiety, confusion, declining blood pressure, tachycardia, and oliguria.

Critical Hemorrhage (Hemodynamically Unstable Patients)

A. Institute antishock therapy immediately.

1. Place patient in the Trendelenburg position (not steep or respiration will be compromised).

2. *Guarantee an adequate airway* (i.e., a plastic oral airway).

3. Insert large-bore (≥18 gauge) IV for *crystalloid replacement* (saline or lactated Ringer's solution).

4. *Obtain blood* from another vein for CBC, platelets, fibrinogen, PT and PTT, fibrin split products, type and crossmatch for 4–6 units of whole blood or packed red blood cells. In severe cases, also consider obtaining fresh frozen plasma, platelet packs, electrolytes, and blood gases.

5. *Consider the necessity of hemodynamic monitoring.*

6. Decide if *vasoactive drugs* are desirable for their pharmacologic effects (e.g., increasing myocardial contractility), or if volume expansion is ineffective. Use dopamine 200 mg in 500 dl saline at 2–5 μg/kg/min increasing to 20–50 μg/kg/min.

B. Insert an *indwelling Foley catheter to measure urinary output* and obtain details of the acute episode.

C. Use the *clot fragility observation test* if serial determinations of fibrinogen levels are not immediately available.

1. Draw venous blood (2–3 ml) into a clean test tube q1h.

2. If clot formation fails to occur within 5–10 min or if dissolution of a formed clot follows gentle shaking, a clotting deficiency due primarily to lack of fibrinogen and platelets is likely.

D. *Examine the abdomen gently.*

1. Measure fundus or mark the uterine apex.

2. Take and record the fetal heart rate frequently and initiate electronic fetal monitoring if available.

3. Determine uterine tone, fetal presentation, and possible engagement of the presenting part (engagement largely excludes total placenta previa).

E. *Decide* whether the patient must be taken to surgery immediately or if blood transfusions and stabilization must be accomplished first.

F. *Ready the patient for surgery* (prepare abdomen, obtain informed consent, notify the operating room, anesthesia department, and neonatal–pediatrics).

G. Continue measuring *vital signs and FHR* every 2–15 min depending on status.

H. *Effect delivery and control of hemorrhage* as soon as practical.

Less Than Critical Hemorrhage (Hemodynamically Stable Patients)

A. Place the patient at *bedrest.*

B. Obtain a *history* of the acute episode and the obstetric history and ascertain the patient's *vital signs.*

C. Do a gentle *abdominal examination.*

1. Measure the fundus or mark the apex.

2. Ascertain the fetal heart rate and initiate electronic fetal monitoring if available. Otherwise, take and record the FHR frequently.

3. Determine uterine tone, uterine irritability, fetal presentation, and the likely station of the presenting part.

D. Start large-bore (≥ 18 gauge) IV and begin *crystalloid maintenance replacement* (saline or lactated Ringer's solution).

E. Obtain blood for CBC, platelets, fibrinogen, PT and PTT, fibrin split products, type and crossmatch for 2–4 units of whole blood or packed red blood cells from another vein.

F. Consider a gentle *vaginal examination,* which is indicated before ultrasonic examination only if

1. Delivery may be imminent,

2. The presenting part is unquestionably engaged,

3. The patient is in active labor.

G. If vaginal delivery is not imminent, *perform an ultrasound examination for placental location* (possible placenta previa) and status (perhaps abruptio placentae). Additionally, the ultrasound examination should include assessment of fetal well-being, estimation of gestational age, and amount and localization of amniotic fluid.

H. In cases of borderline maturity when a few days delay (if possible) may mean the avoidance of respiratory distress, *amniocentesis and subsequent fetal maturity determination* may be useful.

I. *Determine which* of the three *general management options* is most desirable based on the maternal status, fetal status, and probable cause of the bleeding.

1. *Immediate delivery* is indicated when there is fetal or maternal compromise, or persistent heavy bleeding.

2. *Continued labor* is warranted with a mature fetus, active labor (>4 cm), ruptured membranes, bleeding at a controllable rate, or if there are additional complications making vaginal delivery desirable.

3. *Expectant management* is possible in almost 90% of cases, because third trimester bleeding will usually subside within 24 h.

a. Save all pads so that a reasonably accurate estimate of blood loss can be made.

b. Observe the patient carefully for 24 h. If bleeding materially decreases or ceases, and she is not near term, she may be transferred for less intensive observation.

c. If placenta previa has been excluded, perform a gentle cervical visualization and pelvic examination to ascertain the cause of bleeding.

ABRUPTIO PLACENTAE
(Premature Separation of the Placenta, Ablatio Placentae, Accidental Hemorrhage)

DEFINITIONS AND INCIDENCE

Abruptio placentae is defined as *placental separation from a normal implantation site before delivery of the fetus.* It occurs in 1:86 to 1:206 advanced pregnancies, depending on the diagnostic criteria employed and *is responsible for ~30% of all late antepartal bleeding.* About 50% of abruptions occur before labor, but 10%–15% are not diagnosed before the second stage of labor. Abruptio placentae may be classified into three groups by clinical and laboratory findings (Table 11-2).

ETIOLOGY AND IMPORTANCE

The exact *cause* of placental separation *is usually unknown,* although there are a number of common associations. A *previous placental separation* carries a recurrence rate of 10%–17%; following two previous separations, the incidence is >20%. The *hypertensive states of pregnancy* impose a 2.5%–17.9% incidence of abruptio placentae. However, of those cases severe enough to cause fetal demise, ~50% are associated with *hypertensive states of pregnancy* (with one half associated with chronic hypertension and one half associated with pregnancy-induced hypertension). Other frequent predispositions to placental separation include *smoking, uterine overdistention* (e.g., multiple pregnancy, hydramnios), *vascular disease* (e.g., diabetes mellitus, collagen disorders), *microangiopathic hemolytic anemia,* and *uterine anomalies or tumors.* There are direct precipitating causes (in only 1%–5%) of abruptio placentae, including circumvallate placenta, direct uterine trauma (e.g., external version, automobile and other accidents), sudden reduction of amniotic fluid, or short cord.

Table 11-2. Grades of abruptio placentae

Clinical finding	Grade		
	1	2	3
Vaginal bleeding	Slight	Mild to moderate	Moderate to severe, (but may be concealed)
Uterus	Irritable	Irritable, tetanic	Tetanic, painful
Maternal pulse	Normal	Increased	Elevated
Maternal blood pressure	Normal	Maintained, but postural hypotension	Hypotension to shock
Fetal status	Normal	Fetal distress (FHR criteria)	Fetal death
Fibrinogen level	Normal	Reduced (150–250 mg%)	<150 mg% and thrombocytopenia or factor depletion
% of total (approximate)	15	20–40	>45

DIAGNOSIS

The symptoms and signs are variable and are largely predicated on the extent of the problem (Table 11-2). However, the usual *symptoms* of abruptio placentae are *dark red vaginal bleeding* (80%), *uterine irritability* (two thirds), and *lower abdominal or back pain* (two thirds). The erroneous diagnosis of premature labor will be assigned to about 20%. *Fetal distress is present in >50%* of cases.

Because of the protective factors in healthy gravidas, there may be a considerable acute blood loss before anemia develops. Thus, with abruptio placentae, the amount of blood loss is all too frequently out of proportion to the degree of anemia. A peripheral blood smear may reveal schistocytes (suggesting disseminated intravascular coagulation, DIC). Reduced platelet counts and fibrinogen depletion are common in more severe cases. With DIC, elevated levels of fibrin split products will be present.

PATHOLOGY AND PATHOPHYSIOLOGY

Various pathophysiologic mechanisms have been suggested as being operative in abruptio placentae, including *local vascular injury* leading to decidua basalis vessel disruption, an *abrupt rise in uterine venous pressure* leading to intervillous space engorgement and separation, *mechanical factors* (e.g., short cord, trauma, sudden loss of amniotic fluid), and *possible extrinsic initiation of the coagulation cascade* (e.g., trauma with the release of tissue thromboplastin).

Hemorrhage may occur into the decidua basalis or directly retroplacental, from rupture of a spiral artery. In either case, bleeding occurs, a clot forms, and the placental surface cannot provide exchange between mother and placenta. The clot compresses the adjacent placenta, and nonclotted blood courses from the site. In either concealed or external (apparent) bleeding (Fig. 11-1), blood may rupture through the membranes or placenta. The latter has grave significance, for it may lead to maternal–fetal hemorrhage, fetomaternal hemorrhage, maternal bleeding into the amniotic fluid, or amniotic fluid embolus. Occasionally, extensive intramyometrial hemorrhage leads to a purplish, ecchymotic, and indurated uterus (uteroplacental apoplexy, Couvelaire uterus) and loss of contractility.

With severe placental separation there may be DIC. Clinically, the hemorrhagic diathesis consists of widespread petechiae, active bleeding, hypovolemic shock, and failure of the clotting mechanisms. Although not directly observable, fibrin is being deposited in small capillaries, resulting in dire complications, for example: renal cortical and tubular necrosis, acute cor pulmonale, and anterior pituitary necrosis (Sheehan's syndrome).

DIFFERENTIAL DIAGNOSIS

A. *Nonplacental causes of bleeding.* These usually are nonpainful. Rupture of the uterus may cause vaginal bleeding but, if extensive, is associated with pain, shock, and death of the fetus.

B. *Placental causes of bleeding.* Placenta previa is associated with painless hemorrhage and is commonly diagnosed by ultrasonography.

C. *Undetermined causes of bleeding.* In at least 20% of cases, the cause of antepartum bleeding cannot be determined. However, if serious problems can be ruled out, undiagnosed bleeding rarely is critical.

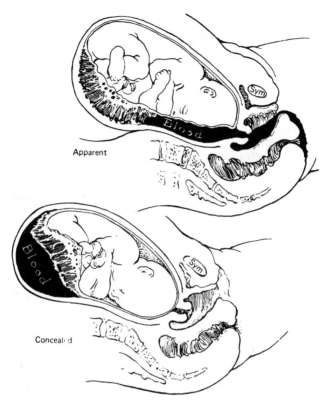

Figure 11-1. Types of premature separation of the placenta. (Redrawn from Beck and Rosenthal, *Obstetrical Practice,* 7th ed. Williams & Wilkins, 1957.)

TREATMENT

A. *Emergency measures.* If deficient, the clotting mechanism must be restored before any attempt is made to deliver the infant. Administer cryoprecipitate, fresh frozen plasma, or fresh blood. Institute antishock therapy. Monitor the fetus continuously.

Rupture the membranes, if possible, irrespective of the probable mode of delivery.

B. *Specific measures*

1. *Grade 1.* When the patient is not in labor, watchful expectancy is indicated, since bleeding ceases spontaneously in many cases. When labor begins, prepare for vaginal delivery in the absence of further complications.

2. *Grade 2.* Anticipate vaginal delivery if labor is expected within about 6 h, especially if the fetus is dead. Cesarean section should be performed if there is persistent evidence of fetal distress, and the infant is likely to survive.

3. *Grade 3.* The patient is always in shock, the fetus has died, the uterus is tetanic, and a coagulation defect may be present. After correction of the coagulopathy, deliver the patient vaginally if this can be done within about 6 h. Vaginal delivery is probably best for the multiparous patient. Otherwise, do a cesarean section.

Surgical Measures

Cesarean section is indicated when *labor is expected to be of long duration* (over 6 h), when *hemorrhage does not respond to amniotomy and* cautious administration of *dilute oxytocin,* and when *early* (not prolonged) *fetal distress is present* and the fetus is likely to survive.

Hysterectomy rarely is indicated. Even a Couvelaire uterus will contract, and bleeding will almost always cease when the coagulation defect is corrected.

PROGNOSIS

Worldwide maternal mortality rates are currently between 0.5% and 5%. Most women die of hemorrhage (immediate or delayed) or cardiac or renal failure. Early diagnosis and definitive therapy should reduce maternal mortality rates to 0.3%–1%.

Fetal mortality rates range from 50% to 80%. About 30% of patients with premature separation of the placenta are delivered at term. Almost 20% of those with abruptio placentae have no fetal heartbeat on admission to the hospital, and in another 20%, fetal distress is soon noted. When maternal transfusion is urgently required, the fetal mortality rate will probably be at least 50%.

Birth is preterm in 40%–50% of cases of premature separation of the placenta. Infants die of hypoxia, prematurity, or delivery trauma.

PLACENTA PREVIA

Placenta previa occurs when the placenta develops low, within the zone of dilatation–effacement of the lower uterine segment. Thus, the placenta precedes the fetus and can block vaginal delivery. Placenta previa complicates 1:200–1:250 pregnancies that continue beyond the 28th week.

The types of placenta previa are *complete,* in which the placenta totally covers the internal os (Fig. 11-2), *partial,* where a portion of the internal os is overlaid by the placenta (Fig. 11-3), and *low-lying,* in which the placenta is just above the os but situated where it may deflect or obstruct the presenting part, e.g., over the sacral promontory (Figs. 11-4 and 11-5).

Painless vaginal bleeding is the presenting complaint in placenta previa. Breech or an abnormal presentation is common because the forelying placenta alters the usual intrauterine space available. Even a small vertex may not engage.

DIAGNOSIS

No laboratory tests will aid in the diagnosis of placenta previa. However, blood studies, e.g., Hgb, Hct, should be obtained periodically because of blood loss and the threat of anemia. The patient should be typed and matched with blood available. X-ray and radioisotope studies to determine the site of the placenta have been abandoned in favor of safer, more accurate ultrasonography.

Ultrasonography. Ultrasonography is the modality of choice for the diagnosis of placenta previa. False negative reports of placenta previa with ultrasonography in early pregnancy are uncommon. Late in pregnancy, it may be difficult to diagnose placenta previa because the presenting part may preclude optimal visualization of the placenta and its relation to the internal cervical os. This can usually be overcome, unless engagement has occurred, by placing the patient in the Trendelenburg position and applying gentle upward traction on the presenting part.

If ultrasonography or another means of diagnosis of placenta previa is unavailable, vaginal examination may be required. In this case, arrange a double setup examination, that is, have the operating room readied for cesarean section because even slight penetration or separation of the placenta may cause hemorrhage.

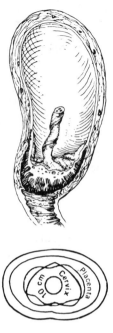

Figure 11-2. Complete placenta previa.

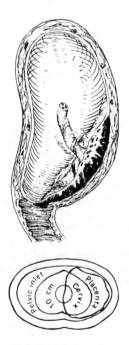

Figure 11-3. Partial placenta previa.

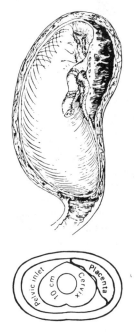

Figure 11-4. Normal placenta.

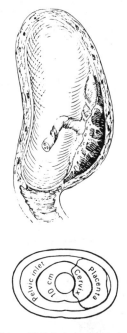

Figure 11-5. Low implantation.

DIFFERENTIAL DIAGNOSIS

Rule out local causes of painless vaginal bleeding, for example, cervical cancer or polyp, by visualization of the cervix, biopsy, or similar means. *Caution:* Do not do a pelvic examination before ultrasonography has excluded placenta previa. Exsanguinating hemorrhage may be induced by vaginal examination of the patient with placenta previa. Even after ultrasonography, penetration of the cervix may be harmful and of no value.

Slight marginal separation of the placenta, impossible to diagnose by ultrasonography or clinically, must be considered, but bleeding probably will cease after bedrest. Since blood loss may be fetal as well as maternal, all gravidas with placenta previa should have a test for fetal blood in the discharge, e.g., APT (potassium hydroxide), Kleihauer-Betke test, identification of nucleated RBC.

COMPLICATIONS

A. *Maternal.* Hemorrhage and shock may follow ill-conceived examination in lieu of ultrasonography. Slight premature separation of the portion of the placenta over the os probably occurs in most cases. Localized placentitis may develop here also. Uterine sepsis before delivery is rare, but postpartum endometritis often complicates placenta previa.

B. *Fetal.* Preterm delivery occurs in ~60% of infants of mothers with placenta previa and is the prime cause of neonatal complications. In addition to early or chronic blood loss, acute fetal bleeding may occur during cesarean section when an anterior placenta previa is torn. Entry below or above the placenta, as indicated by ultrasonography, should minimize the risk. However, the fetal blood loss is directly proportional to the time lapse between laceration of a cotyledon(s) and clamping of the cord.

TREATMENT

Usually, brief hospitalization and expectant management are essential because most gravidas are preterm and bedrest alone will be accompanied by cessation of bleeding within 24 h. The patient or her fetus almost never die during the first occurrence of bleeding (assuming no pelvic examination). Monitor the fetus carefully.

Subsequent bleeding episodes may require continued hospitalization. Delivery should be delayed, if possible, to ensure increased fetal maturity. If ultrasonography was performed before the 30th week, it should be repeated by the 32nd week to determine the placental site, fetal age, and growth.

With rupture of the membranes, labor, or if heavy bleeding occurs, expeditious delivery by the safest means will be necessary. This is necessary regardless of fetal status.

Most primigravidas with placenta previa should be delivered by cesarean section. Some multiparas with partial or low-lying placenta previa can be delivered safely from below unless hemorrhage is marked. Electronic fetal monitoring should be employed in all labors involving placenta previa.

PROGNOSIS

A. *For the mother.* With proper management, the maternal prognosis in placenta previa is excellent. With ultrasonography and expectant therapy, the maternal mortality in the United States has dropped from >1% to <0.2%.

B. *For the infant.* The perinatal mortality rate associated with placenta previa in many hospitals in the United States before expectant treatment was approximately 15% or more than 10 times that of normal term pregnancy. This has dropped, and the rate probably can be reduced to <10% with current management.

PUERPERAL SEPSIS
(See also Shock, p 330).

Any infection in the genital tract that occurs as a complication of abortion, labor, or delivery is termed puerperal sepsis. Streptococci, staphylococci, clostridia, coliform bacteria, and *Bacteroides* are the pathogens most often identified. Cellulitis resulting from vaginal or cervical lacerations may be the site of infection, as may the endometrium, particularly when endometritis occurs in the zone of placental attachment (the equivalent of a large surface wound). Debility (anemia, undernutrition), serious systemic disorders, premature or prolonged rupture of the membranes, protracted labor, and traumatic examinations or delivery predispose to puerperal infection.

The incidence of puerperal sepsis in hospitals in the United States is at least 10%. *Puerperal sepsis is exceeded only by hemorrhage and preeclampsia-eclampsia as a cause of maternal death* in this country.

Clinical Findings

Many genital tract infections are so mild as to cause few or slight symptoms. Others are violent, fulminating, and fatal within a short time.

A. *Symptoms and signs.* Malaise, headache, anorexia, and remittent slight elevations in temperature and pulse generally begin 3–4 days after delivery. Vague discomfort in the perineum or lower abdomen and nausea and vomiting may follow. High fever (childbed fever), rapid pulse, ileus, and localization of pain and tenderness in the pelvis may be observed during the next 1–2 days. The lochia may become foul and profuse. Bacteremic shock may occur. If improvement does not follow after 48–72 h of antibiotic therapy, reexamine the patient: an abscess may be forming.

B. *Laboratory findings.* Polymorphonuclear leukocytosis and an increased sedimentation rate indicate infection. Identification of pathogens from cervical and uterine lochia by culture and sensitivity tests will require 36–48 h.

C. *Ultrasonography x-ray findings.* X-ray studies are not helpful except to exclude gastrointestinal, urinary, or pulmonary problems.

Complications and Sequelae

Genital tract infections commonly progress to peritonitis, pelvic cellulitis, pelvic thrombophlebitis, abscess formation, septicemia, pulmonary embolism, septic shock, and death.

Differential Diagnosis

Febrile complications of the puerperium unrelated to genital tract infection include mastitis, urinary infection, respiratory infection, and enteritis, in that order of frequency.

PREVENTION

Avoidance of puerperal sepsis requires strict aseptic technique during manual examination and delivery. Obstetric trauma should be minimized, since traumatized tissues are susceptible to infection.

TREATMENT

A. *Emergency measures.* Treat septic shock (see p 334).

B. *General measures*

1. Place the patient in the semi-Fowler position. Order a clear liquid diet for at least several days, and administer IV fluids to maintain electrolyte and fluid balance.

2. Administer analgesics, sedative-hypnotic drugs, oxytocics, or laxatives as required.

C. *Specific measures*

1. Initially, give antibiotics in large doses. A reasonable starting antibiotic regimen is ampicillin (2 g IV every 6 h), gentamicin (2 mg/kg IV loading dose), and clindamicin (900 mg IV every 8 h). The maintenance dose of gentamicin is 1.5 mg/kg every 8 h, but peak and trough levels should be monitored. When the results of culture and sensitivity studies are known, continue therapy with the antibiotic of choice in large and repeated doses.

2. For treatment of disseminated intravascular coagulation (DIC), see p 321.

D. *Surgical measures.* Hysterectomy is indicated for serious puerperal infections, e.g., intractable myometritis, a postabortal uterine abscess, infected hydatidiform mole, or myoma. Clipping or ligation of the vena cava and ovarian veins may be life saving in case of repeated (often septic) pulmonary embolization. Pelvic drainage may be necessary. Abscesses may require surgical drainage.

PROGNOSIS

The maternal mortality rate due to puerperal sepsis in the United States is about 0.2%, but in some areas of the world, the mortality rate is vastly greater.

SHOCK

Shock is a syndrome characterized by prostration and hypotension due to diminished circulating blood volume to the point of failure of perfusion of the vital organs.

CLASSIFICATION

The shock syndromes encountered in obstetrics and gynecology may be classified clinically as follows.

1. *Hypovolemic* shock follows hemorrhage, trauma, and dehydration. It is characterized by an absolute or relative decrease in blood volume.

2. *Cardiogenic shock* may result from acute diminution of cardiac output and usually is associated with varying degrees of vasoconstriction (e.g., myocardial infarction, heart failure, paroxysmal tachycardia, myocardial depressant drugs).

3. *Septic shock* most frequently occurs following bacteremia due to gram-negative organisms and their endotoxins.

4. *Toxic shock* (see p 499) is often caused by an exotoxin produced by some coagulase-positive strains of *Staphylococcus aureus.* It is seen most often in menstruating women who use tampons and is characterized by headache, vomiting, diarrhea, fever, rash, and hypotension.

5. *Neurogenic shock,* as seen in simple fainting, spinal anesthesia, and central nervous system injury, is usually associated with peripheral vasodilation.

6. *Metabolic shock* occurs mainly in hypoadrenocorticism. Fluid, electrolyte, and other chemical abnormalities in diabetic acidosis and in acute pulmonary hepatic or renal insufficiency may impair cardiovascular mechanisms and lead to metabolic shock.

7. *Anaphylactic shock* produces marked vasodilatation with relative hypovolemia. This may be due to allergy to medications, sera, or other sensitizing agents.

8. *Drug shock* may follow excessive administration of hypnotic drugs, anesthetics, vasodilators, vasoconstrictors, and other drugs.

9. *Vascular obstructive shock* may occur as a result of blockage of major blood vessels by amniotic fluid, air, or blood clots. Supine hypotension in obstetric patients may be a contributing factor.

Clinical Findings

A. *Impending shock.* A variable period of intense sympathetic activity generally precedes hypotension. Weakness, pallor, cool, moist skin, orthostatic hypotension and tachycardia develop. (*Caution:* Do not confuse with simple fainting.) Fever and shaking chills precede collapse in septic shock. Marked orthopnea, arrhythmia, and severe chest pain are warning signs or cardiogenic shock.

B. *Established shock.* Hypotension (systolic pressure <100 mm Hg) is superimposed on the early signs of impending shock, and tachycardia (>100) usually develops. Thirst, air hunger, severe prostration, and dulling of the sensorium are advanced signs. Coma, cardiac arrest, and death are imminent at this point.

C. *Septic shock.* Chills, high fever, tachycardia, anorexia, and occasional nausea and vomiting are often preceded by a history of infected abortion, traumatic delivery, or recurrent pyelonephritis. Between 3 and 9 h after the first shaking chill, a precipitous drop in body temperature to subnormal levels often heralds shock.

Treatment

Act quickly. Shock is an acute emergency that takes precedence over all other problems except acute hemorrhage, cardiac arrest, and respiratory failure.

Determine the primary cause of shock promptly. A brief history (if available) and the gross physical findings often will permit the differentiation of hemorrhagic, cardiogenic, septic, and allergic shock. Except in neurogenic shock due to fainting—a self-limiting condition treated by placing the patient in the recumbent position and administering stimulant—proceed with antishock measures. Additional therapy may be required for specific problems.

General Measures

1. Place the patient in the recumbent position. Avoid the Trendelenburg position, since it interferes with breathing. Apply military antishock trousers (MAST suit), if available, to patients not bleeding vaginally.

2. Establish an adequate airway and ensure pulmonary ventilation. Administer oxygen by nasal catheter, mask, or endotracheal tube as required, especially when dyspnea or cyanosis is present.

3. Keep the patient comfortably warm with blankets. Do not apply external heat, since this will cause peripheral vasodilatation.

4. Control pain and relieve apprehension. Shock patients often have very little discomfort. A sedative, such as pentobarbital sodium, 0.13 g IV, may be given. (*Caution:* Narcotics are contraindicated for patients in coma, those with head injuries or respiratory depression, and pregnant women who are likely to deliver within 1–2 h.) Avoid overdosage of all drugs.

Fluid Replacement

If superficial veins have collapsed, puncture a large vein, e.g., femoral vein, for temporary infusion before cutdown or perform percutaneous canalization of a major vessel, such as the jugular vein, for infusion and another for monitoring. The latter procedure also provides a direct route for therapy to the heart in cases of extreme blood loss, septic shock, or serious electrolyte imbalance.

Restore adequate blood volume immediately. The most effective replacement fluid for blood loss is usually whole blood, especially if the hematocrit is <35%.

1. *Whole blood.* Whole blood must be correctly grouped and crossmatched for possible transfusion. Treatment in cases of shock may require 4–5 liters of whole blood delivered under pressure in 30 min to restore CVP to 10–13 cm H_2O. Use large needles and multiple infusions if transfusion is needed urgently.

2. *Plasma.* Plasma, serum albumin, and Plasmanate (a reconstituted blood product) are particularly valuable for the treatment of plasma loss. Posttransfusion hepatitis may occur in patients receiving pooled plasma; the risk is about 10%.

3. *Plasma expanders.* Dextran 40 (Rheomacrodex) is a low-molecular-weight dextran that is superior to other dextrans in reducing the viscosity of the blood and maintaining the microcirculation. Administer 1–1.5 g/kg in 10% solution in normal saline IV at a rate of 20–40 ml/min, but do not give more than required to sustain the blood pressure at 85–90 mm Hg. (*Caution:* Patients with cardiac or renal disease may develop pulmonary edema.) Since dextrans interfere with blood typing, blood samples should be obtained before dextran is administered. Dextrans can impair blood coagulation mechanisms and may cause infrequent but serious anaphylactoid reactions.

4. *Saline and dextrose solutions.* Normal saline solution, lactated Ringer's solution, or 5% dextrose may be used as initial therapy or to provide water and electrolytes. The amount necessary to correct acidosis is determined by the blood pH (normal 7.35–7.45) or serum or plasma Pco_2 (normal 24–29 mEq/L). Serial determinations of these values should guide correction.

6. *Adjustment of acid-base balance.* Restore serum sodium, calcium, chloride, etc. to normal values, using periodic blood chemistry determinations as a guide.

Vasoactive Drugs

Vasopressors have almost no place in resuscitation if the patient is in shock. The exception is cardiogenic shock, where a brief use of pressor drugs may increase myocardial contractility and thus improve cardiac function.

The vasoactive drugs should not be considered primary therapy in shock. Volume replacement, correction of hypoxia and fluid and electolyte imbalance, and a search for treatable causes should come first. Unless volume replacement is adequate, the administration of vasodilators may result in prompt failure of the circulation due to a fall in blood pressure and circulatory collapse. Vasodilators are never indicated until the vascular volume has been restored to normal and the CVP is in the high normal range. At that point, use of drugs that dilate the peripheral vasculature may decrease vascular resistance and thus decrease the work of the heart and improve cardiac output and tissue perfusion.

The drug of choice for cardiac resuscitation has been isoproterenol (Isuprel). This drug has two modes of action. It stimulates myocardial contractility and simultaneously lowers peripheral resistance. Give 1–2 mg in 500 ml of lactated Ringer's solution IV at a rate that produces optimal circulatory benefit. Because of its inotropic effect, an increased incidence of cardiac arrhythmias precludes its use if the heart rate exceeds 120/min.

Corticosteroids

Corticosteroids may be beneficial in shock because they support the patient in a serious stress state, aid in the transfer of fluids from intracellular to extracellular compartments, and, in septic shock, block intense sympathomimetic effects of endotoxin and restore vascular tone. They also have a beneficial antiallergic effect.

Treatment of Specific Types of Shock

A. *Cardiogenic shock*. Convert arrhythmias. Digitalis is used to correct myocardial insufficiency. Relieve cardiac tamponade. Administer adrenergic drugs.

B. *Anaphylactic shock*

1. Give epinephrine, 1:1000 solution, 0.1–0.4 ml in 10 ml of normal saline solution slowly IV.

2. Administer diphenhydramine hydrochloride or tripelennamine hydrochloride, 10–20 mg IV, if the response to epinephrine is not prompt and sustained.

3. Give hydrocortisone sodium succinate (Solu-Cortef), 100–250 mg IV over a period of 30 sec, as an adjunct to epinephrine and diphenhydramine. The dosage depends on the severity of the condition. The drug may be repeated at increasing intervals (1,3,6,10 h, and so on) as indicated by the clinical condition.

4. Inject aminophylline, 0.25–0.5 g in 10–20 ml of normal saline slowly IV for severe bronchial spasm. The duration of action is 1–3 h, after which the drug may be repeated.

C. *Hypovolemic shock*. Replace volume, correct hypoxia and fluid and electrolyte balance, and seek treatable causes. Monitor treatment as discussed on page 331.

D. *Septic shock*. Septic shock associated with pregnancy is most often caused by septic abortion, postpartum infections, pyelonephritis, peritonitis, ruptured viscus, and septic thrombophlebitis. During pregnancy, treat septic shock with antibiotics and volume infusion.

Initial volume infusion is accomplished with 2 liters of lactated Ringer's solution. If the systolic blood pressure remains <80 mm Hg, a pulmonary artery catheter should be inserted and volume expansion continued until the pulmonary capillary wedge pressure (PCWP) is ≥14–16 mm Hg. Should the blood pressure fail to respond to volume expansion and if the left ventricular function curve is depressed, begin inotropic therapy with dopamine and digoxin. If there is no improvement in left ventricular function curve, add dobutamine or isoproterenol or both. If the blood pressure fails to respond to this treatment (systolic ≤80 mm Hg) and the systemic vascular resistance index is ≤1500 dynes/sec/cm^{-5}/M^2, phenylephrine may be initiated. If this fails, norepinephrine may be used.

Electrolyte imbalances must be corrected, and administration of oxygen to the mother may be useful. If the site of infection is not known, initiate studies to determine the source.

Evaluation of Antishock Therapy

Observe the patient continuously for clinical and laboratory signs of responses to therapy. Tachycardia subsides, and the skin becomes warm and dry as blood pressure rises above 100 mm Hg.

1. Record blood pressure, pulse rate, and respiratory rate every 15 min.

2. Maintain a fluid intake and output chart, noting time and amount of replacement fluid given and measuring urine output every 30 min. Acute renal failure often is a sequela to deep, unresponsive, or prolonged shock.

3. Monitor PCWP response, especially to initial rapid infusion or transfusion, as a guide both to diagnosis and to subsequent treatment. Try to rapidly achieve and maintain a normal PCWP. Avoid underreplacement or overreplacement of fluids.

4. Auscultate the chest periodically for arrhythmia, rales, muffled tones (cardiac tamponade), or murmurs. Obtain an ECG and appropriate medical consultation in severe cases.

COMPLICATIONS OF LABOR

PRETERM OR PREMATURE LABOR

About 7% of infants born in the United States are preterm, i.e., <37 weeks gestational age. These may or may not be small-for-dates. Preterm labor may be associated with many disorders or diseases (Table 11-3).

Premature delivery is one of the most urgent problems in medicine. The death rate of the low-birthweight neonate is about 40 times that of full-sized infants born at term. Moreover, the association of cerebral palsy with preterm delivery may be as high as 10 times and mental deficiency 5 times that of the term neonate. Visual and hearing deficits, emotional disturbances, and social maladjustments of prematures far exceed those of mature infants.

Continuation of fetal development, in the absence of contradictions, may be imperative. For example, pulmonary matura-tion of a fetus of 24–25 weeks gestational age is so incomplete that the infant probably will die of respiratory distress syndrome or complications of prematurity. However, if the otherwise normal fetus is carried to 33 weeks in utero, it is most likely to survive.

The clinical *definition of premature labor* involves four criteria.

1. A gestation of >20 weeks but <37 weeks

Table 11-3. Conditions associated with premature labor

Primary risk factors
  Multiple gestation
  Previous preterm births
  Uterine or cervical anomalies
  Placenta previa
  Abruptio placentae
  Intrauterine growth retardation
  Premature rupture of the membranes
  Hydramnios
Secondary risk factors
  Previous pregnancy
    Multiple induced abortions
    Cervical or uterine laceration
  Current or previous pregnancy
    Severe pregnancy-induced hypertension
  Current pregnancy
    Malnutrition
    Severe anemia
    Inadequate weight gain during pregnancy
    Pulmonary or systemic hypertension
    Renal disease
    Heart disease
    Substance abuse
      Heavy cigarette smoking
      Alcohol
      Drug abuse
    Peritoneal irritation
      Adnexal torsion or leaking cysts
      Perforated peptic ulcer
      Appendicitis
      Intraabdominal procedures
    Trauma or burns
    Infections (for example)
      Pyelonephritis
      Acute systemic infections
      Fetotoxic infections

2. Regular, painful uterine contractions occurring at least twice every 10 min for at least 30 min

3. Demonstrated cervical effacement or dilatation

4. Intact membranes

Other symptoms may include vaginal bleeding, increased vaginal discharge, and vaginal pressure. Necessary assessments include ascertaining that the maternal health will tolerate therapy, that the membranes have not ruptured, that the fetus is truly premature, that fetal distress is not occurring, and that there is not an abnormal fetal presentation (as so frequently occurs with the premature infant).

The *laboratory studies* include blood for CBC with differential, serum electrolytes, and glucose, urine for analysis and culture and sensitivity, and ultrasonography for fetal size and position and placental location. Amniocentesis may be necessary in borderline cases to determine fetal maturity (LS, Pg, or RST) or to check for fetal infection (bacteria on microscopic analysis). Checking for infection is particularly important, since 7%–26% of premature labors have intrauterine infection.

The following protocol is extremely helpful in management of these patients.

A. *Observation*

1. Observation for 30–60 min with electronic fetal monitoring.

2. Confirmation that the gestational age <37 weeks.

3. Performance of examination and tests to rule out any contraindication to sedation-hydration therapy (Table 11-4). This is very important for suppression of labor in only ~25% of cases, whereas the remaining 75% have either contraindications or do not require tocolysis.

B. *Decisions* regarding the next step *in management* are based on criteria in Table 11-5.

C. *Sedation and hydration*

1. Morphine sulfate 8–12 mg IM (provided there are no allergies, delivery is not imminent, and Narcan is available).

2. Give 500 ml 5% dextrose in 0.5 normal saline (or lactated Ringer's solution 5% dextrose) IV over 30 min.

3. Continue observation of the patient for 1 h, with continuous fetal monitoring.

D. At the end of 1 h, *decisions* are made into which of three *therapy* categories the patient is placed.

1. Cervical effacement and dilatation are progressing. Proceed to first-line tocolytics. Generally, this is only a small percentage of patients.

2. There is no cervical change, but uterine contractions continue. This group should also be placed on first-line tocolytics. This group is usually less than half of the patients, and even if

Table 11-4. Relative contraindications to labor suppression

Mature fetus
Probable lethal fetal defects
Fetal death
Fetal distress (including that occurring with tocolysis)
Chorioamnionitis
Ruptured membranes
Bulging membranes
Cervical dilation of >4 cm and effacement >80%
Polyhydramnios
Erythroblastosis fetalis
Severe intrauterine growth retardation
Severe pregnancy-induced hypertension
Maternal pulmonary or cardiac disease (e.g., pulmonary edema, adult respiratory distress syndrome, cardiac failure)
Maternal hemorrhage (e.g., placenta previa, abruptio placentae, DIC)

---

suppression is currently successful, they still have a risk of subsequent labor and delivery.

3. Uterine contractions cease and there is no cervical change. Observation should continue for 6–12 h. More than half of patients will be in this group, and here, too, there is a continued risk of labor and delivery, but the majority of these patients may be monitored by an outpatient regimen.

E. *Before the use of tocolytic drugs,* begin serial measurement of blood pressure and pulse rate. Obtain baseline ECG and establish a fluid intake and output chart. Continue to monitor the FHR electronically.

F. *Tocolytics*

1. Magnesium sulfate, the safest tocolytic, may be given in a 4–6 g bolus IV over 10 min, followed by an IV infusion of 2 g/h for 6–8 h. Additional fluids should be given by mouth. Monitor vital signs and ECG closely (q30–60 min), and closely watch the deep tendon reflexes and urinary output. Diminution or absence of either indicates the possibility of overdosage. With this program, other serious adverse effects of magnesium administration, e.g., hypotension, sinoatrial or atrioventricular block, or cardiac arrest, are exceptional. However, each time blood is drawn for a magnesium level (q6h), a calcium level also should be determined to ascertain that acute hypocalcemia

Table 11-5. Diagnosis and management of preterm labor based on observation of uterine contractions and cervical change

Uterine contractions	Cervical effacement and dilatation	Diagnosis	Management
No	No	No labor	None
Yes	No	Premature labor	Hydration and sedation
No	Yes	Incompetent cervix	Bedrest, cerclage
Yes	Yes	Premature labor	Tocolytic protocol

has not occurred. The fetus should be minimally affected by this regimen.

Calcium is the antidote for magnesium overdosage and should be administered IV (10 ml of a 10% calcium solution) if magnesium overdosage occurs.

2. Ritodrine is a more effective tocolytic than magnesium sulfate and is FDA approved for tocolysis. Prepare Ritodrine by dissolving 150 mg in 5% dextrose water. This IV solution will yield 0.3 mg/ml. Begin with 0.1 mg/min, gradually increasing by 0.05 mg/min every 10 min until satisfactory uterine inhibition has been achieved. The maximum IV dosage, established mainly by tachycardia, is about 400 mg/min. Ritodrine IV should be continued at effective dosage for at least 2 h after cessation of contractions. Then, it should be slowly reduced over 1–2 h. The maintenance dose of Ritodrine is 20–30 mg orally bid, for weeks if necessary.

Adverse reactions, all dose-related, include hyperglycemia, hypoinsulinemia, and hyperkalemia. Pulmonary edema may occur if Ritodrine is given IV in saline solution, especially with excessive drug dosage or prolonged treatment, or when overhydration occurs or in the presence of infection. Unpleasant cardiovascular, gastrointestinal, or neurologic side affects must be expected, but these usually are mild. Fetal tachycardia may occur with any beta-adrenergic drug therapy. However, with proper selection of patients, correct dosage, and cautiously maintained tocolysis, there should be no harm to the infant.

3. The use of oral or subcutaneous terbutaline has not been cleared for tocolysis by the FDA.

PROLONGED PREGNANCY (POSTDATES)

There is no accurate end point of pregnancy. However, *prolonged pregnancy is defined as one that has continued for ≥ 294 days,* or 14 days beyond the EDC, as calculated from the LMP or other means (280 + 14 = 294 days, or 42 weeks.) About 5% of all pregnancies go beyond 294 days. Prolonged pregnancy may be recidive (a woman who has had one post-date pregnancy has 2 times the likelihood of another). It occurs in fetal anencephaly (due to adrenal hypoplasia and altered hormonal production) and placental sulfatase deficiency and is more prevalent in certain families. However, the cause is not determined in the vast majority.

Among postdate fetuses, 30%–40% are dysmature and are at increased perinatal risk. They may be underweight, with reduced subcutaneous fat, appear wrinkled with peeling skin, and are often meconium stained. Oligohydramnios frequently is an associated finding. These neonates may have or have had fetal distress. However, *the majority of postterm infants appear to be normal* or are macrosomic. Therefore, in the absence of presumed placental insufficiency (causing the fetal alterations noted), fetuses continue to grow slightly even after the EDC. Thus, ascertaining which fetuses are jeopardized and which are not is essential.

Recent studies suggest that the risk after 41 weeks gestation is little different from that at 42 weeks. Therefore, delivery should be considered or careful monitoring initiated.

Evaluation of the Postterm Pregnancy

A. *Accurately date the pregnancy.*

1. The EDC may not yet have been reached! Of course, accurate dating should have been performed prospectively (during the course of pregnancy), but that so often is not the case. Thus, if three of the following four clinical criteria are met, the patient should *not* be considered postdate.

a. Less than 36 weeks have elapsed since a positive pregnancy test.

b. Less than 32 weeks have elapsed since Doppler recording of the fetal heart (FHTs).

c. Less than 24 weeks have elapsed since observed fetal movements.

d. Less than 22 weeks have elapsed since FHTs were noted by auscultation.

2. Two satisfactory *ultrasonographic* fetal biparietal (or other) *measurements,* at least 1 month apart, *can establish gestational age*

by ± 1 week. Therefore, a precise determination is more likely. However, the earlier in gestation the ultrasonic examinations are accomplished, the more accurate dating will be. The EDC cannot be established accurately or confirmed when the fetal biparietal diameter is >9.5 cm by a single ultrasonography.

B. *Fetal surveillance is essential to assess fetal well-being.* Once the due date is past until the 41st week, it may be wise to implement all or part of the surveillance noted below (e.g., weekly instead of biweekly determinations).

1. Clinical parameters include *full maternal evaluation.*

a. Biweekly recording of fundal height and abdominal girth (decreasing uterine contents signals oligohydramnios).

b. Maternal fetal motion counting (Chapter 5).

c. Visualization of the membranes (if possible) through the cervix to determine if meconium has been passed. Meconium is a nonspecific reaction to stress and should not be taken as a sign of fetal distress but as a warning signal that the fetus may be near the limits of placental reserve.

2. *Biweekly biophysical profile testing* or, minimally, biweekly NST.

3. At least one definitive (level III) *ultrasonography,* specifically examining fetal size parameters, fetal organ systems, and the placenta (including grading).

4. *Contraction stress testing* if any parameter is questionable.

5. *Amniocentesis is rarely indicated* but may be useful in the patient who has totally unknown dates and appears without any prospective monitoring. Analysis of the amniotic fluid does not assist in determining the gestational age but can definitively describe fetal pulmonary maturity, even when a sample is contaminated by blood or meconium.

Treatment

The safest time for delivery to occur is 39–41 weeks. After the 41st week, there is steadily rising mortality (e.g., stillborn, uteroplacental insufficiency) and potential morbidity. The *mortality is 5%–7% in infants delivered at or after 42 weeks.* By the 42nd week, the risk is equal to that at <35th week. The exact time for delivery must be individualized. The ideal time for delivery is when the minimal risk of induction is surpassed by the ever increasing risks of postdate gestation. However, it seems unquestionable that delivery by or during the 42nd week is indicated.

A. When definite prolonged pregnancy is confirmed (≥ 42 weeks)

1. Review all the available information to discuss with the gravida and her family.

2. Reconfirm the postdate status, if possible.

3. Induce labor if feasible.

4. About 70% of postterm gravidas have an unripe cervix (low Bishop score) and seem to lack preparation for labor. In these patients, induction of labor often is unsuccessful.

5. In those who have a low Bishop score, consider attempting to enhance the score by preinduction administration of cervical prostaglandin E_2.

B. Monitor the fetus constantly during induction. Dysmature fetuses withstand labor poorly, particularly when oxytocin stimulation is used. They are prone to fetal distress and may die of intrapartum asphyxia.

1. Use electronic fetal monitoring.

2. Observe for meconium on rupture of membranes.

3. Should fetal distress occur, maternal complications intervene, or serial induction of labor fail, cesarean section should be undertaken immediately.

RUPTURE OF THE UTERUS

Uterine rupture, complete or partial, occurs in about 1:1500 deliveries (Figs. 11-6 and 11-7). Complete rupture is through the myometrium and the serosal peritoneum. Rupture may be spontaneous or traumatic. Complete rupture may occur in late pregnancy or during labor in patients who have had classic cesarean section or extensive uterine surgery. Other causes of complete rupture are obstructed labor, oxytocin overstimulation of labor, and operative delivery, e.g., version-extraction. Incomplete or occult rupture during labor may follow partial dehiscence of a low-cervical cesarean section scar or uterine trauma during late pregnancy, e.g., lap-type seatbelt injury. Instrumental perforation of the uterus during induced or incomplete abortion also occurs. Retroperitoneal bleeding may accompany concealed rupture, with late signs and symptoms.

The classic symptomatology of rupture of the uterus is bleeding during labor, suprapubic pain and tenderness, cessation of uterine contractions, disappearance of fetal heart tones, recession of the presenting part, or vaginal bleeding. Hematoperitoneum and hypovolemic shock soon follow. Persistent, uncontrollable uterine bleeding during the third stage of labor in

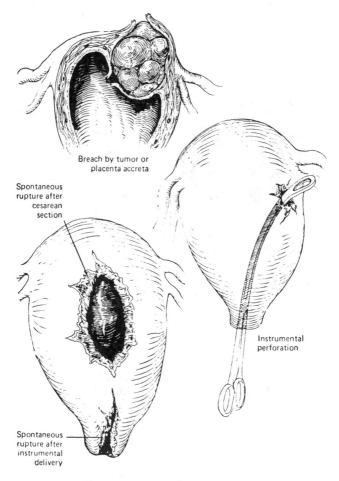

Breach by tumor or
placenta accreta

Spontaneous
rupture after
cesarean
section

Instrumental
perforation

Spontaneous
rupture after
instrumental
delivery

Figure 11-6. Types of uterine rupture.

the absence of cervical or other laceration suggests ruptured uterus.

DIAGNOSIS

If the cervix will admit the examining hand after delivery, uterine exploration usually makes the diagnosis. Ultrasonography

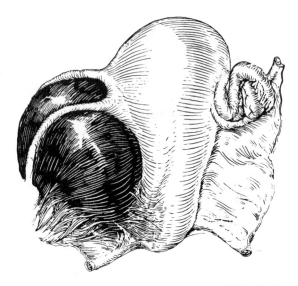

Figure 11-7. Rupture of lower uterine segment with bleeding into the broad ligament.

or x-ray films frequently reveal an abnormal fetal position or extension of fetal extremities in complete uterine rupture.

COMPLICATIONS

Complications of ruptured uterus are hemorrhage, shock, infection, bladder or ureteral injury, thrombophlebitis, disseminated intravascular coagulation, pituitary hypofunction, (e.g., failure to lactate), or death. If the patient survives, infertility or sterility may result.

PREVENTION

Supervise oxytocin induction and stimulation of labor. Avoid difficult vaginal delivery. Do low-cervical, not classic, cesarean sections.

TREATMENT

Ligation of the uterine or internal iliac arteries may check otherwise uncontrollable hemorrhage. Packing of the uterus may temporarily control bleeding. Hysterectomy is the preferred treatment for uterine rupture, but careful repair may be warranted when future childbearing is important.

PROGNOSIS

Rupture of the uterus imposes a maternal mortality of 10%–40% and a perinatal mortality of at least 50%.

Chapter 12

Multiple Pregnancy

Multiple pregnancy involves more than one embryo (fetus) in any one gestation. Two independent mechanisms may lead to multiple gestation: segmentation of a single fertile ovum (identical, monovular, or monozygotic) or fertilization of separate ova by different spermatozoa (fraternal or dizygotic) multiple pregnancy.

In the development of twins (the most frequent and our best model for multiple gestation), monozygotism is constant ($\sim$ 2.3–4/1000 deliveries), whereas dizygotism has certain predispositions. Dizygotic twinning is inherited as a recessive autosomal trait via the female descendants. The father's being a twin has little influence on the rate of twinning in his offspring. Race is of special importance: blacks have the greatest incidence of dizygotic twins (about 50/1000 births in Western Nigeria), whites are intermediate, and Orientals have the fewest ($\sim$ 1–2/1000 births in Japan). Other factors influencing dizygotism include greater maternal height or weight, increasing maternal age (peaks at 35–45), and white mothers of blood group O or A. In developed countries, two of the major causes of multiple gestation are cessation of oral contraception and artificial ovulation induction. The latter is of particular concern. Both the scientific and lay press describe "successes" in which a considerable number of fetuses is conceived. However, delivery is inevitably premature, and intact survivors are uncommon.

In the heterogeneous population of the United States, slightly >30% of twins are monozygotic, and nearly 70% are dizygotic (Fig. 12-1). In such a population, a useful estimate of the *natural frequency of multiple gestation is that twinning occurs $\sim$ 12 per 1000 births* (1:88). Each increase in birth number may then be estimated by raising the ratio 1:88 to the exponential of the birth number minus 1. For example, triplets occur $1:88^{(3-1=2)}$ = 1:7,744; quadruplets occur $1:88^3$ = 1:681,472. In multiple births males predominate (but more die early). *About 75% of twins are of the same sex.* Both are males in $\sim$45% of cases, and both are females in $\sim$30%.

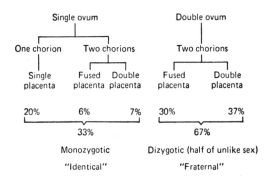

Figure 12-1. Placental variations in twinning. (After Potter.)

Maternal morbidity and mortality are much higher in multiple than in singleton pregnancy. There is increased frequency and severity of anemia, increased occurrence of urinary tract infection, more preeclampsia-eclampsia, hydramnios, and uterine inertia (overdistention), and a greater chance of hemorrhage (before, during, and after delivery).

The perinatal mortality rate of twins is 3 to 4 times higher—and for triplets much higher again—than for singletons because of prematurity and associated difficulties. Indeed, as the number of fetuses rises, their average size and length of gestation decrease. Twins are delivered, on average, at ~36 weeks, triplets at ~32 weeks, and quadruplets at <30 weeks. Moreover, *intrauterine growth retardation (IUGR) is more common in all multiple gestations* (as opposed to singletons.) Congenital abnormalities of all organ systems are as high as 18% among twins (considering both monozygotic and dizygotic). Other *perinatal risks of multiple gestations include abnormal presentation and position, hydramnios, hypoxia because of cord prolapse* (~4%, 5 times more common in multiple pregnancy), *placenta previa, and premature separation of the placenta* after the first twin or operative manipulation. Collision, impaction, and interlocking of twins are additional critical but uncommon complications (Figs. 12-2, 12-3, and 12-4).

Monozygotic multiple fetuses are far more likely to be jeopardized than dizygotic twins. For example, monozygotic twins have 3 times the incidence of serious congenital abnormalities compared to double-ovum twins. Conjoined twins and enhanced early loss of one or both fetuses (probably two thirds of

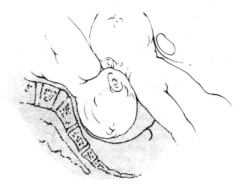

Figure 12-2. Locked twins.

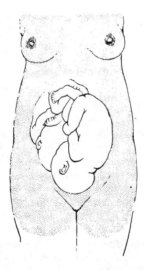

Figure 12-3. Both twins presenting by the vertex.

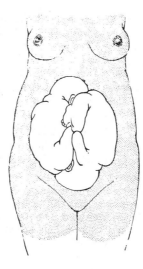

Figure 12-4. One vertex and one breech presentation.

all implanted multiple gestations) result in a single birth. Moreover, a parasitic fetus without a heart (fetus acardiacus) is also a potential problem of monozygous twinning. Other unique monozygotic complications include placental vascular shunts resulting in the *twin-to-twin transfusion syndrome,* in which the smaller but cardiomegalic twin pumps its arterial blood into the lower pressure venous system of the larger, plethoric, and macrosomic twin. Cord abnormalities, more common in monozygous twins, include two-vessel cords and velamentous cord insertion (7% incidence). Cord entanglement in a single monoamniotic sac may occur, and this leads to a ~50% loss. Monozygotic twins are smaller and are more likely to die in utero than dizygotic twins. This may be because a single (monochorionic) placenta is less efficient than a fused dichorionic placenta.

The time of segmentation is crucial to the outcome of monozygotic fetuses. Division before the morula and differentiation of the trophoblast (day 5) lead to separate or fused placentas with two chorions and two amnions. Division after trophoblastic differentiation but before amnion formation (5–10 days) is the pattern of two thirds of all monozygotic twins. This results in a single placenta, a common chorion, and two amnions. Division after amnion differentiation (10–14 days) leads to a single placenta with one chorion and one amnion. Division >14 days results in incomplete twinning. Division just before that (8–14 days) may lead to conjoined (Siamese) twinning.

Monozygotic multiple gestations share the same genetic features, e.g., blood group, histocompatibility, and basic karyotypes. Therefore, skin grafting and organ transplantation are possible and become the ultimate test of monozygotic vs dizygotic twinning. Monozygotic twins are termed *identical,* but they often have considerable phenotypic variation. Dizygotic (*fraternal*) twins may be of the same or different sexes and bear only the resemblance of brothers or sisters. They may or may not have sufficiently similar genetic features to serve as organ donors for each other.

Examination of the placenta and membranes assists in zygosity determination. At delivery, careful inspection and dissection of the placenta(s) and membranes, particularly the membraneous T-septum or dividing membrane between the twins, may reveal microscopic evidence of the probable type of twinning. Monozygotic twins have a thin septum made up of two amniotic membranes only (no chorion and no decidua). Indeed, ~1% of monozygotic twins are monoamniotic. By contrast, dizygotic twins have a thick septum composed of two chorions, two amnions, and intervening decidua (Fig. 12-5). In some circumstances, it is necessary to resort to definitive genetic testing to determine monozygosity or dizygosity.

The early diagnosis of twins is mandatory, and assessment of the placenta is the key.

CLINICAL FINDINGS

The clinical suggestions of multiple pregnancy include the following.

A. A *uterus larger than expected* for the duration of pregnancy (>4 cm than anticipated)

B. *Excessive maternal weight gain* not explained by eating or edema

C. *Hydramnios, iron deficiency anemia*

D. Maternal reports of *increased fetal activity*

E. *Eclampsia-preeclampsia*

F. Uterus containing ≥ 3 *large parts or multiple small parts*

G. Simultaneous auscultation or recording of *two fetal hearts* varying >8 bpm and asynchronous to the maternal heart

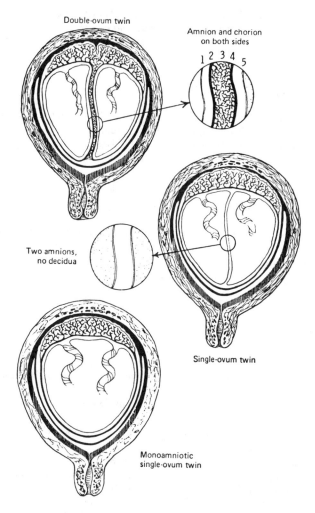

Figure 12-5. Amniotic membranes of twins.

LABORATORY FINDINGS

A. Abnormal *elevation of maternal hCG* or *alpha-fetoprotein* or both

B. Moderate *reduction in HCT (also Hgb and RBC count, i.e., iron deficiency anemia)*

C. *Blood volume increased* over normal pregnancy values

D. Increased incidence of *glucose intolerance*

IMAGING FINDINGS

Multiple pregnancy may be demonstrated by vaginal ultrasonography before 8 weeks, and multiple pregnancy should be routinely detected by other scanning methods at ~10 weeks.

DIFFERENTIAL DIAGNOSIS

Single large pregnancy, hydramnios, hydatidiform mole, abdominal or pelvic tumors complicating singleton pregnancy, and complicated multiple gestation (e.g., triplets) must all be considered in the diagnosis of multiple gestation.

TREATMENT

A. *Prevention of multiple pregnancy*

Currently there are few possibilities for preventing multiple gestation.

1. Use of a barrier type of contraception for the first cycle off oral contraceptives.

2. Administer Clomiphene (initially) if ovulation is to be induced. Clomiphene therapy results in fewer multiple gestations, but dizygous twins still occur in 5%–10%.

3. Avoid the use of human menopausal gonadotropin therapy unless the proper dosage can be established and daily ultrasonography is available for ovulation monitoring.

4. Selective reduction of fetuses (i.e., selective elimination) is a new and controversial technique of elimination of one or more fetuses. This technique employs ultrasonic-guided methods for reducing the number of fetuses with the rationale that intact survival of a few is better than nonintact survival of many. Initial reports support this approach in selected cases.

B. *Avoidance of maternal complications* in multiple pregnancy

1. Diagnose multiple pregnancy early; i.e., order ultrasonography ideally on all and certainly on questionable pregnancies no later than 12–16 weeks.

2. Provide iron and a high-protein, high-vitamin diet; do not limit weight gain.

3. Examine the patient with multiple pregnancy more often than most during pregnancy (individualize, but in most cases twice as often).

4. Limit physical activity to ensure adequate uterine blood flow (e.g., cancel regular exercise programs).

5. Ensure frequent rest periods after the 24th week (e.g., 1 week of bedrest at 26 weeks and again at 32–33 weeks).

6. Anticipate more frequent ultrasound examinations and blood counts. Ultrasound examinations for growth progress may be useful monthly from diagnosis until the 32nd week, when both ultrasonography and BPP on each fetus may be useful on a weekly basis.

7. Deliver all patients with multiple pregnancy in a tertiary medical facility if possible.

8. Stress psychoprophylaxis, and introduce the patient to a support group or provide patient literature concerning multiple gestation.

9. Anticipate increased blood loss at delivery (hemorrhage is 5 times increased over singletons). Seek donors acceptable to the patient in advance.

C. *Prevention of fetal complications* of multiple gestation

1. Avoid prematurity.

a. Maximize maternal antenatal care (as above).

b. Cervical cerclage may delay preterm birth in selected cases.

c. Tocolytic drugs to prevent early birth may be effective (Chapter 11). However, use with great care in multiple gestation because of possible maternal pulmonary edema.

d. Initiate appropriate fetal therapy if early delivery is anticipated (Chapter 11).

2. Ascertain fetal problems early.

a. Order ultrasonic examinations repeatedly to screen for fetal defects, IUGR, fetus-to-fetus transfusion syndrome, and fetal well-being.

b. Use antenatal diagnosis as indicated.

c. Apply individual testing for pulmonary maturity studies (if necessary).

d. If selective reduction is an option, refer the patient to an appropriate center.

3. During labor.

a. Monitor electronically all fetuses separately (in the United States, if fetal monitoring of this type is not primarily available, refer the gravida to a center).

b. Limit maternal analgesia and anesthesia; use psychoprophylaxis or local anesthesia if possible.

c. Ascertain the presentation of both twins by ultrasonography. Identify the presentations. In practice, this nearly always involves one of the three situations outlined in Table 12-1.

d. Start IV lactated Ringer's solution with a large-bore needle.

e. Obtain CBC and blood type. Crossmatch for a minimum of 2 units packed RBC or whole blood.

f. Consider only twins for vaginal delivery. All those of higher birth orders (save in very unusual circumstances) should be delivered by cesarean section.

g. Keep the mother off her back! The degree of aortocaval compression with subsequent hypotension may be profound.

h. Provide proper maternal and fetal oxygenation by oxygen therapy by mask (7 liters/min).

D. *Delivery*

1. Perform cesarean section during labor for monoamniotic twins (10% delivery loss from cord entanglement), any birth number exceeding twins (e.g., triplets), twins <2500 g, or if the first twin is nonvertex (situation C).

2. Deliver all twin gestations (very high risk) in an operating room with full preparation (including maternal abdominal preparation), equipment, and personnel in attendance for cesarean section.

3. Deliver the first fetus vaginally if it presents by the vertex (situation A and situation B).

4. Perform a generous episiotomy to reduce fetal cranial compression.

5. Clamp the cord promptly to prevent the second of monozygotic twins from partially exsanguinating through the first cord.

6. Do a vaginal examination immediately after the first delivery to identify a possible forelying or prolapsed cord and establish the position of the second fetus. If B has continued as a vertex (situation A), perform a second vaginal delivery.

7. If the second fetus is anything but vertex (situation B)

a. Bring the head into the inlet by external guidance (version). If successful, allow labor to proceed for another vertex vaginal delivery.

b. Perform cesarean section immediately if external version is unsuccessful or if the fetus is not a candidate for a vaginal breech delivery.

c. Complete a vaginal breech delivery if the external version is unsuccessful and the fetus is a candidate for a vaginal breech delivery.

8. Cautiously rupture the second sac (if present) late to avoid prolapse of the cord.

9. Employ continuous electronic fetal monitoring.

Table 12-1. Delivery situations according to presentation of twins

Situation	Twin A	Twin B	%
A	Vertex	Vertex	>40
B	Vertex	Nonvertex	~40
C	Nonvertex	Other (any)	~20

10. Should fetal distress supervene (e.g., persistent cord compression or premature separation of the placenta) and the second twin cannot be delivered easily or immediately, perform a cesarean section at once.

11. Remember that the three major preventable causes of morbidity in twins are immaturity, trauma, and manipulative delivery (with associated asphyxia), and prevent their occurrence.

12. Ensure immediate availability of a neonatologist or pediatrician.

E. *Postpartum*

1. Give oxytocin 5–10 units IV slowly but promptly after delivery of the second twin, and start an IV infusion of dilute oxytocin (Chapter 11) if uterine atony becomes a problem.

2. Elevate the uterus out of the pelvis and massage it gently (Chapter 11).

Chapter 13

Hypertensive Disorders During Pregnancy

CLASSIFICATION

The hypertensive disorders of pregnancy have been classified by the American Committee on Maternal Welfare (1985) as follows.

I. *Preeclampsia-eclampsia* (pregnancy-induced hypertension, toxemia, EPH, gestosis)

II. *Chronic hypertension*

A. Primary (essential, idiopathic)

B. Secondary (to some known cause)

1. Renal: e.g., parenchymal (glomerulonephritis, chronic pyelonephritis, interstitial nephritis, polycystic kidney disease), renovascular nephritis

2. Adrenal: cortical-Cushing's disease, hyperaldosteronism, medullary-pheochromocytoma

3. Other: coarctation of the aorta, thyrotoxicosis, etc.

III. *Chronic hypertension with superimposed preeclampsia*

IV. *Transient (atypical, undiagnosed) hypertension* (a nebulous group of patients who develop hypertension in labor or immediately postpartum)

PREGNANCY-INDUCED HYPERTENSION

DEFINITIONS, INCIDENCE, ETIOLOGY, AND IMPORTANCE

Pregnancy-induced hypertension (PIH) is a *disorder of unknown etiology peculiar to pregnant women*. The milder form of the syndrome (preeclampsia) is characterized by hypertension, generalized edema, and proteinuria occurring after the 20th week of pregnancy (usually in the last trimester or early puerperium). Any two of the three signs are diagnostic. The only exception to the 20th week for onset is when PIH is associated with tropho-blastic disease.

Eclampsia, the most fulminating degree of PIH, is character-ized by convulsions or coma, in addition to the other signs and symptoms of preeclampsia. Uncontrolled preeclampsia may prog-ress to eclampsia, with resultant permanent disability or death. Chronic hypertension (CH) alone or with superimposed pre-eclampsia (SIPE) must be differentiated from PIH.

About 8% of all pregnant women in the United States de-velop preeclampsia. However, there is great geographic varia-tion in incidence. Approximately 5% of these cases progress to eclampsia, and about 5% of women with eclampsia die of the disease or its complications. At least 95% percent of cases of PIH occur after the 32nd week, and about 75% of these patients are primigravidas. The incidence is at least doubled with multiple pregnancy, hydatidiform mole, and polyhydramnios. Primigra-vidas of all ages are affected. PIH is more prevalent among blacks and Native Americans than whites. Other factors predis-posing to PIH include age <20 and >35, vascular or renal dis-ease, diabetes mellitus, chronic hypertension, pheochromocy-toma, systemic lupus erythematosus, nonimmune fetal hydrops, malnutrition, and low socioeconomic status. Interestingly, if a multigravida remarries, her chance of having PIH with her next pregnancy is similar to what it would be as a nullipara.

The cause of preeclampsia-eclampsia remains unknown and speculation has been so rife that this disorder has been called a *disease of theories.*

PATHOLOGIC PHYSIOLOGY

A. *Vasospasm.* Arteriolar spasm, consistently observed in the retinas, kidneys, and splanchnic region, promotes hypertension. Furthermore, the normal *refractoriness to angiotensin II (A-II) is lost* weeks before the onset of preeclampsia. In contrast, normal pregnant women lose their refractoriness to A-II after receiving prostaglandin synthetase inhibitors, e.g., aspirin, which impli-cates prostaglandin as a mediator of vascular reactivity to A-II during pregnancy. Moreover, A-II refractoriness can be restored to preeclamptic individuals by drugs that increase levels of cyclic AMP (cAMP), e.g., theophylline. Therefore, *it has been hypothe-sized* (Gant) *that prostaglandin synthesized in arterioles may modulate vascular reactivity to A-II by altering the intracellular level of cAMP in vascular smooth muscle.*

An imbalance between prostacyclin (PGI_2), a vasodilator and inhibitor of platelet aggregation, and thromboxane (TXA_2), a vasoconstrictor and platelet aggregator in preeclampsia, also occurs. The importance of prostaglandins and A-II in the genesis of preeclampsia is emphasized in Speroff's hypothesis of the mechanisms involved (Fig. 13-1).

B. *Sodium and Water Retention*

1. Sodium retention is an adjunct of growth and is normal during pregnancy, but sodium retention, particularly intracellular, is exaggerated in PIH. Nonetheless, sodium retention does not cause this disorder. However, an alteration at the cellular membrane level may inhibit the usual exchange of sodium.

2. Reduced serum levels of albumin and globulin resulting from proteinuria account for the diminished oncotic pressure of the blood despite hemoconcentration.

3. Increased excretion of corticosteroids (including aldosterone) and vasopressin in certain patients suggests increased tissue concentrations of these substances. This results in enhanced sodium and water retention.

C. *Proteinuria.* Degenerative changes in the glomeruli permit loss of protein via the urine. The albumin/globulin ratio in the urine of patients with preeclampsia-eclampsia is approximately 3:1 (vs 6:7 in patients with glomerulonephritis). Here, renal tubular disease contributes only slightly to the leakage of protein.

D. *Hematology.* The hemoglobin and hematocrit are elevated due to hemoconcentration. Severe preeclampsia-eclampsia shares similarities with the disorders of coagulation because disseminated intravascular coagulation (DIC) of varying degrees so frequently occurs. The magnitude of the coagulation defect does not always correlate with the severity of preeclampsia-eclampsia. The alterations may include thrombocytopenia, decreased coagulation factors (especially reduced fibrinogen), and the presence of fibrin split products. Occasionally, evidence of hemolysis (e.g., microangiopathic hemolytic anemia, deformed red blood cells) may be noted in patients with preeclampsia-eclampsia. Microfibrin emboli may occur in the lungs, liver, or kidneys.

E. *Blood Chemistry*

1. Uric acid levels are generally >6 mg/dl. Serum creatinine is most often normal but may be elevated in severe cases.

2. Some serum albumin and globulin are lost via the urine, but blood proteins must also be lost or destroyed in other ways, since proteinuria alone is not sufficient to explain the abnormally low protein levels in severe cases.

3. Acidosis occurs after convulsions.

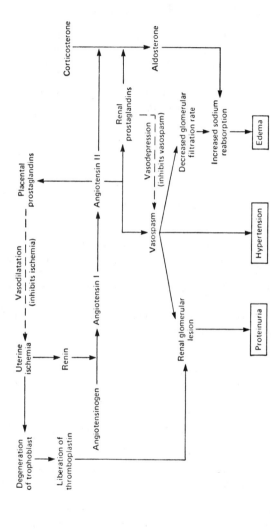

Figure 13-1. Preeclampsia-eclampsia may originate in relative ischemia of the uteroplacental unit, resulting in degeneration of trophoblastic tissue and release of thromboplastin. This may be followed by a com- pensatory response and then by aberration of the renin-prostaglandin system. Dashed arrows indicate inhibitory processes. (Modified from L. Speroff, Toxemia in pregnancy. *Am J Cardiol* 1973;32:582.)

4. Increased sulfobromophthalein retention and elevated levels of hepatic enzymes (e.g., SGOT) indicate hepatic dysfunction.

F. *Placental Clearance of DHEAS*

Placental clearance of dehydroepiandrosterone sulfate (DHEAS), as a measure of placental perfusion, decreases before the onset of preeclampsia.

In summary, *PIH is marked by vasospasm.* Normal pregnancy is marked by sodium and water retention, together with increased blood volume. In preeclampsia, there is enhanced sodium and water retention with a contracted plasma volume. Swan-Ganz catheter studies in preeclampsia reveal normal wedge pressures and normal or elevated cardiac output.

PATHOLOGY

A. *Kidney.* In severe preeclampsia and eclampsia, the only typical lesion is glomerular capillary endotheliosis, i.e., swelling of the glomerular capillary endothelium, narrowing of the capillary lumen, and subendothelial fibrinoid deposition. These abnormalities are totally reversible and disappear by 6 weeks postpartum. In patients with the clinical diagnosis of preeclampsia, renal biopsy reveals *glomerular capillary endotheliosis in ~70%* of primigravidas <25 years, and *~25% have unsuspected renal disease.*

B. *Placenta.* Grossly, no specific placental lesions are typical of preeclampsia-eclampsia, although the placenta is often smaller than normal, and intervillous fibrin deposits (red infarcts) are common. Increased and more severe endarteritis and periarteritis, a thinned and broken syncytium, and calcium and intervillous fibrin deposition may appear (grossly, microscopically, and ultrasonographically) as *premature aging.*

There are two very serious microscopic placental alterations in patients with preeclampsia: the spiral arteries in the myometrium fail to lose their musculoelastic structure, and acute atherosis develops in the myometrial segment of the spiral arteries. This leads to increased vascular resistance and a compromise of the vessel lumen. Thus, the fetus receives less intervillous blood flow.

C. *Fetus.* As a result of the poor intervillous blood flow, *intrauterine growth retardation* may be marked. Fetal death may follow hypoxia or acidosis.

D. *Cardiopulmonary. Pulmonary edema may occur with severe preeclampsia or eclampsia* from cardiogenic or noncardiogenic causes. It is most common postpartum and also may be related to fluid overload and decreased plasma colloid oncotic pressure.

Aspiration of gastric contents may occur as a complication of eclamptic seizures. Death may result from particulate matter obstructing airways or from chemical pneumonitis, leading to the adult respiratory distress syndrome.

Preeclampsia is usually characterized as a hyperdynamic state with increased cardiac output, normal wedge pressure, and normal or slightly elevated systemic vascular resistance.

E. *Gastrointestinal.* In the liver, chronic passive congestion and subcapsular hemorrhages may develop.

CLINICAL FINDINGS: PREECLAMPSIA

Symptoms and Signs

Preeclampsia-eclampsia is characterized by *hypertension, generalized edema, and proteinuria* in the absence of vascular or renal disease. The manifestations develop from the 20th week of pregnancy through the 6th week after delivery.

Hypertension

Hypertension is the key sign in the diagnosis of PIH. Gestational hypertension is a rise in systolic blood pressure of ≥ 30 mm Hg, a rise in diastolic pressure of ≥15 mm Hg, or a blood pressure of ≥140/90. Hypertension also exists with a mean arterial pressure rise of 20 mm Hg. The levels described must occur at least twice, 6 h or more apart, and be based on previously recorded blood pressures.

Occasional patients with hypertension during pregnancy must remain unclassified until studies can be evaluated after the puerperium.

Edema

Edema is the least precise sign of PIH because dependent edema is normal in pregnancy and up to 40% of patients with PIH do not have edema. However, the following criteria may facilitate the diagnosis.

1. Generalized accumulation of fluid in tissues, i.e., >1+ pitting edema after 1 h bedrest

2. A weight gain of ≥2 pounds/week because of the influence of pregnancy

3. Nondependent edema of the hands and face present on arising in the morning

Proteinuria

Gestational proteinuria is often the last sign to develop and is defined as ≥0.3 g/liter in a 24-h specimen or >1 g/liter (1+–2+ by dipstick methods) with urinalysis on random midstream or catheter specimens. Up to 30% of patients with eclampsia will not have proteinuria, but when present, proteinuria signals increased fetal risk (more SGA infants and enhanced perinatal mortality).

If only the noted criteria for preeclampsia are present, it is classified as mild preeclampsia. The *criteria for severe preeclampsia* follow.

A. Blood pressure >160 systolic or >110 diastolic (at bedrest, on two occasions at least 6 h apart)

B. Proteinuria >5 g/24 h (3+–4+ on dipstick)

C. Oliguria (≤500 ml/24 h)

D. Cerebral or visual disturbances

E. Epigastric pain

F. Pulmonary edema or cyanosis

Severe, persistent, generalized headache, vertigo, malaise, and nervous irritability are prominent symptoms in cases of severe preeclampsia. Scintillating scotomas and partial or complete blindness are due to edema of the retina, retinal hemorrhage, or retinal detachment. Epigastric pain, nausea, and liver tenderness are the result of congestion or thrombosis of the periportal system and subcapsular hepatic hemorrhages.

Complications

Maternal complications are related primarily to preeclampsia worsening to eclampsia. The fetal complications are related to acute and chronic uteroplacental insufficiency (e.g., asymmetric or symmetric SGA age fetus, stillbirth, or intrapartum fetal distress) and early delivery (complications of prematurity).

The arresting mnemonic HELLP has been applied to those preeclampsia-eclampsia patients who have hemolysis (H), elevated liver enzymes (EL), and low platelet count (LP). HELLP seems to represent an important subset of patients with fulminating toxemia of pregnancy rather than a new syndrome. Nevertheless, these gravidas deserve special consideration because they usually have an extremely poor perinatal and maternal prognosis without early diagnosis and proper therapy, including prompt expeditious delivery.

[handwritten annotations: Weight   Blood   Hb, WCC, plts, UREA, creat   LFTs, P   Urine   24 hr p, creat, VMA   Urinalysis, mc+s   USS   Growth]

LABORATORY STUDIES
(All Patients with PIH)

1. Hct, or Hgb, WBC
2. Urinalysis, urine culture and sensitivity
3. Serum protein and albumin/globular ratio
4. Serum uric acid and creatinine
5. A 24-h urine collection for
   a. Total protein
   b. Creatinine clearance
   c. Vanillylmandelic acid (if BP varies greatly)
6. Coagulopathy studies
   a. Platelet count
   b. Total fibrinogen
   c. Prothrombin and partial thromboplastin time
7. Liver profile
   a. Bilirubin
   b. Liver enzymes
8. Ultrasonography for possible fetal growth retardation and fetal well-being
9. Also, depending on the gestational age and seriousness of the situation, consider determination of fetal physiologic maturity.

MANAGEMENT

The objectives of treatment of all hypertensive states complicating pregnancy are to prevent or control convulsions, ensure survival of the mother without (or with minimal) morbidity, and deliver a surviving infant without serious sequelae.

General Measures

1. General diet without sodium restriction.
2. Unrestricted fluid intake (but with recorded intake and output).

3. The lateral recumbent position increases renal blood flow, which resolves most edema.

4. Provide high-risk obstetric care and treatment of complications.

5. The keys to treatment are bedrest and delivery.

Those who may be relied on and have very mild preeclampsia (usually only transitory hypertension) may be treated by the following protocol under close supervision as outpatients.

1. Bedrest
2. Every 4 h blood pressure evaluation (while awake)
3. Daily urine dipstick evaluation for proteinuria
4. Minimum twice weekly physician visits
5. Weekly nonstress testing (or other evaluation of fetal well-being)
6. Maternal fetal motion counting
7. Careful patient education concerning signs that would require immediate hospitalization: proteinuria, increasing blood pressure, severe headache, and epigastric pain

Maternal hospitalization may help prevent premature delivery and thus be less expensive (compared to premature neonatal care).

1. Bedrest
2. Daily weights
3. Blood pressures every 4 h
4. Daily urine dipstick for proteinuria
5. 24-h urine twice weekly for
   a. Creatinine clearance
   b. Total protein
6. On admission and weekly thereafter
   a. Liver function studies
   b. Uric acid and creatinine
   c. Electrolytes
   d. Serum albumin
   e. Coagulation profile
7. Ultrasound for gestational age (admission and every 2 weeks)
8. Weekly testing for fetal well-being
9. Glucose tolerance test indicated after 20 weeks gestation if the patient has hyperglycemia or multiple pregnancy
10. Vanillylmandelic acid study required if wide blood pressure fluctuations occur
11. Discharge the patient to home for bedrest if
    a. BP reduction to ≤120/80
    b. Proteinuria ≤150 mg/24 h and normal renal function
    c. No evidence of CNS irritability

12. Deliver when physiologic maturity (amniocentesis and testing) occurs

13. Readmit to hospital for bedrest and possible delivery if relapse occurs

14. If early delivery is required, attempt induction if the cervix is favorable (Bishop score ≥6–7). If induction is not a good option, if labor is delayed, or if fetal distress develops, proceed with cesarean section.

Indications for Delivery

1. Blood pressure criteria
    a. Consistently >100 diastolic for 24 h
    b. A single BP diastolic >110 despite bedrest
2. Laboratory abnormalities
    a. Proteinuria >1 g/24 h
    b. Increasing serum creatinine
    c. Abnormal liver function studies
    d. Thrombocytopenia
3. Maternal complications
    a. HELLP syndrome
    b. Eclampsia
    c. Pulmonary edema
    d. Cardiac decompensation
    e. Coagulopathy
    f. Renal failure
    g. Epigastric pain, cerebral symptoms
4. Fetal abnormalities
    a. Fetal distress
    b. Abnormal NST, CST, or BPP
    c. SGA fetus with growth failure on weekly ultrasonography

Severe Preeclampsia

Severe preeclamptics and their offspring are best cared for in tertiary centers. The goals of management are prevention of convulsions, control of maternal blood pressure, and initiation of delivery.

A. For gestations <25 weeks, consider abortion by prostaglandin E_2 suppositories.

B. For gestations of 25–27 weeks, conservative management

(delaying delivery) may be warranted, but maternal complications (abruptio placentae, eclampsia, coagulopathy, renal failure, hypertensive encephalopathy, and hepatic rupture) and poor perinatal outcomes (stillbirth and neonatal death) occur in the majority of patients.

C. For those ≥28 weeks with a tertiary care nursery available, delivery after short-term maternal stabilization is the treatment of choice.

D. Laboratory assessment should be similar to the mild preeclamptic, but it may be necessary in extreme cases to add electrocardiography and hemodynamic monitoring.

E. Determine fetal pulmonary maturity. Repeat at weekly intervals to accomplish delivery as soon as survival is likely.

F. The severe preeclamptic may be started on magnesium sulfate to help in preventing seizures (see dosage under Eclampsia). Magnesium sulfate prevents seizures by direct CNS action. However, magnesium sulfate decreases acetylcholine release at the neuromuscular junction and causes paralysis at a serum level of ~15 mg/dl. Magnesium sulfate potentiates both depolarizing and nondepolarizing muscle relaxants.

G. The use of corticosteroids to accelerate lung maturity may not harm the fetus, but their effectiveness remains controversial.

H. Prompt delivery must be considered for the indications noted previously.

Prevention

Since there are no known specific causes of preeclampsia-eclampsia, prevention can be achieved only in a general way by providing the highest-quality prenatal care. The diet during pregnancy should be high in protein and contain adequate vitamins and minerals. The patient should be permitted to gain about 12 kg (25 pounds) more than her ideal nonpregnant weight. A moderate salt intake is reasonable. Diuretics should not be used. Alert diagnosis and effective management of prodromal symptoms prevent clinical preeclampsia in the third trimester.

Two preventive measures have been investigated recently, and preliminary reports indicate that both result in a decreased incidence of preeclampsia. One is the use of prenatal aspirin prophylaxis in an attempt to inhibit platelet cyclooxygenase, thus blocking synthesis of thromboxane A_2. Dosages from 80 mg every other day to 150 mg every day have been suggested, but the dose–therapeutic relationships remain unclear. Thus, although promising, the widespread use of aspirin as a preventative is not recommended.

The other preventive measure is prenatal calcium supplements of 600 mg to 1.5 g/day. Those receiving calcium have reduced vascular sensitivity to angiotensin II and at least a 50% reduction in the rate of preeclampsia.

ECLAMPSIA

Definition, Incidence, Associations

A patient with signs of preeclampsia who has a least one convulsion or episode of coma between the 20th week of pregnancy and the end of the 6th week after delivery must be presumed to have eclampsia if other causes can be excluded. Eclampsia occurs in 0.2%–0.5% of all deliveries. The occurrence is influenced by the same factors noted for preeclampsia. Eclampsia is classified according to the time of occurrence of the first convulsion with respect to the time of delivery. Prepartum eclampsia (~75% of total) denotes convulsions before delivery. About 50% of postpartum eclamptic convulsions occur within 48 h of delivery.

Symptoms and Signs

Patients usually have no aura and may have one to several seizures with a variable interval of unconsciousness. The seizures are of the tonic-clonic type and are marked by apnea. Hyperventilation (to compensate for the respiratory and lactic acidosis) is common after the seizure. Fever is a poor prognostic sign. Tongue biting is common, and other complications include aspiration, head trauma, broken bones, and retinal detachment.

Laboratory Findings

1. A chest x-ray to rule out aspiration is mandatory for the patient who has had a seizure.

2. If the patient has not been evaluated previously, the studies noted should be obtained.

3. Eclampsia is associated with proteinuria of 3+ to 4+, hemoconcentration, a greatly reduced blood CO_2 combining power, and increased serum uric acid, blood nonprotein nitrogen, and blood urea nitrogen levels.

4. *Special examinations.* Ophthalmoscopic examination may reveal papilledema, retinal edema (increased sheen), retinal detachment, vascular spasm, arteriovenous nicking, and hemorrhages. Repeated examination is helpful in determining improvement or failure of treatment in preeclampsia-eclampsia.

Differential Diagnosis

1. *Convulsions* may be due to hypertensive encephalopathy, epilepsy, thromboembolism, drug intoxication or withdrawal, trauma, hypoglycemia, hypocalcemia (of parathyroid or renal origin), hemolytic crisis of sickle cell anemia, or the tetany of alkalosis, as well as eclampsia.

2. *Coma* usually follows the convulsions of eclampsia, but it may occur without convulsions. Other causes of coma (in descending order of probability) are epilepsy, syncope, alcohol or other drug intoxication, acidosis or hypoglycemia (diabetes), stroke, and azotemia.

Management

Emergency Management

A. *Guarantee immediate maternal well-being.*

1. Insert an oral airway or padded tongue depressor to minimize tongue biting and to guarantee an airway.

2. Initiate suctioning of the oropharynx as soon as it can be ascertained that the patient will not bite the suction catheter.

3. Gently restrain the patient to prevent bony or soft tissue injury.

4. Administer oxygen.

B. *Control seizures.*

1. Magnesium sulfate is usually given in a 4–6 g IV loading dose followed by IV infusion of 1.5–2 g/h, attempting to reach a therapeutic level of 4.8–8.4 mg/dl. When magnesium sulfate is being administered, a urinary catheter is usually desirable to ascertain that adequate urinary output is occurring. Magnesium sulfate is largely excreted by the kidneys, and the drug may reach dangerous levels if urinary output is impaired.

2. If seizures recur >20 min after the loading dose and therapeutic levels are confirmed, consider diazepam 5–10 mg IV or up to 250 mg amobarbital (be aware of their effect on the fetus and neonate).

C. *Control hypertension* (usually only initiated for diastolic >110 and with a goal to bring the diastolic to 90–100). Labetalol may be given every 10 min: 20 mg first dose, 40 mg second dose, 80 mg subsequent doses (to a maximum 300 mg or until blood pressure is controlled). Diazoxide, sodium nitroprusside, trimethaphan, and nitroglycerin also have been used acutely to lower blood pressure. However, each had side effects that must be weighed carefully.

General Measures

A. *Hospitalize the patient* in a single, darkened, quiet room at absolute bedrest, with bedrails in place for protection during convulsions. Provide special nurses around the clock, and allow no visitors.

B. *Do not disturb the patient for unnecessary procedures* (e.g., enemas, tub baths). Leave the blood pressure cuff on her arm. Turn the patient on her side to prevent inferior vena cava syndrome or aspiration of vomitus.

Keep at hand a padded tongue blade to be placed between the patient's teeth during convulsions, a bulb syringe and catheter or suction machine to aspirate mucus or vomitus from the mouth, glottis, or trachea, and an oxygen cone or tent (masks and nasal catheters produce excessive stimulation).

C. *Have available typed and crossmatched whole blood* for immediate administration because patients with eclampsia often develop premature separation of the placenta and hemorrhage. They are susceptible to shock also.

D. *Laboratory tests.*

1. Insert a retention catheter to accurately measure the amount of urine passed (50–100 ml/h is desirable).

2. Determine quantitatively the protein content of each 24-h urine specimen until the 4–5 postpartum day.

3. Creatinine clearance tests may indicate impending renal failure. Sulfabromophthalein retention and greatly elevated levels of hepatic enzymes may presage liver failure. Coagulation studies may suggest DIC.

E. *Physical examination.*

1. Check the blood pressure hourly during the acute phase and every 2–4 h thereafter. Evaluate fetal heart tones every time the mother's blood pressure is obtained.

2. *Perform ophthalmoscopic examination* daily. Examine the face, extremities, and especially the sacrum (which becomes dependent when the patient is in bed) for edema.

F. A *patient* undergoing stabilization for delivery *should remain NPO.*

G. *Measure and record fluid intake and output* for each 24-h period. If the urine output exceeds 700 ml/day, replace the output plus insensible fluid loss (approximately 500 ml/day) with salt-free fluid (including parenteral fluids). Give 200–300 ml of 20% dextrose in water 2–3 times daily during the acute phase to protect the liver, to replace fluids, and to aid in nutrition. Do not give 50% glucose, since it will sclerose the veins. Use no sodium-containing fluids (e.g., physiologic saline, Ringer's solution).

H. *Delivery is mandatory* once the gravida has been stabilized. Deliver the infant by the safest, most expeditious method. Cesarean section is preferred for primigravidas, but induction by rupture of the membranes and vaginal delivery may be appropriate for some multiparas. Note if meconium is present in amniotic fluid. The method of delivery should be individualized. Indications for cesarean section have been liberalized, but cesarean section may be lethal for a patient with continuing convulsions or coma. Seizures and insensibility should be absent for a period of ~4 h before cesarean section is performed on a maternal indication.

I. *For cesarean section, well-controlled epidural or caudal anesthesia may be employed.* Spinal anesthesia is a bad choice because it may cause sudden, severe hypotension. After delivery, give thiopental anesthesia during abdominal closure. If an anesthetist is not available, procaine, 0.5 or 1% (or its equivalent), can be used for local infiltration of the abdominal wall. For vaginal delivery, pudendal block is preferred.

J. *Continue postpartum magnesium sulfate* for at least 24–48 h. Phenobarbital (120 mg/day) may be used in patients with persistent hypertension and no spontaneous postpartum diuresis. If the diastolic blood pressure is consistently >100, consider the administration of a thiazide diuretic and methyldopa or other antihypertensives.

Complications

Early

Convulsions increase the maternal mortality rate 10-fold and the fetal mortality rate 40-fold. The causes of maternal death due to eclampsia are (in descending order of frequency) circulatory collapse (cardiac arrest, pulmonary edema, shock), cerebral hemorrhage, and renal failure. The fetus usually dies of hypoxia, acidosis, or placental abruption. Blindness or paralysis (due to retinal detachment or intracranial hemorrhage) may persist in patients who survive eclampsia.

About 30% of patients who develop premature separation of the placenta have one of the hypertensive disorders. Approximately half of such patients will be found to have hypertensive disease and about one quarter will have preeclampsia-eclampsia.

Postpartum hemorrhage is common in patients with hypertensive syndromes during pregnancy. Toxic delirium in patients with eclampsia, either before or after delivery, poses serious medical and nursing problems. Injuries incurred during convulsions include lacerations of lips or tongue and fractures of the vertebrae. Aspiration pneumonia may also occur. Renal or hepatic failure and DIC are rare maternal complications.

Preterm delivery with all attendant neonatal morbidity and mortality is a marked risk with preeclampsia-eclampsia.

Late

Fifteen to thirty-three percent of patients with severe preeclampsia or eclampsia (without known preexisting hypertensive or renal disease) suffer a recurrence of preeclampsia-eclampsia with subsequent pregnancies. If, however, their problem was not preeclampsia but undiagnosed chronic hypertensive cardiovascular disease, the rate of recurrence is nearly 100%. Permanent hypertension, the result of vascular damage, may occur as a result of severe preeclampsia-eclampsia in 30%–50%.

Prognosis

For the Mother

The outlook for patients with preeclampsia is good if eclampsia does not ensue. Death from preeclampsia is <0.1%. If eclamptic seizures develop, 5%–7% of these patients will die. The causes of death include intracranial hemorrhage, shock, renal failure, premature separation of the placenta, and aspiration pneumonia. Moreover, chronic hypertension may be a sequel of eclampsia.

Chronic hypertension may be present before conception or <20 weeks gestation, or hypertension may persist for >6 weeks postpartum. Superimposed preeclampsia on chronic hypertension is defined by ≥30 systolic or ≥15 diastolic increase from previous levels with either nondependent edema or proteinuria.

For the Infant

Perinatal mortality has been as high as 20%. Most of these infants are preterm. However, with early diagnosis and proper therapy, this loss probably can be reduced to <10%.

CHRONIC HYPERTENSION

DEFINITION AND INCIDENCE

It is often difficult to distinguish chronic hypertension from preeclampsia, especially when the patient registers late in pregnancy (Table 13-1). The correct diagnosis can be made by renal biopsy, but this carries a considerable risk during pregnancy. Moreover, the exact diagnosis may be academic, for (as noted previously) ~25% of patients with preeclampsia have underlying renal disease and ~20% of patients with the clinical diagnosis of chronic hypertension and superimposed preeclampsia have renal disease.

Chronic hypertension occurs in 0.5%–4% of pregnancies (averaging 1.5%). Approximately 80% of chronic hypertension is idiopathic, and 20% is due to renal disease. Common associations include >30 years of age, obesity, multiparous, diabetes mellitus, nonwhite, and family history of hypertension.

DIAGNOSIS

Signs

1. Documented hypertension before conception
2. Hypertension <20 weeks gestation or >6 weeks postpartum

Laboratory Evaluation

Hypertensive patients should be evaluated as soon as feasible in pregnancy. The following baseline laboratory studies (in addition to the customary prenatal laboratory tests) are recommended in addition to the tests for preeclampsia.

Table 13-1. Differential diagnosis of chronic hypertensive cardiovascular disease and preeclampsia

Features	Hypertensive disease	Preeclampsia
Onset of hypertension	Before pregnancy; during first 20 weeks of pregnancy	After 20th week of pregnancy (exception: trophoblastic tumors)
Duration of hypertension	Permanent; hypertension persists beyond 3 months postpartum	Hypertension usually absent at 6 weeks postpartum; always by 3 months postpartum
Family history	Often positive	Usually negative; may be positive
Past history	Recurrent toxemia	Psychosexual problems common
Age	Usually older	Generally teenage, early 20s
Parity	Usually multigravida	Usually primigravida
Habitus	May be thin or brachymorphic	Usually eumorphic
Retinal findings	Often arteriovenous nicking, tortuous arterioles, cotton wool exudates, hemorrhages	Vascular spasm, retinal edema; rarely, protein extravasations
Proteinuria	Often none	Usually present (see definition); absent at 6 weeks postpartum

From RR de Alvarez. In R.C. Benson, ed., *Current Obstetric & Gynecologic Diagnosis & Treatment*, 4th ed. Lange, 1982.

1. SMA-6 or SMA-12
2. Urine culture and sensitivity
3. 24-h urine collection for creatinine clearance (decreased in 5%–10% of patients, who will also have elevated serum creatinine and proteinuria) and total protein
4. Chest x-ray films (rule out cardiomegaly because those with increased heart size are at greater risk of superimposed preeclampsia, pulmonary edema, and arrhythmias)
5. Electrocardiogram (expect left ventricular hypertrophy in 5%–10% of patients)

Management

Obstetric patients with chronic hypertensive cardiovascular or renal disease should be managed similarly to those with preeclampsia. Many of the former will have superimposed preeclampsia, and it may not be possible to decide what the basic problem actually was until at least 3–4 months after delivery, when appropriate tests and studies should be ordered.

If the diastolic BP exceeds 100 mm Hg, start antihypertensive drug therapy to prevent maternal stroke or cardiac failure. The aim should be maintenance of BP at 80–90 mm Hg. Whether or not uterine blood flow is autoregulated is still undecided. If it is, antihypertensive therapy is not likely to decrease blood flow. On the other hand, if uterine blood vessels are always fully dilated and the flow is not autoregulated, lowering of the maternal BP should decrease uterine blood flow—possibly harmful to the fetus. Hence, antihypertensive drugs must be used cautiously because they carry an uncertain risk–benefit ratio.

Methyldopa, a popular antihypertensive drug, has been used during pregnancy. However, the drug is responsible for contraction of the blood volume in chronic hypertension-preeclampsia after recent diuretic therapy. Therefore, it may not be the drug of choice in many preeclamptic patients.

Diazoxide, a direct arteriolar vasodilator, acts more rapidly than hydralazine. It is not effective until the patient becomes hypotensive. However, the dose may overshoot, to the detriment of the fetus particularly. Diazoxide is not a favored drug in obstetrics.

Beta-blockers may cause hypoglycemia and respiratory depression. Moreover, these drugs blockade the tachycardiac response of neonates of mothers on beta-blocker therapy. Alternative drugs probably are safer and are a least as effective in late pregnancy.

Fetal Assessment

Fetal activity determinations and nonstress and stress tests are important assessment parameters because they may indirectly indicate reduced uterine blood flow and placental function, which may become critical factors in preeclampsia-eclampsia. Determine fetal maturity (LS ratio or rapid surfactant test), and monitor the fetal status closely to properly plan delivery.

CHRONIC HYPERTENSION WITH SUPERIMPOSED PREECLAMPSIA

Patients with chronic hypertension with superimposed preeclampsia (about one third of all chronic hypertensives in pregnancy) on hospitalization may seem to stabilize but then deteriorate rapidly. One of the complications is premature separation of the placenta, noted in >10% of patients with chronic hypertension (>10 times the incidence in normal pregnancy). Other problems include thrombocytopenia, oliguria, and retinal detachment.

Even if chronic hypertensive patients have apparently normal renal function, the incidence of superimposed preeclampsia is 15%–30%. If there is renal insufficiency, almost all these patients will develop preeclampsia-eclampsia.

Intrauterine growth retardation is a major fetal hazard if preeclampsia is superimposed on chronic hypertension. Prematurity is often another problem because preterm delivery may occur spontaneously or by necessity.

Preeclampsia is superimposed on chronic hypertensive disease in at least 50% of cases. The seriousness of the preeclampsia-eclampsia is directly related to the severity of the underlying cardiovascular disorder. Fetal growth may be retarded, probably because of reduced uterine blood flow and placental dysmaturity (premature aging). The perinatal mortality rate is much higher than that in normal pregnancies or in preeclampsia-eclampsia not associated with chronic hypertensive cardiovascular disease.

Use diuretics only when absolutely necessary, but not for the treatment of pregnancy-induced hypertension. If diuretics are given at all, carefully monitor the electrolytes and platelet count.

Chapter 14

Medical and Surgical Complications During Pregnancy

CARDIOVASCULAR DISEASES

CARDIAC ARREST

Cardiac arrest is cessation of heart action. Ventricular standstill (asystole) and ventricular fibrillation are the immediate causes, but the underlying etiologies are most frequently acute myocardial hypoxia or alteration in conduction or both. In obstetrics and gynecology, cardiac arrest occurs during induction of anesthesia and during operative surgery or instrumented delivery. Cardiovascular disease increases the risk of cardiac arrest, and hypoxia and hypertension are contributory causes. Cardiac arrest may follow shock, hypoventilation, airway obstruction, excessive anesthesia, drug administration or drug sensitivity, vasovagal reflex activity, myocardial infarction, air and amniotic fluid embolism, and heart block.

Cardiac arrest occurs in ~1:800 to 1:1000 operations and is apt to occur during minor surgical procedures as well as during major surgery. It occurs in ~1:10,000 obstetric deliveries, usually operative, complicated cases. Fortunately, it is possible to save at least 75% of patients when cardiac arrest occurs in the well-managed and well-equipped operating or delivery room.

CARDIOPULMONARY RESUSCITATION (CPR)

CPR is used for treatment of asphyxia or cardiac arrest (Fig. 14-1).

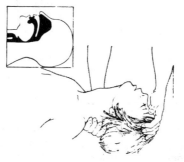

(1) Open airway by positioning neck anteriorly in extension. Inserts show airway obstructed when the neck is in resting flexed position and opening when neck is extended.

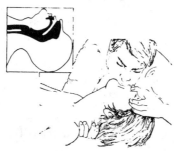

(2) Rescuer should close victim's nose with fingers, seal mouth around victim's mouth, and deliver breath by vigorous expiration.

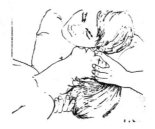

(3) Victim is allowed to exhale passively by unsealing mouth and nose. Rescuer should listen and feel for expiratory air flow.

Figure 14-1. Technique of mouth-to-mouth insufflation.

Phase I: First Aid (Emergency Oxygenation of the Brain)
Basic life support must be instituted within 3–4 min for optimal
effectiveness and to minimize permanent brain damage. Do not
wait for confirmation of suspected cardiac arrest. Call for help,
but do not stop preparations for immediate resuscitation.

Step 1: Place patient supine on a firm surface (not a bed).

Step 2: Determine whether the patient is breathing. If the patient is not breathing, take immediate steps to open the airway. In unconscious patients, the lax tongue may fall backward, blocking the airway. Tilt the head backward and maintain it in this hyperextended position. Keep the mandible displaced forward by pulling strongly at the angle of the jaw.

If Victim Is Not Breathing

Step 3: Clear mouth and pharynx of mucus, blood, vomitus, or foreign material.

Step 4: Separate lips and teeth to open oral airway.

Step 5: If steps 2–4 fail to open airway, forcibly blow air through mouth (keeping nose closed) or nose (keeping mouth closed) and inflate the lungs 3–5 times. Watch for chest movement. If chest movement does not occur immediately and if pharyngeal or tracheal tubes are available, use them without delay. Tracheostomy may be necessary.

Step 6: Feel the carotid artery for pulsations.

    a. If Carotid Pulsations Are Present

    Give lung inflation by mouth-to-mouth breathing (keeping patient's nostrils closed) or mouth-to-nose breathing (keeping patient's mouth closed) 12–15 times per min—allowing about 2 sec for inspiration and 3 sec for expiration—until spontaneous respirations return. Continue as long as the pulses remain palpable and previously dilated pupils remain constricted. If pulsations cease, follow directions in step 6b.

    b. If Carotid Pulsations Are Absent

    Alternate cardiac compression (closed chest cardiac massage, Fig. 14-2) and pulmonary ventilation as in step 6a. Place the heel of one hand on the sternum just above the level of the xiphoid. With the heel of the other hand on top of it, apply firm vertical pressure sufficient to force the sternum

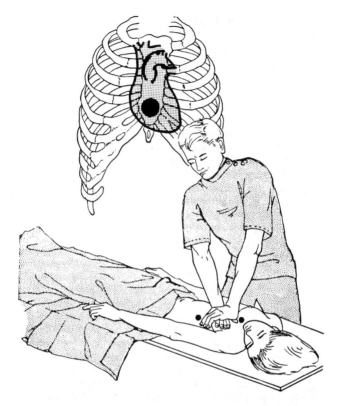

Figure 14-2. Technique of external cardiac massage. Heavy circle in heart drawing shows area of application of force. Circles on supine figure show points of application of electrodes for defibrillation.

about 4–5 cm (2 inches) downward (less in children) about 80–100 times/min. After 5 sternal compressions, alternate with 1 quick, deep lung inflation. Repeat and continue this alternating procedure until it is possible to obtain additional assistance and more definitive care. Resuscitation must be continuous during transportation to the hospital. Open heart massage should be attempted only in a hospital. When possible, obtain an ECG, but do not interrupt resuscitation to do so.

Phase II: Restoration of Spontaneous Circulation

Until spontaneous respiration and circulation are restored, there must be no interruption of artificial ventilation and cardiac massage while steps 7–13 are being carried out. The physician must make plans for the assistance of trained hospital personnel, cardiac monitoring and assisted ventilation equipment, a defibrillator, emergency drugs, and adequate laboratory facilities. Three basic questions must now be considered.

What is the underlying cause, and is it correctable? What is the nature of the cardiac arrest? What further measures will be necessary?

Step 7: Provide for intubation, administration of 100% oxygen, and mechanically assisted ventilation. A cutdown for long-term IV therapy and monitoring should be established as soon as possible. Attach ECG leads and take the first of serial specimens for arterial blood gases and pH. Promote venous return and combat shock by elevating legs, and give IV fluids as available and indicated. The use of firmly applied tourniquets or military antishock trousers (MAST suit) on the extremities may be of value to occlude arteries to reduce the size of the vascular bed.

Step 8: If a spontaneous effective heartbeat is not restored after 1–2 min of cardiac compression, have an assistant give epinephrine, 0.5–1 mg (0.5–1 ml of 1:10,000 aqueous solution) IV every 5 min as indicated. Epinephrine may stimulate cardiac contractions and induce ventricular fibrillation that can then be treated by DC countershock (see step 11).

Step 9: If the victim is pulseless for more than 10 min, give sodium bicarbonate solution, 1 mEq/kg IV, to combat impending metabolic acidosis. Repeat no more than one-half the initial dose every 10 min during cardiopulmonary resuscitation until spontaneous circulation is restored. Monitoring of arterial blood gases and pH is required during bicarbonate treatment to prevent alkalosis and severe hyperosmolar states.

Step 10: If asystole and electromechanical dissociation persist, continue artificial respiration and external cardiac compression, epinephrine, and sodium bicarbonate. Monitor blood H, gases, and electrolytes.

Step 11: If ECG demonstrates ventricular fibrillation, maintain cardiac massage until just before giving an external defibrillating DC shock of 200–300 J for 0.25 sec with one paddle electrode firmly applied to the skin over the apex of the heart and the other just to the right of the upper sternum. Monitor with ECG. If cardiac function is not restored, resume massage and repeat shock at intervals of 1–3 min.

Step 12: Thoracotomy and open heart massage may be considered (but only in a hospital) if cardiac function fails to return after all of the above measures have been used.

Step 13: If cardiac, pulmonary, and central nervous system functions are restored, the patient should be observed carefully for shock and complications of the precipitating cause.

HEART DISEASE

Congenital heart disease is the principal cardiovascular problem complicating pregnancy in the United States. Rheumatic heart disease is less a problem today than a generation ago because of better rheumatic fever prophylaxis, improved health care, and advances in cardiovascular surgery. Syphilitic carditis has all but disappeared in pregnancy. Women with collagen disorders, e.g., Marfan's syndrome, or those with prosthetic heart valves are prone to cardiac problems during pregnancy. Reported incidences of heart disease vary from 0.5% to 2% of obstetric patients but probably are lower in the general population because only referral centers are likely to report their experience.

Heart disease is a major cause of maternal death, but maternal and perinatal mortality rates are only slightly increased if the disability is minimal.

Functional Classification of Heart Disease

For practical purposes, the functional capacity of the heart is the best single measurement of cardiopulmonary status.

Class I: Ordinary physical activity causes no discomfort.

Class II: Ordinary activity causes discomfort and slight disability.

Class III: Less than ordinary activity causes discomfort or disability; patient is barely compensated.

Class IV: Patient decompensated; any physical activity causes acute distress.

Eighty percent of obstetric patients with heart disease have lesions that do not interfere seriously with their activities (classes I and II) and usually do well. About 85% of deaths ascribed to heart disease complicating pregnancy occur in patients with class III or IV lesions (20% of all pregnant patients with heart disease). Nevertheless, much can still be done to improve the prognosis for the mother and infant in these unfavorable circumstances.

Pathologic Physiology

The effects of pregnancy on certain circulatory and respiratory functions are reviewed in Chapter 4.

Three major burdens on the heart are associated with pregnancy: cardiac output is increased by ~40%, the heart rate is accelerated by 10–15 bpm, and the plasma volume is expanded by 45%–50%. These unavoidable stresses must be considered in appraising the patient's ability to undergo pregnancy, delivery, and the puerperium.

By the 12th week of pregnancy, increased physiologic factors, especially blood volume increase, may produce systolic flow murmurs. These, together with the third heart sound often noted during pregnancy, can lead to a false diagnosis of heart disease. Cardiac arrhythmias, e.g., atrial fibrillation or flutter, common in women with mitral valve or congenital heart disease, may be a serious sign of cardiopathy.

In addition to these physiologic burdens, there are avoidable or treatable medical liabilities, e.g., anemia, obesity, hyperthyroidism, thyroid disease, infection, and emotional and physical stresses. Youth, adequate functional cardiac reserve, stability of the cardiac lesion, and an optimistic, cooperative attitude are important assets that do much to improve the cardiac patient's chances for a successful confinement.

Labor, delivery, and the early puerperium impose the following specific physiologic burdens on the maternal heart.

During Labor and Delivery

1. The *heart rate slows with each contraction* and returns to the resting level between contractions. The alteration is less in the lateral recumbent as compared to the supine position.

2. *Oxygen consumption increases* intermittently with uterine contractions, approaching that of moderate to severe exercise.

3. *Tachycardia during the second stage* may result from distention of the right atrium and ventricle by blood from the uterus and from the effect of straining.

During the Puerperium

1. *Cardiac output increases slightly* for ~1 week after delivery. Elimination of the placenta, contraction of the uterus, and reduction of the pelvic circulation suddenly make more blood available to the heart.

2. A *decrease in plasma volume* (*and increase in hematocrit*) occurs for about 12 h after delivery. A second marked decrease in plasma volume, with an accompanying reduction in the amount of total body water, persists for 7–9 days. These changes are due to postpartal diuresis.

Treatment

Determine the functional cardiac status (class I–IV) before the third month if possible and again at 7–8 months. Obtain consultation with a cardiologist for all class II–IV patients early in pregnancy. Restrict physical activity to necessary duties only, with fatigue as a limiting factor. Make certain that the patient obtains assistance with essential household duties (child care, laundry, cleaning, and marketing). Help the patient and her family to understand the medical problem and allay her fears, anxiety, and tension. Periods of maximal cardiac stress occur at 14–32 weeks, during labor, and, particularly, during the immediate postpartum period. Especially good rapport and medical control must be maintained at these times.

General Medical Measures

1. Correct anemia, hyperthyroidism, and obesity as indicated.

2. Limit sodium after 8–12 weeks in pregnant cardiac patients.

3. Avoid warfarin anticoagulant during pregnancy because of possible teratologic effects.

4. Treat cardiac complications, such as congestive failure, pulmonary edema, infective endocarditis, and arrhythmia, as in the nonpregnant patient. Diuretics may be used, but not to the point of hyponatremia. Avoid hypokalemia.

4. Prevent and treat preeclampsia-eclampsia.

5. Treat all infections specifically, promptly, and vigorously. Intercurrent respiratory, gastrointestinal tract, or urinary tract infections can be serious.

Individualize Therapy by Classification

1. *Class I–II.* The great majority of these patients who are asymptomatic or who have only mild distress with their usual activities can continue in pregnancy with minimal restriction or intervention other than close medical supervision. Severe activity-induced symptoms indicate cardiac decompensation, in which case hospitalization, treatment for cardiac failure, and bedrest until delivery are necessary.

2. *Class III.* In selected cases, pregnant patients with mitral stenosis who develop marked cardiac symptoms with average activity may be candidates for mitral valvulotomy up to the eighth month. Generally, in the absence of an operable lesion, severe activity limitation or bedrest until term is recommended.

3. *Class IV.* All gravidas up to about the 14th week of pregnancy with severe functional incapacity at rest, who do not have an operable cardiac abnormality, should consider abortion. If the lesion is not correctable, sterilization should also be considered. In some cases, cardiac surgery during pregnancy may be necessary. If the incapacity takes place in late pregnancy, it may be possible to prolong the pregnancy by maximal medical intervention to a premature but viable delivery.

Specific Delivery Measures

1. *Vaginal delivery is preferred* for patients with heart disease, except where there are obstetric indications for cesarean section. However, coarctation or aneurysm of the aorta contraindicates vaginal delivery, and numerous other patients will also require cesarean section on an individualized basis.

2. Manage the third stage of labor carefully to limit postpartum bleeding. *Do not administer ergot* preparations (which have a pressor effect), but give oxytocin if necessary after delivery for uterine atony.

3. *Lower the patient's legs promptly after delivery* (or deliver with the legs down) to reduce drainage of peripherally pooled blood into the systemic circulation.

4. *Anticipate* the possibility that some patients who have experienced no cardiac symptoms during pregnancy or labor may go into *shock or acute cardiac failure* immediately after delivery because of sudden engorgement of the splanchnic vessels. Treat for hypovolemic shock and acute cardiac failure.

5. Class I or II patients may breastfeed.

6. Prescribe cautious, brief, early ambulation of class I–III patients provided the medical course is otherwise uncomplicated.

7. Class II–IV patients must remain in the hospital after delivery until cardiovascular function is stable.

8. Before discharge, ascertain that the patient is returning to a controlled home situation where adequate rest in a nonstressful milieu will be possible.

9. Recommend contraception and urge sterilization, particularly for class II–IV patients with continuing disease or life-threatening conditions.

Surgical Measures

1. *Therapeutic abortion* may be indicated in 5%–8% of cases of heart disease complicating pregnancy. Patients who have had cardiac failure in a previous pregnancy will usually have failure again with another pregnancy and should consider abortion or sterilization or both. Abortion is seldom beneficial after the fourth month but may be considered.

2. If the cardiac lesion is severe enough to warrant abortion and if surgical treatment is not feasible, *sterilization* probably is indicated. If the patient is not sterilized, strict pregnancy prevention must be employed.

3. *Mitral valvotomy* is indicated only in patients with severe stenosis of the mitral valve who have insufficient cardiac reserve, even with ideal supportive therapy, to withstand the stress of pregnancy. In general, such patients will have had cardiac decompensation in a previous pregnancy despite the best care.

4. Even in the best of circumstances, *open heart surgery* during pregnancy *carries marked maternal and fetal risks.* Thus, it should be undertaken only when other possibilities have more morbidity and mortality.

Prognosis

Maternal Death

Cardiovascular disease is the sixth leading cause of maternal death (after infection, preeclampsia-eclampsia, hemorrhage, trauma, and complications of anesthesia). The maternal mortality rate for all types of heart disease is 0.5%–2% in large medical centers in the United States, and heart disease accounts for 5%–8% of all maternal deaths.

Perinatal Mortality

The perinatal mortality rate (including fetal deaths due to therapeutic abortion) largely depends on the functional severity of the mother's heart disease. Approximate rates are shown.

Mother's Functional Disability	Perinatal Mortality Rate
Class I	~5%
Class II	10%–15%
Class III	~35%
Class IV	>50%

Perinatal Morbidity

The *incidence of congenital defects* is greater among infants delivered of women with congenital and syphilitic heart disease than among those delivered of women with normal hearts, but rheumatic and other types of heart disease do not (without other factors) increase the incidence of fetal anomalies. Other forms of perinatal morbidity depend on the circumstances of the pregnancy and delivery and may include the sequelae of hypoxia and acidosis.

PERIPARTUM CARDIOMYOPATHY

This uncommon myocardial disorder, which causes cardiac failure 1–5 months postpartum, has an unknown etiology. It is potentially critical and most often affects multiparas with no evidence of prior heart disease. It seems predisposed by multiple gestation and preeclampsia-eclampsia. It must be distinguished from other cardiac disorders.

Dyspnea and chest pain with usual activity are the most common initial *symptoms*. A holosystolic murmur (mitral insufficiency) develops. Cardiac catheterization reveals cardiomegaly (ventricular dilatation) and low output cardiac failure with pulmonary hypertension. Pericardial effusion is never present.

Therapy includes digitalis, treatment of pulmonary edema, medical consultation, extended bedrest, and possibly anticoagulant therapy (to minimize embolization). Patients who respond and whose heart size returns to normal within 6 months have a good prognosis but should be aware that peripartum cardiomyopathy may recur after subsequent pregnancy. For those who do not respond within 6 months, the disease is all too frequently fatal. Cardiac transplantation may be lifesaving in some patients. Postmortem findings include focal myocardial degeneration and mural thrombi but no coronary disease.

TRAUMA DURING PREGNANCY

Physical trauma, especially that involving automobile accidents, affects thousands of pregnant women yearly in the United States. *The primary diagnostic concern is to differentiate traumatic shock from drug or substance abuse and from posteclamptic coma.* The physiologic changes of pregnancy may mimic symptoms of shock in gravid accident patients (e.g., increased respiratory rate, hyperventilation, increased pulse rate, and potentially lower blood pressure). Moreover, because of the physiologic anemia of pregnancy, a slightly low HCT may not be a good indication of blood loss. Obviously, it is impossible to detail therapy for the many trauma situations that might complicate pregnancy. However, certain elements of managing the pregnant trauma patient warrant emphasis.

Emergency and Supportive Treatment

A. *Resuscitate, ensure the airway, and give oxygen* if the patient is unconscious.

B. Pregnant women are prone to regurgitation with aspiration of gastric contents. *Insert a nasogastric tube with suction* if the patient is obtunded to avoid gastric fluid aspiration.

C. *Monitor the vital signs,* and check for CNS, abdominal, or other injuries.

D. *Treat shock very aggressively* (it is poorly tolerated by the fetus).

1. While blood studies are being done, the patient is being assessed, and IVs are started, an autotransfusion may be achieved by wrapping the legs with elastic bandages and elevating the legs. MAST trousers may be lifesaving in massive trauma.

2. In late pregnancy, ascertain that the inferior vena caval syndrome is not compounding the problem by elevating the right hip or placing the patient in a lateral recumbent position.

3. Start IV fluids, usually lactated Ringer's solution. Even transient hypovolemia should be avoided, since it poses special fetal risk.

E. *Ascertain fetal well-being* (regardless of the gestational age).

1. An electronic fetal monitoring device will assist in ascertaining fetal well-being as well as determining uterine contractions.

2. Additional information may be obtained by a BPP.

3. Real time ultrasonography is necessary in even the earliest gestations to ascertain the fetal status and detail any potential problems (either preexisting or secondary to the trauma).

F. Promptly *transfer patient to a perinatal center,* even for seemingly minor injuries.

G. Anesthesia or cesarean section may further jeopardize the accident victim. However, prompt *abdominal delivery may be necessary* to save the mother with a ruptured viscus or internal hemorrhage. Additionally, an uncontrollably distressed fetus will require immediate rescue.

H. The tissue thromboplastin released from blunt trauma all too frequently leads to initiation of the clotting cascade, with development of abruptio placentae. Thus, *observe carefully any mother with trauma for 24–48 h* to ascertain that abruptio placentae is not occurring.

I. Best results are achieved by a team approach, with consultation with a trauma surgeon and neonatologist.

HEMATOLOGIC DISORDERS

ANEMIA

The physiologic alterations discussed in Chapter 3 and certain of the pathologic changes possible during pregnancy make the determination of anemia difficult. Not only do blood values during pregnancy differ from those in the nonpregnant patient, but these factors also vary as a function of the length of pregnancy.

In every evaluation of clinical and laboratory data, the following questions must be answered: (1) Is *anemia* present? (2) Is there evidence of *iron deficiency?* (3) Are *megaloblasts* present in the blood smear? (4) Are there signs of *hemolysis?* (5) Is there *bone marrow deficiency?*

Iron Deficiency Anemia (IDA)

IDA is the most common anemia in pregnancy. About 95% of pregnant women with anemia have IDA due to excessive menses or iron deprivation often from previous pregnancies. It is also the most likely anemia of undetermined type, regardless of cell morphology.

Pregnancy increases the gravida's total iron requirements. Of ~1 g (4–5 mg/dl) of elemental iron needed, 300 mg is for the fetus and placenta and 700 mg is added to the maternal hemoglobin. About 200 mg of iron is lost in bleeding during and after delivery. Fortunately, some 500 mg of iron from leftover (metabolized) maternal RBCs is returned to iron stores postpartum. Therefore, the *mother loses about 500 mg of iron with each viable pregnancy.* Repeated pregnancies, especially with a short interval between, can result in severe iron deficiency. Many women, anemic before pregnancy, never catch up during gestation or afterward because their iron stores remain low.

Laboratory Findings

Hgb may be ≤5g/dl
RBC ≤2.5 million/μl
Mean corpuscular volume (MCV) = ≤80 mm^3 (microcytosis)
Mean corpuscular Hgb concentration ≤93 (hypochromia)
Serum iron ≤60 mg/dl
Total iron-binding capacity ≥300 mg/dl
Transferrin saturation ≤15%
Bone marrow: stain faint or negative for iron

Differential diagnosis includes microcytic anemia (thalassemia) or anemia of chronic debilitating disease, e.g., sprue.

Complications of uncorrected IDA include maternal infections and low-birth-weight infants. Severe IDA is associated with increased maternal and perinatal morbidity.

Treatment

A. *Oral iron.* Ferrous sulfate 325 mg tid (180 mg elemental iron per day).

B. *Parenteral iron.* For intolerance to oral iron or poor absorption, parenteral iron 250 mg for each gram of Hgb below normal (normal in women 12–16 g/dl) is advised. Iron dextran (Imferon) contains 5% metallic iron (50 mg/ml). Give 50 mg (1 ml) IM initially, then 100–250 mg IM twice weekly until the total dose has been given. *Note:* Inject deeply with a 2-inch needle into the upper outer quadrant of the buttock using a Z technique; i.e., draw the skin and then the superficial musculature to one side or the other to prevent leakage and tattooing of the skin.

Prognosis

The symptomatology of the IDA will resolve with correction of the anemia. Improvement following the use of parenteral iron is usually only slightly more rapid than with oral medication.

Prevention

The total pregnancy iron requirements of 800 mg cannot be met by adequate diet alone. Therefore, daily elemental iron prophylaxis for all gravidas of 60 mg/day is recommended. Ferrous rather than ferric iron is preferable because the former is better absorbed and is cheaper.

Folic Acid Deficiency Anemia (Pernicious or Megaloblastic Anemia of Pregnancy)

Pernicious anemia of pregnancy is caused by folic acid—*not* vitamin B_{12}—deficiency. Unusual in the United States, the reported incidence of folic acid deficiency anemia (FADA) abroad is 1:400–1:1200 deliveries. Folic acid deficiency is most common in multiparas >30 or in individuals on inadequate diets. Other *predispositions to FADA* include multiple pregnancy, preeclampsia-eclampsia, sickle cell anemia (whose bone marrow requirements for folic acid are increased), and epileptics on prolonged treatment with primidone (Mysoline) or phenytoin (Dilantin), both antifolate drugs.

The usual *symptomology* (and signs) includes lassitude, anorexia, and mental depression. Pallor may not be marked. Glossitis, gingivitis, emesis, or diarrhea may occur, but there are no abnormal neurologic signs.

Laboratory Findings

Serum folate is low.
Increased segmental PMN leukocytes are prominent.
The Hgb may be ≤4–6 g/dl and the RBCs may be ≤2 million/dl.

The MCV is normal or increased.
Bone marrow hyperplasia with megaloblasts is typical.
Serum iron levels are high.
Serum vitamin B_{12} levels are normal.

Differential Diagnosis

FADA is uncommon in the reproductive years, but vitamin B_{12} anemia is not. Both disorders evoke megaloblastosis. Strict vegetarians may develop vitamin B_{12} anemia but not FADA. In FADA, serum vitamin B_{12} values and gastric HCl are normal, but they are low in true pernicious anemia.

Complications

Secondary infections, placental separation, and bleeding often occur with FADA. Increased maternal morbidity and perinatal mortality are recognized, although the fetus does surprisingly well even when the mother's anemia is severe.

Treatment

Give folic acid, 5–10 mg/day orally or parenterally, until a hematologic remission is achieved. Megaloblastic anemia of pregnancy does not usually respond to vitamin B_{12} even in large doses. *Administer iron* orally as indicated. Prescribe a high-vitamin, high-protein diet. Transfusions are rarely necessary, and therapeutic abortion and sterilization are not indicated for FADA.

Prognosis

FADA during pregnancy is not apt to be severe unless it is associated with systemic infection or preeclampsia-eclampsia. If the diagnosis is made at least 4 weeks before term, treatment often can raise the hemoglobin level to normal or nearly normal. The *outlook for mother and infant is good* if there is adequate time for treatment. Spontaneous remission usually occurs after delivery. Anemia usually recurs only when the patient becomes pregnant again.

Drug-Induced Hemolytic Anemia

Drug-induced hemolytic anemia during pregnancy or the puerperium may occur in individuals with the inborn error of metabolism, glucose-6-phosphate dehydrogenase deficiency (G6PD) in erythrocytes. This X-linked trait affects 12% of black men and 3% of black women. The trait is sex-linked and of intermediate dominance. Whites, mainly of Mediterranean or Middle East origin, may develop either an acute or a chronic hemolytic anemia due to G6PD in which both the RBC and WBC lack the enzyme.

The anemia develops after diabetic acidosis, viral or bacterial infections, ingestion of fava beans, exposure to naphthalene (moth balls), or after treatment with oxidant drugs (including primaquine, nitrofurantoin, or sulfonamides). The anemia may affect either mothers or their neonates and is a self-limited, acute, moderately severe, hemolytic anemia.

Prevention

Education of those likely to be predisposed to induced hemolytic anemia will avoid or decrease the problem.

Laboratory Tests

Obtain a G6PD test.

Treatment

Discontinue the drug or toxic substance. Treat infection vigorously. Give iron supplements. Transfusion is rarely necessary.

Prognosis

Recovery with proper therapy is likely.

Sickle Cell Disease

Sickle cell anemia is an *autosomal recessive disorder* in which the homozygous individual (sickle cell anemia) has a preponderance of Hgb S (as contrasted to the usual Hgb A). Hemoglobin S is less soluble in deoxygenated form, and the erythrocytes sickle (deform) at low oxygen tension and especially at low pH. Heterozygous carriers (sickle cell trait) have both Hgb A *and* Hgb S. Those with sickle trait have RBC sickling in vitro (a useful test) but do not manifest the sickling in vivo (with rare exception), as do those with sickle cell anemia (homozygous individual). Sickle cell disease occurs almost exclusively in blacks. In the United States, 8%–10% of African Americans have sickle cell trait, and 1:500 has sickle cell anemia.

The substitution of only a single amino acid, *valine,* for glutamic acid at the sixth position on each of two hemoglobin β chains distinguishes the sickle cell hemoglobin molecule from Hgb A. The oxygen-carrying capacity and survival time of the sickle cell RBC are adversely affected by this anomaly. In vivo the tendency for the RBC to sickle depends primarily on the state of Hgb oxygenation, temperature, levels of non-S hemoglobin, and intraepithelial Hgb concentration. With sickle cell disease, intravascular sickling begins with oxygen saturation of <85% and is almost complete at 38% oxygen saturation. Patients with sickle cell trait (Hgb A and Hgb S) show no sickling until the oxygen saturation is <40%.

Sickled cells are more rigid and may block the blood flow in the microvasculature. This causes resistance to blood flow, impeding RBC passage. Adherence of RBC to vascular endothelium and vascular stasis causes further deoxygenation and platelet aggregation, local hypoxia, worsening acidosis, and accelerated sickling, and, eventually, tissue infarction occurs. All organs can be involved, especially those with turbid flow and high oxygen extraction, e.g., the spleen, bone marrow, and placenta. Pain and edema are common in ischemic tissue (vaso-occlusive crisis). Until the RBC has become irreversibly sickled because of a damaged membrane, the sickled erythrocyte can return to its rounded shape when hypoxic or acidic conditions are neutralized. Sickle cell crises, often precipitated by infection, dehydration, fever, or exposure to cold, may last for hours or days.

With sickle cell disease during gestation, anemia is accelerated (a complication in ~50%) and often has a folic acid overlay, the frequency of painful crises is increased, urinary tract infections and pyelonephritis are increased, and thrombosis or visceral or orthopedic pain is quite frequent. Other complications include hematuria, leg ulcers, bone infarction, osteomyelitis, cholecystitis, and cardiopathy. Overtreatment with iron may result in hemochromatosis. Acute sequestration of sickled RBC is evidenced by a rapidly falling Hgb, even ≤3 g/dl. Marrow aplasia may be a sequel to a crisis.

Sickle cell disease is inimicable to pregnancy. *The fetus is at considerable risk because of the maternal complications.* Moreover, genetic counseling is crucial. For example, if both parents have sickle cell trait, the offspring's chance is 1:4 of having sickle cell anemia, and one half of offspring will be carriers. If one parent has sickle cell disease and the other has only Hgb A, all of the offspring will have sickle cell trait.

Laboratory Findings

The Hgb may fall to 7–8 g. The *reticulocyte count will be elevated.* Population screening for sickling is useful for carrier detection but does not differentiate between the different hemoglobins that may be involved (S, C, or D) or separate sickle cell trait and sickle cell disease. The definitive test is *hemoglobin electrophoresis.*

Treatment

Obstetric patients in sickle cell crisis should be referred to a tertiary hospital where *automated erythrocytopheresis* is available as soon as feasible. This technique removes both Hgb S-containing RBCs and irreversibly sickled cells by extracorporeal differential centrifugation. The patient's own plasma, including leukocytes, platelets, and clotting factors, is simultaneously returned together with buffy coat-poor, washed donor RBCs. All of this can increase Hgb A concentration rapidly, and hypovolemia is minimized.

To avoid crisis antenatally, *a high hemoglobin must be maintained.* The concentration of Hgb S should be <50% to prevent crisis. Thus, *transfusions are often necessary.* Indeed, if erythrocytopheresis is not available for crisis, partial exchange transfusion will interrupt a sickle cell crisis during pregnancy. This temporarily diminishes erythropoiesis, improves oxygen-carrying capacity of the circulating blood, and reduces the concentration of Hgb S by substituting Hgb A-containing RBC for Hgb S-containing cells.

Patients with sickle cell disease should be offered maximal obstetric care. If this is unavailable, strict contraception is recommended until their circumstances can be maximized. If maternal complications are too life-threatening, sterilization should be considered. Cesarean section should be performed on obstetric indications.

Prognosis

Before modern treatment modalities, maternal mortality was as high as 25% in sickle cell anemia but should be <5% today. Transfusions decrease the severity of pain during crises and benefit the fetus indirectly. Perinatal growth retardation is common. Almost half of all pregnancies of women with sickle cell anemia end in perinatal death unless maximal obstetric care is given.

THROMBOEMBOLIZATION

Thrombophlebitis and Phlebothrombosis

Thromboembolization (TE) is a common complication of pregnancy antepartum (0.2%), postpartum (0.6%), and following cesarean section (1%–2%). Unfortunately, pulmonary embolism (15% mortality) occurs in about half of those with documented deep vein thrombosis (DVT), and only 5%–10% are symptomatic before the pulmonary embolism! Fortunately, DVT is uncommon without predisposing factors, including postpartum endomyometritis (or other severe infection), previous TE, severe superficial thrombophlebitis, major venous varicosities, operative delivery, difficult or prolonged labor, anemia, hemorrhage, heart disease, obesity, heavy smoking, enforced bedrest (e.g., a fracture), and cancer.

The *pregnant woman's predispositions to TE* include stasis, vascular damage, and hypercoagulability. Venous thrombi usually develop in relatively small veins and then extend centrally (they are almost always in the lower extremities or pelvis) as far as the inferior vena cava. The usual *symptoms and signs* (erythematous, tender, firm vein) *are usually absent with DVT*. However, if larger proximal veins are involved, swelling of the affected leg, pain, tenderness, local cyanosis, and fever may occur. If the iliofemoral system is involved, there is acute swelling of the leg, pain about the hip, vaginal bleeding, and possibly pain over the femoral triangle. Homans' sign is of little value.

Compression stockings or pantyhose are of some preventive value. However, in those at risk, *prophylaxis* is best accomplished using heparin 5000 units bid to tid (depending on the patient's size and stage of pregnancy—one third more is required from the beginning of the third trimester). Preoperatively, subcutaneous heparin (5000 units 2 h before surgery, repeated 12 h after surgery, then bid until the patient is ambulatory) is preventive.

If the condition is even considered, *initiate diagnostic studies:*

directional Doppler ultrasound, venography, or various tests for thrombosis. Superficial venous thrombophlebitis is treated with limb elevation, moist heat, and nonsteroidal anti-inflammatory agents.

Heparin is the drug of choice for acute therapy of DVT; 25,000–30,000 units/24 h may be given IV (continuously or intermittent bolus) or intermittently subcutaneously. This therapy must be monitored carefully because bleeding is a major side effect (5%). Other side effects include thrombocytopenia, fat necrosis, and (over long term) osteoporosis.

Monitoring heparin's activity is primarily accomplished by activated partial thromboplastin time (the goal is 1.5–2 times the control), but coagulation time, thrombin clotting time, and heparin assay may be useful. Heparin should not be administered if the platelets are ≤50,000 μl. Protamine (1 mg/100 units of heparin) will rapidly counteract heparin's effects.

Oral anticoagulants (warfarin) usually are contraindicated during pregnancy because of possible teratic effects (nasal hypoplasia, skeletal abnormalities, and multiple CNS problems). It is concentrated in the breast milk and is thus problematic to the newborn but may be useful for long-term postpartum therapy in the nonbreastfeeding mother.

Septic Pelvic Thrombophlebitis (SPT)

SPT occurs in 1 in 2000 deliveries and is defined as *clotting in pelvic veins due to infection*. It is predisposed by infection (e.g., prolonged rupture of the membranes), operative delivery, malnourishment, and systemic disease. It most commonly occurs 2–3 days to 6 weeks postpartum. Even with modern therapy, the mortality approaches 10%.

The usual clinical presentation is a picket-fence fever (from normal up to 41°C) in spite of adequate anaerobic and aerobic organism antibiotic coverage. The pelvic examination is usually normal, but about one third of patients will have palpable veins in the vaginal fornices or parametrial or lower abdominal areas. The pulse and the respiratory rate may be rapid. In untreated cases, 30%–40% will have septic pulmonary embolism.

The *differential diagnosis* includes pyelonephritis, appendicitis, meningitis, SLE, TB, malaria, typhoid, sickle cell crisis and adnexal torsion. *Treatment* is heparin and broad-spectrum antibiotics. Within 48–72 h, the fever should resolve, but heparin should be continued for 7–10 days. Surgery is only indicated if medical management fails, if septic emboli occur during therapy, if the patient has puerperal sepsis and pulmonary infarction, or if medical therapy is contraindicated. In such cases, percutaneous placement of a vena caval filter often is all that is necessary. However, occasionally it is necessary to ligate the ovarian veins.

LEUKEMIA, LYMPHOMA, AND HODGKIN'S DISEASE

Leukemia affects the leukopoietic tissues (lymphatic, myeloid, or monocytic) and may be acute or chronic. Lymphomas affect the lymphoreticular system and are subdivided into Hodgkin's disease and non-Hodgkin's lymphoma. All types usually occur after the childbearing age, so *these conditions are an uncommon pregnancy complication.*

A normochromic, normocytic anemia occurs in leukemia and Hodgkin's disease. Moderate thrombocytopenia and marked leukocytosis must be expected. Bleeding and premature delivery are common. The perinatal mortality rate is high and may depend on the necessary maternal therapy. Several cases of possible transfer of leukemia or Hodgkin's disease to the offspring have been reported and mandate careful follow-up. Approximately 85% of Hodgkin's relapses occur <2 years. Thus, if another pregnancy is planned, it is recommended to defer it until the mother's stability is determined. Definitive discussion of these unusual conditions is beyond the purpose of this text.

RENAL DISEASES

URINARY TRACT INFECTION

The urinary tract is especially vulnerable to infection during pregnancy because of *ureteral dilatation, urinary stasis,* and *ureterovesical reflux.* The *trauma of labor and delivery* and *urinary retention after delivery* may also initiate or aggravate infection in the urinary system. *Escherichia coli* is the offending organism in ~80% of cases.

Asymptomatic bacteriuria occurs in at least 3% of all pregnant women, and intercurrent pyelonephritis can be expected in >30% of these patients without prophylactic treatment. By way of contrast, symptomatic urinary tract infection will develop in only 1%–2% of pregnant women without antecedent bacteriuria. Up to an additional 5% will develop urinary tract infections after delivery. Chronic pyelonephritis, a major contributor to death in older women, often follows recurrent acute urinary tract infections during successive pregnancies. Symptomatic urinary tract infection is responsible for a considerable increase in the incidence of premature rupture of the membranes and premature delivery and its resultant morbidity and mortality.

The diagnosis should be based on urinalysis and culture of a catheterized or clean-catch specimen of urine. If the culture reveals >100,000 colonies/ml, treatment is required. Sensitivity tests to determine response to the various antiinfective agents are desirable. An initial urinary infection may be treated with ampicillin (250 mg qid) or nitrofurantoin (100 mg orally qid). Change to other drugs as dictated by the results of laboratory studies, but treat for 2 weeks.

Repeat urinary culture after completion of therapy is useful to ascertain therapeutic effectiveness. If urine cultures are not available, use one of the nitrite tests, or a stained smear of the centrifuged sediment of a catheterized or clean-catch specimen may be examined for bacteria each week for 3 weeks. If no bacteria or pus cells are seen and the patient is asymptomatic, she probably is cured.

For urgency and frequency, give pyridium 100 mg qid. Force fluids (if indicated) and acidify the urine (vitamin C or cranberry juice). Give analgesics, laxatives, and antipyretic drugs as indicated.

If obstruction is present, urethral or ureteral catheterization may be necessary. Ureteral obstruction usually resolves after delivery, but if it is permanent, surgical repair may be required. If response to chemotherapy and ureteral catheterization is inadequate, nephrotomy may be necessary, particularly during the second trimester and before fetal viability.

GLOMERULONEPHRITIS

An initial attack of acute glomerulonephritis is rare during pregnancy. Most obstetric problems developing to glomerulonephritis involve chronic forms of the disease. *There is no evidence that pregnancy aggravates glomerulonephritis.*

Infertility, abortion, premature delivery, fetal death in utero, premature separation of the normally implanted placenta, and placental dysmaturity occur more frequently in women with glomerulonephritis than in normal women. Nephritis causes hypertension, predisposes to preeclampsia-eclampsia, and is associated with a high incidence of perinatal mortality and morbidity. Fetal growth and activity must be carefully monitored.

The medical treatment of glomerulonephritis is the same whether or not the patient is pregnant. Corticosteroids may be harmful, and antibiotics are ineffective. Therapeutic abortion may be justified for acute, severe exacerbations of glomerulonephritis with renal insufficiency.

Glomerulonephritis may be an indication for cesarean section when placental dysmaturity or preeclampsia-eclampsia occurs.

URETERAL STONE

Ureteral stone is more common during pregnancy than otherwise because hypercalciuria occurs during pregnancy when calcium and vitamin D are supplemented, because the renal pelvis and ureter dilate in response to high levels of steroid sex hormones, and because minor (physiologic) obstructive uropathy is characteristic of pregnancy. Small, previously retained stones are thus permitted to enter the proximal ureter. Most ureteral stones are passed in the urine, albeit painfully. Others become impacted. Sudden, agonizing pain in the costovertebral angle and flank with radiation to the lower quadrant and vulva, urinary urgency, and hematuria without (initially) pyuria or fever are characteristic of ureteral stone. Intravenous urography may demonstrate partial obstruction and the stone.

Symptomatic therapy with analgesics and antispasmodics is always indicated and may be best given parenterally. Retrograde catheter manipulation may dislodge the stone and permit it to pass, or the stone may be extracted transurethrally. If such efforts are unsuccessful and progressive hydronephrosis develops, remove the stone by extraperitoneal ureterolithectomy irrespective of the patient's obstetric status. Lithotripsy during pregnancy is contraindicated.

GASTROINTESTINAL DISORDERS

PEPTIC ULCER

Pregnancy generally exerts an ameliorating effect on peptic ulcer, but hemorrhage or perforation may occur during or shortly after pregnancy. Pregnancy offers no protection to aggravation of peptic ulcer by anxiety. Exacerbation of peptic ulcer in the puerperium may be a result of a rise in gastric acidity during lactation.

Medical treatment is the same as for the nonpregnant woman, but cimetidine and other histamine receptor antagonists are pregnancy class B drugs (use only if clearly needed, as there are promising animal studies but no well-controlled studies in pregnant women). Surgery should be reserved for emergencies.

HIATAL HERNIA

Hiatal hernia, or partial protrusion of the stomach or esophagus (or both) through the diaphragm, develops in patients with a weakened or congenitally widened diaphragmatic crux because of increases in intraabdominal pressure during pregnancy. With gestation, there is progressive enlargement of the uterus with elevation of the stomach by the uterine fundus. Hiatal hernia occurs more frequently in multiparas and in older or obese pregnant women. About 15% of all pregnant women develop symptomatic hiatal hernia.

Persistence of nausea and vomiting beyond midpregnancy, progressive pyrosis, and eructation during recumbency are typical findings. The sensation of substernal pressure may be severe and is relieved by erect posture but aggravated by lying down.

Conservative treatment is usually adequate to carry the patient through pregnancy and delivery. Prescribe a bland diet, small meals, antispasmodics, and antacids (calcium products are preferred), and caution the patient against lying flat or exercising immediately after eating or drinking. Prevent unnecessary increases in intraabdominal pressure by prescribing laxatives for constipation, by restricting lifting, and by the use of low forceps delivery so that the patient will not have to bear down during the second stage of labor. The patient should sleep in a semireclining position. Obese women should not gain extra weight. The great majority of hiatal hernias resolve soon after delivery, with dramatic relief. Thus, surgery is rarely necessary.

BOWEL OBSTRUCTION

Mechanical obstruction of the intestine (most frequently the small bowel) occurs in about 1:6000 pregnancies. About one quarter of cases occur during the second trimester, when the enlarging uterus displaces the bowel sufficiently to stretch adhesions. Mechanical obstruction should be considered as a cause of ileus in women with one or more abdominal scars. Other causes of obstruction include incarceration of a loop of intestine in an external or internal hernia, volvulus, and intussusception. Symptoms of bowel obstruction include nausea, vomiting, and persistent abdominal pain.

Laparotomy is indicated without delay. The maternal mortality rate may be as high as 10% if treatment of septic closed-loop obstruction is delayed. *Fluid and electrolyte imbalance must be corrected early.* (*Note:* Hypokalemic alkalosis can cause convulsions that may be confused with eclamptic seizures.) Broad-spectrum antibiotics should be given parenterally if infection occurs.

ADYNAMIC ILEUS

Mild adynamic ileus may be present for 1–3 days even after normal delivery or longer after cesarean section. Other obstetric and gynecologic conditions that may cause adynamic ileus are intraperitoneal, or retroperitoneal hemorrhage and infection, pyelonephritis, nephroureterolithiasis, torsion of the adnexa, bladder atony, and hypokalemic acidosis. Older women seem more prone to adynamic ileus than young ones.

Adynamic ileus in obstetric and gynecologic patients almost always responds to withholding oral food and fluids, correction of fluid and electrolyte imbalance by means of parenteral fluids, intestinal (nasogastric) decompression, and evacuation of the rectosigmoid colon by enemas. In more difficult cases, gastric suction usually will suffice. If ileus is marked, a long intestinal tube (Werner, Miller-Abbott) should be inserted to decompress the small bowel.

APPENDICITIS

Appendicitis occurs in about 1:1200 pregnancies (Fig. 14-3). Management is more difficult than when the disease occurs in nonpregnant persons because the appendix is carried high and to the right, away from McBurney's point. Hence, the traditional localization of pain does not usually occur. The distended uterus

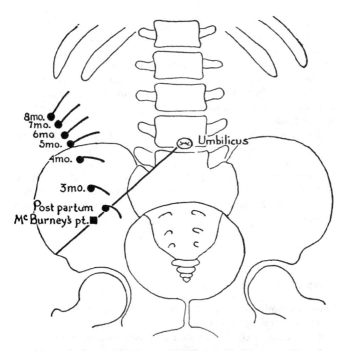

Figure 14-3. Diagram showing the level of the appendix at the various months of pregnancy (Baer). (From A.C. Beck and A.H. Rosenthal, *Obstetrical Practice*. 7th ed. Williams & Wilkins, 1957.)

displaces the colon and small bowel, uterine contractions prevent abscess formation and walling-off, and the intestinal relationships are disturbed. In at least 20% of obstetric patients with appendicitis, the correct diagnosis is not made until the appendix has ruptured and peritonitis has become established. Delay may lead to sepsis, premature labor, or abortion.

Early appendectomy is indicated. If the diagnosis is made during labor or near term, cesarean section and appendectomy should be done to minimize peritonitis. Therapeutic abortion is never indicated. If drains are necessary, they should be transabdominal, never transvaginal. With early diagnosis and appendectomy, the prognosis is good for the mother and infant, but if intraabdominal abscesses occur, labor may cause subsequent rupture, with massive sepsis.

INFLAMMATORY BOWEL DISEASE

The cause of this group of diseases (regional enteritis or Crohn's disease, ulcerative colitis, and granulomatous colitis) remains unknown. Young women are most commonly affected, and the peak incidence is in the second and third decades. In the absence of pelvic abscesses, fertility is unaffected. Crohn's disease increases abortion by 25%, but ulcerative colitis and granulomatous colitis do not enhance the rate of abortion. In general, pregnancy is not contraindicated, nor does pregnancy generally exert an untoward influence on inflammatory bowel disease. However, when conception coincides with active ulcerative colitis, 50%–75% of patients will suffer a severe relapse during pregnancy or in the puerperium. When colitis has its onset during pregnancy, more than half of the patients will suffer a hectic course, and a few will die. When colitis has its onset during the puerperium, most patients will have a very severe, often protracted course.

In severe, fulminating cases, colitis induces intractable bloody diarrhea, fever, fluid and electrolyte imbalance, collapse, toxicosis, and death. When the disease becomes chronic, malnutrition and invalidism are associated with remissions and exacerbations of diarrhea.

There is no specific treatment. Dietary, symptomatic, and supportive medical measures, corticosteroids, and sulfasalazine are usually employed during pregnancy. Although, the last two are possible teratogens, that small risk is usually preferable to acute exacerbations. Sulfasalazine may cause neonatal hyperbilirubinemia, and if it is used, maternal folic acid should be administered.

BILIARY AND HEPATIC DISORDERS

Choledocholithiasis and Cholecystitis

Severe choledocholithiasis and cholecystitis are *uncommon during pregnancy* despite the fact that the smooth muscle relaxation of pregnancy (due to progesterone) is predisposing and women have an increased tendency to form gallstones (one third of all women over age 40 have gallstones). When acute gallbladder inflammation or biliary colic does occur, it is usually in late pregnancy or, more often, in the puerperium. About 90% of patients with cholecystitis have stones.

When cholecystitis occurs, *treatment* with antibiotics, IV fluids, and nasogastric drainage may be all that is required. Meperidine or atropine is effective in alleviating pain and ductal spasm. Gallbladder surgery in pregnant women should be attempted only in extreme cases (e.g., obstruction) because it greatly increases the perinatal mortality rate (up to about 15%). Cholecystostomy and lithotomy may be all that is feasible during advanced pregnancy, with cholecystectomy deferred until after delivery. On the other hand, withholding surgery when it is definitely needed may result in necrosis and perforation of the gallbladder and peritonitis. Intermittent high fever, jaundice, and right upper quadrant pain may indicate cholangitis due to impacted common duct stone.

Cholestatic Jaundice of Pregnancy

Cholestatic or recurrent jaundice of pregnancy is an uncommon disorder of successive pregnancies that is caused by an *inherited deficiency in liver metabolism.* Hepatic excretory insufficiency is apparently provoked by estrogen. Cholestatic jaundice of pregnancy is characterized by itching, gastrointestinal complaints, and jaundice during the last trimester of pregnancy. The symptoms disappear within 2 weeks after delivery but tend to recur in subsequent advanced pregnancies. The levels of most liver enzymes are only slightly elevated, and the results of hepatic function tests are normal.

The *diagnosis* of cholestatic jaundice of pregnancy requires the exclusion of other liver disorders, e.g., viral hepatitis, drug toxicity, and cholecystitis. A history of jaundice during a previous pregnancy or with use of oral contraceptives is most helpful diagnostically. *Treatment is symptomatic.* Jaundice and itching may be reduced by administration of ion exchange resins, which absorb bile salts.

Cholestyramine may be beneficial. However, it absorbs fat-soluble vitamins and may even induce bleeding due to malabsorption of vitamin K. Thus, vitamin K supplementation should be given to both mother and newborn. This disorder is limited to the duration of pregnancy (or estrogen therapy).

Acute Fatty Liver of Pregnancy

This rare (1:13,000) disease in the past had maternal and perinatal mortality of 75%–85%, but this is currently down to ~20%. It is a maternal multisystem disorder with hepatitis a prominent manifestation and usually occurs >35 weeks and does not tend to recur with subsequent pregnancy. The *symptoms* include severe nausea, vomiting, hematemesis, abdominal pain, jaundice, stupor, and progressive hepatic insufficiency. Disseminated intravascular coagulation or renal failure may be associated late problems.

Acute fatty liver must be *differentiated* from toxic or viral hepatitis, cholestatic liver dysfunction, cholecystitis, and pancreatitis. *Effective supportive therapy is the only known treatment.*

Viral Hepatitis

Three types of viral hepatitis (A, B, and C) affect females of all ages. The incidence is 0.2% in pregnancy when the manifestations, although similar, may be more severe and prolonged (especially in advanced pregnancy). Maternal and perinatal prognosis is quite different in the three types. Table 14-1 details characteristics of the three types.

Treatment for all three generally consists of supportive medical measures as for the nonpregnant patient. Certain other generalizations may be useful. Operative intervention is to be avoided, if possible. Anesthetics, analgesics, and sedatives that may be hepatotoxic must be avoided. A very low prothrombin concentration may lead to hemorrhage, which should be treated with oral or parenteral vitamin K. The maternal and fetal risks are low (except as noted later) if adequate nutrition is maintained. Terminate pregnancy only in case of impending or actual hepatic coma. Deterioration may justify cesarean section for the viable infant.

If obstetric care is good, the *maternal mortality rate* is approximately that of nonpregnant women with viral hepatitis. It is wise to allow more than 1 year to elapse between hepatitis and subsequent pregnancy. By this time, liver function tests should return to normal values unless serious complications have developed. The fetal effect of chronic active hepatitis depends on the extent of maternal disease (loss is high with poor liver function or esophageal varices). Treatment with immunosuppressants and corticosteroids does not preclude pregnancy.

Hepatitis A (*infectious hepatitis*) is usually quite benign during pregnancy, with only enteric isolation, supportive treatment, and careful monitoring of liver enzymes being necessary. Hepatitis A antibody is useful for detection. The rate of perinatal (fetal or neonatal) transmission is low, and maternal and perinatal morbidity is little affected in developed countries, although there is enhanced loss in undeveloped areas. Gamma globulin prophylaxis is effective protection for pregnant women exposed to hepatitis A.

Table 14-1. Characteristics of viral hepatitis

	Hepatitis A	Hepatitis B	Hepatitis C (non-A, non-B)
Virus	RNA (27 nm)	DNA (42 nm)	RNA (30–50 nm)
Incubation (days)	15–50	45–160	18–100
Source	Enteric (fecal-oral), close family or contacts	Parenteral (body fluids), blood, saliva, vaginal secretions, semen	Parenteral (body fluids)
Laboratory diagnosis	HA Ab (IgM, IgG)	HBsAG, HBcAb, HBsAB, HBeAg	HCAb
Perinatal transmission	Low	Active 0–28 weeks <10% 29–40 weeks 65% Carrier HBeAG+ 75–95% HBeAg− <5% HBcAg+ <5%	Unknown
Newborn	Rare 14–30 days	Active 30–120 days Mild disease Carrier 30–120 days Severe disease (death possible)	Unknown
Carrier development (maternal)	0	5%–10%	50%
Carrier development (infant)	None	Frequent	Unknown
Sequelae	None	Chronic active hepatitis	Chronic active hepatitis

Hepatitis B (serum hepatitis) occurs in about 1:500 pregnancies. Vertical transmission may be prevented by hepatitis B immune globulin and hepatitis B vaccine. Detection is by screening with hepatitis B surface antigen (HBsAg) and the hepatitis B surface antibody (HBsAb). HBsAb indicates a noninfectious state. HBsAg without HBsAb is the chronic carrier state, with a high likelihood (75%–95%) of vertical transmission. When HBsAg is detected, it is imperative to ascertain if the e antigen is present. The maternal course is unaltered, but prematurity is increased. Care must be taken not to infect the newborn at delivery. When the mother is HBsAg positive and HBsAb negative, the neonate should have HBsAg and HBsAb studies drawn and receive both hepatitis B immune globulin and the hepatitis B vaccine immediately. If antigenicity studies can be obtained rapidly, hepatitis B vaccine may be delayed up to 7 days of age. If the baby is HBsAg negative, the original dose is given and is then repeated 1 month later. The third dose is given 6 months after the original dose.

Hepatitis C (non-A, non-B) is diagnosed after ruling out hepatitis from other sources (especially infections, e.g., mononucleosis, cytomegalovirus, Epstein-Barr virus). Immune globulin is indicated for the newborn of a mother with active disease to decrease the infectious morbidity.

ABDOMINAL HERNIAS
(Intestinal)

As pregnancy advances, the enlarging uterus fills the lower abdomen, displacing the intestines, so that nonadherent bowel may recede from an inguinal aperture. However, pregnancy permanently enlarges umbilical and incisional hernial rings. The uterus also shields incisional and other weak points from herniation. Hence, many abdominal hernias reduce spontaneously during pregnancy. A few irreducible (adherent) ones become incarcerated. Femoral and pelvic hernias are uncommon but are often overlooked in obstetric patients.

The patient with a large hernia should not strain in labor or delivery. Low forceps usually suffice, and cesarean section is not indicated for delivery. Elective surgery for repair of an abdominal hernia should be delayed until after pregnancy, but emergency operation for the relief and correction of an incarcerated hernia may be performed during pregnancy.

DERMATOLOGIC COMPLICATIONS

Pregnancy has a sparing effect on most dermatoses. With few exceptions, *skin disorders during pregnancy and the puerperium are similar to those in nonpregnant women.*

Dermatologic disorders induced by pregnancy include abnormalities of pigmentation (e.g., chloasma), herpes gestationis, noninflammatory pruritus of pregnancy, angiectids or vascular spiders, and erythema palmare. Dermatologic disorders usually aggravated by pregnancy include *Candida* vulvovaginitis, acne vulgaris (early in pregnancy), erythema multiforme, dermatitis herpetiformis, granuloma inguinale, condylomata acuminata, pemphigus, neurofibromatosis, and systemic lupus erythematosus. It is unlikely that malignant melanoma is aggravated by pregnancy. Pregnancy is likely to have a beneficial effect on acne (late in pregnancy), psoriasis, and seborrheic dermatitis.

CHLOASMA (MELASMA)

Chloasma consists of blotchy, petal-shaped, yellowish brown pigmented patches symmetrically distributed over the forehead, nose, and malar prominence. These become confluent to form the *mask of pregnancy.* Chloasma usually fades soon after delivery. Only cosmetic treatment is required. Hydroquinone cream (Eldoquin), 2%, applied nightly may limit the development and speed the clearing of chloasma, but skin may develop a grayish color.

HERPES GESTATIONIS

This serious disease affecting about 1:4000 gravidas is the *most common skin disorder that affects the fetus.* The cause of herpes gestationis is unknown, but it may be a variation of dermatitis herpetiformis. It is not related to the herpesvirus, and the nomenclature is unfortunate. The intensely burning, pruritic, occasionally painful urticarial papulovesicular eruption involving the buttocks, extensor surfaces of the arms and legs, back, and upper abdomen begins during or after the fifth month of pregnancy. Occasionally, it is noted early postpartum. Fetal death may occur during any period. The fatal pathophysiologic sequence is unexplained.

Grouped vesicles on inflammatory bases are typical. The

bullae of herpes gestationis form an annular pattern around the edge of the lesions, in contrast to those of erythema multiforme, whose bullae are centrally located. The lesions leave small pigmented scars on healing. A high eosinophil count in blood and vesical fluid is usual. Biopsy shows subepidermal bullae, increased eosinophils, and deposits of complement in the basement layer of the skin with immunofluorescent staining. *Corticosteroids are useful but not curative.*

NONINFLAMMATORY PRURITUS OF PREGNANCY

The cause is not known. No cutaneous lesions can be seen, but the patient experiences *intense itching all over the body.* Areas excoriated by scratching may become infected.

A papular pruritic dermatosis of pregnancy with a high fetal mortality rate, associated with abnormally elevated hCG levels, has been described and must be differentiated from the benign noninflammatory pruritus of pregnancy. *Symptomatic therapy* is advised for the latter.

Pruritus may result from cholestatic jaundice of pregnancy (p. 404). In this condition, no rash develops but minute bilirubin deposits in the skin cause itching.

ERYTHEMA PALMARE

This benign disorder is a dusky thenar and hypothenar vascular engorgement of the skin of the hands noted 4–6 weeks after the onset of pregnancy. The erythema disappears during the early puerperium. It is based on genetic predisposition and provoked by hyperestrogenism (as are vascular spiders).

VASCULAR SPIDERS OR SPIDER ANGIOMAS

These are small, red, pulsating (arteriolar) telangiectatic points in the skin over the face, neck, thorax, and arms. Most vascular spiders develop during the second and third trimesters of pregnancy and fade almost to invisibility after delivery. They reappear during subsequent advanced pregnancies. In most instances, these angiomas have only minor, temporary cosmetic significance, but the possibility that cirrhosis and hereditary hemorrhagic telangiectasia (and their complications) may be related must be kept in mind.

PRURITIC URTICARIAL PAPULES AND PLAQUES OF PREGNANCY

This intensely pruritic cutaneous eruption of late pregnancy is of unknown origin. *Symptoms* include numerous erythematous urticarial papules and myriads of minute plaques that first appear on the abdomen and then spread to involve the thighs and, at times, the buttocks and arms. Tissue biopsy of the lesions aids in the *differential diagnosis,* which includes herpes gestationis, prurigo gravidarum, and papular dermatitis of pregnancy. *Corticosteroid therapy* is moderately beneficial, but the dermatitis improves rapidly after delivery. Occasional patients have slight subsequent itching of the hands, sometimes during menses. The infants are free of skin abnormalities. Because of the small number of patients followed, the probability of recurrence of the disorder in subsequent pregnancies is uncertain.

CONNECTIVE TISSUE DISORDERS

RELAXATION OF THE PELVIC JOINTS
(Pregnancy Pelvic Arthropathy)

Considerable relaxation of the pelvic joints, the result of increased steroids and relaxin, is normal during pregnancy, but about *1:100 suffers from pelvic joint pain and ~1:1500 is seriously incapacitated.* Normally, considerable separation of the pubis (allowing vertical movement with ambulation) and instability of the sacroiliac joint occur with some instability and, occasionally, pain. This joint relaxation is progressive during the second trimester and early part of the third trimester. Undue mobility persists until after delivery. Joint stability may not return to normal until several months postpartum.

Pelvic arthropathy is presumed to be due to an exaggeration of this normal alteration of elasticity of connective and collagen tissues. However, the extent of disability is not always directly related to the degree of joint instability. This condition is most frequently associated with obesity or multiple pregnancy. Occasionally, it may be simply an unmasking of a previously underlying disorder.

The usual *symptoms* include extreme pain in the sacroiliac and pubic joints on standing, walking, and turning. Prolonged sacroiliac backache may be a sequela to sacroiliac arthropathy of pregnancy. *Orthopedic* (and occasionally *neurologic*) *consultation* is useful to ascertain that other conditions have been excluded or properly managed.

Treatment for pelvic arthropathy consists of limitation of activities, analgesics, and a sturdy, fitted girdle that gives support by snug encirclement of the sacrum, symphysis, and greater trochanters. Every precaution must be taken to avoid exaggerated positions, marked traction, and sudden movement of the patient during delivery.

SYSTEMIC LUPUS ERYTHEMATOSUS

Systemic lupus erythematosus (SLE) affects principally females and develops most frequently during the childbearing years. It is an uncommon but often extremely serious complication of pregnancy. Pregnancy does not consistently influence the course of this disorder: ~50% remain unchanged, a few cases improve, but the rest have exacerbations (especially during the puerperium). However, if comparable time intervals are contrasted with nonpregnant patients with acute SLE, the probability of an exacerbation is 1–3 times greater in the first half, 1–2 times greater in the second half of pregnancy, and >600 times during the puerperium.

Moreover, *SLE patients have a marked increase in pregnancy wastage.* Spontaneous abortion is increased about threefold. Premature labor (and delivery) and preeclampsia-eclampsia are increased. There is an enhanced possibility of the newborn having congenital heart block.

Corticosteroids may relieve the symptoms and reduce the number and intensity of acute exacerbations. Prednisone, 30–50 mg (or equivalent) daily orally in 4 divided doses, may be required for treatment of an acute attack. After improvement has occurred, the drug dosage may be gradually reduced to withdrawal or to a maintenance dose of about 10 mg/day. Even prolonged use during pregnancy and the puerperium has not demonstrated teratic activity sufficient to preclude usage. Occasionally, *antineoplastics* may be necessary. Patients must avoid overactivity and exposure to the sun and other sources of ultraviolet light. Pigmented emollient cosmetic lotions opaque to ultraviolet light may be applied over facial lesions. *Analgesics and physical therapy* may be given for musculoskeletal discomfort.

The *maternal mortality rate* is approximately 20%, and the *perinatal mortality rate* is about 30% in acute disseminated SLE. The mortality rates in chronic SLE depend on the duration and severity of the disease. The postdelivery period may be the most critical. Thus, corticosteroids should not be discontinued too early. Pregnancy rarely exacerbates SLE so severely that therapeutic abortion is justified. Cesarean section should be performed only for clear-cut obstetric indications.

Barrier-type contraception is usually recommended. Oral contraceptives may trigger an exacerbation of SLE. With steroids, the likelihood of infection is increased with intrauterine devices. Surgery may induce exacerbation of SLE, and this must be weighed when considering sterilization.

NEUROLOGIC DISEASES

The effect of neurologic diseases on pregnancy is rarely critical. For example, pregnancy is not an absolute contraindication to urgent neurosurgery for the evacuation of a subdural hematoma, removal of an intracranial tumor, or treatment of an intracranial aneurysm. Neurologic disorders are only rarely so serious as to require interruption of pregnancy. However, certain neurologic diseases may be aggravated by pregnancy (e.g., chorea gravidarum or Sydenham's chorea, severe nonspecific polyneuritis, and herniation of an intervertebral disc).

Consider sterilization only when the woman's life and health will be jeopardized by subsequent pregnancy or when there is a significant likelihood of transmission of serious hereditary disorders.

EPILEPSY

Epilepsy has no demonstrable effect on the clinical course of pregnancy, but recurrent attacks of grand mal or petit mal epilepsy and psychomotor seizures may be activated or intensified during pregnancy. They are more frequent during the last trimester in women who are hypertensive, proteinuric, and edematous. Convulsive seizures may be associated with alkalosis, fluid and electrolyte imbalance, cerebral hypoxia, cerebral edema, hypoglycemia, or hypocalcemia. Epilepsy may be difficult to differentiate from eclampsia, but an accurate history of seizures in the nonpregnant state is most helpful. However, the burden of proof is on the physician who claims that convulsions in the third trimester of pregnancy do not indicate eclampsia.

When seizures occur for the first time in a woman during pregnancy, a careful neurologic examination, including electro-encephalographic studies, is indicated.

Proper *management of the acutely seizuring patient* is crucial.

1. Prevent aspiration of gastric contents by placing the patient on her side (never on her back).

2. Extend the head and hold the tongue out to ensure a clear airway.

3. Slip an oral airway (or soft mouth gag) between her jaws so that she will not bite her tongue.

4. Gently restrain the patient to prevent injury.

5. If convulsions continue, give diazepam (Valium), 5–10 mg IV initially (repeated if necessary at 10–15 min intervals to a maximum dose of 30 mg), or phenytoin (Dilantin), 150–250 mg IV at a rate not exceeding 50 mg/min. IV sodium amobarbital also may be used, but rapid administration should be avoided because pulmonary edema and right heart failure may result in the patient with eclampsia. (*Caution:* Because of their depressive central nervous system effects, do not administer narcotics or general anesthetics unless absolutely necessary to control re-peated seizures.)

Longer-term management of epileptics during pregnancy in-cludes avoiding fluid retention and adequate anticonvulsant ther-apy. Acetazolamide (Diamox) may be used as a diuretic. The most commonly used anticonvulsant, phenytoin (Dilantin) may be mildly fetotoxic. Thus, its use during pregnancy must be weighed against the risk. Other alternatives include phenobarbi-tal, diazepam (Valium), and chlordiazepoxide (Librium).

Idiopathic epilepsy has a *hereditary pattern*. The risk of having an infant with epilepsy is 2%–3% if one parent has epilepsy. It is 20%–25% if both parents are afflicted.

HERNIATED INTERVERTEBRAL DISC

Herniation of the nucleus pulposus of a lumbar intervertebral disc is more frequent during pregnancy because the estrogens, pro-gestogens, and relaxin cause the intervertebral disc's fibrous rings to weaken and swell the nuclei pulposi, hypervascularization of the back and pelvic nonosseous tissues contributes to relaxation of back support, and the equilibrium of the lumbosacral joint is disturbed during pregnancy by the increase in volume and weight of the abdominal contents. There are no obstetric complications due to disc hernia, but *disability and even paralysis may occur in extreme, neglected cases.*

Temporary or permanent relief usually follows *medical management:* bedrest, traction, sedatives, and analgesics. Back strain or injury should be avoided during pregnancy and the puerperium, and obese patients should lose weight. Severe, recurrent, or progressive pain and incapacity may require surgery, but this is rarely necessary during pregnancy.

CEREBROVASCULAR ACCIDENTS

The higher incidence of vascular accidents during pregnancy than in the nonpregnant state may be partially explained by collagen changes in the blood vessels during pregnancy. Recurrent subarachnoid hemorrhage may be an indication for abortion or cesarean section. Hypertension of preeclampsia-eclampsia, IV administration of ergot (pressor) preparations, and increased intracranial pressure with straining during the second stage of labor may account for rupture of congenital cerebral aneurysms, arteriovenous malformations, or thrombosed cerebral veins.

MULTIPLE SCLEROSIS (MS)

The incidence of MS is 2–3:1000 pregnancies. Physiologic changes during pregnancy do not influence the development or the course of multiple sclerosis. Multiple sclerosis per se does not affect the course of pregnancy (including labor). However, sequelae (e.g., bladder dysfunction and stasis with subsequent infections) are frequent. Spinal anesthesia should be avoided when spinal cord disease is present. Vaginal delivery is preferred. Pregnancy is not contraindicated after several years remission.

MYASTHENIA GRAVIS

Myasthenia gravis, a metabolic disorder involving acetylcholine use at the myoneural junction, affects motor function, causing muscle weakness, particularly of the face, tongue, throat, neck, arms, and respiratory muscles. The peak prevalence of myasthenia gravis is at ~25 years. Pregnancy may complicate the disorder, although some patients undergo remission during pregnancy. *With proper management, most myasthenic patients complete pregnancy safely, and congenital myasthenia gravis is rare.*

Infections may precipitate onset or relapse and must be treated aggressively during pregnancy. Symptoms of relapse include easy fatigability, intermittent double vision, drooping of the upper eyelids, facial muscle weakness, and in more serious cases, upper arm weakness and breathing difficulty. Neostigmine (Prostigmine) is beneficial. If edrophonium chloride (Tensilon) is used, it should be given cautiously IV. However, since edrophonium may precipitate uterine contractions, it is (if possible) avoided.

Myasthenic patients usually tolerate labor well. Meperidine is the obstetric analgesic of choice. Local anesthesia is preferred. If general anesthesia is required, nitrous oxide, oxygen, and cyclopropane usually are the best combination. Oxytocin may be given, but muscle relaxants are contraindicated. Myasthenic patients must be carefully supervised postpartum because relapses often occur during the puerperium.

An occasional newborn may have myasthenia gravis and require neostigmine treatment for 1–2 months. Complete recovery is the rule.

Chorea Gravidarum

Sydenham's chorea (St. Vitus' dance) that recurs or develops for the first time in young women during pregnancy is often associated with acute rheumatic fever. Although very rare, it may be a serious complication of pregnancy. If usually appears early after the first missed period and, curiously, often vanishes following termination of pregnancy. Treatment is similar to that of Sydenham's chorea in the nonpregnant patient.

ENDOCRINE AND METABOLIC DISEASES

Diabetes Mellitus

Diabetes mellitus is a metabolic disorder affecting carbohydrate, protein, and fats with the potential for long-term degenerative alterations. *It is one of the three* (anemia and urinary infections) *most frequent medical complications of pregnancy* (1:325–350 in the United States) and so adversely affects pregnancy as to be an important contributor to maternal and perinatal morbidity. Although maternal death is rare with modern treatment, the perinatal mortality rate may be as high as ~5%.

Pregnancy is diabetogenic. Manifestations of this include gestational diabetes, intensification of overt diabetes, increased insulin requirements, and the enhanced occurrence of metabolic complications (e.g., ketoacidosis).

There are two major types of diabetes mellitus. *Type I, insulin-dependent diabetes,* is usually of juvenile onset and is associated with deficient insulin secretion. The pathogenesis is multifactorial. *Type II diabetes* is generally late onset and has elevated serum insulin levels, and the tissues are insensitive to insulin. Type II also has a strong hereditary component, usually developing in adults who are overweight or pregnant. It is useful to classify (especially for purposes of management and counseling) diabetics according to the system of White (Table 14-2).

Effect of Diabetes Mellitus on Pregnancy and Delivery

Infertility and abortion are increased (2–3 times) *in poorly controlled diabetics.* Rigid control of the glucose removes these risks. Maternal fluid and electrolyte balance is easily disrupted. Both the mother and the infant may be edematous. The incidence of polyhydramnios is 10 times the general incidence. Preeclampsia-eclampsia is much more frequent (30%–50%), especially with prepregnancy vascular sclerosis and hypertension.

The 3 times increase in congenital abnormalities found in the offspring of uncontrolled diabetics is also lowered by proper glucose control. The *most common abnormalities* are cardiac, but the most increased abnormality (it almost never occurs except in diabetic pregnancies) is the caudal regression syndrome. Premature labor and delivery are common in the more advanced classes (>C), and the likelihood of an excessively large fetus (>4000 g) is greater in classes A and B. The risk of fetal death is heightened, particularly after the 36th week, because of maternal glucose instability (with possible acidosis) and placental insufficiency. Dystocia and operative delivery are more frequent, and fetal mortality and morbidity rates are consequently increased.

The incidence of early neonatal death from respiratory distress syndrome or hypoglycemia (due to hyperplasia of fetal islets of Langerhans) is increased.

Table 14-2. Classification of pregnant diabetics

Class	Characteristics
A	Diabetic based only on an abnormal glucose tolerance testing
B	Onset of diabetes after age 20; duration of diabetes 10–19 years; no vascular disease
C	Onset of diabetes between ages 10–19; duration of diabetes 10–19 years; no vascular disease
D	Onset of diabetes age <10; duration of diabetes ≥20 years; vascular disease, including calcification of leg vessels
E	Same as group D, plus calcification of pelvic vessels
F	Same as group E, plus nephropathy (often Kimmelstiel-Wilson intercapillary nephrosclerosis)
H	Coronary artery disease
R	Malignant proliferative retinopathy

After J. Hare and P. White, Gestational diabetes and the White classification. *Diabetes Care* 3:394, 1980.

Clinical Findings

Diabetic screening in all women is desirable but is mandatory in the following circumstances: a family history of diabetes, a previously unexplained premature, stillbirth, or hydramnios, a prior newborn weighing >4000 g (9 pounds), or a previous term-sized infant with respiratory distress syndrome. Obesity or glucosuria before the 20th week or recurrent glucosuria after the 20th week should be investigated.

The current diabetic screening is to administer a 50 g oral carbohydrate load and draw a blood glucose in 1 h. If that level is >150 mg/dl, the test is positive and other (more definitive) testing is necessary. A normal fasting blood glucose level does not rule out diabetes. Moreover, fasting blood glucose levels may be slightly elevated or the postprandial blood glucose may be elevated in other diseases besides diabetes (e.g., liver disease). Fasting glucosuria suggests diabetes but is less reliable during pregnancy because of the lowered renal threshold for glucose. Lactose, which may give false positive tests for glucose, may be excreted in the urine during the last 4–6 weeks of pregnancy and during the postpartum period. For these reasons, glucosuria is less diagnostic than hyperglycemia.

When the diabetic screen is abnormal or if the signs and symptoms are suggestive, a *glucose tolerance test* is performed. The generally accepted normal values for whole blood glucose in the oral glucose tolerance test (100 g glucose load) are fasting level, 90 mg/dl; 1 h, 165 mg/dl; 2 h, 145 mg/dl; 3 h, 125 mg/dl. A glucose tolerance test containing one or more above-normal values is abnormal. Before glucose tolerance testing, place the patient on a high-carbohydrate intake for at least 48 h because carbohydrate restriction decreases tolerance.

Caution: It is unnecessary and possibly harmful to perform a glucose tolerance test on a patient whose initial blood glucose level is ≥200 mg/dl. Proceed to therapy for diabetes.

In pregnancy, the fasting blood glucose level is often slightly low, yet the oral glucose tolerance curve may be of the diabetic type. These changes are most marked after the sixth month. Following delivery, glucose tolerance tests return to nonpregnant values within 72 h. Thus, if delivery events indicate a glucose tolerance test as being desirable, it should be done <48 h.

Treatment

A. *Emergency Measures*

1. *Diabetic acidosis and coma.* Admit the patient to a hospital and obtain medical consultation. Determine blood glucose, pH, CO_2 combining power, serum electrolytes. Treat with insulin as for any patient with diabetic acidosis or coma.

2. *Insulin shock.* If the patient is comatose and it is not possible to rapidly differentiate between diabetic coma and insulin shock, treat first for insulin shock by giving 20–40 ml of 50% glucose in water slowly IV. Determine the cause and make the necessary adjustments of insulin or food.

B. *Antenatal Care*

1. *Maximize therapy before pregnancy occurs.* Evaluate the patient as a candidate for pregnancy before conception and optimize health and control.

2. *Fingerstick dextrose determinations.* Obtain before breakfast, before lunch, before dinner, and before bed. It is inappropriate to attempt to regulate pregnant diabetics (because of their special and rapidly changing status) with urine testing. Blood glucose should be maintained with a mean of 100 mg/dl ± 10 mg/dl. The maximum must not exceed 120 mg/dl.

3. a. *Adjust diet* to the ideal nutritional state depending on the patient's height, weight, and build. The goal is not weight reduc-

tion but prevention of both fasting and postprandial hyperglycemia. Diet is usually according to the American Diabetic Association (ADA) guidelines. Generally, diabetics should have 35 kcal/kg unless obese, in which circumstances no less than 30 kcal/kg should be given. There are innumerable formulas for calculation of the distribution of calories, but it is important to have ~ 50% carbohydrates, at least 100 g of protein, and the rest fat. For example, a woman whose ideal weight is 60 kg (132 pounds) should have a daily diet of 2100 kcal (35 × 60). The caloric value of carbohydrate and protein is 4.1 kcal/g, and that of fat is 9.3 kcal/g. Thus, a sample dietary composition follows.

50% carbohydrate = 1050 kcal/4.1 kcal/g = 256 g
25% protein = 525 kcal/4.1 kcal/g = 128g
25% fat = 525 kcal/9.3 kcal/g = 56 g

It is also important to divide the calories into meals that release the nutrients in a regular fashion. Currently, 2/9, 2/9, 2/9, 2/9, 1/9 is favored.

b. Give *vitamins, minerals, and dietary supplements* individualized to the patient's needs.

4. Consider and obtain the necessary *consultations*. In most circumstances, the patient, internist, and obstetrician should work in close cooperation.

5. Overt diabetics require insulin, and the *insulin requirement is usually greater during pregnancy*. Diet and insulin must be regulated by blood glucose determinations as noted previously. Oral hypoglycemic agents, which are teratogenic, should not be used during pregnancy. The combination of insulin is usually an intermediate and short-acting, and they are usually given in 2–3 doses/day to enhance precision. The NPH/regular insulin ratio should be 2:1 in the morning and 1:1 in the evening, and the morning total should be twice the evening total.

For example, a total of 90 units/day should be divided as 40 units NPH and 20 units regular in the morning, and 15 units NPH and 15 units regular in the evening.

6. The *routine evaluation* of diabetics should include either skin testing for tuberculosis or a chest x-ray. The ocular fundi must be evaluated, renal function determined, and a periodic series of screening for urinary tract infection (increased 3 times) instituted. In the classes with vascular involvement, an ECG is mandatory at any age.

7. *Fetal monitoring*

a. Use ultrasonography early to determine gestational age, fetal viability, and possible defects as soon as pregnancy is confirmed, then at 4–6 week intervals until biophysical profile monitoring is undertaken.

b. Begin NST or BPP monitoring for fetal well-being at 27 weeks.

C. *Labor and Delivery*

1. *Consider elective delivery* when the LS ratio and Pg indicate pulmonary maturity. Nearly all may have vaginal delivery if the vertex is presenting and other details are favorable. Cesarean section is indicated if the fetus weighs 4000–4500 g or if presentation is abnormal.

2. When signs of *fetal distress* develop, terminate pregnancy by the most expeditious means. If the pulmonary maturity testing does not indicate fetal maturity, the decision to deliver the infant or continue observation becomes a calculated risk.

3. The usual insulin dose is not given on the day of delivery, and *insulin by infusion* is used to treat the hourly monitored blood glucose.

D. *Neonatal Care*

1. *At delivery*

a. Clamp the cord immediately (avoids hypervolemia).

b. Obtain cord blood for pH, blood gases, and glucose.

c. A neonatologist or pediatrician should be present at delivery.

2. *Immediate care* (including resuscitation) should be the same as any other delivery, with special attention to respiration, cardiac, neurologic, drying, warming, and getting to a controlled environment as soon as possible.

3. *Admit to an observation nursery.* Perform frequent blood sugar determinations (q 30–60 min) in the first 2–3 h, with continued blood sugar determination before feedings for the first 12–24 h. Blood glucose <45 mg/dl is defined as hypoglycemia, and oral glucose should be administered. Immediate IV glucose therapy is required for hypoglycemia <30 mg/dl or if the hypoglycemia is not rapidly responsive to the oral glucose load.

4. *Observe respirations,* turn the infant frequently, and stimulate breathing when necessary.

5. *Observe for tremor or convulsive movements.* These may be due to hypocalcemia, in which case give 10% calcium gluconate, 100 mg/kg slowly IV, after a blood specimen is drawn for calcium and glucose determinations.

E. *Postpartum Management*

Carefully evaluate the mother's diabetic status during the puerperium, since *extraordinary changes occur.* For example, one third of the late pregnancy dose of insulin is usually all that is needed the day after delivery.

Prognosis

Joint management by an internist, obstetrician, and pediatrician will result in lower maternal and perinatal mortality and morbidity. The *maternal mortality rate* with modern therapy should be <0.2%. Deaths are due to diabetic coma, preeclampsia-eclampsia, infection, nephropathy, cardiac complications, dystocia, and embolism. Neglect and improper treatment are the main contributory causes of virtually all maternal deaths. An increase of diabetic retinopathy and nephropathy occurs in most patients during pregnancy.

Factors influencing fetal survival are the severity of diabetes, control of diabetes during pregnancy, placental function, placental bleeding, preeclampsia-eclampsia, polyhydramnios, and interruption of pregnancy <34th week or after the 38th week of gestation. The perinatal mortality rate even with modern therapy is <5%. Fetal anomalies occur in ~4% of infants but are more frequent when polyhydramnios is present. In general, vaginal delivery is safer than cesarean section for the fetus (except for the macrosomic fetus).

Pregnancy termination may be justified in certain instances of diabetic retinopathy, retinitis proliferans, severe vascular (usually cerebral or coronary) disease, or Kimmelstiel-Wilson disease.

THYROID DISORDERS

THYROTOXICOSIS

Thyrotoxicosis does not increase the hazard of spontaneous abortion or fetal anomalies but does increase the incidence of premature delivery, postpartum hemorrhage, cardiovascular complications secondary to myocardial stress, psychosis, liver damage, and thyroid storm. Preeclampsia-eclampsia may occur slightly more often in women with toxic goiter. *Overtreatment of thyrotoxicosis* during pregnancy may result in maternal and fetal hypothyroidism and may cause maldevelopment and goiter in the infant.

Treatment

A. *Emergency Measures.* All pregnant patients with moderate or marked thyrotoxicosis should be *hospitalized at bedrest and given propranolol and possibly sedatives.*

B. *Specific Measures. Individualize treatment* according to the degree of toxicity and the duration of pregnancy. Toxic goiter during pregnancy may require antithyroid drug therapy (e.g., propylthiouracil or equivalent, 0.1 g PO tid or qid). To avoid resultant hypothyroidism, levothyroxine (Synthroid) should be given. Subtotal thyroidectomy must not be attempted until the patient has become euthyroid following medical treatment and is rarely necessary during pregnancy. Iodides are used before surgery but can damage the fetal thyroid gland. Therapeutic abortion is almost never required. Toxic goiter is not an indication for labor induction or cesarean section.

C. *Treatment of Complications.* Levothyroxine (Synthroid) should be administered whenever hypothyroidism develops, immediately before and for several weeks after thyroidectomy, or when the patient receives a thiourea compound.

D. *Neonatal.* If a congenitally athyroid or markedly hypothyroid infant does not receive thyroid or one of its analogs promptly, followed by continuation of the maintenance dose to ensure euthyroidism, normal mental and physical development cannot be expected.

Prognosis

The prognosis is excellent for mother and fetus if normal thyroid function can be achieved promptly and then maintained.

Hypothyroidism

Slight thyroid deficiency is common, and although replacement therapy is not harmful, it seldom is indicated. More severe deficiency causes abortion, premature labor, and congenital fetal anomalies. Hashimoto's disease is by far the most common cause of hypothyroidism in the general population. Women with moderate to severe degrees of hypothyroidism are relatively infertile, and sterility is the rule in myxedema.

Treatment

Pregnant women with early hypothyroidism may be treated initially with relatively large doses of *thyroid supplement,* levothyroxine (Synthroid). Start with doses of 0.05–0.1 mg/day, and increase weekly to the limit of tolerance (~0.3 mg/day), adjusting to maintain the optimal effect. The optimal dosage may be estimated on the basis of the serum T_3 and T_4, but clinical judgment is often very accurate. *Thyroid overdosage causes nervousness, tremors, tachycardia, insomnia, sweating, vomiting, diarrhea, and weight loss.*

The nonspecific use of thyroid medication must be condemned.

Prognosis

With prompt, adequate, and continued thyroid replacement, the prognosis is excellent for mother and infant. If a hypothyroid infant does not receive prompt replacement therapy, irreversible mental and physical retardation is to be expected.

AUTOIMMUNE THYROID DISEASE

Autoimmune mechanisms are responsible for only about 10% of all clinical thyroid disorders. However, they play a major role in two thirds of the most serious thyroid diseases: Graves' disease and Hashimoto's disease or thyroiditis. Autoantibodies do not appear to play a role in the development of thyroid cancer.

Predisposition to autoimmune disease is inherited (50% concordance in identical twins, about 10% in fraternal twins or siblings). Autoimmune disease never appears at birth, and its appearance follows a random distribution over time. Currently, there is no effective method of antigenically treating autoimmune thyroid disease. All one can do is to correct the hyperthyroid or hypothyroid state and maintain normality.

Postpartum transient autoimmune thyroiditis (of Amino) is an interesting variant. In the last trimester of pregnancy, there usually is an amelioration of the autoimmune process followed by a rebound (thyrotoxicosis) after delivery. Antithyroid drugs should control the problem but contraindicate breastfeeding.

PARATHYROID DYSFUNCTION AND TETANY

Pregnancy normally causes a slight (secondary) hyperparathyroidism. Severe, chronic hyperparathyroidism causing osteitis fibrosa cystica is rare during pregnancy except in patients with long-standing renal disease. The most serious problems relating to parathyroid dysfunction during pregnancy are hypoparathyroid tetany and muscle cramps. Tetany is usually associated with a calcium deficiency, phosphate excess, or lack of vitamin D and parathyroid hormone. In established hypoparathyroidism, hypocalcemia is a dilutional phenomenon during pregnancy. The requirements for vitamin D and calcium in parathyroid disease may be greater than in nonpregnant women.

Tetany may follow infection or the hypocalcemia that sometimes occurs during lactation, or it may be seen during the latter months of pregnancy if calcium supplements are inadequate. Of course, hyperventilation during labor may precipitate tetany.

Tetany of the newborn is unusual in breastfed infants but may occur transiently if the infant's phosphate intake is excessive, e.g., if too much cow's milk rather than formula is given or as a result of relative hypoparathyroidism in the neonatal period.

INFECTIOUS DISEASES

All systemic infectious diseases of the mother, if severe enough, can complicate pregnancy by causing fetal injury, death of the fetus, or premature labor and delivery. High fever, septicemia, and toxicosis are usually responsible. Most maternal infectious diseases (e.g., pneumonia, scarlet fever, and typhoid fever) are not responsible for fetal anomalies. However, the so-called TORCH infections (toxoplasmosis, rubella, cytomegalovirus disease, herpes simplex) and syphilis may be devastating to the fetus.

Toxoplasmosis

Toxoplasmosis, a multisystem disease caused by the protozoan *Toxoplasma gondii,* is a serious threat to the fetus. Serologic evidence of *T. gondii* infection is present in almost 25% of women in the United States. Most cases are chronic and probably pose little risk to the fetus. The acute case may lead to fetal infection with marked sequelae.

The major vector in the United States remains unclear. The infection may be obtained from consumption of undercooked meat. Cats have been overemphasized as a vector. Only about 1% of cats hunting and consuming rodents harboring *T. gondii* are infected at any one time. If infection occurs, the cat sheds oocytes in the feces for only about 2 weeks. During this time, human inoculation must occur by hand-to-mouth contact of cat fecal material.

Toxoplasmosis, usually asymptomatic in adults, resembles cytomegalovirus disease in the infant. Severe perinatal toxoplasmosis is associated with growth retardation, microcephalus or hydrocephalus, microphthalmia, chorioretinitis, central nervous system calcification, thrombopenia, jaundice, fever, and death.

Routine antenatal screening for antibodies to T. gondii has been recommended. The Sabin-Feldman dye test and the indirect immunofluorescence test are diagnostic of toxoplasmosis. Both tests give positive results 2–3 weeks after infection and for years thereafter. Thus, without sequential tests, an acute infection cannot be distinguished from a chronic one. The diagnosis of toxoplasmosis in a newborn is supported by elevated IgM in cord blood.

Treatment of toxoplasmosis during pregnancy is problematic. Pyrimethamine currently is the drug of first choice against *T. gondii.* However, this drug may be teratogenic, especially during the first trimester. If the newborn is treated with pyrimethamine, folinic acid supplementation will be required to reduce the toxicity of the drug. Sulfadiazine often is used additionally. Sulfonamide therapy is effective but must be discontinued before delivery. Sulfonamide drugs have a greater albumin-binding affinity than bilirubin, which may rise after delivery to critical levels. Even exchange transfusion of the newborn may be necessary to avoid kernicterus.

A cat should not be a hazard if minimal precautions are taken—frequent handwashing and occasional soaking of litter boxes with ammonia solution. Pregnant women should cook meat well or freeze meat for at least 4 h before consumption to destroy *T. gondii* tissue cysts. Women at high risk for toxoplasmosis, e.g., veterinarians, butchers, or those with many cats, should be screened periodically for the disease.

The *outlook for the neonate with congenital toxoplasmosis is serious to grave.* Encysted (intramuscular) focus of *T. gondii* can not be eradicated and may cause recrudescence of the disease. If a woman has an affected child, subsequent progeny probably will be unaffected.

Exanthematous Diseases

Most of the exanthematous diseases are caused by viruses, which invariably gain access to the fetus via the placenta (Table 14-3).

Table 14-3. Exanthematous diseases in pregnancy

Disease	Effect of disease on pregnancy	Effect of disease on offspring
Rubeola (measles)	Abortion; premature labor if disease is severe	May be born with rash
Varicella (chickenpox)	Severe, disseminated epidemic type may be fatal to mother due to necrotizing angiitis	Virulent infection may cause fetal death in utero; newborn may be born with pocks
Rubella (German measles)	Occasional early abortion	Congenital anomalies if disease occurs during first trimester

The effect on pregnancy and the fetus depends on the virulence of the virus, the mother's resistance to the disease, and the stage of fetal development. Fetal immunity depends largely on maternal active immunity (e.g., rubella) or passive immunity (e.g., immune serum globulin administration). High fever or toxicosis may cause increased uterine contractility and loss of the pregnancy. Viral placentitis and viremia followed by fetal death in utero may lead to abortion or premature delivery.

Rubella (German Measles)

The rubella virus is *extremely teratogenic.* Many infants are abnormal and maldeveloped if the mother contracts rubella during the *first trimester of pregnancy.* Excluding patients affected during epidemics, the risk of congenital anomalies occurring during the first 3 months of pregnancy declines from almost 50% (first month) to about 10%. After the first trimester, the danger of anomalies is negligible, but vision or hearing defects or both are common.

Fetal defects include cataracts, congenital heart disease, dental dysplasia, deafness, and mental retardation. It may take 1–2 years to be certain of the extent of infant defects. There is some evidence that an abnormal child may be born of a mother who has previously been vaccinated but contracts a subclinical form of the disease when reexposed during pregnancy. Thus, rubella screening titers (specific serum hemagglutinating antibody) are

considered routine in antenatal care to demonstrate the susceptibility to rubella.

Prophylactic immune serum globulin may prevent the rash
but not the viremia of rubella, even when given before exposure
to the disease. Therefore, the virus remains a significant threat to
the fetus. This has led to the recommendation that immune serum globulin is rarely indicated in pregnancy.

Attenuated rubella virus vaccine will confer *active immunity*
for a prolonged but uncertain period. Because the vaccine can
potentially infect the fetus, it is recommended that immunization
should be carried out in women only if they are not pregnant and
pregnancy can be avoided for 3 months after vaccination. Although this remains a good guideline, when vaccination has occurred during pregnancy, there have been few, if any, demonstrable teratic effects. Reactions to the vaccine may include mild
fever, local soreness at the site of injection, and arthralgia.
Spread of the virus to others is not a problem.

CYTOMEGALOVIRUS (CMV) DISEASE

Most cases of CMV disease are clinically inapparent. In some
adults, the symptoms are like those of infectious mononucleosis.
The disease is usually sexually transmitted. During pregnancy,
the only sign may be mild leukorrhea. Specific virus-neutralizing
and complement-fixing antibody reactions indicate that most
women have (at some time) sustained this infection. About 20%
of adults do not have neutralizing antibody to cytomegalovirus
and thus are considered susceptible for acute infections.

There is now evidence that CMV is much more prevalent
during pregnancy than was thought and causes severe anomalies
in ~10,000 infants in the United States per year. CMV is recovered from 15%–20% of women examined in public health clinics
and from the semen of men who have had numerous sexual
partners. The virus can be cultivated from the salivary glands of
10%–25% of healthy individuals, from the cervix of 10% of
healthy women, from the urine of 1% of all newborns, and sometimes from breast milk. This carrier state probably explains subsequent cases occurring in the same family.

*Cytomegalovirus disease is usually acquired by the fetus during
early intrauterine life.* In the newborn, the disease produces
erythroblastosis and thrombocytopenia that lead to scattered
hemorrhages. Chorioretinitis, periventricular necrosis with calcification, microcephaly, and sclerosis of the bones are often noted

at birth. Early jaundice beginning on the first or second day, melena, hematemesis, and hematuria develop. The antemortem diagnosis can be made by identification of cytomegalic inclusion cells in the gastric washings, cerebrospinal fluid, or fresh urine. Culture of CMV is proof of the diagnosis. The direct and indirect serum bilirubin are elevated, but the Coombs test is negative. Death may occur soon after birth as a result of interstitial pneumonitis, focal hepatitis, or adrenocortical failure.

There is no cure. Corticosteroids and supportive therapy together with immune serum globulin may be helpful. When the obviously infected infant survives, marked developmental and psychomotor deficiencies and hepatosplenomegaly usually are present. Hearing loss is frequent in the more numerous cases of clinically inapparent CMV.

Sexually Transmitted Diseases

Herpes simplex (p 495), syphilis (p 590), and gonorrhea (p 586) are discussed on the pages indicated.

Poliomyelitis

Poliomyelitis, which exerts an unfavorable effect on pregnancy and the puerperium, has been virtually eradicated in the United States, but it is still a serious problem in developing countries. Pregnant women have a greater incidence of poliomyelitis than nonpregnant women of comparable ages. Approximately 67% of pregnant women who contract poliomyelitis are between ages 20 and 29, and ~75% are parous.

Pregnancy aggravates poliomyelitis, and the disease in turn increases the risk of abortion and fetal loss. Rare congenital anomalies are ascribed to poliomyelitis. The infant may show growth retardation if the mother contracts poliomyelitis in the early months of pregnancy. The fetus may contract poliomyelitis during its passage through the birth canal.

Salk vaccine contains killed virus. *Sabin vaccine* is an attenuated live virus preparation. Either can be given whether the patient is pregnant or not, but it is preferred to give the vaccine to nonpregnant women. Immune serum globulin may assist in protecting the exposed infant against poliomyelitis. If the newborn survives but has acquired the disease, flaccid paralysis may be present.

The maternal mortality rate in pregnancy complicated by poliomyelitis is markedly increased. The later in pregnancy the disease is contracted, the higher the morbidity and mortality rates for both mother and infant.

PULMONARY TUBERCULOSIS

Tuberculosis of the bronchi, lungs, and pleura is not directly affected by pregnancy. Tuberculous pregnant women are slightly more prone to spontaneous abortion and premature delivery than other women. Tuberculous endometritis is exceptional. Interruption of pregnancy because of pulmonary tuberculosis is almost never justified now that antituberculosis drugs are available. Infants born of tuberculous mothers are no more likely to develop the disease than others provided they are separated from the infected mother and unfavorable environment at birth.

However, it is important to discourage pregnancy in women with active tuberculosis and to maintain close medical supervision of those tuberculous women who do become pregnant. Institute follow-up study of all women with a history of treated tuberculosis, and be alert to the possibility of reactivation of tuberculosis during each pregnancy. Advise deferring pregnancy (and prescribe contraception, if acceptable) until tuberculosis has been inactive for at least 2 years if minimal, 3 years if moderately advanced, and 5 years if far-advanced.

In patients who have had tuberculosis, order *chest x-rays* after the fifth month, immediately after delivery, and 6 months after delivery. The *management* of the pregnant patient with tuberculosis requires the collaboration of the pulmonary physician and the obstetrician. The *treatment* of tuberculosis includes rest (physical and emotional), hospitalization if the disease is moderate or advanced, and chemotherapy. The reader is referred to other texts for details of treatment.

MALARIA

Malaria may cause infertility, abortion, or premature labor and delivery. Infants of mothers with malaria are often smaller than average. Approximately 10% of infants born of women with demonstrable parasitemia will have plasmodia in cord blood.

Malarial relapses often occur during pregnancy for unknown reasons. A renewal of attacks is common during the puerperium or after hemorrhage and infection. Labor is frequently prolonged and hazardous for obstetric patients with malaria. These women become fatigued sooner, and operative delivery is required more often. The parasite is not transmitted in the milk, but lactation should be discouraged in women with clinical evidence of malaria.

The severity of maternal malaria is reflected in the stillbirth rate, which rises as pregnancy approaches term, and the vitality of newborns who do survive is temporarily reduced.

No antimalarial drug is completely safe for use during pregnancy. If a pregnant woman must be treated for malaria, other texts should be consulted for details of treatment.

LISTERIOSIS

Maternal listeriosis may be responsible for abortion and fetal disease or death depending on the severity of the infection and the duration of pregnancy. Encephalitis and granulomatosis of the newborn are described. Pregnant women suffering from a septic form of this disease may have only malaise, but they may transmit the infection to the fetus either transplacentally or when the fetus is exposed to the organisms in the lower genital canal during birth.

A *diagnosis* of listeriosis during pregnancy is difficult but can be made by complement-fixation or fluorescent antibody tests of leukorrheic discharges. A positive complement-fixation test in high dilution is almost invariably present in acute maternal infection. Gram-positive rods should be sought in the meconium of the newborn to diagnose listeriosis early.

Treat the mother and child with large doses of ampicillin or erythromycin.

Chapter 15

Operative Obstetrics

ANESTHESIA*

PREGNANCY ALTERATIONS MOST INFLUENCING ANESTHESIA

Anesthesia management is markedly influenced by pregnancy. Pregnancy-induced physiologic alterations may be compounded by labor, pregnancy-associated conditions (e.g., pregnancy-induced hypertension), or intercurrent disease states of the mother or fetus (e.g., diabetes, isoimmunization).

Cardiovascular Alterations

At term, cardiac output is increased by 30%–40% above non-pregnant levels in the absence of aortocaval compression. Increased cardiac output speeds the onset of inhalation anesthetics. Uterine involution leads to an autotransfusion of ~500 ml. Thus, there is potential for fluid overload with volume loading.

Pulmonary Alterations

Parturients have a diminished functional residual capacity despite increased total lung capacity, increased oxygen consumption, and diminished oxygen saturation. Little apnea may produce significant hypoxia. Therefore, supplemental O_2 is recommended with either regional or general anesthesia. There is a decrease in physiologic dead space and a decreased gradient between arterial and end-tidal CO_2 tensions. Thus, with general anesthesia, the end-tidal CO_2 levels should be maintained several torr higher than in the nonpregnant patient.

*Modified from M.L. Pernoll and J. Mandel, Cesarean section. In: J.S. McDonald, ed. *Bonica's Text of Obstetrical Anesthesia.* In press.

Gastrointestinal Alterations

Term parturients have increased intragastric volumes, decreased gastric pH, accentuated intragastric pressure, and delay in gastric emptying. Thus, there is enhanced risk of gastric aspiration, and aspiration of gastric contents may cause maternal death.

PREOPERATIVE PREPARATION

Laboratory Determinations

For the *normal patient undergoing anesthesia,* determination of HCT or Hgb is necessary, but a differential count contributes little to management. The history and physical examination are generally sufficient predictors of derangements of electrolytes and the coagulation profile. In the majority of patients, a preoperative ECG is unnecessary, and although chest x-ray carries little fetal risk, it should be obtained only if the history and physical examination suggest its necessity.

The population of patients requiring cesarean section includes a higher proportion of *high-risk pregnancies* than those delivered vaginally. For operative patients, *individualized studies are required.* For example, diabetics will need a serum glucose determination. Preeclamptics may exhibit coagulation defects in the coagulation cascade and platelet function, and assessment may require the usual platelet count, fibrinogen, prothrombin, and partial thromboplastin times as well as an Ivy bleeding time.

For the anticipated cesarean section patient, type blood for ABO/Rh and screen for unexpected significant antibodies. Patients who have active bleeding (e.g., placenta previa or abruptio placentae), preeclampsia, overdistention of the uterus, coagulopathy, or prolonged labor or who required oxytocin stimulation are at risk of hemorrhage and should have at least 2 units of packed red cells available. In response to concerns about HIV, many obstetricians advise gravidas to have 1–2 units of blood drawn during pregnancy, usually in the late second or early third trimester and stored for autotransfusion if necessary.

Fasting

The practice of maintaining patients NPO past midnight before elective cesarean section or major anesthesia should lower intragastric volume and raise pH, thus reducing the risk of gastric aspiration.

Intravenous Hydration

Fasting, emesis, or insensible loss may directly diminish intravascular volume, aortocaval compression may cause inadequate venous return in parturients, and complications (e.g., toxemia and hemorrhage) may be present. Therefore, *volume repletion* is an important part of anesthetic management of any parturient. This is even more pressing if the use of sympatholytics is anticipated.

The use of glucose in volume expansion has been controversial. Addition of 25 or 57.5 g of dextrose produces a significant rise in maternal and cord glucose concentrations, with a noticeable increase in fetal insulin levels and decrease in fetal glucagon levels. These changes are accompanied by a significant incidence of neonatal hypoglycemia at 2 h of age and an increase in the incidence of neonatal jaundice. Use of 7.5 g of dextrose was not associated with such effects nor was administration of glucose at rates <6 g/h. It seems prudent not to deprive the parturient of maintenance glucose infusion but not to use solutions containing 5% dextrose for acute volume loading. Dextrose administration of <6 g/h or 7.5 g acutely should be considered safe.

Acid Aspiration Prophylaxis

Acid aspiration prophylaxis is mandatory for a gravida undergoing a general anesthetic. The nonparticulate antacid, sodium citrate, when given <1 h preoperatively, is effective in raising gastric pH >2.5. Although cimetidine and ranitidine—type 2 histamine (H_2) antagonists—also are capable of raising gastric pH, sodium citrate is the treatment of choice because of the simplicity of use and lower cost.

Premedications

With the exception of acid prophylaxis, *premedication of obstetric patients is rarely necessary or desirable.* However, when it is required, the relative safety of the benzodiazepine diazepam in doses <10 mg has been confirmed. Anticholinergics are also used for obstetric premedication because these drugs blunt bradycardic responses to succinylcholine, diminish oral secretions, and possibly decrease gastric volume. Atropine 0.01 mg/kg and glycopyrrolate 0.005 mg/kg do not significantly affect the fetal heart rate, but with administration of larger doses of atropine, tachycardia may occur. Glycopyrrolate produces anti-sialagogic effects with less maternal tachycardia and sedation. Hence, it may be preferable.

Miscellaneous

Informed consent for the procedure must be obtained before the patient receives medication. Establish a secure, large-bore IV route (preferably with a ≥18-gauge needle) preoperatively.

For cesarean section, place an indwelling catheter in the bladder. Surgically prepare the abdomen after administration of a regional anesthetic but before administration of a general anesthetic. To control blood loss immediately after delivery, have sufficient oxytocin available for rapid infusions and to add to subsequent IV solutions.

CHOICE OF ANESTHETIC TECHNIQUES

Which anesthetic technique should be used is determined by many factors, including the procedure to be done, the length of time anticipated for the procedure, the discomfort the procedure is likely to evoke, the effect of anesthetic agents on the mother and fetus, the urgency for the procedure (e.g., cesarean section), the contraindications, and patient preference. The question of the best anesthesia for cesarean section is further clouded because studies of maternal and fetal outcome with general and regional anesthesia have not provided unequivocal evidence of superiority of any technique. It is impossible to conclude that one anesthetic technique will be optimal for all situations. *The patient's desire for or against a given anesthetic is an important determinant.* Most patients prefer to be awake during delivery. Thus, epidural anesthesia is used in about 40% of cesarean sections in the United States.

Epidural anesthesia may be preferable to general anesthesia in patients for whom it is an option. Epidural anesthesia benefits intervillous blood flow. This increases with the sympathetic block to the point of hypotension. However, when hypotension occurs, intervillous blood flow declines precipitously. Nonetheless, maternal stress response should not be a problem with epidural anesthesia to T6. Although genital herpes may not affect epidural anesthesia administration, administration of an epidural through an area of active lesions or to a patient with active HSV-2 viremia is contraindicated because of consequences of herpetic encephalitis. *Contraindications to epidural or spinal anesthesia include coagulopathies and intercurrent infection.* When maternal demise occurs with regional anesthesia, it is usually from errors in technique, vascular or subarachnoid injection, inadequate volume repletion, or unsuspected cardiac disease. When emergency cesarean section is indicated, time considerations may prevent the use of epidural anesthesia.

General anesthesia is more commonly employed in emergencies because it takes less time. However, general anesthesia (because of aspiration) is associated with a greater incidence of maternal mortality and may be responsible for slightly more blood loss than regional anesthetics. A 20% reduction in intravillous blood flow occurs with induction of general anesthesia in healthy parturients. No disease state provides an absolute contraindication to all forms of general anesthesia, however.

Anesthetics cannot be compared by fetal effects. Cord pH may be lower after regional anesthesia, but the fetus may exhibit higher Apgar scores and shorter times to sustained respiration. There is little difference in neonatal neurobehavioral outcome after epidural vs general anesthesia except in cases of maternal hypotension. A prolonged interval from induction to delivery is associated with poorer fetal outcome under general anesthesia. This is not the case with subarachnoid anesthesia.

Epidural Anesthesia

The single greatest risk of epidural anesthesia is hypotension. The incidence is ~30% with labor and 36% without labor, and the hypotension occurs from aortocaval compression and sympathetic block. Hydration and left uterine displacement do not entirely eliminate hypotension. A patient may appear to be in no distress while significant hypotension is developing. Thus, the blood pressure must be monitored carefully following induction of epidural anesthesia.

The toxicity of local anesthetics may be influenced by numerous factors in the gravida undergoing epidural anesthesia. Pregnancy has been demonstrated to diminish the dose of bupivacaine necessary to produce cardiovascular collapse, hypoglycemia diminishes the dose of bupivacaine necessary for cardiovascular collapse, and cimetidine but not ranitidine has been shown to interfere with hepatic clearance of lidocaine. Thus, ranitidine is recommended for parturients who undergo epidural anesthesia when H_2 blockade is desired. Since propranolol interferes with lidocaine and bupivacaine metabolism, exercise caution in administration of multiple doses of bupivacaine or lidocaine to patients receiving this medication. Preeclampsia also diminishes lidocaine clearance.

Greater safety may be obtained by slow induction of epidural anesthesia. A 20-min interval between doses of bupivacaine does not limit subsequent spread. Time permitting, give an initial 10 ml dose, with an interval of at least 10 min before a subsequent injection. This technique also allows assessment of the adequacy of catheter placement.

Fetal toxicity of local anesthetic agents is affected by the same factors influencing maternal toxicity. Fetal acidosis, e.g., from maternal hypotension, hypoxia, or uteroplacental insufficiency, increases fetal local anesthetic levels by ion trapping. Thus, the relative merits of available anesthetic techniques need careful evaluation.

Various local anesthetic agents have been used extensively for epidural anesthesia: bupivicaine, lidocaine, 2-chloroprocaine, and mepivacaine. Recently, the safety of the first three drugs has been questioned.

Epidural 2-chloroprocaine has been associated with persistent neural blockade and adhesive arachnoiditis. Since 1983, the FDA has recommended that 0.75% concentration of bupivacaine not be used in obstetrics because it had been associated with toxic reactions, including maternal deaths. Therefore, it is advised that ≤ 5 ml of any bupivacaine solution be injected in the period required to manifest premonitory signs of a toxic reaction (30–60 sec). The use of epinephrine in obstetric epidural anesthesia is controversial.

Epidural administration of narcotics has become almost routine practice in many institutions. Fentanyl 50–100 fg added to the local anesthetic can improve both quality and duration of anesthesia. Fetal depression has not followed these small doses.

It is imperative that the ability to deliver oxygen under positive pressure, suction, and the equipment and drugs necessary for tracheal intubation be available at the location where any anesthetic is administered. Standards of monitoring adhered to in the operating room should apply to the patient undergoing epidural anesthesia, including an ECG and blood pressure monitor.

Generally the *left lateral recumbent position* to displace the uterus favorably is preferred for initial catheter placement and induction of anesthesia, although the sitting position is also acceptable. Place obese patients in a slightly head-up position during induction, but do not inject such patients in the sitting position.

Special training and detailed technical knowledge are necessary to undertake epidural anesthesia. The exact location of an epidural catheter is uncertain (e.g., 3–10/10,000 are subarachnoid). Thus, before administration of the therapeutic dose, employ a test dose of the anesthetic. Usually the test dose consists of a combination of epinephrine and local anesthetics to detect intravascular and subarachnoid catheter placement, respectively.

Management of Complications

Unintended dural puncture occurs in 1%–3% of obstetric epidurals. Following this event, the incidence of *postlumbar puncture headache* is 30%–78%. Instillation of 30–60 ml of preservative-free saline or 5 ml of the patient's blood through a subsequent successful epidural catheter is suggested.

The first preventive or therapeutic measure for *hypotension* is left uterine displacement or left lateral recumbency. Adequate volume repletion with crystalloid should rapidly follow. Should this fail, ephedrine is the agent of choice because it is cardiotonic and does not depress uterine blood flow.

Subarachnoid injection of local anesthetic in quantities intended for the epidural space has been associated with significant morbidity and mortality. Such occurrences are rare, but the absence of CSF flowing from the epidural needle does not guarantee it is extradural.

1. If an impending total spinal or convulsion is suspected, withdraw the needle immediately.

2. Rapidly institute supportive measures, for example, cardiopulmonary resuscitation.

a. Assure the airway, preferably by endotracheal intubation.

b. Ventilate with 100% O_2.

c. Support circulation with positioning, fluids, and ephedrine as needed.

3. Following the patient's stabilization, consider the consequences of the large volume of local anesthetic in the subarachnoid space, particularly if 2-chloroprocaine was the agent.

Toxic levels of local anesthetics may occur by either cumulative absorption of local anesthetics injected into the epidural space or by unintended intravascular injection. Toxicity is usually manifested by generalized seizures, but cardiovascular collapse may follow bupivacaine administration. The toxic reaction is often accompanied by prodromal symptoms, e.g., tinnitus and perioral numbness. If these are noted, give oxygen immediately. A small dose of thiopental (50–100 mg) may be preventive. Consider immediate induction of general anesthesia if prodromal symptoms intensify. Promptly begin CPR if a generalized seizure or cardiovascular collapse ensues.

Assess the fetal status promptly. If the fetus is delivered immediately, local anesthetic levels may be elevated due to ion trapping. Hence, prepare to provide cardiopulmonary resuscitation and supportive measures for the neonate also.

Almost 20% of patients will experience some discomfort while undergoing cesarean section with epidural anesthesia. This can almost always be predicted by *careful assessment of the quality of the block.* Reassurance and emotional support may be adequate, but if unsuccessful, give general anesthesia. Nitrous oxide in concentrations below 50%, and fentanyl (1 fg/kg) should be safe adjuncts.

Droperidol is effective in ameliorating nausea and vomiting after spinal and epidural anesthesia. Metaclopromide, 0.15 mg/kg given immediately after umbilical cord clamping, also significantly reduces nausea without sedation.

Shivering frequently occurs in patients undergoing epidural anesthesia. This may be controlled by warming IV and local anesthetic solutions and applying radiant heat to the gravida's face and chest. If that fails, give meperidine 25–50 mg for relief.

Subarachnoid Anesthesia

Subarachnoid anesthesia is more likely to create supine hypotension than epidural anesthesia, probably due to the greater extent and speed of onset of the sympathetic block. Correct the fall in cardiac output and blood pressure by turning the patient to the left lateral decubitus position or by left uterine displacement. Either of these is essential in the safe conduct of subarachnoid anesthesia. As with epidural anesthesia, the laboring patient undergoing subarachnoid anesthesia is at lower risk for hypotension than one not in labor. This is due to the transient autotransfusion with uterine contractions.

Volume preloading can only reduce the risk of hypotension. It may be more effective when combined with uterine displacement, however. Excepting patients who are at risk for volume overload, preloading with approximately 1000 ml of crystalloid will also increase safety. Despite these measures, up to 50% of patients will manifest significant hypotension and should be treated with IV ephedrine.

Because of the much lower dosages involved, local anesthetic toxicity and placental transfer of local anesthetics are not problems with subarachnoid anesthesia.

Although frequently used for subarachnoid anesthesia, *tetracaine may result in inadequate anesthesia.* Combining *tetracaine with procaine* (instead of glucose) yields a solution of greater baricity, resulting in greater patient comfort and reduced supplemental analgesia requirements.

Bupivacaine has been used as 0.5% isobaric, 0.5% hyperbaric, and 0.75% hyperbaric solutions, but analgesia may be incomplete in hyperbaric 0.5% doses of <12.5 mg.

Hyperbaric lidocaine provides rapid onset but relatively brief duration of anesthesia. It also carries a high incidence of dysphagia due to high blockade; thus, subarachnoid lidocaine (especially for cesarean section) has been discouraged.

The duration of tetracaine and bupivacaine is adequate for virtually all cesarean sections. Hence, the addition of epinephrine is usually unnecessary.

With single-dose subarachnoid anesthetic, control of spread is achieved by baricity, volume of injection, and patient position. Cerebrospinal fluid dynamics are altered at term, particularly during labor, due to engorgement of the epidural veins, and *hyperbaric solutions should be used for obstetric subarachnoid anesthesia.* The anesthetic may be induced with the patient in right lateral decubitus position if she is turned to the left in approximately 1 min. When technical considerations prevent this, the sitting position may be used, but anesthetic onset will be delayed.

Management of Complications

The complications of spinal anesthesia are similar to those of epidural anesthesia. *Postlumbar puncture headache* is greater, even when using 25-gauge needles. Treatment is as noted previously. *Hypotension and high levels of blockade* also occur more frequently. However, with reduced dosage, local anesthetic toxicity is rarely seen. Treatment for hypotension and high blockade levels is as with epidural anesthesia.

General Anesthesia

Adequate maternal and fetal oxygenation are the most important physiologic alterations in both induction and maintenance of general anesthesia. Intubation, while perhaps more difficult, is even more critical because of the risks of aspiration. General anesthesia during pregnancy should not be undertaken without endotracheal intubation.

Induction Agents

Thiopental is used extensively for induction of anesthesia for cesarean section. However, it is well recognized that smaller doses must be used for the pregnant patient. Doses of 4–7 mg/kg are not associated with diminished Apgar scores, but with larger doses, neonatal depression may occur. Pregnant patients eliminate thiopental faster than nonpregnant women, whereas neonatal elimination is significantly slower than in normal adults.

Breast milk and feeding should not be affected by a single dose of 5 mg/kg thiopental for anesthetic induction.

Muscle Relaxants

Muscle relaxants are used for both *induction and maintenance of general anesthesia.* Induction of general anesthesia implies rapid sequence induction. Therefore, it is useful to provide light anesthesia and allow surgical exposure. The commonly employed agents may all be given safely before cord clamping. Magnesium sulfate administration renders parturients particularly susceptible to muscle relaxants, however.

In the first 10 weeks of pregnancy, plasma cholinesterase activity falls rapidly and remains low, putting >10% of patients at risk for prolonged duration of *succinyldicholine-induced muscle relaxation.* Prolonged paralysis occasionally occurs with succinyldicholine. Therefore, monitoring the degree of neuromuscular blockade should be performed even after a single intubating dose.

Administration of succinyldicholine may have a number of unpleasant side effects (e.g., muscle fasciculations, myalgias, and increased intragastric pressure), and preadministration of a small dose of nondepolarizing muscle relaxant is often used in nonpregnant patients as a preventative. However, *pretreatment is not recommended for pregnant patients* because the advantage is less and they are more likely to develop drug complications.

Although succinyldicholine continuous infusion was used

widely for maintenance of muscle relaxation during cesarean section, *it has largely been replaced by the short-acting non-depolarizing agents, atracurium and vecuronium.*

Placental transfer of *curare* may occasionally cause neonatal depression.

Pancuronium has been used for maintenance of muscle relaxation in cesarean section. An umbilical venous/maternal venous ratio of 0.22 has been determined for this drug. However, this value increases with prolongation of the incision-to-delivery interval. Fortunately, neonatal depression associated with pancuronium is rare.

Atracurium provides good maintenance of muscle relaxation in cesarean section with minimal neonatal effects at doses of ~0.3 mg/kg. It does not cross the placenta in significant quantities. It may become acceptable as an induction agent when succinylcholine is contraindicated.

The maternal venous/umbilical venous ratio for maintenance *vecuronium* is 0.11, and its neonatal half-life is 36 min. Maternal clearance is increased in pregnancy; thus, there is rapid blockade resolution. In doses of 0.04 mg/kg, adverse neonatal effects are not found for vecuronium or pancuronium (by Agpar or neuro-adaptive scores). After further study, this drug may become acceptable when succinyldicholine must be avoided.

Maintenance Agents—Narcotics

All narcotics cross the placenta. Thus, narcotics were discouraged for obstetric anesthesia. Newer, short-acting narcotics, such as fentanyl 1 fg/kg administered within 10 min of delivery, produce no appreciable neonatal effect, however. Attenuation of the hypertensive response to intubation in pregnancy-induced hypertension may be achieved by fentanyl 200 fg plus droperidol 5 mg or alfentanil 10 fg/kg administered 1 min before induction of general anesthesia.

The practice of administering small doses of narcotics during induction of general anesthesia should be reserved for those patients in whom the benefits of diminution of cardiovascular response to intubation outweigh the risks of a depressed neonate. Consult and ensure the availability of *naloxone* and staff capable of managing the apneic newborn.

Following delivery, there is no contraindication to the administration of narcotics, and fentanyl in doses up to 5 fg/kg permits diminution of the inhalational anesthetic.

Inhalational Agents

Inhalational agents cross the placenta as a function of time and concentration. However, inhalational agents permit adequate anesthesia at lower concentrations of nitrous oxide. This permits the use of a higher F_{IO_2} and provides greater safety.

Halothane, enflurane, and isoflurane are all used for maintenance of cesarean section anesthesia, have an acceptable incidence of maternal recall, and are not associated with depression of uterine blood flow. However, all three agents cause dose-dependent depression of uterine contractility. Currently, isoflurane is used most frequently.

Nitrous oxide crosses the placenta rapidly, with a fetal/maternal ratio of 0.8 after 3 min. Prolonged administration of high concentration nitrous oxide has been associated with poor perinatal outcome. Limit concentrations of nitrous oxide to 50%, and if delivery has not been effected within 15 min, discontinue nitrous oxide. Avoid nitrous oxide in the severely compromised fetus, and ensure normocarbia and uterine displacement.

Agents for Control of Blood Pressure

The treatment of choice for *hypotension* is (1) relieve aortocaval compression, (2) restore intravascular volume, and (3) use ephedrine when necessary.

Hypertension, most frequently a problem during intubation, is brief and not serious for the normal parturient. When acute, either due to pregnancy-induced hypertension or coexisting cardiovascular disease, consider short-acting narcotics. These attenuate the response to intubation but may induce hypoventilation in the neonate. Nitroglycerine infusion obtunds the hypertensive response without adverse neonatal effects. However, this must be used with caution because of increased intracranial pressure. Nitroprusside has been used without cyanide toxicity for the acute management of transient hypertension. However, discontinue nitroprusside if the patient is resistant to the drug or if tachyphylaxis develops.

Technical Considerations

Rapid sequence induction is the induction of choice for general anesthesia for pregnant patients. Since cricoid pressure is an accepted practice in such cases and preparation for the management of regurgitation is routine, the only distinction between the rapid sequence and the deliberate sequence is the avoidance of positive pressure mask ventilation. Positive pressure ventilation by mask may produce gastric distention and regurgitation. Nevertheless, application of cricoid pressure prevents gastric inflation, assuring no airway obstruction.

Apply pulse oximetry routinely. For those parturients exhibiting desaturation during induction of general anesthesia, apply gentle (<35 cm H_2O) ventilation by mask and cricoid pressure.

We favor the following procedure for *cesarean section*. Routinely administer sodium bicitrate 30 ml before induction. Following preoxygenation, perform rapid sequence induction with thiopental 1.0 mg/kg and succinyldicholine 1.0 mg/kg. Accomplish intubation with a tracheal tube of appropriate size. Maintain oxygen 50%, nitrous oxide, and isoflurane 0.5%–1.0%. Following return of twitch, continue muscle relaxation with atracurium or vecuronium. After clamping of the umbilical cord, decrease isoflurane to 0.25%, or discontinue this and give fentanyl <5 fg/kg. This reverses neuromuscular blockade. Then extubate the patient following sustained head lift and responsiveness.

Airway management during pregnancy may be complicated by edema of preeclampsia, bearing down during the second stage of labor, or weight gain in pregnancy. Do not attempt to intubate with a tube >7.0 mm. However, a series of smaller endotracheal tubes should be available in the event of an inability to pass the selected size endotracheal tube.

Failed endotracheal intubation is evident in the majority of avoidable maternal deaths associated with anesthesia. This applies in about 1 in 300 cesarean sections. Successful management of failed intubation requires a concerted plan of action of which mask ventilation with cricoid pressure is an accepted component.

LOCAL ANESTHESIA

Local infiltration anesthesia for major obstetric surgery (e.g., cesarean section) has never been widely used and is so rare today that few obstetricians and surgeons have learned the technique. There are few, if any, absolute contraindications to other anesthetics or absolute indications for local anesthesia. The procedure takes more time than other anesthetic techniques. Additionally, in an attempt to relieve pain, toxic levels may be reached.

CESAREAN SECTION

Cesarean section is the transabdominal delivery of a viable fetus (with placenta and membranes) through a uterine incision. If the fetus is *previable,* the same procedure is termed *abdominal hysterotomy. Primary* describes the first cesarean, and *repeat cesarean* section is used to describe any cesarean section after the first. The various types of cesarean section used are *lower uterine segment* (or low segment—incision in the lower uterine segment), *classic* (incision in the uterine corpus), *extraperitoneal* (the uterus is entered without incising the peritoneum), and *cesarean hysterectomy* (cesarean section followed by hysterectomy). Several other descriptive terms are used: elective (vs mandatory), transverse (incision at right angle to the uterine long axis), and vertical (incision corresponds to the long axis of the uterus).

INCIDENCE

In 1965, the U.S. cesarean delivery rate was ~4.5%; by 1985, it was ~22.7%. The current indications for cesarean section include ~48% repeat cesareans, ~29% dystocia, 16% fetal distress, 5% breech, and 2% other complications. Regrettably, the medicolegal climate in the United States may be largely responsible for the increasing use of cesarean section.

CONTRAINDICATIONS

There are few contraindications to cesarean section in the presence of a valid indication. These contraindications include pyogenic infections of the abdominal wall, *an abnormal fetus incompatible with life, a dead fetus* (except to save the life of the mother), and *lack of appropriate facilities, equipment and supplies, or personnel.*

INDICATIONS

Cesarean section is warranted when vaginal delivery imposes risks exceeding that of cesarean section to the mother or fetus.

The indications may be absolute or relative and are summarized in Table 15-1.

OPERATIVE PROCEDURES

Lower segment cesarean section is the procedure of choice because there is less blood loss, the scar is less likely to rupture in a subsequent labor (and delivery), and there is less chance of bowel adhesions to the incisional site. The *classic cesarean section* is only employed for specific indications. *Extraperitoneal* is a more problematic variation of the lower segment cesarean section and is rarely used today. Vaginal cesarean section has been abandoned. *Cesarean hysterectomy* is also only used for very specific indications.

Surgical Principles

The principles of hemostasis, accurate tissue apposition, avoidance of tissue necrosis, minimizing suture material, reducing operating time, and avoiding infection will influence outcome beneficially.

Elective Procedures with Cesarean Section

Carefully consider elective procedures coincident with cesarean section. These include operating time, need for transfusion, infection potential, and so on. *Tubal ligation* is the most frequent coincident procedure and rarely is medically contraindicated. *Incidental appendectomy* (the second most common elective procedure with cesarean section) may be accomplished safely if the appendix is readily accessible and there are no other complicating factors. *Pedunculated myomas* can be ligated and removed, but excision of other myomas nearly always leads to hemorrhage.

Abdominal Incisions

The *choice of abdominal incision* for cesarean section is predicated on the type of uterine incision planned and whether or not access to the upper abdomen is necessary. To perform a lower

Table 15-1. Common indications for cesarean section

Repeat cesarean section
Dystocia
 Fetopelvic disproportion
  Pelvic (*Passage* insufficiency)
   Bony pelvis
    Pelvic inlet (usually anterior-posterior <10 cm)
    Midpelvis (usually ischial spines <9.5 cm)
    Outlet (very unusual and then almost never seen in the absence
     of other pelvic contractures)
   Soft-tissue obstruction
    Low-lying placenta (especially posteriorly implanted)
    Uterine leiomyomas
    Ovarian tumors
    Other genital tract neoplasia (rare)
 Fetal complications (the *Passenger*)
  Normal fetus
   Macrosomia (>4000 g)
   Malposition and malpresentation
    Breech unfavorable for vaginal delivery
    Deflexed head
    Transverse or oblique lie
    Brow
    Posterior mental position
    Shoulder presentations
    Compound presentations
  Anomalous fetus
   Meningomyelocele
   Hydrocephalus
   Sacrococcygeal teratoma
   Miscellaneous fetal anomalies
  Multiple gestation
   Twins
    Twin A any presentation except vertex
    Twin B not suitable for vaginal delivery
    Failure of intrapartum external version
    Fetal distress (even if Twin A has been delivered vaginally)
    All monoamniotic twins
   Triplets or greater number
Abnormalities of labor (the *Powers*)
 Primary uterine inertia
  Prolonged latent phase (unusual, but >20 h in a nullipara and
   >14 h in a multipara)
  Protraction disorders
   Protracted active phase dilatation (nulligravida <1.2 cm/h,
    multigravida <1.5 cm/h)

(*continued on next page*)

Table 15-1. (*Continued*)

Protracted descent (nulligravida < cm/h, multigravida <2 cm/h)
Arrest disorders
Prolonged deceleration phase (nulliparas ≤3 h, multiparas ≤1 h)
Secondary arrest of dilatation (no dilatation for ≥2 h)
Active phase arrest of descent (≥1 h)
Failure of descent in the deceleration phase or second stage (≥1 h)
Uterine inertia due to fetopelvic disproportion
Failed induction
Fetal distress
Uteroplacental insufficiency
Cord accidents
Metabolic acidosis
Obstetric hemorrhage (maternal or fetal or both)
Abruptio placentae
Placenta previa
Ruptured uterus
Vasa previa
Infections
Severe chorioamnionitis
Active maternal genital herpes
Some cases of genital condylomata acuminata
Maternal and/or fetal complications potentially adversely influenced by labor or vaginal delivery or both
Antepartal testing indicative of labor intolerance
Cervical dystocia
Medical
Fulminant preeclampsia-eclampsia
Diabetes (only occasionally indicated)
Erythroblastosis
Severe maternal heart disease
Other debilitating conditions
Surgical
Cervical or uterine scarring of extent that may rupture with labor (e.g., extensive myomectomy, trachelorrhaphy)
Cervical cerclage
All abdominal cervical cerclages
Certain vaginal cerclages (e.g., cannot remove)
Serious maternal problems (eg, vesicovaginal or rectovaginal fistula)
Prior extensive vaginal plastic operations
Carcinoma of the cervix

uterine segment cesarean section, enter the abdomen through a lower abdominal transverse (Pfannenstiel) or a vertical abdominalincision. There is a *better cosmetic result with the transverse incision,* and the patient may wear a bikini swim suit without the scar showing. In addition, healing proceeds faster, the incision is less painful, and there is less risk of hernia formation (the action of the abdominal muscles tends to pull the incision together, not apart). The primary advantages of the vertical incision are more rapid performance than for a transverse incision and better access to the upper abdomen.

Transverse Abdominal Incisions

For best cosmetic results, make the symmetric incision about 2 cm superior to the symphysis pubis to curve slightly cephalad laterally. Divide the subcutaneous tissues similarly and obtain hemostasis. After transversely incising the rectus fascia, grasp the midline raphe and separate the underlying tissues by sharp dissection. Retract the rectus muscles (and pyramidalis, if present) laterally and enter the attenuated posterior fascia and parietal peritoneum transversely or vertically by sharp dissection.

To close the peritoneum, begin the transverse incision closure with a running 0 or 00 polyglycolic suture. Approximate the rectus muscles in the midline and close the fascia with interrupted or running 0 to 00 polyglycolic suture. Approximate the subcutaneous tissues and close the skin appropriately.

Vertical Abdominal Incision

The abdomen is usually entered through a low vertical midline incision, although a transverse abdominal incision occasionally may be used for a *classic cesarean section.* The midline incision usually follows the linea nigra and extends from the umbilicus to the symphysis pubis. After incision of the subcutaneous tissues, sharply incise the midline raphe and enter the parietal peritoneum by sharp dissection.

The vertical incision is usually closed with the peritoneal layer sutured with a 0 to 00 polygycolic suture. The fascial tissues are closed with interrupted 0 absorbable or nonabsorbable sutures. Following reapproximation of the subcutaneous tissue, the skin is closed.

Lower Segment Cesarean Section

After the peritoneum is entered, identify the veriscouterine peritoneal fold and incise the uterine peritoneum transversely ~1 cm from the bladder attachment. Remove the areolar connections between the bladder and the lower uterine segment for 3–4 cm by blunt dissection, and retract the bladder toward the symphysis pubis, exposing the lower uterine segment. The lower uterine segment is an anatomic area extraordinarily influenced by late pregnancy and labor; e.g., without labor, it is located far down in the pelvis, but after full dilatation, it may be one-third the distance to the umbilicus. Thus, judgment is necessary to properly locate the uterine incision. Carefully enter the lower uterine segment transversely by sharp dissection. Extend the incision laterally, curving cephalad with bandage scissors. Visualize and avoid the uterine vessels just beyond the limits of the incision.

Use a vertical incision in the midline of the lower uterine segment for more access to the uterus. The major problem with this incision is extension into the myometrium of the uterine corpus.

Next, deliver the fetus, the placenta, and membranes. Explore the uterine cavity with a laparotomy pad over the gloved hand to ensure the removal of the placenta and membranes. Close the uterine incision in two running or interrupted layers using 0 or 00 absorbable suture (e.g., polygycolic). Replace the bladder over the area of the incision. Close the visceral peritoneum using a running suture with 000 or 0000 absorbable suture.

Classic Cesarean Section

The *indications for classic cesarean section are placenta previa, transverse or oblique fetal lie, and when rapid delivery is essential.*

The classic cesarean section is the simplest to perform. Make a vertical incision in the lower portion of the uterine corpus (above the vesicouterine fold) through the visceral peritoneum into the myometrium. After the uterine cavity is entered extend the incision caudally and cranially using bandage scissors. Effect the delivery of the infant, the placenta, and the membranes. Repair the incision with three layers of absorbable suture (e.g., polyglycolic). Close the two deeper layers with a running or interrupted 0 or 00 and the superficial layer with a running (or baseball) 00 or 000 suture.

Extraperitoneal Cesarean Section

Extraperitoneal cesarean section avoids entering the peritoneal cavity. This procedure may have had advantages before extensive use of antibacterial agents but *it is rarely used today.*

Cesarean Hysterectomy

The indications for cesarean hysterectomy include inability to control bleeding (e.g., from uncontrollable atony, from the placental implantation site of a previa), rupture of the uterus (with repair impractical), placenta accreta, massive infection of the uterus involving tissue necrosis, and uterine or cervical tumors (e.g., uterine leiomyomas, cervical carcinoma in situ). *Subtotal hysterectomy* (i.e., leaving the cervix) is reserved for cases (usually hemorrhage) in which the patient's well-being is threatened by the significant operative time and risk of total hysterectomy.

Cesarean hysterectomy is technically the same as other hysterectomy except for the size of the uterus, the friability of tissue, and the extraordinary vascularity. Over two thirds of cesarean hysterectomy patients require transfusion, and morbidity remains high.

Intraoperative Control of Bleeding

The *blood loss from an average vaginal delivery is ~500 ml, whereas that from an uncomplicated cesarean is ~1200 ml.* The effect of this on the gravida may be appreciated by noting the HCT on the third postpartum day when the early hemodynamic alterations have begun to stabilize. The vaginally delivered patient will have increased her HCT by about 3, whereas the average postcesarean patient will have decreased her HCT by approximately 3.

Intraoperative *blood loss may be decreased* by meticulous surgical hemostasis, exteriorization of the uterus (through the abdominal incision) for removal of the placenta (and membranes) or repair of the uterine incision, and postdelivery administration of oxytocin. Administer the latter slowly IV (5–10 IU) immediately after delivery of the newborn or immediately after delivery of the placenta. Then, add 10–20 IU to each liter of fluid until the uterus is well contracted.

COMPLICATIONS

Maternal Mortality

The *maternal mortality rate of cesarean section is* 40–80/100,000, which is >25 *times that of vaginal delivery.* Indeed, infectious morbidity and mortality are 80 times higher than that of vaginal delivery. However, those having cesarean delivery may be at higher relative risk because of factors necessitating the procedure. Anesthetic complications contribute 10% to the overall maternal mortality. However, both low-risk patients and high-risk patients may be affected. Thus, anesthesia has consistently remained the fifth or sixth cause of maternal mortality.

Intraoperative Maternal Morbidity

Intraoperative surgical complications with cesarean section are >11% (~80% minor and 20% major). *Major complications include* bladder injury, laceration into cervix or vagina, laceration in the corpus uteri, laceration through the isthmus into the broad ligament, laceration of both uterine arteries, intestinal injury, and trauma to the infant with sequelae. Complications are higher in emergency (~19%) than in elective (~4.2%) cases. *Minor complications include* blood transfusion, injury to the infant without sequelae, minor laceration of the isthmus, and difficulty in delivering the infant.

The risk factors in emergency cesarean section but not in elective cesarean include station of the fetal presenting part (very low or very high), labor before surgery (no labor or very lengthy labor enhances risk), low gestational age, rupture of fetal membranes (with labor) before surgery, previous cesarean section, and skill of the operator. Although uncommon, massive venous air embolus may complicate cesarean section. Measures to decrease the possibility of venous air embolus include adequate prehydration and avoidance of extreme Trendelenburg position.

Postoperative Maternal Morbidity

Postoperative morbidity following cesarean section is ~15%, of which ~90% is infectious (endometritis, urinary tract and wound sepsis). Complications are more likely after emergency (~25%) than elective cesarean section (~5%). Predispositions to postoperative morbidity are duration of ruptured membranes before surgery, duration of labor before surgery, anemia, and obesity.

Factors most significantly associated with the risk of postoperative infection include rupture of the membranes for ≥8 h, labor for ≥12 h with cervical effacement and dilatation to ≥4 cm, multiple vaginal examinations, low socioeconomic status, and complicating medical conditions. The use of prophylactic antibiotics materially decreases infectious morbidity and mortality. In <2% of postcesarean patients, infections will become life threatening because of septic shock, pelvic abscess, or septic pelvic thrombophlebitis.

Other factors enhancing risk due to infection include a lack of prenatal care, maternal age (the very young are at increased risk), malnutrition, lower gestational age, longer preoperative hospital stays, and systemic illnesses (e.g., diabetes, systemic lupus erythematosus, chronic renal disease). The number of vaginal examinations that place the patient at risk for infection may be 3–7. There are conflicting data about the effect of intrauterine catheter monitoring on the risk of postcesarean section infectious morbidity.

Common noninfectious cesarean postoperative complications (<10% of the total) include paralytic ileus, intraabdominal hemorrhage, bladder paresis, thrombosis, and pulmonary disorders (e.g., pneumonia).

Perinatal Mortality and Morbidity

Cesarean section carries less risk for the infant than a complicated vaginal delivery, and thus, by inference, perinatal mortality and morbidity are decreased. This may apply to certain conditions. However, there is no proof that the current high cesarean section rate has generally enhanced mental performance or reduced the overall incidence of neurologic abnormalities of those delivered by cesarean section.

Iatrogenic prematurity from elective repeat cesarean has been a major concern. Nonetheless, with currently available means of fetal assessment, including ascertaining gestational length (e.g., early pregnancy testing, early ultrasound examination) or defining fetal pulmonary maturity (e.g., LS ratio, phosphatidylglycerol) before elective cesarean section, iatrogenic prematurity has been markedly decreased.

Prophylactic Antibiotics

Prophylactic antibiotics with all cesarean sections may lower the infectious morbidity. However, ~20% of women will still require systemic antibiotic therapy for postoperative uterine infection, and some serious postoperative pelvic infections still occur. Yet even using current risk criteria, ~50% of cases that become infected will not have been identified. Finally, although prophylactic antibiotics do significantly reduce febrile morbidity and endomyometritis, the data are less conclusive for wound and urinary infections. Nonetheless, the use of prophylactic antibiotics for the risk groups is well accepted.

Preoperative maternal antibiotics may result in therapeutic levels in the fetus. This complicates the evaluation of the newborn at risk for sepsis. Thus, except in extreme cases, antibiotics are usually administered IV after the cord is clamped or after the uterine wound and peritoneal cavity are lavaged with an antibiotic solution.

The usual microorganisms involved in postcesarean endometritis are group B streptococci, aerobic gram-negative bacilli, anaerobic gram-positive cocci, and anaerobic gram-negative bacilli.

Prophylactic antibiotics should be effective for the contaminating organisms, inexpensive, nontoxic, and clinically effective. Prophylactic antibiotics should not be one of the few antibiotics reserved for the treatment of specific severe infections or a drug used against bacterial pathogens with acquired resistance. Although many antibiotics have been studied for their prophylactic efficacy, first and second generation cephalosporins are probably the best. If more than one agent is used, they should be tailored to cover both anaerobic and aerobic organisms. There is no single agent or combination of agents that can be designated the treatment of choice.

PREVENTION OF UNNECESSARY CESAREAN SECTION

While cesarean section delivery rates continue to rise, there are increasing reports of methods that could decrease the number of cesarean sections. These include vaginal birth following cesarean section, use of active management of labor, antepartum external version to decrease the number of breech presentations, vaginal birth for selected breech presentations, and the selective use of forceps.

Particularly noteworthy are increasing trends for vaginal birth after cesarean (VBAC), which has been demonstrated to be both effective and relatively safe. It may be anticipated that two thirds of those women who had a prior cesarean section will undertake a trial of labor if it is offered, and ~80% will achieved a vaginal delivery. With vaginal birth there will be less maternal morbidity due to uterine dehiscence (~2%) or uterine rupture (0.3% with repeat cesarean and 0.5% with VBAC). Hence, if there is no urgent or continued indication for cesarean section, vaginal delivery should be chosen, and the policy of "once a cesarean section, always a cesarean section" should be abandoned.

Chapter 16

Gynecologic History and Examination

HISTORY

It is common practice to obtain much of the history by paramedical personnel, interactive computer activities, or a patient questionnaire completed before seeing the physician. Hence, important positive and negative findings may be reviewed with the patient before the physical examination.

AGE, MARITAL STATUS, GRAVIDITY, AND PARITY

CHIEF COMPLAINT

The patient's main problem(s) in her own words listed in her order of seriousness comprise the chief complaint.

PRESENT ILLNESS

The patient's health at the onset of illness and the symptoms in sequence of development form the present illness. As much detail (e.g., facts, dates) as is possible is included, documenting what, where, when, why, how, and to what degree each complaint affects her.

Past History

Menstrual history: The age and character of the menarche (or menopause) should be described. The last menstrual period (LMP), previous menstrual period (PMP), and last normal menstrual period (LNMP), if relevant, should be recorded. Also, the regularity, duration, amount of bleeding (number of perineal pads or tampons), pain, mucous discharge, and intermenstrual or postcoital spotting should be recorded.

Gynecologic history: Record the following. Gravida (G), the number of previous pregnancies; para (P), the number of previous term pregnancies; abortions (Ab), the number of pregnancies terminated (spontaneously or electively) before 20 weeks gestation or 500 g; premature deliveries (Pre), the number of pregnancies terminated between 21–35 weeks gestation or 500–2499 g; living children (LC), the number of children currently living, with twins noted in parenthesis at the end of the sequence. Often, this is recorded in a summary with just the numbers in the sequence noted; e.g., 4,2,1,2,4 (Twins 1 pr.) would mean the woman had been pregnant 4 times, had 2 term pregnancies, had 1 abortion, had 2 premature births, and has 4 living children (here, the twins were premature but survived). In some patients, a more detailed obstetric history is indicated, including dates of all pregnancies, their duration, character and duration of labor, method of delivery (with type of uterine incision if cesarean birth). Complications, weight and sex of infant(s), stillbirths, abortions, neonatal complications, and current status of living children should be noted also.

Medical and surgical history: Record medical allergies (e.g., penicillin, iodine, horse serum) as well as important nonmedical allergies (e.g., shrimp). Record any excessive bleeding potentially indicative of a coagulopathy. A summary of the patient's childhood and later illnesses in chronologic order together with complications and the treatment prescribed for each is important. Record operations and injuries, with dates and outcome. Record all medications (prescription, proprietary).

Family history: Age, health, and cause and date of death of first through third degree relatives (often a brief pedigree is the best demonstration of this material) should be recorded. Also note familial or hereditary abnormalities, diseases, bleeding tendencies, occurrence of cancer, tuberculosis, diabetes mellitus, syphilis, heart disease, hypertension, and nervous or mental disorders.

Sexual history: Current and past contraception usage should be recorded, as well as libido and the frequency of coitus. Additional notes should be made about the duration of present marriage or living arrangement, patient's assessment of the relationship, age and health of spouse/partner, former marriages or relationships (when and how long) and degree of compatibility, vaginal and pelvic infections, and sexually transmitted diseases (including HIV).

Social history: The patient's occupation, avocation(s), and travel (especially abroad or in the tropics) should be assessed for hazards. Reactions to others may be assessed tangentially by questions relating to successes, failures, and participation in social or religious organizations.

Personal history (habits): Sleep pattern, exercise habits, and alcohol, tobacco, and drug usage should be noted.

SYSTEM REVIEW

A positive or negative comment for each portion of this category will aid in health assessment (do not repeat the symptoms referable to the chief complaint).

General: Comment on the patient's health, present weight, average weight, weight before present illness, reason for weight loss or gain, skin disorders, and change in hair pattern.

Head and neck: Pain, tenderness, swelling, restriction of neck, and trauma should be noted.

Eyes: Vision with and without glasses, double vision, irritation, swelling of the lids, and prominence of eyes deserve comment.

Ears: Record pain, buzzing, discharge, and patient's assessment of hearing.

Nose: Obstruction to nasal passages, bleeding, discharge, and change in ability to smell require recording.

Mouth: General condition of the teeth, gums, tongue, bleeding, and chewing difficulties should be noted.

Throat: Speech difficulties, swallowing, or voice changes are notable.

Cardiovascular: Skin color (pale, ruddy, dusky), edema, precordial or substernal pain, irregular or labored heartbeat, and shortness of breath at rest or with exercise should be recorded.

Respiratory: List any of the following: cough, wheezing, sputum, hemoptysis, chest pain with breathing, chills, fever, and night sweats.

Gastrointestinal: The patient's appetite, thirst, digestive difficulties (e.g., nausea, vomiting, preprandial or postprandial pain, hematemesis, food intolerance), jaundice, and frequency, character, and color of stools should be assessed.

Urinary: Urinary frequency, nocturia, oliguria, dysuria, hematuria, urethral discharge, sores, swelling, and other urinary alterations should be recorded.

Neuropsychiatric: Strength, ability to work, skin sensations, ataxia, dizziness, tremor, headaches, "spells" or "fits," acuity of memory, and strange occurrences should be explored if warranted.

PHYSICAL EXAMINATION

VITAL SIGNS

The patient's weight, height, blood pressure, pulse, temperature, and respirations must be noted.

GENERAL

The patient's appearance, ability to ambulate, attitude, and color of skin are often recorded.

HEAD AND NECK

Skull size and shape, hair (amount, color, and texture), tumors, and tenderness may be useful.

Eyes: Prominence of the eyes or lids as well as the size, shape, pupillary reaction to light, character of conjunctiva and sclera, fundi, and ocular movements should be assessed.

Ears: The external ear, external auditory canal, and tympanic membrane should be examined, and discharge, cerumen, tophi, tenderness, or other abnormalities must be noted.

Nose: Any deformity, septal deviation, septal erosion, obstruction, tenderness, discharge, or tenderness over the sinuses requires comment.

Neck: Swelling, pulsations, tracheal deviations, thyroid, lymph nodes, retractions, and abnormal masses should be noted.

Mouth and throat: The lips, gums, tongue, dentition, tonsils, and oropharynx should be examined.

Thorax

The general size, shape, symmetry, and spinal integrity may bear notation.

Breasts: The size, shape, equality, masses, tenderness, scars, and nipple discharge should be noted (see next section for discussion).

Heart: The point of maximal impulse at the apex, abnormal pulsations, retractions, or venous distention in the neck or in other veins should be noted. Auscultation of the heart should be accomplished.

Lungs: Inspect the chest to reveal the equality of inspiration and expiration. Palpate to reveal muscle tone, tenderness, and tactile fremitus. Percussion should reveal resonance, cardiac silhouette, diaphragmatic exclusions, and gastric tympany. Auscultation reveals the quality and intensity of breath sound, rales, fremitus, and friction rubs.

Abdomen

Note the size, shape, and abdominal contour as well as masses, visible peristaltic waves, prominent veins, and herniation. Palpation may indicate the thickness of the abdominal wall, the liver edge, the spleen and any tenderness, rigidity, masses, hernias, and the presence or absence of a fluid wave. Percussion should confirm organ position or masses. Auscultation will reveal the presence of peristaltic tones.

Back

The back should be checked for kyphosis or scoliosis. Costovertebral angle tenderness should be noted.

Extremities

Size, shape, color, and movements of the hands should be visualized, and condition of the fingers and nails should be noted. The size, color, condition, and movement of the legs should be assessed. The peripheral vascular system may be appraised by palpating the radial, femoral, distal pedal, posterior tibial, and popliteal arteries for thickness and resilience.

NERVOUS SYSTEM

Cerebral function, cranial nerves, cerebellar function, motor and sensory systems, and reflexes should be reported.

PELVIC EXAMINATION

A proper pelvic examination records visual inspection and palpation of the external genitalia, Bartholin's, urethral, and Skene's glands (BUS), introitus, vagina, and cervix. The bimanual examination includes palpation of the uterus, ovaries, and uterine tubal areas. The rectovaginal examination must include palpation of vagina, rectum, and rectovaginal septum as high as the cul-de-sac (see next section for details).

IMPRESSION (ANALYSIS)

List probable diagnoses for each problem (in same order of chief complaint).

PLAN

Record a plan for each problem, i.e., diagnosis and therapy. Note any tests performed in the office (e.g., wet mount and Pap smear) and indicate other testing the patient is to have (e.g., mammography) and when she will be seen again. Indicate any counseling or instructions given to the patient.

SIGNATURE

Include time and date of notation.

GYNECOLOGIC EXAMINATION

Increasingly, obstetrician–gynecologists are providing the entire spectrum of primary health care for women. Thus, it is proper to determine if the patient is seeing you for her entire health care or if she is to have only gynecologic consultation or treatment. The depth of the general workup and health care advice may then be appropriately designed. If the patient is to be seen for gynecologic complaints only and is already under the care of another primary physician, the gynecologic examination may be more specific and complete, with particular reference to the chief complaint.

The gynecologic evaluation devotes particular attention to examination of the breasts, abdomen, and pelvis. The general examination and appropriate laboratory studies should be performed. An appraisal of other body systems should be done more frequently than the usual standards when indicated by the history or unusual physical findings. Do not dismiss a patient following the initial workup without a tentative diagnosis depending on signs and symptoms.

BREAST EXAMINATION

The breast examination has three components: breast self-examination (BSE), physician examination, and mammography.

Breast Self-Examination (BSE)

After age 20, BSE is recommended on a monthly basis for all women. Women who do BSE as recommended discover breast disease significantly earlier, and death from breast cancer can be avoided or delayed by early diagnosis and prompt therapy. Moreover, BSE is simple, costs nothing, and is painless. Despite these advantages, only approximately one third of women perform BSE monthly, and of those, only about half do this correctly.

Since BSE is more often and better performed if taught by a nurse or a physician, the time of examination is an ideal opportunity to teach BSE and discuss its significance.

1. Most information will be gained in a menstruating woman immediately after menses when hormonal changes in the breast are at a minimum. In nonmenstruating women, it is often most convenient for them to choose a time when they have another monthly duty (e.g., paying bills) to remind them of BSE.

2. The examination is begun in the upright position with good direct light. Looking in a mirror, she should inspect the breasts carefully, first with her arms at the sides and then raised above her head. She should seek abnormalities of contour or symmetry, skin changes, masses, retraction, or nipple alterations.

3. Palpation of the supraclavicular and axillary regions should be performed next. She should be looking for changes from previous examinations, masses, nodes, or other abnormalities.

4. The patient should then recline, with a towel or small pillow beneath the back on the side of the breast being examined (to rotate the chest so that the breast may be symmetrically flattened against the chest wall). Next, using the flat of her fingers, she should systematically palpate each quadrant of the breast by pressing against the chest wall. Finally, the areola and the area beneath the nipple should be palpated and the nipples compressed for evidence of secretion. Again, she should be looking for changes from previous examinations, lumps (masses), and any other abnormalities.

5. Should anything raise concern, she should immediately consult her physician.

6. Many women find keeping a simple sketch as a record of the findings from month to month to be a useful way to detect change.

Physician Breast Examination

A complete physician breast examination is recommended every 2–3 years for women age 20–40 (Figs. 16-1, 16-2, 16-3). Women >40 should have at least annual examinations. The physician should proceed as follows.

1. With the patient sitting in good light with her arms at the side, perform a visual inspection. Ask her to press her hands on her hips (to tense the pectoralis muscles), and continue the inspection. With her arms raised above her head, examine both breasts and the axilla. Finally, have the patient bend forward from the erect position to reveal irregularities or dimpling when the breasts fall forward. The physician must look for the same abnormalities as the patient (i.e., asymmetry, masses, nipple retraction, skin retraction, or other changes). Often oblique light is helpful to confirm surface dimpling

2. With the patient sitting, ask her to extend her arms 60°–90°. Carefully palpate each axilla using the flat of the fingers of the right hand for the left axilla and the left hand for the right

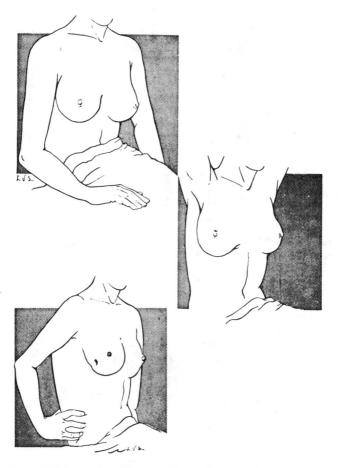

Figure 16-1. Inspection of breasts. Observe breasts with patient sitting, arms at sides and overhead, for presence of asymmetry and nipple or skin retraction. These signs may be accentuated by having the patient raise her arms overhead. Skin retraction or dimpling may be demonstrated by having the patient press her hand on her hip in order to contract the pectoralis muscles. (From J.L. Wilson. In: J.E. Dunphy and L.W. Way, eds., *Current Surgical Diagnosis & Treatment,* 4th ed. Lange, 1979.)

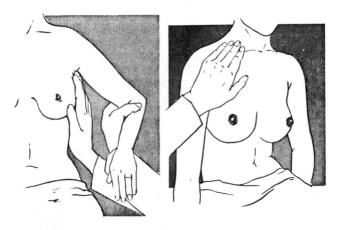

Figure 16-2. Palpation of axillary and supraclavicular regions for enlarged lymph nodes. (From A.E. Giuliano. In: L.W. Way, ed., *Current Surgical Diagnosis & Treatment,* 6th ed. Lange, 1983.)

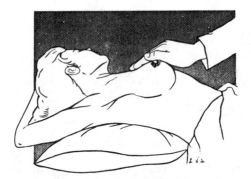

Figure 16-3. Palpation of breasts. Palpation is performed with the patient supine and arm abducted. (From A.E. Giuliano. In: L.W. Way, ed., *Current Surgical Diagnosis & Treatment,* 6th ed. Lange, 1983.)

axilla. Both the supraclavicular and infraclavicular lymph node areas must be carefully palpated. Ask the patient to lean forward for bimanual palpation of each breast using the flat of the fingers. Both side-to-side and upper-to-lower palpation may be necessary depending on the configuration of the breasts.

3. With the patient supine and arms above the head, again inspect the breasts. Reexamine the axilla with the patient's arms slightly extended and palpate the breasts between the examining fingers. Finally, with the woman's arms relaxed at the sides, carefully palpate each breast quadrant by compression against the chest wall. Palpate one breast at a time, holding the fingers flat against the breast and carefully feeling with gentle pressure. Gently compress the areas beneath the areola and nipple with the thumb and index finger to detect masses and to express fluid. Should a nipple discharge be present, it should be smeared on a slide and fixed for cytologic examination.

Observe breast consistency for thickened or firm zones. Identify the cordlike duct structures and any shotty or nodular masses. Determine whether masses are fixed to the skin or chest wall.

When a breast mass is identified, the presumptive diagnosis is usually established by mammography. It may be necessary to aspirate a cyst or biopsy to confirm the diagnosis.

Mammography

High-quality mammograms should be obtained with ≤ 0.3 rad exposure. This technique has been demonstrated to correctly identify ~89% of cancers (41.6% of which were not detectable clinically). The American Cancer Society guidelines for mammographic screening of asymptomatic women are widely accepted.

1. Baseline mammogram for all women age 35–40
2. Mammography at 1–2 year intervals from age 40 to 49
3. Annual mammograms for women ≥ 50 years

High-risk women (e.g., previous breast cancer, mothers or sisters with bilateral or premenopausal breast cancer, and those with histologic abnormalities associated with subsequent breast cancer—Chapter 17) should have biannual examinations and annual mammography. Such a screening program will identify >6 cancers per 1000 asymptomatic women. Moreover, the tumors will be detected earlier (80% have negative axillary nodes vs 45% not screened). Approximately 40% of early breast cancers can be discovered only by mammography, and ~40% can be detected only by palpation. Thus, both modalities are crucial.

ABDOMINAL EXAMINATION

Observe the abdomen with the patient sitting, and then examine in the dorsal recumbent position with knees slightly flexed to improve abdominal relaxation. Note the contour (flat, scaphoid, or protuberant), and inspect the abdomen for respiratory movement, prominence or enlargement of internal organs, asymmetry, scars, and significant skin changes (e.g., striae, rashes). Note the escutcheon pattern as well as other hair distribution. Conduct auscultation in each of the quadrants.

Palpate the abdomen gently for evidence of tenderness, herniation, or masses. Feel for deep masses or sensitivity, especially over the cecum, colon, and bladder. Identify the liver by percussion and palpate its edge. Examine the gallbladder and epigastric region. Check for splenic enlargement. Muscle guarding and abdominal rigidity may indicate infection. Gentleness is essential. Always progress from areas of less tenderness to the areas of discomfort. With hematoperitoneum, the guarding increases as the pressure of palpation is increased. Rebound tenderness is a sign of peritoneal irritation and must be investigated further. Employ auscultation in all four quadrants.

PELVIC EXAMINATION

With the patient in the lithotomy position and appropriately draped, the examination usually begins with the physician seated. Surgically clean gloves are used. It may be desirable to have a female attendant present as a chaperone and assistant. The pelvic examination consists entirely of inspection and palpation.

Inspection

Observe the labial development, hair distribution, and abnormalities. By gentle lateral traction separate the labia majora and inspect the clitoris. The glans may be exposed by slight traction on the foreskin. Both labia minora should then be inspected. Separate the labia to visualize the urethral meatus. Observe the vaginal orifice for vaginal discharge and the status of the hymen. Inflammation, cysts, or tumors may be seen in the region of Bartholin's glands. Inspect the fossa navicularis for discharge, scars (e.g., episiotomy), or lesions (e.g., condylomata). Inspect for skin changes over the perineum, thighs, mons veneris, and perianal region. Note and record the presence of masses and tender areas. Describe discernible external genital lesions (e.g., inflamed, hypertrophied, atrophied, or ulcerated areas).

Speculum Examination

Warm the speculum with tap water. Lubrication of the speculum is rarely necessary and may confuse vaginal cytology, bacterial smears or cultures, and wet preparations for *Trichomonas, Candida,* and *Gardnerella vaginalis.* Use a good light source, preferably daylight or a blue-white spotlight. A single-blade speculum is advantageous to view the vaginal surface (e.g., searching for a vesicovaginal or rectovaginal fistula). The Kelly air vaginoscope is especially useful for examination of the very young or when the introitus is atrophic (Fig. 16-4).

To facilitate speculum insertion, ask the patient to relax and then to bear down slightly as with a bowel movement. This reduces muscular resistance while you introduce the speculum carefully and obliquely. Spread the labia with the gloved fingers of one hand, insert the gloved index finger of the same hand slightly into the vagina, and depress the perineum slightly. Asking the patient to loosen the muscle being pressed on may facilitate relaxation.

Do not insert the speculum directly into the vagina but downward and inward at approximately 45° to avoid the urethra. Visualize the vaginal canal while inserting and opening the speculum. To avoid a traumatic encounter with a vaginal obstruction, mass, or friable lesion, continue observation as the speculum is advanced. As the blades of the bivalve speculum approach the cervix, open the instrument so that the blades slip into the anterior and posterior fornices to fully expose the cervix. The blades may be fixed in the open position by tightening the screw lock.

Examine the cervix carefully. Determine the color, size, contour, and surface characteristics and the zone of the squamocolumnar junction. Note lacerations, displacement, size and configuration of the external os, distortion or ulceration, type and amount of discharge, blood, or fluid present in the cervical canal, and the character of the endocervix (through a patulous os).

Before digital examination, obtain a clean scraping of the squamocolumnar junction and the endocervix. Additionally, obtain vaginal mucus from the posterior vagina fornix and from the cervical canal for cytologic examination. Fix the smear on the slide immediately. Touch or gently wipe ulcerations or friable lesions with a cotton-tipped applicator for evidence of contact bleeding. Biopsy suspicious lesions or apply topical therapy at

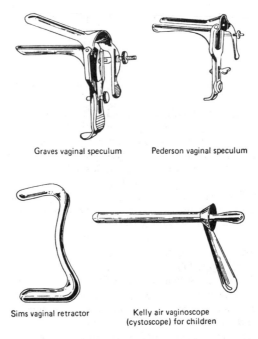

Graves vaginal speculum   Pederson vaginal speculum

Sims vaginal retractor   Kelly air vaginoscope
(cystoscope) for children

Figure 16-4. Vaginal specula and vaginoscope. These come in various sizes.

this point. This may be deferred until after bimanual examination, however.

Slowly remove the speculum from the vagina to facilitate inspection. Note the color, the presence or absence or rugae, the apparent thickness of the mucosa, and any abnormalities (redness, ulceration, or tumors). When cystocele, rectocele, or descensus is suspected, insert a single blade of the speculum up or down and have the patient bear down so that the degree of relaxation or herniation can be determined. Strip Skene's glands and the distal urethra distally after removal of the speculum. Observe and make smears or cultures or both of expressed discharge.

Palpation

Digital examination is easiest with the patient in the lithotomy position and the examiner standing with one foot on a step or low stool and the elbow on that knee to brace the examining arm and hand. Insert the gloved, lubricated index finger gently but deliberately into the vagina. Again, apply slight downward pressure at the fourchette (and ask the patient to relax) to reduce tension. After a pause to enhance relaxation, slip the middle and forefinger of the examining hand into the vagina.

Palpation of Structures of Introitus

Note tenderness, masses, and thickening. With the thumb external and the palm turned downward, feel for enlargement and sensitivity of Bartholin's gland. Investigate the lower vaginal wall for abnormalities. Feel the urethra for relaxation, local dilatation, masses, and tenderness.

Palpation of Cervix

Lightly outline the cervix with the fingers to determine its size, position, contour, consistency, and dilation. Move the cervix to stretch the uterosacral and transverse cervical ligaments. This usually will reveal the degree of freedom of the cervix. Deliberately move the cervix up and down to elicit tenderness on motion.

Palpation of Bladder Base

Feel beneath the bladder to determine sensitivity, relaxation, or masses. Slight tenderness and a suggestion of thickening over the normal ureter at or near its insertion into the bladder are normal.

Bimanual Examination

The foregoing procedures require only one unaided hand. In bimanual examination, the other hand is used on the abdomen to outline the deeper pelvic structures. Hold the abdominal hand palm down on the abdomen with the fingers together and slightly flexed. Press firmly with the flat of the fingers against the abdominal wall. Generally, the vaginal fingers are used to elevate structures for palpation through the abdominal wall. Ideally, use first one hand and then the other in the bimanual examination. Masses in the right pelvis may be palpated more easily with the right hand, and vice versa. The patient, with mouth open, should take shallow, rapid breaths to avoid tensing the abdominal wall.

Palpation of Uterus

Attempt to depress the fundus of the uterus with the abdominal hand while the fingers of the hand in the vagina are resting against the cervix and lower portion of the corpus. Relaxation of the vaginal walls and fornices may permit palpation of much or all of the cul-de-sac and of the posterior aspect of the uterus. A normally free uterus usually can be brought well downward and forward by the abdominal hand. This makes possible vaginal palpation of both the anterior wall and the uterine fundus. Determine the uterine position, size, consistency, contour, and mobility as well as the patient's discomfort on manipulation. Gently explore the posterior fornix and uterosacral ligaments for masses, fullness, fluctuation, and sensitivity. Acute tenderness in this region may inhibit examination.

Palpation of Adnexa

Turn the hand in the vagina so the palm is upward, Insert the two examining fingers slightly posteriorly but high into one of the lateral fornices. Sweep the abdominal examining hand downward over the fingers in the vagina to attempt to feel the ovary and tube between the hands.

The ovary usually lies just lateral to the uterus near its midportion. If the ovary is not felt initially, check the cul-de-sac, the lateral pelvic wall, or the space anterior to the uterus for a displaced, possibly adherent ovary and tube. The ovary is normally slightly tender, distinguishing it from nontender masses, such as fecal material within the bowel. Rectovaginal examination may permit the best delineation of the ovary. Observe the position, size, consistency, contour, and mobility of each ovary, and note any unusual tenderness.

Ordinarily, the uterine tube is not sensitive, but it is so delicate that a normal tube cannot be palpated. Tenderness, swelling, or a cordlike thickening between the ovary and the uterus indicates tubal disease. Inflammation or tumor may convert the tube into an enlarged mass that may be mistaken for an ovarian tumor.

Salpingitis, endometriosis, or cancer may involve one or both adnexa so extensively that these structures and the uterus become a single mass filling the entire true pelvis. The cul-de-sac may be filled or obliterated, thus altering gynecologic landmarks.

Rectovaginal Examination

Rectovaginal examination should be performed routinely even though all of the internal genital structures have been palpated properly on vaginal evaluation. Anal abnormalities, lesions of the rectovaginal septum, and even sacral masses may be felt only on rectovaginal examination. This examination is invaluable in children, virgins, and elderly women, in whom the vaginal introitus is so small that only a single finger can be inserted. Rectovaginal examination is much preferred to rectal examination only because the second finger reaches farther when the first finger is in the vagina, and rectovaginal septal abnormalities may be discovered.

With the patient and the examiner positioned as for bimanual vaginal examination, insert the lubricated second finger of the examining hand to the anus. Insert the distal half of the finger into the anal canal while the patient bears down slightly to relax the anal sphincter. When the examining finger has been inserted a short distance, introduce the forefinger into the vagina. The perineal body will then be between the two fingers. Encourage the patient to relax by adopting a gentle, slow, deliberate manner. Finally, reach as high as possible in the pelvis with the tips of both the vaginal and rectal fingers and palpate bimanually, as with the vaginal examination. The rectal finger should be swept about the circumference of the bowel and the patient asked to bear down. Fully 50% of all large bowel polyps and cancers should be located within the range of this examination.

To demonstrate a rectocele, bring the rectal finger back to the perineal body, removing the vaginal finger. As this is done, the rectal pouch will be entered, and its protrusion into the vagina may be evident at the introitus. The patient may be able to see a rectocele herself, demonstrated if she holds a mirror at the appropriate angle.

Feces from the rectal examination may be tested for the presence of occult blood. This is particularly important in women ≥45 years of age, when rectal carcinoma becomes more prevalent.

LABORATORY STUDIES

Smears or Cultures

Bacteria

Obtain specimens for bacterial smears or cultures using a sterile cotton-tipped applicator. Fluid exudate may be obtained from the urethral meatus, Skene's and Bartholin's ducts, the vaginal walls, the posterior vaginal fornix, and the cervical os. Using bacteriologic technique, apply the applicator directly to the culture medium or to a transfer medium. Avoid heating and drying the sample. When gonorrhea is suspected, inoculate a sterile chocolate agar or blood agar plate or use Transgrow medium. Prepare smears by spreading the discharge in a thin layer on a clean glass slide. If it is to be used for staining, it may be air dried. If it is to be used for other techniques (e.g., immunofluorescent identification of herpesvirus or *Chlamydia*), it must be handled according to the methods recommended for that technique.

Trichomonas vaginalis

Examine separate wet mount preparations from the posterior fornix, the cervical os, and the urethral meatus. Moisten a clean cotton-tipped applicator with normal saline, and swab the site of exudation or touch the applicator to the discharge. Transfer a drop of the exudate to a polished slide and apply a clean coverslip. Immediately examine microscopically for trichomonads (while still warm). This technique is also useful for examining other pathogens in a wet mount (e.g., *Gardnerella*). If these organisms are not identified in the wet smear, careful inspection of the stained exfoliative vaginal cytologic smear (Papanicolaou) generally will reveal their presence. It is rarely necessary to prepare cultures. However, should culture be necessary, use aerobic methodology with Trichosel or Difco's hash medium (B-1016T, a modified trypticase medium, not requiring addition of serum).

Candida albicans

For demonstration of *Candida*, the technique is similar to that for trichomonads, but apply 1–2 drops of 10% aqueous potassium hydroxide to the discharge to be viewed on the slide. This dissolves the epithelial, inflammatory, and red blood cells. The mycelia, hyphae, and spores will be prominently displayed. The material most likely to show mycelia is the white plaque of vaginal thrush, which must be rubbed from the mucosa with a moist cotton applicator. In questionable cases of *Candida,* it is necessary to culture vaginal fluid on Sabouraud's or Nickerson's medium.

Urine

Collect a midstream, clean-catch urine specimen (or catheterize the patient if necessary) in a sterile container. Use sterile technique and equipment after thoroughly cleansing the urethral meatus with a mild antiseptic solution.

Cytologic Examination

The cytologic examination (Papanicolaou or Pap smear) is a cancer screening technique. When cytology is positive for premalignant or malignant cells, further diagnostic procedures (e.g., colposcopy, cervical biopsy, conization, endometrial biopsy, or D & C) must be performed to determine the diagnosis. However, a positive cytology is ~95% accurate in the diagnosis of cervical carcinoma.

The patient should not have douched for >24 h before obtaining a cytologic specimen and must not be menstruating. During the speculum examination when the cervix is first exposed, a specially designed small plastic or wooden spatula is used to lightly scrape the squamocolumnar junction. Endocervical cells are obtained separately, as are exfoliated cells in the vaginal pool. The material from each site is immediately placed on separate slides, and a preservative spray or solution is applied.

Laboratories report findings to the physician through one of several systems. Purely descriptive terminology is best, and, increasingly, laboratories are reporting smear interpretation by the Systematized Nomenclature of Medicine (SNOMED) classification. This describes the type of cells, estrogen effect, inflammatory changes, and presence or absence of atypical cells. Some laboratories also use the traditional classification according to degree of deviation from normal: class I—normal cells, class II—slightly abnormal, usually inflammatory change (a repeat test is generally recommended after therapy or in <6 months), class III—cellular abnormality, usually atypia (indicating the need for colposcopy), class IV—distinctly abnormal cells, possibly malignant (usually requiring colposcopy and biopsy), class V—malignant cells (necessitating directed biopsy).

How frequently cervical cytologic screening should be obtained is currently debated. However, yearly evaluations are recommended. More frequent examination is indicated for women with previously abnormal cytologic studies, women with more than one sexual partner (or an uncircumcised partner), women with a history of sexually transmitted disease, and those with genital condylomata or herpes. In addition to premalignant and malignant changes, the cytologic smear is useful for the detection of viral infections (e.g., herpes simplex, condylomata acuminata) and folic acid and vitamin B_{12} deficiencies.

Chapter 17

Diseases of the Breast

COMMON BENIGN BREAST DISEASES

MAMMARY DYSPLASIA
(Fibrocystic Breast Disease, Chronic Cystic Mastitis)

Mammary dysplasia is the most common breast disorder—~50% of women between 30 and 50 years of age are affected, but it is uncommon in postmenopausal women. Mammary dysplasia is characterized by bilateral, painful, usually multiple breast masses. *Fluctuation in mass size and discomfort* occur rather quickly and *are usually related to the menstrual cycle,* with the most pain and largest size occurring during the premenstrual interval. Indeed, it is the pain, size fluctuation, and multiplicity of masses that are most useful in distinguishing this process from carcinoma and fibroadenoma. Mammography is often used for the *clinical diagnosis* and women ≥25 years with mammary dysplasia should have baseline mammography. Biopsy may be necessary for suspicious lesions or if the breasts are too dense to adequately visualize the lesions. Ultrasonography may assist also in the differentiation of cystic vs solid lesions.

Microscopically, cysts (both macroscopic and microscopic) are derived from terminal ducts and acini. Papillomatosis, adenosis, fibrosis, and ductal epithelial hyperplasia may occur. Because estrogen promotes growth of mammary ducts and periductal stroma, *estrogen is presumed to be a causative factor.* The improvement normally seen during pregnancy and lactation suggests that progesterone may help to alleviate the disorder. Although not necessarily part of the process, if epithelial dysplasia occurs, it is more likely to lead to breast cancer.

Treatment is largely symptomatic. Advise the patient to perform monthly breast self-examination. It is useful for her to keep a schematic representation of the lesions, so that if changes other than those of the mammary dysplasia occur, she can promptly report this to her physician. The patient should *avoid trauma* (e.g., apply good support while jogging) and *wear a supportive and protective brassiere both night and day.* Analgesics may assist in relief of pain. Long-term restriction of dietary methylxanthines (e.g., caffeine) may relieve some women. Unconfirmed reports suggest that vitamin E may help to alleviate symptomatology.

Breast cysts occasionally reach a size requiring aspiration under local anesthesia. The aspirated fluid should be examined cytologically. If no fluid is obtained or if the fluid is bloody or if a mass persists, biopsy is indicated. In the past, low-dose androgens were used for therapy of the disorder, but undesirable (virilizing) side effects often developed. *Medroxyprogesterone acetate* 5–10 mg orally daily for 5–10 days at the end of each cycle may be beneficial. Similarly, *low-dose oral contraceptives* may give relief but no cure. *Danazol* often gives marked relief, but objectionable side effects may develop. *Tamoxifen* 10 mg bid by mouth may be useful. *Bromocriptine* (a dopamine-receptor agonist that inhibits prolactin secretion) 2.5 mg bid may relieve the mastalgia.

Mammary dysplasia virtually disappears at the menopause. However, the prognosis until that time must be guarded and vigilance maintained to rule out breast carcinoma. Therefore, these patients must be followed carefully and indefinitely.

Fibroadenoma of the Breast

Fibroadenoma of the breast is a common, *benign, usually unilateral* (10%–15% bilateral), *solid* (firm), *discrete, usually solitary, and nontender mass* that commonly develops at 20–40 years of age. Fibroadenomas generally are 1–5 cm in diameter. This tumor is more frequent and tends to occur at an earlier age in blacks than whites or Orientals. Fibroadenomas are composed of both fibrous and glandular tissue. Tumor growth is stimulated by pregnancy, and regression (often with calcification) occurs postmenopausally. Fibroadenomas must be *differentiated from mammary dysplasia and breast carcinoma. Treatment* is excision under local anesthesia.

Cystosarcoma phyllodes (giant mammary myxoma) is a type of breast fibroadenoma with unusually proliferative cellular stroma. It may grow rapidly to large size. Cystosarcoma phyllodes is rarely malignant but may recur if incompletely excised. Hence, a wide margin of excision is essential.

Other Nonpuerperal Benign Breast Disease

Intraductal papillomas characteristically occur in the *perimenopausal interval* with a bloody, serous, or turbid nipple discharge.

Although a tumor is rarely palpable, it frequently is possible to determine the involved duct by palpably initiating the discharge. The workup includes mammography and cytologic examination of the fluid. The *differential diagnosis* must include *galactorrhea and breast cancer.* Treatment generally is excisional biopsy of the involved duct. Histologically, intraductal papillomas vary from the clearly benign to the anaplastic with invasive tendencies.

Fat necrosis is presumably related to *trauma,* although only about one half of patients with fat necrosis recall an injury. Ecchymosis, skin retraction, or local tenderness may or may not be present. The mass is usually tender. Generally, the mass resolves slowly, and only occasionally is biopsy required to rule out malignancy.

Mammary duct ectasia usually occurs in the fifth decade. It is characterized by ductal dilatation, inspissation of breast secretion, and chronic intraductal and periductal inflammation, with plasma cell predominance. Nipple retraction from scarring may occur, and enlarged axillary glands are frequent. Once differentiated from breast cancer, *no therapy* is necessary.

Galactocele is cystic dilatation of a duct with thick, inspissated milky fluid, present during or shortly after lactation. Galactocele indicates ductal obstruction. Diagnosis is facilitated by mammography, and needle aspiration is usually curative.

Macromastia, occasionally unilateral, has its onset at puberty, although it may develop with pregnancy or even after menopause. The cause of macromastia is unknown. The disorder does not predispose to cancer. *Therapy* includes tamoxifen or surgical reduction (often not curative).

Breast abscess in the nonlactating woman is very rare. Thus, biopsy of any indurated tissue is prudent.

Benign breast diseases are summarized in Table 17-1.

PUERPERAL MASTITIS

Puerperal mastitis is usually marked by *unilateral, often localized inflammation, with fever, localized pain, tenderness, and segmental erythema.* Often a fissured nipple (entry site of the bacteria) still exists. The usual causative agent is hemolytic *Staphylococcus aureus.* Hence, penicillinase-resistant antibiotic therapy (e.g., oxacillin, cephalothin) must be used. Primigravidas are more often affected. Puerperal mastitis tends to occur in two epidemiologic types, epidemic and sporadic. In the *epidemic* type, the infection often can be traced to a carrier, and this type tends to fulminate.

Table 17-1. Types, incidence, and peak years of benign breast diseases

Type	Incidence (%)	Peak (years)	Symptoms
Mammary dysplasia	~50	30–50	Bilateral, painful, solid or cystic masses with cyclic variability
Fibroadenoma	2–3	20–40	Usually unilateral (10%–15% bilateral), firm, discrete, solitary, nontender mass
Intraductal papillomas	3–5	45–55	Bloody, serous, or turbid nipple discharge from a duct without palpable mass
Fat necrosis	>5	Any age	Half give a history of trauma, ecchymosis, skin retraction, or local tenderness
Mammary duct ectasia	~1	50–60	Tender, bilateral masses, possible nipple retraction, enlarged axillary glands
Macromastia	<0.1	Puberty	Diffuse enlargement with continued growth
Galactocele		Perilactation	Cystic ductal dilatation
Breast abscess	~2	Lactation	Unilateral, localized inflammation, fever, pain, tenderness, segmental erythema, caused by *Staphylococcus aureus;* in absence of lactation, must be biopsied

Therefore, intensive therapy is required. Weaning, antibiotic therapy, suppression of lactation, cold packs to the breast, and a brassiere worn day and night are recommended.

In the *sporadic* type of puerperal mastitis, the infant (the most frequent source of the infecting organism) may continue to nurse. By decreasing engorgement, the likelihood of abscess formation is decreased. A nipple shield may assist in controlling discomfort. Antibiotic therapy is the same as for the epidemic type.

In either type, if antibiotic therapy is initiated before suppuration, the infection is usually controlled within 24 h. If the infection advances to form an abscess, surgical drainage will be required.

CARCINOMA OF THE BREAST

One of every 9–11 American women will develop breast cancer at some time during her life. The mean and median age of breast cancer occurrence is 60–61 years. The *etiology remains unknown.* Risk factors for breast cancer, based largely on the patient's past and family history, are listed in Table 17-2. Unopposed estrogen may increase the risk for breast cancer, but the oncotic effect is not as well correlated as it is for endometrial carcinoma. Although there is some controversy, oral contraceptives do not appear to enhance the risk of breast cancer.

Most breast carcinoma arises from the epithelial lining of the breast ductal system. If the origin of the cancer is the large or intermediate-sized ducts, it is termed *ductal* (~90%); if it arises from the epithelium of the lobular terminal ducts, it is termed *lobular.* Several histologic subtypes of breast cancer have been identified (Table 17-3). However, 70%–80% are nonspecific infiltrating ductal carcinomas, and the histologic type has little bearing on prognosis, as projected by tumor staging. Breast cancer is *multicentric;* i.e., more than one malignant focus can be identified in the same breast in 40% of patients and in the opposite breast in ~2% of patients. There is a 5%–8% incidence of cancer occurring later in the opposite breast.

Breast cancer occurs in the upper outer quadrant in ~45% of cases, in the central zone (periareolar or subareolar) in ~25%, in the upper inner quadrant in ~15%, in the lower outer quadrant in ~10%, and in the lower inner quadrant in ~5%. Lymphatic dissemination is the rule, with the axillary regional lymph nodes involved about twice as frequently as the internal mammary nodes. Unfortunately, *hematogenous spread* of breast cancer frequently

Table 17-2. Risk factors in breast cancer

High risk factors
  Previous breast cancer
  Breast cancer in mother or sister
Moderate risk factors
  Age >40 years
  Menarche <12 years
  Menopause >50 years
  First pregnancy >35 years
  Nulliparity
  Cancer of the endometrium or ovary
  Severe mammary dysplasia (when accompanied by proliferation
    changes, papillomatosis, or atypical hyperplasia)
  Breast cancer in aunt or grandmother
Symptoms indicating risk
  Lump in breast
  Nipple discharge
  Ulceration of the nipple
  Recent onset of pain in one breast

occurs, most often to *bone, liver,* or *lungs.* Nodal metastases are present in ~1% of patients with noninfiltrating cancers.

CLINICAL FINDINGS

Screening

The screening processes of self-examination, physician examination, and mammography are discussed in Chapter 16.

Symptoms and Signs

About 90% of breast abnormalities are discovered by the patient, and about 5% are found during a physical examination for other reasons. The initial finding, in the great majority of breast cancers (66%), is a *firm or hard, nontender, fixed mass with ill-defined margins* (due to local invasion). In about 11%, a painful breast mass is the presenting sign. Nipple discharge (9%), local

Table 17-3. Histologic types of breast cancer*

Type	%
Infiltrating ductal (not specified)	70–80
Medullary	5–8
Colloid (mucinous)	2–4
Tubular	1–2
Papillary	1–2
Invasive lobular	6–8
Noninvasive	4–6
Intraductal	2–3
Lobular in situ	2–3
All others	<1

*After A.E. Giuliano, The breast. In *Current Obstetric and Gynecologic Diagnosis and Treatment,* 6th ed., M.L. Pernoll and R.C. Benson, eds. Appleton & Lange, 1987.

edema (4%), nipple retraction (3%), and nipple crusting are the other usual presentations. Initial symptomatology involving ulceration, itching, pain, enlargement, redness, or axillary adenopathy is infrequent.

Special Clinical Forms of Breast Cancer

Paget's carcinoma accounts for 1%–3% of all breast cancers. It usually occurs as a pruritic or burning eczematoid ulceration of the nipple, although the nipple may not be grossly involved, and nipple discharge is only occasionally present. Paget's carcinoma is a particular form of intraductal carcinoma arising in the main excretory ducts of the breast. It usually is well differentiated and multicentric, with extension to the skin of the nipple or areola. Although in about two thirds of patients the underlying carcinoma may be palpated, there is great danger that this lesion may be treated as a dermatologic lesion, with the usual risk of metastases and the harm of delaying treatment.

Inflammatory carcinoma is the most virulent type and accounts for <3% of breast cancers. It occurs as a rapidly enlarging, usually diffuse, and sometimes painful mass, with induration of the surrounding tissues. The overlying skin is often red, warm, and possibly edematous due to infiltration of malignant cells in subdermal lymphatics. The disease is rarely curable because metastases occur early and are widely distributed.

Breast cancer during pregnancy or lactation accounts for only 1%–2% of all breast cancers and complicates approximately 1 in 3000 pregnancies. However, it is difficult to diagnose (secondary to the physiologic changes), and the overall survival rate is low when compared to nonpregnant rate. Axillary metastases are present at diagnosis in 60%–70%, and for them the 5-year survival is 30%–40%. However, if the cancer is confined to the breast, the 5-year survival is ~70%. Delay posed by pregnancy and lactation must be avoided to preserve the mother's life.

Laboratory Findings

With extensive metastases, expect an elevated sedimentation rate. Hypercalcemia is a frequent observation in advanced breast cancers. Liver or bone metastases cause elevated alkaline phosphatase levels. Carcinoembryonic antigen (CEA) may serve as a marker for recurrent breast cancer.

Mammography and Other Imaging Techniques

Mammography has greatly increased the diagnosis of small, even occult, cancers (see also Chapter 16). Mammography may identify some breast cancers up to 2 years before they reach palpable size. The primary limitations of mammography are that it may not reveal clinical cancer in a very dense breast (e.g., the young woman with mammary dysplasia) and that it may not reveal medullary type cancer. The indications for mammography are summarized in Table 17-4.

Because of the incidence of early metastases, *radiographs* of the chest, lumbar spine, pelvis, and skull should be part of a breast cancer workup. Additionally, *bone scans* may be necessary in some cases and may be a part of follow-up.

Ultrasound scanning may be useful in visualizing palpable focal masses in women <30 years (thus reducing the need for radiation). Ultrasound is also helpful in the differentiation of cystic from solid masses and in demonstrating potentially malignant solid tissue adjacent to or within a cyst.

Although other imaging techniques (thermography, transillumination, and MRI) are used occasionally, they lack the large database of mammography and are less widely employed.

Table 17-4. Indications for mammography

1. To screen at regular intervals (see Chapter 16)
2. To assess a questionable or ill-defined breast mass or other suspicious breast change
3. To evaluate each breast at intervals when a diagnosis of potentially curable breast cancer has been made
4. To search for an occult breast cancer from an unknown primary in women with metastatic disease in the axillary nodes or elsewhere
5. To appraise women with large breasts that are difficult to examine
6. To reassure women with cancerophobia

DIFFERENTIAL DIAGNOSIS

The differential diagnosis of breast cancer includes (in decreasing order of frequency) *mammary dysplasia, fibroadenoma, intraductal papilloma, duct ectasia, and fat necrosis.*

SPECIAL PRETHERAPY WORKUP

Biopsy

The *definitive diagnosis* of cancer requires analysis of tissue. Thus, mammography cannot be a substitute for biopsy. The *indications* for breast biopsy include a persistent breast mass, bloody nipple discharge, exzematoid nipple changes, and suspicious or positive mammography results. About 30% of cases considered strongly suggestive of cancer will be found to be benign on biopsy. In contrast, about 15% of abnormal foci thought to be benign will be diagnosed as malignant on biopsy.

Needle biopsy (under local anesthesia) may be used to aspirate tumor cells or obtain a small tissue core. False-negative needle biopsies occur in 15%–20% of cancers. *Open biopsy* is more conclusive and preferably is performed as a separate procedure (often under local anesthesia) before definitive therapy, and there has been no demonstrable adverse effect from a 1–2 week delay. Occasionally, when mastectomy is contemplated for a very suspicious lesion, the open biopsy may be assessed by frozen section and definitive therapy immediately performed under the same anesthetic. The indications for open breast biopsy are summarized in Table 17-5.

Hormone Receptor Site Analysis

Obtain *estrogen* and *progesterone receptor assays* on every breast cancer patient at the time of initial diagnosis. This information is invaluable for hormonal management of patients with recurrent or metastatic disease and may even provide some prognostic assistance. For example, with recurrence or metastases, ~60% of patients with estrogen receptors in their original cancers will respond to hormone therapy, whereas <10% of estrogen receptor-negative patients will respond. Patients with estrogen receptors in their tumors have a more favorable course following mastectomy than those with estrogen receptor-negative tumors. Postmenopausal patients have a higher incidence of estrogen receptor-positive tumors (~60%) than do premenopausal patients (~30%).

The synthesis of progesterone receptors is estrogen-dependent, and progesterone receptors have been found in ~40% of estrogen receptor-positive tumors. When both types of receptors are present, ~80% of patients with recurrent or metastatic disease respond to hormone therapy.

There is no significant relationship between hormone receptor site activity and chemotherapy responsiveness.

Staging

Clinical and histologic staging are of great prognostic significance and are used in designing the treatment plan. Table 17-6 details staging and crude 5-year survival.

Table 17-5. Indications for open breast biopsy

1. Suspicious mammographic abnormalities
2. Clinically suspicious mass, regardless of mammographic findings
3. A cystic mass that does not completely collapse on aspiration or contains bloody fluid
4. Serous or serosanguineous nipple discharge that is not galactorrhea

TREATMENT

Therapeutic options include surgery, radiation therapy, chemotherapy, endocrine therapy, and combinations of these methods.

Surgery

The major surgical procedures and the extent of each are summarized in Table 17-7.

Table 17-6. Clinical and histologic staging of breast carcinoma and relation to survival

Clinical staging (American Joint Committee)	Crude 5-year survival (%)
Stage I	85
Tumor <2 cm in diameter	
Nodes, if present, not believed to contain metastases	
Without distant metastases	
Stage II	66
Tumor <5 cm in diameter	
Nodes, if palpable, not fixed	
Without distant metastases	
Stage III	41
Tumor >5 cm *or*	
Tumor any size with invasion of skin or attached to chest wall	
Nodes in supraclavicular area	
Without distant metastases	
Stage IV	
With distant metastases	10

Histologic staging	Crude survival (%)	
	5 years	10 years
All patients	63	46
Negative axillary lymph nodes	78	65
Positive axillary lymph nodes	46	25
1–3 positive axillary lymph nodes	62	38
>4 positive axillary lymph nodes	32	13

From A.E. Giuliano. In *Current Obstetric and Gynecologic Diagnosis and Treatment,* 7th ed. M.L. Pernoll, ed. Appleton & Lange, 1991.

Radical mastectomy, which is very effective for local control of cancer, is extremely disfiguring. Moreover, it does not appear to offer an advantage over less radical surgery combined with radiation therapy. Following any of the more radical surgeries, physical therapy is advisable, principally to limit edema of the arm.

Radiation Therapy

Although initially radiation therapy was used after surgery when the axillary nodes were positive, it is now increasingly employed as part of primary therapy for small tumors in conjunction with segmental mastectomy and axillary node sampling. For patients with small primary tumors, less than total mastectomy combined with radiotherapy may be as effective as the more radical operations.

Usually 4500–5000 rad are delivered by external beam to the breast and anterior chest wall (including the internal mammary chain). If lymph nodes are positive, the ipsilateral supraclavicular and axillary nodes also are irradiated. When more radiation is necessary to a localized area, the site may be enhanced with interstitial iridium-192. Major complications of such ther-

Table 17-7. Summary of surgical treatments for breast cancer

Procedure	Extent of surgery
Radical mastectomy	En bloc removal of the breast, pectoral muscles, and axillary nodes
Extended radical mastectomy	In addition to the above also includes the internal mammary nodes
Modified radical mastectomy	En bloc removal of the breast, underlying pectoralis major fascia (but not muscle), and axillary lymph nodes
Simple mastectomy	Removal of the entire breast
Segmental mastectomy	Removal of the area involved, e.g., partial mastectomy, quadrant excision, or lumpectomy (often combined with axillary node sampling)

apy (arm edema or weakness, radiation pericarditis, and soft tissue necrosis) occur in ~2% of patients.

Chemotherapy

Overall, *~75% of patients with breast cancer succumb in <10 years.* Thus, the assumption holds that many patients with breast cancer already have disseminated disease at the time of diagnosis. Therefore, chemotherapy is used as an adjunct to initial therapy, with the objective of eliminating occult metastases responsible for late recurrences. There are numerous regimens, but the most extensive and favorable clinical experience has been with *cyclophosphamide, methotrexate,* and *fluorouracil* (CMF). Such adjuvant chemotherapy improves survival (~20%) and lengthens the disease-free interval in premenopausal women, especially those with one to three positive nodes. The effect in postmenopausal women is less beneficial.

Endocrine Therapy

In the past, oophorectomy, adrenalectomy, and hypophysectomy were used to decrease or eliminate estrogen stimulation of breast cancer, especially in postmenopausal women. Although, the last two procedures have largely been abandoned, oophorectomy is still often used to reduce estrogen exposure of the tumor in premenopausal women. However, *tamoxifen* (an antiestrogen) is rapidly becoming the most commonly used agent in endocrine therapy. Overall, about one third of patients respond, but the response with estrogen receptors in the tumor is ~60%, and with both estrogen and progesterone receptors, the response is ~80%. By contrast, only 5%–10% of receptor-negative tumors respond to tamoxifen therapy.

Psychologic Therapy

Sensitivity to the patient's psychologic needs during the workup and therapy is crucial. Full discussion regarding the rationale of therapy and its cosmetic and emotional effects is necessary. Reconstructive surgery as well as prosthetics must be considered. Support groups (e.g., The Service Committee of the American Cancer Society's program Reach to Recovery) or psychiatric intervention may be useful.

Current Therapy Summary

Although breast cancer therapy is currently in transition and several crucial conclusions are not available, certain guidelines are useful. Potentially curable lesions may be treated by partial mastectomy plus axillary lymphadenectomy and radiation therapy or by modified radial mastectomy. If in the premenopausal patient axillary nodes are involved, adjuvant chemotherapy is prudent. Radical mastectomy should be reserved for cases of advanced local disease with tumor invading the pectoralis muscle. Extended radical mastectomy is justified for patients with medial lesions without signs of distant spread. Receptor-positive breast cancers may benefit from endocrine therapy.

FOLLOW-UP CARE

Follow-up care should be lifelong and has two objectives: *to detect recurrence(s)* and *to observe the other breast for evidence of carcinoma.* Every month, the patient should examine her own breast(s). Mammography should be obtained annually or when any change is detected. During the first 3 years, when metastases are most likely, physician examinations are performed every 3–4 months. Between 4 and 5 years, examination is performed every 6 months. After 5 years, examinations are continued at 6–12 month intervals.

The use of estrogen or progestational agents in women free of disease after primary breast cancer therapy is probably inadvisable, particularly if the primary cancer was hormone receptor positive. However, recent evidence indicates that this is not the risk previously thought and that hormonal replacement may, in some instances, be undertaken. Pregnancy following treatment of breast carcinoma carries less risk than previously indicated. Currently, particularly in stage I or II cases, some authorities are recommending deferring pregnancy for at least 2 years. If a complete evaluation is negative at that point and the patient is knowledgeable concerning the risks, pregnancy may be undertaken. It has been suggested that such a protocol does not enhance the chance of death from breast carcinoma. It seems prudent to individualize recommendations for hormonal replacement therapy or pregnancy after breast cancer following consultation with the team caring for the patient and perhaps with oncologic centers.

Palliative therapy of disseminated breast cancer is beyond the scope of this handbook. The interested reader is referred to an excellent summary by A.E. Giuliano (The breast, in *Current*

Obstetric Gynecologic Diagnosis and Treatment, 7th ed. M.L. Pernoll, ed. Appleton & Lange, E. Norwalk, CT, 1991).

PROGNOSIS

The mortality rate for breast cancer patients exceeds that for age-matched controls by nearly 20 years. Thus, 5-year follow-up information is less useful than in other tumors, and 10-year surveillance is necessary.

Survival is most reliably correlated with the stage of breast cancer (Table 17-5). If the disease is localized to the breast, without regional spread (by microscopic analysis), 5-year survival may approach 90%. When breast cancer involves the axillary nodes, the 5-year cure rate is 40%–60%, and the 10-year clinical cure rate is only ~25%.

Other possible beneficial correlations to survival include presence of estrogen and progesterone receptors and older age (breast cancer seems to be more malignant in younger women). The least favorable anatomic site for breast cancer is the median portion of the inner lower quadrant.

Chapter 18

Disorders of the Vulva and Vagina

COMMON VULVOVAGINAL INFECTIONS ASSOCIATED WITH LEUKORRHEA

Leukorrhea is a usually whitish vaginal discharge that may occur at any age and affects virtually all women at some time. Although some vaginal discharge (mucus) is physiologic and nearly always present, when it becomes greater or abnormal (bloody or soils clothing), is irritating, or has an offensive odor, it is considered pathologic. Pathologic discharge is often coupled with vulvar irritation. Commonly, the pathologic conditions are due to infection of the vagina or cervix. Other causes may include uterine tumors, estrogenic or psychic stimulation, trauma, foreign bodies (retained tampon), excessive douching (especially with irritating medications), and vulvovaginal atrophy (hypoestrogenism).

Vulvovaginal disorders constitute the major reason for office gynecology visits. These disorders are heavily influenced by the physiologic alterations summarized in Table 18-1. Estrogen and progesterone influence the nonkeratinized squamous epithelium of the vagina and vulva. Without hormonal influence, the epithelium is thin and atrophic and contains little glycogen, and the vaginal fluid has a high pH. By contrast, with adequate estrogen and progesterone, cellular glycogen content increases and the pH decreases (partially due to breakdown of glycogen to lactic acid). During their reproductive lives, most women harbor three to eight major types of pathogenic bacteria at any given time (Table 18-1).

Physiologic vaginal secretions consist mainly of cervical mucus (a transudate from the vaginal squamous epithelium) and exfoliated squamous cells. Lesser amounts are contributed by the metabolic products of the microflora, exudates from sebaceous sweat glands, Bartholin glands, and Skene glands, and small amounts of endometrial and oviductal fluid. When there is

Table 18-1. Summary of the hormonal influence, vaginal pH, and usual (predominant) vaginal organisms at different times of a female's life

Time of life	Hormonal influence	Vaginal pH	Usual predominant vaginal organisms	
Birth	Estrogens Progesterone	3.7–6.3	Anaerobic and aerobic	
Infant	None	6.0–8.0	Gram-positive cocci and bacilli	
Puberty– Reproductive	Estrogen Progesterone	3.5–4.5	Aerobes (%)	
			Lactobacillus	(70–90)
			Staphylococcus epidermidis	(30–60)
			Diphtheroids	(30–60)
			Alpha-hemolytic *Streptococcus*	(15–50)
			Group D *Streptococcus*	(10–40)
			Nonhemolytic *Streptococcus*	(5–30)
			Escherichia coli	(20–25)
			Beta-hemolytic *Streptococcus*	(10–20)
			Anaerobes (%)	
			Bacteroides fragilis	(5–40)
			Bacteroides species	(1–40)
			Peptococcus	(5–60)
			Peptostreptococcus	(5–40)
			Clostridium	(5–15)
			Veillonella	(10–15)
Menopause	Little or none	6.0–8.0	Gram-positive cocci and bacilli	

little hormonal stimulation (e.g., prior to puberty and postmenopausally), vaginal secretions are scant and the genital tract is less resistant to infection. Physiologic events enhancing the amount of cervical mucus and vaginal discharge occur as a result of sexual or other emotional stimulation, ovulation, pregnancy, and with the excessive estrogen produced by feminizing ovarian tumors.

The normal vaginal flora is most likely to be interrupted during nonphysiologic conditions with the symptomatology noted. The most common organisms causing leukorrhea include *Trichomonas vaginalis* (protozoon), *Candida* (yeast), *Gardnerella* and *Chlamydia* (bacterial). Helminths (e.g., *Oxyuris*) may cause leukorrhea in children. Leukorrhea is unusual in genital gonorrhea or tuberculosis.

Investigation of vaginal discharge involves collection of historical information (what, when, where, why, and to what degree), examination of the vulva, vagina, and cervix, assessment of the discharge (texture, color, odor), and preparation of a saline wet mount (see p 472). In the majority of infections, it is not necessary to perform a culture for confirmation of diagnosis.

TRICHOMONAS VAGINALIS

Trichomonas infection generally is manifest as a diffuse vaginitis with varying vulvar involvement. *T. vaginalis* infections result in marked pruritus with variable edema and erythema. Numerous red points (strawberry patches), which rarely bleed, may be scattered over the vaginal surface and cervical portio. The cervix, urethra, and bladder may be secondarily infected. The leukorrhea is characterized as thin, yellow-green, and occasionally frothy, with a fetid odor. The discharge has a pH of 5–6.5. On saline wet mount, the unicellular flagellate may be observed moving about in a field of many leukocytes. The trichomonads are pear shaped and smaller than epithelial cells but larger than white cells.

T. vaginalis is almost always a sexually transmitted infection. It causes 20%–25% of infectious vaginitis and is responsible for up to 3 million cases a year (USA). The source often can be traced to the male partner, who may harbor the flagellate beneath the prepuce or in the urethra or urethral prostate, yet remain asymptomatic. Moreover, ~25% of females harboring *T. vaginalis* are also asymptomatic, although some may have urinary frequency and dyspareunia. *T. vaginalis* vaginitis is frequently followed by chronic bacterial cervicitis.

The *treatment* for trichomoniasis is oral metronidazole (a single 2 g dose, 1 g q12h × 2, or 250 mg tid for 5–7 days). The side effects of metronidazole include nausea, occasional vomiting, a metallic taste, and intolerance to alcohol. It should not be taken during the first trimester of pregnancy. It is necessary to treat both partners. Men usually are treated with metronidazole 2 g PO or 1 g q12h × 2. In cases of sensitivity to metronidazole, topical clotrimazole is used.

CANDIDA ALBICANS

Candida albicans and related pathogens, *Candida glabrata* and *Candida tropicalis*, are natural fungal inhabitants of the bowel and are also found on the perineal skin. Thus, vaginal contamination from these sources is common. *C. albicans* is also found in the vaginal flora of ~25% of asymptomatic women. Candidal infections occur when vaginal flora abnormalities take place (e.g., a decrease in lactobacilli), and 80%–95% are caused by *C. albicans*. With *Candida* infections, there is generally more vulvar pruritus than with *Trichomonas* infections but less burning. The usual symptomatology includes vaginal discharge, vulvar pruritus, burning, and dyspareunia. *Candida* vaginitis commonly leads to dermatitis of the vulva and thighs. Symptomatology generally begins in the premenstrual phase of the cycle, but ~20% of women with *Candida* are asymptomatic. Unlike bacterial or protozoal vaginitis, *Candida* infections are not considered a sexually transmitted disease and are not commonly associated with mixed infections or sexually transmitted diseases. At particular risk for developing candidiasis are diabetics, oral contraceptive users, those who have recently taken antibiotics, and pregnant women.

Vaginal discharge due to *Candida* infection has a cottage cheese appearance, usually without odor. White, curdlike collections of exudate often are present, and some are lightly attached to the cervical and vaginal mucosa. When these are removed, slight oozing occurs. There may be both erythema and edema of the vulva and vagina. The discharge with *Candida* infection has a pH of 4–5. Mixing the secretions with a drop of 10%–20% KOH microscopically reveals the characteristic mycelia and hyphae, with only a moderate leukocyte response. Should culture be necessary, it may be accomplished using Nickerson's or Sabouraud's medium.

The *treatment* for *C. albicans* infection is topical 2% miconazole nitrate, 1 applicator or vaginal suppository at bedtime for 3–7 days. Alternatively, clotimatzole or butoconazole vaginal suppositories or cream may be used nightly for 7–14 days. If *C. albicans* recurs (a frequent occurrence), the patient should have a glucose screening examination for carbohydrate intolerance. It is also worthwhile to inquire about the possibility of a sexual partner with *Candida* infection about the prepuce. Finally, it is crucial to recognize that *C. glabrata* and *C. tropicalis* are resistant to the imidazoles and may be the cause of recurrent infections. The discharge must be cultured, and treatment is topical gentian violet q3–4d × 2–3. Boric acid (600 mg in gelatin caps) inserted high in the vagina bid and douching qhs with povidone-iodine may be useful therapeutic adjuncts.

GARDNERELLA VAGINALIS

Gardnerella vaginalis is normally found in the respiratory tract. However, it is present in ~30% of normal women's vaginal flora. The organism is a gram-negative bacillus that is ordinarily found in the presence of anaerobic bacteria (e.g., *Bacteroides* and *Peptococcus*). It is likely that sexual transmission occurs because 90% of male partners are infected. *Gardnerella* usually produces a characteristic copious, gray discharge that is malodorous (fishy). In contrast to *Trichomonas* or *Candida* infections, pruritus or burning is usually minimal (<20% of patients), as is vulvar involvement.

The ph of *Gardnerella* discharge is usually 5–5.5. On microscopic examination, *G. vaginalis* appears as a heavy clouding of the saline wet mount, with the epithelial cells being dusted with bacteria (clue cells). The addition of 10% KOH releases amines, producing further enhancement of the fishy odor. Few white blood cells are present in the discharge.

The *treatment* for *G. vaginalis* infection is metronidazole 500 mg bid for 7 days. Alternate therapy is cephradine 500 mg qid for 7 days. Elective treatment of the sexual partner is desirable.

CHLAMYDIA TRACHOMATIS

Chlamydial infections are caused by the obligate intracellular bacterium, *Chlamydia trachomatis*. Other closely related infections are lymphogranuloma venereum, inclusion conjunctivitis, urethritis, cervicitis, salpingitis, proctitis, epididymitis, and pneumonia of the newborn. *C. trachomatis* infection may be the most prevalent sexually transmitted disease in the United States, affecting >3 million persons annually. It is often asymptomatic

(~60%–80% of infected women and ~10% of infected men). The organism is best detected by enzyme-linked amino acids in a fluorescein-conjugate monoclonal antibody test. The infections usually begin as mucopurulent, often odorous or pruritic discharges, and the principal site of infection is the cervix. *Chlamydia* can be eradicated from the vagina and cervix by tetracycline or erythromycin 500 mg PO qid for 7 days.

COMMON VULVOVAGINAL VIRAL INFECTIONS

HERPES SIMPLEX VIRUS (HSV)

HSV infections of the genital tract are a sexually transmitted disease. Type 2 HSV accounts for ~90% of infections, and 10% are type 1. This DNA virus has an incubation period of 3–22 days, and even primary attacks may be asymptomatic, although most patients complain of fever, malaise, anorexia, local genital pain, leukorrhea, dysuria, or even vaginal bleeding. Typical genital lesions are multiple vesicles that progress to shallow ulceration often surrounded by redness or erythematous patches. Painful bilateral inguinal adenopathy is usually present during the primary infection. If the urethra or bladder is affected, dysuria or urinary retention may result. The lesions gradually heal without scarring (7–10 days) unless bacterial superinfection occurs.

The diagnosis is usually made on the typical appearance of vesicles and ulcers. Cytologic smear of the ulcers or vesicles demonstrates classic multinucleated giant cells with acidophilic intranuclear inclusion bodies. Definitive culture may be obtained from the fluid of unruptured vesicles using Hanks medium. However, false negative cultures are frequent. Serologic diagnosis is possible, and use of the gamma globulin or macroglobulin response may determine if the attack is recurrent or primary.

Affected individuals harbor the virus indefinitely. Recurrent lesions may be triggered by emotional distress, exposure to the sun, or a variety of other stimuli. After the primary lesion, the patient frequently develops paresthesias in the affected region before a recurrence (the virus resides in specialized nerve endings during latent intervals). Recurrent lesions account for much of the morbidity but are not as painful as the primary lesions.

Genital herpes during pregnancy is hazardous to the fetus. Serial cultures for the detection of asymptomatic viral shedding have been very disappointing as a diagnostic technique during pregnancy. It is recommended that an infant not be delivered through the birth canal with active lesions. Although cesarean section does not guarantee that the infant will not be infected, it may be undertaken if it is <4 h after rupture of the membranes. Delivery through an infected birth canal with active lesions poses ~50% chance of the neonate developing neonatal herpes. Of those infected ~50% die and ~25% have permanent neurologic sequelae. Additionally, HSV type 2 has been suggested (but not proven) as etiologic in cervical dysplasia.

Currently, *there is no cure for herpes simples viral infections.* Symptomatic measures include hot sitz baths, douching with Burrow's solution, and oral or parenteral acyclovir. Local or oral acyclovir may shorten the course of an initial attack but has little effect on recurrences. General rules for prevention of dissemination include covering small lesions situated away from the oral or vaginal orifices with occlusive dressing during sexual contact, the use of condoms and the application of contraceptive cream or foam. A partner may become infected despite these precautions. If a regular partner has had genital herpes or has not been infected despite prolonged exposure, precautions are probably not necessary.

Human Papillomavirus (HPV)

A member of the Papovavirus group, human papillomavirus causes *condylomata acuminata.* The virus is sexually transmitted, commonly affects both partners, and affects the same age group as other venereal diseases. This DNA virus causes easily discernible, raised, papillomatous lesions of the vulva as well as less discernible lesions of the vagina and cervix. The lesions are much more florid in patients who are diabetic, pregnant, taking oral contraceptives, or immunosuppressed. The most common complaints concern the lesions themselves, but vaginal discharge or pruritus may be present.

The vaginal or cervical lesions are occasionally exophytic or papillomatous (wartlike) but may also be flat, spiked, or inverted. The flat condylomata are white lesions with a somewhat granular surface and a mosaic pattern (some with punctuation) on colposcopy. The papillomatous condylomata is a raised white lesion with fingerlike projections, often containing capillaries. The spiked condyloma is a hyperkeratotic lesion with surface projection and prominent capillary tips. Inverted condylomata grow into cervical glands and, thus, do not occur in the vagina.

Subtypes 6 and 11 are primarily responsible for genital warts. Cytologic smear or biopsy of vaginal or cervical lesions reveals koilocytes, which are superficial or intermediate cells characterized by an enlarged perinuclear cavity that stains only faintly. Biopsy often is necessary to distinguish cervical condylomata from dysplasia.

Treatment in nonpregnant patients generally consists of weekly applications of podophyllin (25% in tincture of benzoin). If after 4–6 weeks this is not successful, cryosurgery, electrocautery, or laser therapy may be necessary. Podophyllin should not be used during pregnancy, and if it is used within 6 weeks of biopsy, the pathologist must be notified because bizarre changes occur that could alter the diagnosis. During pregnancy, cryosurgery is most commonly used for therapy of condylomata. If vaginal or introital lesions are present, consider cesarean section because of the possibility of bleeding from the very friable lesions as well as the possibility of the fetus acquiring laryngeal papillomatosis (infection of the vocal cords by papillomavirus) during the birth process.

MOLLUSCUM CONTAGIOSUM

Molluscum contagiosum is an autoinoculable virus with an incubation period of 1–4 weeks. Asymptomatic pink to gray, discrete, umbilicated epithelial skin tumors <1 cm in diameter develop generally on the vulva. The histologic picture is that of numerous inclusion bodies in the cell cytoplasm. Each lesion must be *treated* by desiccation, freezing or curettage, and chemical cauterization of the base.

OTHER VULVOVAGINAL INFECTIONS

BARTHOLIN DUCT CYST AND ABSCESS

The Bartholin duct is susceptible to infectious occlusion because of its length and narrowness. Infectious organisms (often *Neisseria gonorrhoeae* with secondary streptococci, staphylococci, or *Escherichia coli*) become pocketed within the passage to form an abscess. The inflammation usually resolves, but permanent occlusion of the distal duct causes retention of mucus produced by the gland, and a cyst develops. The process is usually unilateral and occurs in up to 2% of women. The gland is almost never seriously involved with the ductal infection, but in older women acquiring a mass in the Bartholin area, carcinoma (see p 510) must be excluded.

Clinical manifestations include acute pain, tenderness, and dyspareunia. Surrounding tissues (at the junction of the mid and lower thirds of the labia minora) become inflamed and edematous. The introitus may be distorted, and a fluctuant mass usually is palpable. Rarely are systemic symptoms reported or signs of infection noted. Smears and cultures may reveal a specific bacteriologic diagnosis. However, by the time the process is seen, the culture usually will not be reliable.

The *differential diagnosis* includes inclusion cysts, large sebaceous cysts, hidradenoma, congenital anomalies, primary malignancy, and metastatic cancers.

Treatment consist of drainage of the infected cyst or abscess, preferably by marsupialization (Fig. 18-1). This procedure best affords permanent fistula formation. Other procedures (e.g., simple incision and drainage) frequently lead to recurrence. Marsupialization is feasible under local anesthesia, and fine interrupted polyglycolic acid sutures are generally employed. If considerable surrounding inflammation is present, broad-spectrum antibiotics should be given until appropriate antibiotics for organisms in the abscess pus (determined by culture at the time of surgery) can be determined. Bedrest, local dry or moist heat or both, and analgesics should be used as indicated. Prognosis is good with marsupialization. With other treatment, recurrent infection and cystic dilation are likely. Rarely, it is necessary to surgically excise the entire gland. Although in all cases it is desirable to biopsy an area for pathologic section, this becomes crucial in the perimeno-

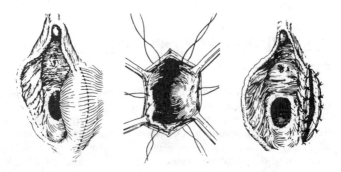

Figure 18-1. Marsupialization of Bartholin cyst.

pausal or postmenopausal woman because of the risk of Bartholin carcinoma.

HIDRADENITIS

Hidradenitis is a refractory infection of the apocrine sweat glands usually caused by staphylococci or streptococci. It is analogous to cystic acne, and symptoms are soreness and local swelling, edema, cellulitis, and suppuration of the groin. Involvement of apocrine glands establishes the diagnosis. *Treatment* consists of hot, wet packs, drainage, and specific antibiotics chosen on the basis of culture and sensitivity testing. Excision may be necessary, but the wound must be allowed to heal by secondary intention.

TOXIC SHOCK SYNDROME (TSS)

Toxic shock syndrome generally occurs in previously healthy women of childbearing age (usually 12–24 years). The incidence is currently ~5/100,000 menstruating women per year. TSS is characterized by abrupt onset of high fever (≥102°F), a diffuse macular erythematous rash (sunburnlike) over the face, trunk, and proximal extremities, and hypotension (systolic <90 mm Hg). Additionally, there is involvement of three or more of the following systems: gastrointestinal (vomiting and watery diarrhea), muscular (tenderness), mucous membranes (nonpurulent conjunctivitis, sore throat), renal (failure), hepatic (failure), hematologic (thrombocytopenia), and central nervous system (nuchal rigidity, headaches, confusion). Renal failure and cardiac failure are manifestations in severe cases and generally occur within <48 h of onset.

Coagulase-positive *Staphylococcus aureus* has been isolated from the vagina of victims, but blood cultures are negative. The cause is most likely an exotoxin (exfoliatin) produced by some strains of staphylococci. TSS begins (95% of cases) within 5 days of the onset of menses in which tampons are used, and superabsorbent tampons appear to be linked to causation. Other potential sources of TSS include delivery, diaphragm usage, surgery, soft-tissue abscess, pyelonephritis, and osteomyelitis.

The *laboratory workup* must include a CBC with differential count, electrolytes, UA, BUN, creatinine, liver function studies, blood culture, throat culture, and vaginal culture. A lumbar puncture should be performed if signs of meningitis are present, and the CSF should be analyzed and cultured. The *differential diagnosis* includes Kawasaki disease (in children), scarlet fever, Rocky Mountain spotted fever, leptospirosis, gram-negative sepsis, and measles.

Treatment includes removal of a tampon if present (as well as culture for penicillinase-producing *S. aureus*), admission to a critical care unit for intensive (often invasive) monitoring, correction of fluid and electrolyte deficiencies (sizable deficits occur from third spacing), corticosteroid therapy (methylprednisolone 30 mg/kg or dexamethasone 3 mg/kg as a bolus, repeated q4h prn), antistaphylococcal antibiotics (beta-lactamase-resistant antibiotics, e.g., nafcillin, oxycillin, or methicillin 1 g IV q4h or vancomycin 500 mg IV q6h if penicillin allergy exists), and management of renal and cardiac insufficiency. It may be necessary to give blood and blood products (packed RBCs, fresh frozen plasma, platelets). Corticosteroids shorten the fever duration and reduce the severity of illness. Dopamine infusion may be necessary (2–5 μg/kg/min) if fluids do not correct hypotension. Naloxone may be used in persistent hypotension for its antiendorphin activity. Since gram-negative sepsis is in the differential diagnosis, an aminoglycoside should be given until gram-negative sepsis is ruled out. For both vancomycin and the aminoglycoside, drug levels must be carefully monitored.

Complications include adult respiratory distress syndrome (ARDS), intractable hypotension, and hemorrhage from disseminated intravascular coagulation, any of which can be fatal. Mortality from TSS is 3%–6%. Desquamation, especially of palms and soles occurs 1–2 weeks after onset of TSS. There is a 30% recurrence rate, especially in the first 3 months after the attack. The recurrences are reduced to ~5% by administration of antistaphylococcal antibiotics in the initial episode. If a woman recovers from TSS, she should forego the use of tampons until cervicovaginal and nasal cultures for *S. aureus* are negative twice at 4 week intervals and then avoid tampon use at night.

FURUNCULOSIS

Furuncular abscesses caused by staphylococcal infections are termed furunculosis or *boils*. Symptoms usually include throbbing pain and regional tenderness. Pustular areas require incision and drainage, with culture of the pus. *Treatment* includes segregation, topical moist heat periodically, and systemic antibiotics (e.g., cephalosporin).

TUBERCULOSIS

Vulvovaginal tuberculosis, rare even in developing countries, is manifest by chronic, minimally painful, exudative sores that are reddish, raised, moderately firm and nodular, with central apple jellylike contents. Later, ulcerative, undermined, necrotic, discharging lesions develop. There is some tendency toward healing with heavy scarring, but induration and sinus formation are common in the scrofulous type of infection. The *differential diagnosis* includes cancer and sexually transmitted diseases. Demonstration of *Mycobacterium tuberculosis* is necessary for diagnosis. *Treatment* consists of antituberculosis chemotherapy.

VULVAR INFESTATIONS

PEDICULOSIS PUBIS

Pthirus pubis (crab louse) is transmitted by sexual contact or from bedding or clothing. The eggs are laid at the base of the pubic, axillary, or scalp hair. When the eggs hatch, the lice attach to the skin and cause intense itching. Close observation reveals minute, pale brown insects and their ova attached to hair shafts near the skin. The *treatment* consist of 1% gamma benzene hexachloride cream/lotion or shampoo (not recommended for pregnant or lactating women) or pyritherans applied to the infestation and adjacent hair areas. Retreatment may be required in 1 week. It is necessary to treat all contacts and sterilize infected bedding and clothing.

SCABIES

Sarcoptes scabei causes intractable itching and excoriation of the surface in the vicinity of minute skin burrows where the parasites have deposited ova. The mite is transmitted directly from person to person. Treatment is 1% gamma benzene hexachloride cream/lotion from the neck down overnight, washing off thoroughly after 8 h, or 10% crotamiton cream or lotion applied from the neck down twice nightly and washed off thoroughly after the second application. With this infestation, contacts must be treated, and all infected clothing and bedding must be sterilized.

ENTEROBIASIS (PINWORMS)

Enterobius vermicularis is a short, spindle-shaped roundworm that commonly infects children. The usual symptomatology is nocturnal perianal itching, which leads to excoriation. The usual diagnostic technique is a short strip of cellophane pressure-sensitive tape applied to the perianal region and then spread on a slide. This reveals the adult worms or ova in >90% of cases. *Therapy* is a single oral dose of mebendazole 100 mg.

BENIGN VULVAR LESIONS

ECZEMA

Eczema is a nonspecific, common, pruritic, moist dermatitis characterized by excoriation and crusting with later lichenification. Eczema is often a contact dermatitis caused by irritants in soap, bath oils, or deodorant medications, dyes in clothing, or allergy to wool or silk. Sensitivity tests and the exclusion of other dermatitis aid in diagnosis. General *treatment* depends on elimination of the irritant. Therapy is Burrow's solution followed by steroid creams (e.g., 0.5% hydrocortisone bid).

PSORIASIS

Pruritic, reddened, slightly elevated lesions (without the typical silvery scale seen on elbows and knees) are seen in body folds. The elbows and knees are frequently affected by the scaly lesions, however. Psoriasis is a chronic, often familial, disorder of unknown etiology. Exacerbations often occur in winter, and *treatment* includes improving hygiene and 0.5% hydrocortisone cream applied bid. More extensive lesions require dermatologic consultation.

BENIGN NEOPLASIA

A number of benign tumors may involve the vulvovaginal area. These are generally characterized as either cystic or solid. The cysts include epidermal cysts, sebaceous cysts, and apocrine sweat gland cysts. A cyst of epidermal origin may arise from trauma or occlusion of pilosebaceous ducts. These tend to be small, solitary, lined with squamous epithelium, and filled with sebaceous material as well as desquamated epithelial cells. Most are asymptomatic.

Cysts of the sebaceous or sweat glands are frequently multiple and almost always involve the labia majora. They are asymptomatic unless infection develops. Apocrine sweat glands become functional after puberty. Then, occlusion of the ducts results in an extremely pruritic, microcytic disorder, Fox-Fordyce disease. Should the apocrine glands become infected by streptococci or staphylococci, the process termed hidradenitis supprativa occurs.

Less common cysts or pseudocysts include Skene duct cysts, urethral diverticula, inguinal hernia, occlusion of a persistently patent vaginalis (canal of Nuck), dilation of mullerian duct vestiges, and supernumerary mammary tissue.

The most worrisome benign vulvar solid tumors are pigmented nevi. Because nearly all vulvar nevi are of the junctional type, they may give rise to malignant melanomas. Thus, vulvar pigmented nevi should be viewed more cautiously than elsewhere on the body. All small pigmented lesions of the vulva are suspect and should be removed with a 0.5–1 cm margin. Other benign solid tumors usually are incidental findings and, like the cystic tumors, usually are provisionally diagnosed by clinical examination. If therapy is required, excisional biopsy is usually sufficient.

An acrochordon (or skin tag) is a small, flesh-colored, polypoid tumor composed of fibrous epithelial elements and is never malignant. Mesodermal vulvar tumors are infrequent, although leiomyomas arise from the round ligament and fibromas and lipomas also occur. Neurofibromas are usually small lesions that arise from the neural sheath and are of little consequence unless associated with general neurofibromatosis (von Recklinghausen disease).

VULVAR DYSTROPHIES

Disorders of vulvar epithelial growth and nutrition produce numerous nonspecific gross changes collectively termed vulvar dystrophies. These abnormalities are divided into hypertrophic, atrophic, and mixed types. Generally, the lesions are circumscribed or diffuse white lesions of the vulva and do not have a uniform microscopic appearance throughout. Therefore, multiple biopsies are necessary. The toluidine blue test and colposcopy may assist in detailing areas most suitable for biopsy. The malignant potential of vulvar dystrophies is <5%. Table 18-2 is the International Society for the Study of Vulvar Disease classification of vulvar dystrophies.

Treatment of atrophic dystrophies is topical 2% testosterone proprionate in petrolatum bid for 1 week, then daily, gradually decreasing to one to two applications per week. Androgenic side effects may occur—thus the amount used should be minimal. Control of itching is accomplished by removal of any source of irritation (e.g., nylon panties, use of strong soaps), intermittent Burrow's solution wet dressings (bid or tid), and topical fluorinated corticosteroid (e.g., 0.025%–0.1% triamcinolone acetonide) bid for 1–2 weeks. Because these latter compounds may cause vulvar atrophy and contracture, the dose must be decreased as symptoms subside. Surgical repair is indicated in cases of lichen sclerosis with severe constriction of the vulva at the posterior fourchette.

Hypertrophic Dystrophies

Chronic vaginal infection or other chronic irritation may cause benign epithelial thickening and hyperkeratosis. In the acute

Table 18-2. Classification of vulvar dystrophies adopted by the International Society for the Study of Vulvar Disease

	Clinical features	Histologic features
Lichen sclerosis	Pruritic, thin, parchment-like atrophic area; introital stenosis	Thin, loss of rete homogenization; inflammatory infiltrate
Hyperplastic*	Pruritic, thick, gray or white plaques on skin or mucosa	Acanthosis, hyperkeratosis, inflammatory infiltrate
Mixed*	Areas compatible with both forms may be present at the same time	(See above)

*Atypia may accompany hyperplastic dystrophy and is graded as mild, moderate, or severe.

phase, this lesion may be red and moist, often with evidence of secondary infection. Following subsequent epithelial thickening and maceration, a raised white lesion (lichen simplex chronicus or neurodermatitis) often develops, which may involve any of the external genital area. Diagnosis is afforded by multiple biopsy assessment. Characteristically, hyperkeratosis and acanthosis with thickening of the epithelium and elongation of the rete pegs occur. If advancement to atypical hyperplasia or carcinoma in situ occurs, expect pleomorphism and loss of epithelial cellular polarity. The patient must be reexamined periodically to rule out advancement to frank cancer. Surgical excision of more advanced lesions is indicated.

ATROPHIC DYSTROPHIES

Lichen sclerosis et atrophicus (LSA) is a cutaneous degenerative disorder of unknown cause. The vulva is most frequently affected, but the skin of the back, axillas, beneath the breast, neck, and arms also may be affected. The topical disease can occur in most age groups but is most common in white women >65 years. In the perineal area, LSA classically involves the vulvar, perineal, and perianal areas in an hourglass pattern. The skin is white, thin, and wrinkled, and there may be surface atrophy of the labia minora and majora. The chief symptom is pruritus.

Microscopically, LSA is distinguished by hyperkeratosis, epithelial atrophy, and flattening of the rete pegs. Beneath the epidermis is a homogeneous, collagenous, acellular, pink-staining zone. Below this lies a concentration of plasma cells. Cellular pleomorphism and loss of epithelial cell polarity are typical. Although the lesion appears atrophic, the rate of cellular turnover is higher than in normal skin or many hypertrophic lesions. Thus, there is an enhanced rate of malignancy.

Treatment of hypertrophic and atrophic lesions involves eliminating infection and the cautious use of estrogenic creams or topical corticosteroids and testosterone (e.g., 1% hydrocortisone and 2%–3% testosterone tid to qid). Treat carcinoma in situ or invasive cancer in a dystrophic area definitively. Lesser vulvar intraepithelial neoplasias (VIN I or mild dysplasia, VIN II or moderate dysplasia) should be treated conservatively to relieve symptoms. However, arrange close follow-up for signs of progression.

VULVAR CARCINOMA IN SITU

SQUAMOUS CELL CARCINOMA

A vulvar carcinoma in situ (CIS) is diagnosed when the full epithelial thickness is replaced by hyperchromatic cells with poorly defined cellular boundaries. Increased cellular density, abnormal mitoses, multinucleated cells, and increased nuclear/ cytoplasmic ratios may also be noted. Chronic infections, granulomatous disease, and the vulvar dystrophies have long been associated with enhanced susceptibility to vulvar CIS. There is increasing evidence that papillomavirus infections may play a major role in the etiology of VIN. VIN is most often found in women >40 years of age. However, with evidence of papillomavirus, the median age falls to ~31 years. The progression rate from VIN to carcinoma appears to be low.

CIS of the vulva is likely to be located posterior to the vaginal orifice in the vulvar and perineal areas. VIN III (severe dysplasia and CIS), like the vulvar dystrophies and VIN I and II, is most frequently multifocal, and contiguous areas may be affected. For example, with vulvar CIS the following may be affected: anus (22%), clitoral glans (18%), vagina (10%), and urethral meatus (2%).

The symptoms of vulvar CIS usually are nonspecific, e.g., mild irritation or itching. The gross appearance of the vulva with CIS is variable (white patches, reddish nodules, dystrophic areas, pigmented nevi). Biopsy is mandatory to establish the diagnosis. Because the lesions are usually discrete and multifocal, the toluidine blue test or colposcopy or both are helpful to identify the correct area(s) for sampling. Colposcopic examination will not reveal the characteristic tissue and vascular patterns often found on the cervix (see p 732), but it is useful in identifying white or pigmented lesions for biopsy.

The toluidine blue test, which stains nuclei in the superficial epithelium, is not diagnostic of CIS, but the dye is a useful adjunct. Aqueous 1% toluidine blue is applied to the vulva, and after drying for >1 min, the excess is gently removed with a cotton swab moistened with 1% acetic acid. The areas retaining a blue color are the ones to be biopsied. Although exfoliative cytology may be useful in ulcerated lesions, it is of much less value for vulvar than for cervical lesions because the thick keratinized skin does not shed cells readily.

Biopsy is easily accomplished using a 4–5 mm Keyes dermal punch after local anesthesia has been administered. The dermal thickness is penetrated, the specimen is elevated, and the underlying stroma is incised. Bleeding may be controlled using pressure or Monsell's solution (ferrous subsulfate) or silver nitrate.

Therapy for CIS requires the removal of all vulvar VIN together with any condylomata acuminata. Currently, the therapeutic modalities include laser vaporization, topical 5-fluorouracil (5-FU), and surgery. Carbon dioxide laser treatment allows healing in 2–3 weeks without scarring. Ablation is usually to a depth of 3–4 mm under local or general anesthesia. More than one therapy session may be necessary for very extensive lesions. The use of 5-FU will successfully eliminate CIS in ~75% of patients, but it causes vulvar edema, and severe pain may be reported for ~6 weeks. Wide local excision has all but been replaced by laser therapy. Should surgical therapy be necessary, wide local excision, a skinning vulvectomy, i.e., removal of the superficial vulvar skin and replacement with a split-thickness graft while preserving the clitoris, and simple vulvectomy are options. Prognosis for patients with CIS is good with all modes of therapy.

PAGET'S DISEASE

This rare vulvar intraepithelial lesion, which most often affects postmenopausal Caucasian women, is associated with other vulvar disorders (31%) or more distant carcinoma or CIS. The latter group approaches 30% of cases and includes the breast, cervix, rectum, urethra, and skin. Therefore, identification of vulvar Paget's disease mandates a thorough search for other cancers.

Vulvar Paget's disease may be confused with other chronic pruritic vulvar lesions. Paget's disease is typically a velvety, red skin discoloration that comes to resemble eczema with secondary maceration and the development of white plaques. It is slowly growing but may spread to the perineum, perianal area, or thighs. The primary symptom is pruritus. Biopsy is mandatory, and Paget cells on microscopy are pathognomonic (it is equivalent to Paget's disease of the breast).

Extramammary Paget's disease is an in situ lesion that warrants simple vulvectomy with careful pathologic examination, including the surgical margins. Local recurrence is a major problem, and repeated local surgical excisions may be necessary. However, progression to adenocarcinoma is rare. Women with vulvar Paget's disease posttherapy should have an annual breast evaluation (Chapter 17), vulvar evaluation, cervical cytologic study, and screening for malignant gastrointestinal disease.

CANCER OF THE VULVA

Cancer of the vulva occurs primarily in postmenopausal women. There is usually a long history of vulvar irritation, with itching, local discomfort, and possibly bloody discharge. Whereas early lesions may appear as chronic vulvar dermatitis, the late lesions appear as nodules, exophytic lesions, or hard ulcerated areas. *Diagnosis* requires biopsy.

Vulvar tumors are 85%–90% epidermoid in origin. Nonetheless, cancer of the vulva may arise also from the urethra, glandular elements of the vulva, or mucosa of the lower third of the vagina. Vulvar cancers are intraepithelial or invasive. Vulvar cancer is the fourth most common female genital cancer (after endometrial, cervical, and ovarian cancer) and accounts for ~5% of gynecologic malignancies. The patient with vulvar malignancy is predisposed also to other malignancies; 22% will have another primary tumor (most commonly of the cervix). The average age of patients with vulvar cancer is 65, and >50% of afflicted women are >50 years.

The cause of vulvar cancer is unknown, although HSV type 2 and HPV are possible etiologic agents. Preexisting genital condylomata are the sites of ~5% of vulvar cancers. Although most patients with vulvar cancer give no history of predisposing conditions, many other local disorders may be present, e.g., hypertrophic and atrophic vulvar dystrophies, chronic granulomatous disorders (especially lymphogranuloma venereum, syphilis, and granuloma inguinale), chronic irritation, extramammary Paget's disease, pigmented moles, irradiation, and intraepithelial carcinoma. Associated etiologic factors include poor hygiene and lack of proper medical care. The mean age of patients with vulvar CIS is ~10 years less than patients with invasive cancer.

Cancers of the vulva are diagnosed most often (in order of frequency) in the labia majora, the prepuce of the clitoris, the labia minora, Bartholin gland, and the vaginal vestibule. Vulvar cancer usually begins as a surface growth, with ulceration and extension downward and laterally. Slow growth is typical, and although metastases are unpredictable, the malignant cells may remain in the regional lymph nodes for some time before further dissemination. Eventual metastases occur via lymphatic channels of the vulva to the superficial and deep inguinal or femoral nodes and the external iliac and obturator nodes. Since the lymphatics of the vulva cross, tumor cells may spread from one side to the other.

TYPES OF VULVAR CANCER

Epidermoid Vulvar Cancer

Epidermoid cancer most frequently involves the anterior half of the vulva and arises in the labia (major and minor) in 65% of patients and in the clitoris in 25%. Over one third of tumors are midline or bilateral. There is no positive correlation as to frequency of metastases between the gross appearance, exophytic (cauliflower-like), ulcerative lesions, or red velvety tumors. The primary determinant of metastases and subsequent outcome is tumor size. However, histologic grading is pertinent to potential metastasis if the tumor is <2 cm.

Typical grade I epidermoid carcinomas of the vulva are composed of well-differentiated spicule or prickle cells, many forming keratin pearls. Occasional mitoses are seen. Malignant cells invade the subepithelial tissues, and leukocytes and lymphocytes infiltrate the stroma and tissues adjacent to the tumor. Grades II and III epidermoid cancers are composed of increasingly poorly differentiated cells. Verrucous carcinoma, a variant of epidermoid cancer, grossly resembles condylomata acuminata. Local spread is common, but lymphatic metastasis in elderly patients is uncommon.

Malignant Melanoma

Malignant melanoma, comprising 6%–11% of all vulvar carcinomas, is the second most common type of vulvar cancer. Melanomas, extremely aggressive malignancies, usually arise from pigmented nevi of the vulva. Melanomas predominantly affect postmenopausal white women. Malignant melanomas most frequently involve the labia minora or the clitoris. Generally, malignant melanomas are single, hyperpigmented, raised, nontender, ulcerated lesions that bleed easily. All malignant melanomas spread early by the venous system. Also, local recurrences are frequent. *Treatment* is similar to that for squamous cell carcinomas.

Basal Cell Carcinoma

Basal cell carcinomas are ulcerative lesions composed of small, rounded, basophilic malignant cells derived from the innermost layer of the epidermis. The cells are arranged in irregular groups and often penetrate the underlying connective tissue. Occasional mitoses are observed, but there is no keratinization. Unlike keratinizing squamous cell carcinoma, basal cell carcinomas metastasize infrequently and late. However, local recurrence is common. Basal cell carcinomas account for 2%–3% of vulvar cancers, and they almost always arise in the skin of the labia majora. The usual *treatment,* is wide local excision because the tumor does not metastasize readily. However, ~20% recur. One exception to therapy is the basal–squamous cell type tumor, which requires treatment similar to that for invasive squamous cell carcinoma.

Bartholin Gland Carcinoma

Although the cure rates are the same, stage by stage, for Bartholin gland carcinoma and squamous cell carcinoma, two factors make Bartholin gland carcinomas more dangerous. Generally, the diagnosis of cancer of the Bartholin gland is delayed because it is slightly less accessible than cervical cancer and may be interpreted as a Bartholin cyst. Additionally, because the tumors have access to the lymphatic channels draining the rectum, they may metastasize directly to the deep pelvic lymph nodes. Nonetheless, *therapy* for Bartholin gland carcinoma is similar to that for squamous cell carcinoma.

Vulvar Sarcomas

Sarcomas of the vulva represent <2% of vulvar cancers. The most common of these stromal cell cancers are leiomyosarcoma and fibrous histiocytoma. Adenocarcinomas of the vulva (except those of Bartholin origin) are extremely rare. Metastatic cancers to the vulva may come from other genital tract tumors or from the kidney or urethra.

CLINICAL FINDINGS

Pruritus is the most common symptom of ulcerated vulvar cancer. A *lump* may be present for months or years before the patient consults a physician. A *sore* (ulceration), *odorous discharge,* and *bleeding* usually occur later, but in postgranulomatous cases, these signs often occur early. *Lymphadenopathy* is always suggestive of metastasis. *Pain,* a late symptom, depends on the tumor's size and location as well as the presence or absence of infection. On physical examination, *nodular, ulcerative lesions,* especially those occurring in postmenopausal women and those containing granulomatous or leukoplakia changes, are particularly suggestive of vulvar cancer.

Staging

Staging is summarized in Table 18-3.

Diagnostic Procedures

In the workup of vulvar carcinoma, obtain CBC (with differential and HCT), BUN, AST, lactic dehydrogenase, and electrolytes. It is useful also to have a UA, chest x-ray, and IVP. An ECG should help identify patients at risk from anesthesia or operative procedures. A repeat biopsy should be obtained if the first is inadequate. Toluidine blue dye may be used to determine better sites for biopsy. Colposcopy may demonstrate the need for multiple biopsies and detail suspicious areas. Lymphangiography is indicated for cancer in stages II–IV (Table 18-3). Cystoscopy, colposcopy, proctoscopy, or barium enema is required if the symptoms suggest involvement of pelvic organs by the tumor or injury to pelvic organs during therapy. A liver scan is required for malignant melanoma.

TREATMENT

The primary treatment of vulvar cancer (except in those previously noted instances requiring local excision) is radical vulvectomy and regional lymphadenectomy. The operative extent may be modified according to the medical condition of the patient or by the site or extent of the cancer.

Lymphadenectomy may involve unilateral or bilateral deep or superficial inguinal lymph node areas. Cloquet's node is the highest deep inguinal lymph node beneath the inguinal ligament, and it must be submitted for a frozen section examination. If

Table 18-3. Staging of carcinoma of the vulva*

Cases should be classified as carcinoma of the vulva when the primary site of the growth is in the vulva. Tumors present in the vulva as secondary growths from either a genital or extragenital site should be excluded from registration, as should cases of malignant melanoma.

FIGO Nomenclature

Stage 0	Carcinoma in situ.
Stage I	Tumor confined to vulva—2 cm or less in diameter. Nodes are not palpable or are palpable in either groin, not enlarged, mobile (not clinically suspicious of cancer).
Stage II	Tumor confined to the vulva—more than 2 cm in diameter. Nodes are not palpable or are palpable in either groin, not enlarged, mobile (not clinically suspicious of cancer).
Stage III	Tumor of any size with (1) adjacent spread to the urethra and any or all of the vagina, the perineum, and the anus, and/or (2) nodes palpable in either or both groins (enlarged, firm, and mobile, not fixed but clinically suspicious of cancer).
Stage IV	Tumor of any size (1) infiltrating the bladder mucosa or the rectal mucosa or both, including the upper part of the urethral mucosa, and/or (2) fixed to the bone or other distant metastases. Fixed or ulcerated nodes in either or both groins.

TNM Nomenclature

1.1	Primary tumor (T)	
	TIS, T1, T2, T3, T4	
		See corresponding FIGO stages.
1.2	Nodal involvement (N)	
	NX	Not possible to assess the regional nodes.
	N0	No involvement of regional nodes.
	N1	Evidence of regional node involvement.
	N3	Fixed or ulcerated nodes.
	N4	Juxtaregional node involvement.
1.3	Distant metastasis (M)	
	MX	Not assessed.
	M0	No (known) distant metastasis.
	M1	Distant metastasis present.
		Specify_____

*American Joint Committee for Cancer Staging and End-Results Reporting; Task Force on Gynecologic Sites: Staging System for Cancer at Gynecologic Sites, 1979.

metastatic disease is present, an ipsilateral extraperitoneal deep pelvic lymphadenectomy should be performed eliminating the common iliac, external iliac, hypogastric, presacral, and obturator lymph nodes. Contralateral lymph node dissections are usually done if the ipsilateral lymph nodes are positive.

Anemia and metabolic and cardiovascular diseases should be treated intensively before surgery. Preoperatively, broad-spectrum antibiotic therapy for several days may be beneficial if local infection is present. Additionally, minidose heparin prophylaxis (5000 U SC bid or tid) started preoperatively and continued postoperatively is useful to prevent deep venous thrombophlebitis.

Topical fluorouracil (2%–5% bid) has been used for treatment of vulvar CIS. Radiotherapy is not a primary treatment but may be of great value in the treatment of a cancer recurrence, particularly basal cell carcinoma. Radiation also is useful in instances of known incomplete surgery or for palliation of inoperable cancer. Paget's disease and malignant melanoma do not respond well to radiation.

Routine follow-up involves examination every 3 months for 2 years and every 6 months thereafter. Five-year survival is ~60% after surgical treatment of invasive squamous cell carcinoma. With tumors <2 cm diameter, the incidence of nodal metastasis is 10%–15%, and when nodal metastasis occurs, the 5-year survival rate is 15%–30%. Operative mortality rate is ~5%, and death may be due to cardiovascular complications, primary or secondary hemorrhage, infection, or venous thrombosis.

CANCER OF THE VAGINA

Cancer of the vagina is usually asymptomatic and is most often revealed by abnormal vaginal cytology. Early in its course, there may be painless bleeding from an ulcerated tumor. In late cases, expect pain, bleeding, weight loss, or local swelling. Squamous cell carcinoma represents ~85% of primary vaginal cancers. The rest (in decreasing frequency) includes adenocarcinomas, sarcomas, and melanomas. Primary cancer of the vagina represents ~1%–2% of gynecologic malignancies and usually develops about 10 years after the menopause.

Two special vaginal carcinomas are noteworthy: clear cell carcinoma and sarcoma botryoides. Clear cell carcinoma of the cervix or vagina occurs in females age 10–30 years whose mother received diethylstilbestrol during early pregnancy. The tumor is

Table 18-4. Staging of carcinoma of the vagina*

Preinvasive carcinoma

Stage 0   Carcinoma in situ, intraepithelial carcinoma.

Invasive carcinoma

Stage I	Carcinoma limited to the vaginal wall.
Stage II	Carcinoma has involved the subvaginal tissue but has not extended to the pelvic wall.
Stage III	Carcinoma has extended to the pelvic wall.
Stage IV	Carcinoma has extended beyond the true pelvis or involved the mucosa of the bladder or rectum. Bullous edema as such does not permit allotment of a case to stage IV.
Stage IVA	Spread of carcinoma to adjacent organs.
Stage IVB	Spread to distant organs.

*American Joint Committee for Cancer Staging and End-Results Reporting; Task Force on Gynecologic Sites: Staging System for Cancer at Gynecologic Sites, 1979.

multicentric but is most commonly found in the upper third of the vagina. Sarcoma botryoides occurs most frequently in young children. In all cases, however, loose connective tissue and rich vascular lymphatic circulation favor rapid growth and early cancer dissemination. Tumors of the lower vagina metastasize in the same manner as vulvar cancer, whereas those in the upper vagina spread like cervical cancer.

Painless bleeding is the initial manifestation in ~50% of cases of carcinoma of the vagina. Primary vaginal carcinoma must be distinguished from extensions of the vulvar or cervical cancer and cancer metastasis from the urinary tract, gastrointestinal tract, or ovary. Staging is summarized in Table 18-4.

The preferred *treatment* is radiation. Radical surgery (exenteration) should be reserved for vaginal cancers near the introitus, for sarcomas, and for definitely localized cancers involving the urethra or bladder. Prognosis depends on the type, location, extent of the tumor, and treatment response. With adequate treatment, the 5-year survival in stage I and II of carcinoma is 70%–75%. Few malignant melanomas respond to treatment. Adequate survival data are not available for sarcoma of the vagina, but the prognosis for most patients is poor.

Chapter 19

The Cervix

ANOMALIES OF THE FEMALE GENITAL TRACT

Malformations of the female genital tract affect nearly 10% of girls and women. Known genetic problems cause ~20%, about 5% are due to chromosome aberrations, and approximately 10% are due to environmental causes. Multifactorial inheritance (e.g., a combination of environment and genetics) probably accounts for the rest.

Anomalies of the vulva and labia are rare. They include bifid clitoris (occurs with bladder exstrophy), congenital vaginal prolapse, and vulvar duplication (seen with duplication of the urinary and intestinal tracts). Occasionally, one labia is much larger than the other. If therapy is required, surgical excision is easily accomplished.

Anomalies of the hymen occur frequently, as it is the most variable structure of the genitalia. The variations include imperforate hymen, variation of orifice diameter, more than one orifice, thickening of the membrane, or a median ridge between two orifices. The imperforate hymen requires opening or early complications of mucocolpos or hematocolpos will occur. Later complications may include endometriosis and adenomyosis.

Vaginal anomalies include transverse and longitudinal vaginal septa. Transverse vaginal septa are discussed on p. 15–16. Longitudinal vaginal septa are commonly associated with cervical or uterine anomalies or both. A double vagina is found in association with duplication of the cervix. When asymptomatic, these defects require no therapy. One of the more common associations of total vaginal agenesis is the Rokitansky sequence (p. 616).

Uterine anomalies usually occur as a result of failure of mullerian fusion. The potential defects include subseptate uterus, arcuate uterus, bicornuate uterus, unicornuate uterus, rudimentary uterine horn, uterus didelphys, duplex cervix, cervical atresia, and septate vagina. The most serious complications of these defects are problems of reproduction. Various surgical corrections are feasible but are beyond the scope of this text.

Fallopian tube anomalies are rare. They include aplasia, atresia, and duplication (particularly distal).

The most common *ovarian anomalies* include anomalous ovarian descent, in which the ovary may be in the inguinal canal or the labia majora. Complete ovarian agenesis occurs if the primordial gonads do not form. Agonadism is the formation of the ovaries, followed by degeneration. These and other ovarian anomalies, including gonadal dysgenesis, are discussed in Chapter 21. In Turner's syndrome (45,XO), the patients have height and weight <3rd percentile, broad chest and small nipples, webbed neck, aortic coarctation, prominent epicanthal folds, nevi, and short fourth metacarpals. Karyotyping should be performed in all dysgenetic patients. The presence of a Y chromosome increases the incidence of neoplasia in the genital ridge.

Clinically, most genital tract anomalies confront the physician at the time of birth or at the menarche (Chapter 1). At birth, ambiguous genitalia or other problems of sexual identification must be resolved (Chapter 1) to obviate sexual misassignment. This is usually accomplished by careful physical examination, pelvic ultrasound, hormonal assessment, and karyotype. Some problems of sex identification may be described as female or male pseudohermaphroditism or true hermaphroditism. Female pseudohermaphroditism is masculinization of a female fetus in utero. The most common abnormality is clitoral enlargement, although varying labial fusion, hypospadiac urethral meatus, and a malpositioned vaginal orifice may be present also. Female pseudohermaphroditism may be fetal in origin (congenital adrenal hyperplasia) or maternal (exogenous androgens, exogenous androgenic progestins, or secondary to functional ovarian tumors or tumors of the adrenal gland).

Male pseudohermaphroditism is seen most often in the androgen insensitivity syndrome (testicular feminization syndrome) in which the karyotype is 46,XY but the individual appears female. This is an X-linked genetic disorder. Another possible cause (albeit rare) is genetic mosaicism.

True hermaphroditism (rare) occurs when there is dual gonadal development. Some of these individuals are genetic mosaics, but most are 46,XX. The degree of masculinization depends on the amount of testicular tissue present.

Intrauterine exposure to diethylstilbestrol (DES) or analogs is associated later with clear cell carcinoma of the vagina or cervix. Other vaginal abnormalities include vaginal adenosis, incomplete septa, fibrous bands, and segmental vaginal narrowing. Intrauterine exposure to DES also causes uterine deformity (T-shaped uterus with hysterography), and cervical abnormalities, including incompetent cervix, complete or incomplete circular sulcus, recessed areas surrounding the external os, portio vaginalis completely covered by columnar epithelium, pseudopolyp formation due to localized, eccentric hypertrophy of endocervical tissue, and rough or smooth anterior cervical lip protuberances. The end result of these defects (cancer not included) is a higher than expected reproductive wastage.

CERVICAL EVERSION

The squamous epithelial covering of the cervix normally extends to or just within the external os. Thus, when the *endocervical columnar epithelium replaces the squamous epithelium on the external cervix,* it is termed an eversion. This is a physiologic process that occurs when hormonal factors cause endocervical hypertrophy and hyperplasia. The resultant increased tissue has only the opportunity for expansion to the exterior. Although the process may enhance the amount of vaginal discharge, the columnar epithelium is not as resistant to trauma or infection as is squamous epithelium. Hence, this process contributes to cervicitis. Cervical eversion does not require topical therapy, only observation to differentiate it from an *erosion* or ulceration (localized loss of the cervical mucosa).

When the abnormal hormonal stimulus is not present, the condition reverts to or toward normal. However, another process of resolution is that of *squamous metaplasia* of the columnar epithelium. As this superficial epidermidization occurs, deeply infolded columnar epithelia may remain unchanged. The gland openings are often narrowed to form mucous collections, termed *Nabothian cysts.* Their appearance is usually sufficient to differentiate them from the other cystic cervical lesions (e.g., mesonephric cysts or endometriosis). *Mesonephric cysts* are remnants of the wolffian duct and are present deep in the stroma external to the external os. They may reach 2.5 cm in diameter and contain a ragged cuboidal epithelium. They usually require no therapy. *Endometriosis* is manifest on the cervix as small (generally <2 mm) reddish to purple to nearly black cysts on the ectocervix. Patients with cervical endometriosis are more likely to have internal endometriosis also. Biopsy of the lesion should reveal the endometrial glands, stroma, and perhaps old blood. Therapy is cauterization or excision.

CERVICITIS

Nonspecific chronic cervicitis probably affects at least *50% of all women* at some point in life. Eversion (with trauma and infection) and puerperal lacerations are probably the two major *etiologic factors,* although, poor hygiene, diminished resistance to infection, and irritation (e.g., retained tampon) also may be causative. The three most common organisms cultured are staphylococci, streptococci, and chlamydia. However, many other vaginal organisms may cause the problem. Rarely, very unexpected organisms (e.g., *Corynebacterium diphtheriae*) cause cervicitis. The usual *symptomatology* is leukorrhea (purulent discharge, often with a disagreeable odor) or vulvar–vaginal irritation (itching or burning). However, backache, lower abdominal pain, dyspareunia, dysmenorrhea, dysuria, and postcoital spotting may also occur. The *clinical signs* depend on the stage of the infection. When acute (hours to 2 days), the cervix is reddened, and the discharge indicates acute inflammation. During this stage, the cervix is tender when moved. After the acute stage, the signs of chronic cervicitis are those of chronic infection: a pus-laden cervical mucus, friable and vascular surface tissue, gland infection, and cervical hypertrophy.

The *cervical cytology* may be obscured by infection, and it is often necessary to resolve the infection before a meaningful cervical cytologic study can be obtained. The usual workup includes investigation for the common causes of vaginitis and cervicitis (*Trichomonas vaginalis, Candida albicans,* and *Gardnerella vaginalis*), monoclonal immunofluorescent stains for *Chlamydia,* and culture for *Neisseria gonorrhoeae.* Both herpes simplex and human papillomavirus may infect the cervix.

The *differential diagnosis* of cervicitis includes an early neoplastic process, chancre, chancroid, tuberculosis, and granuloma inguinale. Specific *therapy* (Chapter 22) is administered for the causative organism(s). Local therapy (vaginal acidification, removal of irritants, improved hygiene) is beneficial. Local surgical therapy (incision, excision, coagulation, and conization) is infrequently applied, but cryosurgery is commonly used to treat a severe chronic infection. Complete healing generally requires 2–3 months, with reestablishment of normal mucosa. Colposcopy is especially useful in evaluation of atypical cases or those with unusual findings.

CERVICAL INJURIES

Cervical lacerations due to childbirth are common. Gross lacerations occur in any quadrant. These are of varying length, may bleed extensively, and can contribute to both immediate and delayed postpartum hemorrhage. They should be repaired at the time of delivery. Nonapparent submucosal separation of the fibrous connective tissue stroma may occur at the level of the internal cervical os and later become apparent as an *incompetent cervix.* Although nonobstetric cervical lacerations may occur with instrumentation (e.g., D & C), they are unusual and, except for cases of postmenopausal atrophy, chronic inflammation, or extreme fibrosis, are largely preventable.

Other cervical injuries may include perforation (self-induced or iatrogenic) and ulcerations from tampons or pessaries. Annular detachment is rare but may occur when the external os fails to dilate and the prolonged pressure of the fetal head causes vascular infarction.

Cervical stenosis may be of congenital, inflammatory, or neoplastic origin but most commonly is postsurgical (electrocoagulation, cryotherapy, laser vaporization, or conization). Dysmenorrhea may result, and complete occlusion may cause hematometra. *Therapy* is careful surgical dilation.

CERVICAL NEOPLASIA

BENIGN (CERVICAL POLYPS)

Cervical polyps are relatively common in the reproductive age group. There are two primary types of cervical polyps, *endocervical* and *ectocervical.* The majority are endocervical polyps, which are small, usually pedunculated (but occasionally sessile) tumors, composed of proliferative columnar epithelium with a vascular and connective tissue supporting structure. They originate from the endocervix and may occur at the external os as red, soft, friable tumors a few millimeters to several centimeters in diameter and on a stalk that can be 1 cm or more in length. Polyps may cause discharge or abnormal bleeding. Occasionally, a submucous uterine or cervical leiomyoma on a pedicle will occur at the cervix.

Local inflammation may play a fundamental role in the formation of cervical polyps. Occasionally, polyps arise from the cervical portio. These ectocervical polyps are covered with squamous epithelium and are more often sessile, fibrous, and less likely to bleed than endocervical polyps.

Local complications of polyps include torsion, necrosis of the tip, and infection. Although metaplasia is common, anaplasia is rare. Cervical cytology often indicates inflammatory atypia. The *differential diagnosis* must include products of conception, endometrial polyps (adenocarcinoma or sarcoma), and a prolapsed leiomyoma. *Malignant transformation of a polyp is uncommon* (<1%). The usual *therapy* is polypectomy, which may be accomplished by avulsion (often with simultaneous torsion) or excision. The base is often curetted or electrocoagulated. *Recurrence is common,* not because polyps per se are recidive but because the factor(s) that caused the primary episode persist.

CERVICAL DYSPLASIA AND CANCER

The incidence of cervical cancer has decreased remarkably over the past 50 years, and it is now the *sixth* most common cancer in women. The decrease is the result of screening (cervical cytology, the Papanicolaou smear) and prevention (therapy for preinvasive disease). Nonetheless, between 1% and 2% of all women >40 years will develop cervical cancer. The average age at diagnosis is 45–47 years, but the disease can occur much earlier. *Squamous cell carcinoma* constitutes 87% of cases, and nearly all the rest are *adenocarcinoma or adenosquamous carcinoma.* Sarcomas and other malignancies are rare.

Cervical cancer is the end result of progressive cervical epithelial alterations, most commonly (~90%) occurring at the squamocolumnar junction. The exact etiology is unknown, but *risk factors* for the continuum of cervical dysplasia and cancer are multiple sexual partners, early first coitus (<20 years), young age at marriage, young age of first pregnancy, high parity, lower socioeconomic status, and smoking. Human papillomavirus (types 16 and 18, especially with aneuploidy) and possibly herpesvirus type 2 are *causative agents* in the development of cervical dysplasia, which may terminate in cancer over time.

Cervical Intraepithelial Neoplasia (CIN)

The process whereby cervical cancer usually occurs begins with cervical intraepithelial neoplasia. CIN may occur soon after early sexual activity (teen years), with a peak incidence by 25–35 years. CIN affects 1.2%–3.8% of nonpregnant women. If CIN is untreated, carcinoma in situ (CIS) appears at about 30–40 years. The degree of CIN is determined by the extent to which the neoplastic cells involve the full thickness of the cervical epithelium. *CIN I* (*mild dysplasia*) indicates that the neoplastic cells are confined to the lower third of the epithelium. In *CIN II* (*moderate dysplasia*), the neoplastic cells occupy up to two thirds of the epithelial thickness, and *CIN III* (*severe dysplasia*) comprises undifferentiated neoplastic cells extending almost to the surface. CIN III also includes CIS, in which the undifferentiated neoplastic cells extend the full thickness of the epithelium. CIN may follow three courses: regression, persistence, or progression to invasive cancer. The risk of progression increases with increasing anaplasia. Spontaneous regression rarely occurs once CIS is established.

Certain gross changes (e.g., a white surface patch) may suggest CIN, but colposcopy will often aid in the diagnosis. Suggestive colposcopic findings include coarse mosaicism and punctation. Ultimately, *diagnosis* depends on colposcopically directed biopsy or cervical conization. At the time of biopsy or conization, a thorough endocervical curettage should be performed.

CANCER OF THE CERVIX

Although >95% *of cancers of the cervix can be cured,* about 80,000 women in the United States die of this disorder each year. Earlier diagnosis and proper therapy will continue to reduce this loss.

Pathogenicity

Most incipient cancers of the cervix develop slowly, passing through dysplasia to acute malignancy. It has been estimated that the *transition from CIS to invasive cancer requires approximately 7 years.* Most cancers of the cervix develop in the cellularly active intraepithelial layer at the squamocolumnar junction.

Initial stromal invasion to even 2 mm beyond the basement membrane is a localized process requiring months to years. However, beyond this point, lymphatic or hematogenous penetration and metastases occur. Lymphatic spread of malignant disease to the regional lymph nodes (parametrial, hypogastric, obturator, external iliac, sacral) is far more frequent than spread via the bloodstream, e.g., to the lungs or brain.

The more pleomorphic or extensive the cancer, the more likely are nodal metastases. If squamous cell carcinoma is confined to the cervix (*stage I*), pelvic lymph node metastases occur in 15%–20% of cases. Once the parametrium is involved (*stage IIB*), carcinoma will be present in the lymph nodes in ~35% of cases. Paraaortic lymph node inclusion of cervical cancer must be expected in about half of patients with *stage III* lesions.

Pathology

About 87% of cancers of the cervix are of the squamous type. The rest include adenocarcinomas, adenosquamous carcinomas, and occasional sarcomas.

Epidermoid cancers of the cervix are graded according to predominant cell type. The degree of differentiation expressed as grades 1–3 roughly parallels the malignant potential of epidermoid carcinoma of the cervix.

In *grade* 1, the well-differentiated carcinomas, there are many well-keratinized epithelial cells, often in pearls or clusters, with identifiable intercellular bridges and <2 mitoses per high-power field (hpf). Overall, minimal variation in the size and shape of tumor cells is evident.

In *grade* 2, there are infrequent epithelial pearls, moderate keratinization, occasional intercellular bridges, 2–4 mitoses/hpf, and moderate variation in the size and shape of tumor cells.

In *grade* 3, expect no epithelial pearls, only slight keratinization, and no intercellular bridges. More than 4 mitoses/hpf is usual, with marked variation in the size and shape of the tumor cells. Occasional small, elongated, closely packed tumor cells are present together with numerous giant cells.

Undifferentiated malignant squamous cell tumors metastasize earlier than do well-differentiated cancers, but the latter also respond well to radiation therapy. Tumor cells near or involving blood vessels increase the risk of hematogenous spread, which worsens the prognosis. In contrast, collections of lymphocytes surrounding tumor cells indicate a reduced likelihood of metastases and a better prognosis.

Adenocarcinomas of the cervix, derived from glandular elements of the endocervix, are tall, columnar, secretory cells arranged in an adenomatous pattern supported by stroma cells. An uncommon but often virulent adenocarcinoma arises from mesonephric (wolffian) duct remnants within the cervix. This tumor is composed of small cuboidal, slightly irregular cells in a poorly defined glandular pattern.

Adenocarcinomas of the cervix are graded as well-differentiated, moderately differentiated, and poorly differentiated. Considerable variability in various areas makes more precise grading impossible. Regrettably, adenocarcinomas of the cervix usually are concealed within the cervical canal and, therefore, are rarely diagnosed until they are ulcerated, i.e., advanced.

During pregnancy, marked changes in the endocervix occur, including hypertrophy and hyperplasia of glandular cells. These changes, evident on biopsy or curettage, may be surprising. However, gestational changes should not be permitted to confuse the diagnosis of cancer.

Clinical Findings

Signs and Symptoms. There are no signs or symptoms of noninvasive cancer of the cervix. However, periodic testing, e.g., cytologic assessment by Pap smears, colposcopy, and biopsy, and a high index of suspicion must be applied.

Postcoital spotting or blood-tinged leukorrhea is often an early sign of ulcerative cervical cancer. Hence, metrorrhagia is the most common sign of invasive cervical malignancy.

Bladder or rectal discomfort or dysfunction and fistulas are late manifestations of cancer of the cervix. Pain, often unilateral and radiating to the hip, may develop with advanced cervical cancer when the ureter becomes partially occluded or when the sacral nerves are involved by the tumor. Anemia, anorexia, and weight loss are signs of advanced malignant disease.

Staging. Staging, or the plotting of the probable extent of malignant cervical disease, is essential for treatment and prognosis. Numerous staging schemes have been suggested, and the International Classification of Cancer of the Cervix (Table 19-1) is the one most commonly used.

Diagnosis

Biopsy and the microscopic assessment of tissue obtained are essential for the diagnosis of cancer or its elimination. Where to biopsy is especially important.

Because necrosis and inflammatory elements are present in

Table 19-1. International classification of cancer of the cervix*

Preinvasive carcinoma

Stage 0   Carcinoma in situ, intraepithelial carcinoma.

Invasive carcinoma

Stage I   Carcinoma strictly confined to the cervix (extension to the corpus should be disregarded).

IA   Microinvasive carcinoma (early stromal invasion).

IB   All other cases of stage I. (Occult cancer should be labeled "occ.")

Stage II   Carcinoma extends beyond the cervix but has not extended onto the pelvic wall. The carcinoma involves the vagina but not the lower third.

IIA   No obvious parametrial involvement.

IIB   Obvious parametrial involvement.

Stage III   Carcinoma has extended to the pelvic wall. On rectal examination, there is no cancer-free space between the tumor and the pelvic wall. The tumor involves the lower third of the vagina. All cases with hydronephrosis or nonfunctioning kidney.

IIIA   No extension onto the pelvic wall.

IIIB   Extension onto the pelvic wall and/or hydronephrosis or nonfunctioning kidney.

Stage IV   Carcinoma extended beyond the true pelvis or clinically involving the mucosa of the bladder or rectum. Do not allow a case of bullous edema as such to be allotted to stage IV.

IVA   Spread of growth to adjacent organs (i.e., rectum or bladder with positive biopsy from these organs).

IVB   Spread of growth to distant organs.

*American Joint Committee for Cancer Staging and End-Results Reporting; Task Force on Gynecologic Sites: Staging System for Cancer at Gynecologic Sites, 1979.

Note: The interpretation of the physical and microscopic findings is to some extent subjective, and the personal opinion of the examiner unavoidably influences the staging of various cases. This is especially true with stages II and III. Therefore, when the results of therapy for carcinoma of the cervix are being reported, all cases examined should be reported so that the reader can determine what series of cases in his or her own experience the data apply to. In reporting the results of therapy for stage II carcinoma at a given institution, the statistics for stage III should be included so that the reader may compare the reported results with a more surely comparable series of cases at another institution.

bleeding, presumably invasive cancer of the cervix, biopsies from an ulcerative area may be useless or difficult to interpret. Therefore, obtain biopsies from the edge of the lesion, where normal and malignant tissue offer a contrast. This may be facilitated by the Schiller test.

Schiller Test

Aqueous solutions of iodine stain the surface of the normal cervix brown because normal cervical epithelial cells contain glycogen. Areas of cancer within the epithelium over the cervix do not contain glycogen, and these remain unstained when Schiller's solution or Lugol's solution is applied. Hence, biopsy of Schiller-positive areas as well as granular, nodular, or papillary lesions usually will confirm invasive cancer when it is present.

Colposcopy

Colposcopy may identify possible early invasive carcinoma in an area of CIN. Directed biopsies from such suspicious sites may reveal early stromal invasion. Colposcopically directed punch biopsies and light curettage of the endocervix may obviate a more extensive cone biopsy of the cervix. However, frank invasion usually produces ulceration and bleeding, and colposcopy then becomes unnecessary for biopsy.

Complications

Metastases to regional lymph nodes occur with increasing frequency from stage I (about 15%) to stage IV (at least 60%).

Extension occurs in all directions. Most commonly, the tumor grows laterally in the base of the broad ligments on one or both sides. The ureters often are obstructed lateral to the cervix. Hydroureter and hydronephrosis impair kidney function. Almost two thirds of patients with carcinoma of the cervix die of uremia when ureteral obstruction is bilateral. Perivascular, perineural, and lymphatic channels facilitate cancer spread.

Cervical carcinoma may *invade the uterus* by direct surface extension up the cervical canal. Downward extension often involves the vagina.

Invasion of the rectum is by posterior extension from the cervix along the uterosacral ligaments.

Anterior progression is followed by invasion of the bladder in stages III and IV.

Pain and swelling in the leg, particularly the upper thigh, may indicate lymphatic occlusion or obstruction of the venous return by carcinoma.

Pain in the back and in the distribution of the lumbosacral plexus indicates chronic infection or neurologic involvement by extending cancer.

Pelvic infections may complicate cervical carcinoma. Obstruction of the cervical canal may require drainage of a pyometra and chemotherapy to resolve infection.

Death due to hemorrhage occurs in about 10%–20% of cases of extensive invasive carcinoma of the cervix. Protracted bleeding causes anemia.

Vaginal fistulas involving the gastrointestinal and urinary tracts are particularly discouraging. Incontinence of urine and of feces are major complications, particularly in debilitated individuals.

Metastasis to the liver is common, but spread to lung or brain is rare.

Differential Diagnosis

Eversion and redness around the cervical os caused by infection, irritation, or hormonal imbalance are smooth, soft, and minimally irregular. Unlike *carcinoma,* eversion is not exudative and does not bleed easily.

The small, hard chancre of *primary syphilis* is a shallow, oval, or circular ulceration with a glistening surface and a firm edge and base. There is minimal serous discharge, and bleeding is uncommon. *Treponema pallidum* may be identified by darkfield examination of the thin exudate. Serologic tests for syphilis are positive.

The characteristics of *chancroid* (soft chancre), *granuloma inguinale, lymphogranuloma venereum,* and *cervical tuberculosis* are described elsewhere.

Abortion of a cervical pregnancy results in a soft, nontender, deep, freely bleeding cavity, usually within the cervical canal. Biopsy of the tissue lining the cavity will usually disclose trophoblastic debris but no cancer cells.

Metastatic choriocarcinoma or other secondary cancer must be considered in the diagnosis, as well as rare conditions, such as *actinomycosis, amebiasis,* and *schistosomiasis.*

Prevention

The incidence of cervical cancer should be reduced by (1) improved personal hygiene, including prevention and prompt treatment of vaginitis and cervicitis, male circumcision in infancy, precoital washing of the penis, and habitual use of condoms, (2) avoidance of intercourse at an early age and limiting the number of consorts, (3) regular periodic cytologic screening of all women, especially parous women in low socioeconomic groups and those who have had numerous sexual partners, and (4) prompt treatment of suspicious cervical lesions.

Treatment of Cervical Dysplasia

A. *Mild or Moderate Dysplasia.* Many CIN I or II lesions regress (approximately 60% and 30%, respectively) or persist (approximately 25% and 5%, respectively), and only a minority progress to CIN III (approximately 15% and 20%, respectively). Therefore, it is reasonable to follow such patients with medical therapy (to treat HPV or bacterial infections) and serial cytologic studies every 6 months. Cryosurgery, laser therapy, loop electrosurgical excision procedure (LEEP), and electrocoagulation are the methods most often used to treat CIN I or II.

B. *Moderate to Severe Dysplasia (CIN III).* CIN III lesions require cryotherapy, laser, LEEP, or definitive surgical therapy. If there is extension up the cervical canal, conization is required initially.

C. *Severe Dysplasia (CIS).* The most effective method of treatment of CIS, and the one usually recommended for women >40, is total abdominal hysterectomy with a wide vaginal cuff. Whether to remove the ovaries is a decision that must be based on the patient's age, the status of the ovaries, and family history of cancer.

Cervical conization may be considered for patients who desire pregnancy or who are reliable and can be carefully supervised. In either case, cervical smears every 6 months are recommended.

Treatment of Cervical Cancer

A. *Emergency Measures.* Vaginal hemorrhage originates from gross ulceration and cavitation in stage II–IV cervical carcinoma. Ligation of bleeding points and suturing are impractical. Styptics, such as negatol (Negatan), 10% silver nitrate solution, or acetone, are effective, although later slough may result in further bleeding. Vaginal packing or radiation (if tolerance permits) is helpful. Embolization or ligation of the uterine or hypogastric arteries may be lifesaving.

B. *General Measures.* Admit the patient to the hospital for thorough study and rest before therapy is begun.

The basics of a *cervical cancer workup* include hemogram (anemia or infection), liver function tests (liver metastases or liver disease), BUN (impaired renal function or ureteral obstruction), cystoscopy (bladder invasion), sigmoidoscopy (bowel invasion), ultrasonography (to detect tumor masses), chest x-ray (pulmonary disease or metastases), intravenous urograms (obstruction), skeletal survey (metastases), and a barium enema (bowel invasion or disease). Additionally, a pelvic and abdominal CT scan or MRI will assist in detailing local metastases.

Eradicate vaginal, urinary, or pelvic infections before surgery or radiation. Correct anemia and improve nutrition. Keep debilitated patients in the hospital for supportive therapy during radiation treatment, and readmit discharged patients if radiation is poorly tolerated.

Control pain with such analgesics as acetaminophen with codeine 8 or 15 mg qid as necessary. Give diphenoxylate (Lomotil) 2.5 mg, loperamide (Imodium) 2 mg, or paregoric 4–8 ml qid as necessary for diarrhea. For urinary frequency and dysuria, give Pyridium, 100 mg q6h as necessary.

C. *Local Measures.* During radiation therapy, plain warm water douches may aid in comfort and hygiene.

D. *Treatment According to Stage*

1. *Stage IA* (*microinvasive carcinoma*) (depth of invasion <3 mm). Total extrafascial abdominal hysterectomy with a wide vaginal cuff is current therapy. Patients with invasion >3 mm have a small but definite likelihood of lymph node metastasis. Therefore, they should be treated as for stage IB.

2. *Stage IB.* External supervoltage radiation and intracavitary and forniceal cesium or radium therapy or radical hysterectomy and pelvic lymphadenectomy probably are equally effective in the treatment of stage IB carcinoma. The latter often is favored in young, otherwise healthy, slender patients. The ovaries need not be removed unless they are abnormal or the woman is perimenopausal. Older patients, obese patients, and those who have serious medical problems are best treated by radiation.

3. *Stages IIA and IIB.* With rare exceptions, stage II cervical cancer should be treated by radiation. In some centers, pretreatment laparoscopy or laparotomy for biopsy of paraaortic lymph nodes may be done in stage IIB patients. If the nodes are cancer-positive (~15%), paraaortic extended-field radiation therapy should increase survival, although complications may be more

frequent and severe. Even when cancer-containing nodes are found beyond the pelvis, the original staging must remain the same.

4. *Stages IIIA and IIIB.* Radiation therapy is used for all stage III cases. Pretreatment paraaortic lymph node sampling is important. However, these nodes will be positive in 30%–50% of patients. Hence, extended-field therapy may be beneficial.

5. *Stage IV.* Supervoltage external radiation therapy to the whole pelvis is best for almost all stage IV patients. If the cancer has extended anteriorly or posteriorly without spread elsewhere, anterior or posterior exenteration may be chosen as primary therapy.

Treatment must be individualized for cervical stump cancers, bulky or barrel-shaped cancerous cervices, and laterally recurrent lesions.

Chemotherapy using cisplatin may be appropriate if the patient fails to respond to conventional therapy. Neurosurgery for relief of pain may be considered in selected cases.

E. *Radiation Therapy.* Radiation is generally considered to be the best treatment for invasive carcinoma of the cervix. X-ray radium, ^{60}Co, the cyclotron, linear accelerator, or other sources of radiation may be used. All stages of cancer may be treated by this method, and there are fewer medical contraindications to radiation than to radical surgery. Optimal results have been achieved with the use of externally applied supervoltage radiation combined with intracavitary and paracervical vaginal radium.

The *objectives* are destruction of primary and secondary carcinoma within the pelvis and preservation of tissues not involved in the cancer. The amount of radiation required to destroy cancer varies from patient to patient. A safe cancericidal dose for cervical carcinoma is about 7000 rad to point A and about 5000 rad to point B (see p 530) administered over a period of 4–5 weeks.

Although it is impossible to administer adequate homogeneous radiation to destroy cancer throughout the pelvis without damaging vital structures, such as the bowel, bladder, ureters, and blood vessels, the cervix can be treated intensively because it has a high tolerance to radiation. The cervix and vagina can tolerate 24,000 rad, but the bladder and ureter will be seriously injured by doses higher than 7000 rad and the bowel by doses higher than 4000–5000 rad. Major blood vessels have approximately the same tolerance to radiation as the intestine. Therefore, dosage is determined by the radiosensitivity of both cancer cells and noncancerous tissue. In practice, the experienced oncologist or radiologist applies as much radiation as possible to the cancer within a reasonable time, with particular concern for the neighboring organs.

When vaginal contractures, a cervical stump, or the patient's condition precludes radium therapy, external radiation may be used alone. Cesium or radium alone is often used when the cancer is small and medical or surgical problems contraindicate protracted external radiation therapy.

1. *Manchester method of radiation therapy for cervical cancer.* The Manchester model, one of the most logical and popular methods, emphasizes the importance of calculating the radiation dosage as delivered to two precise points in the pelvis. *Point A* is defined as lying 2 cm lateral to the central canal of the cervix and 2 cm above the lateral fornix in the axis of the uterus (approximately the point where the uterine artery crosses the ureter). *Point B* lies 5 cm lateral to the central canal of the cervix and 2 cm above the lateral fornix (at the pelvic side wall). Point B represents a lymph node focus adjacent to the iliac vessels. This point is a pelvic focus for metastatic cancer from the cervix.

Rubber applicators for carrying radium tubes in tandem are available in three lengths for the deep, average, and shallow uterus. Paracervical rubber ovoids for radium application are designed so that the distance of the radium from points A and B can be varied by changing the amount of radium used, the thickness of the three graduated ovoids, and rubber spacers. The dosage depends on the amount of radium inserted and the distribution employed. By using both intrauterine and paracervical radium applicators, the maximal dose of radiation is applied to the area of greatest benefit and least risk. This is far more effective than a radium tandem placed in the cervix alone or radium placed only in the vagina.

The *optimal predetermined dosage from cesium or radium alone to point A is 7000 rad.* This dosage is delivered in two sessions of 2–3 days each, the first preceding external radiation therapy and the second following it. Treatment is more effective if external radiation therapy is also used. An external radiation dose of 3000 rad is given through two anterior and two posterior ports to the parametrium (point B) within 4 weeks.

2. *Treatment of cervical cancer during pregnancy* This is variable and requires great individualization, but one plan is noted here.

a. *First trimester.* Deliver 6000 rad of external radiation to the pelvis through each of four ports. Concurrently, give two courses of intracervical and paracervical radium and await spontaneous abortion.

b. *Second trimester.* Deliver intracervical and contracervical radium. In 7–10 days, perform an abdominal (classic) hysterectomy. Two weeks after surgery, begin 6000 rad of external radiation and then give a further course of intracervical and contracervical radiation during the last week of external radiation.

c. *Third trimester.* Perform classic cesarean section when the infant is viable. In 7–10 days, begin 6000 rad of external radiation and then give two courses of intracervical and paracervical radium 1 week apart, the first during the last 7–10 days of external radiation.

F. *Surgical Measures* (see also *Treatment According to Stage*). Total hysterectomy with removal of a wide vaginal cuff is the surgical treatment of choice for women over age 40 with in situ carcinoma of the cervix. Deep conization of the cervix may be acceptable for younger women who wish to have more children, but this is a calculated risk even when the woman understands the need for vaginal cytologic smears every 6 months for an indefinite time.

Radical total hysterectomy (Clark-Wertheim or Okabayashi) together with pelvic lymphadenectomy is performed for treatment of stage I and stage IIA cervical carcinoma by surgeons skilled in the technique required for this exacting procedure. The 5-year survival rate with operation is as good as that for radiation therapy in selected cases. Obesity, advanced age, and serious medical problems that are likely to complicate surgery or convalescence greatly reduce the number of candidates for elective cancer surgery. In general, the hazards of the operation exceed those of radiation therapy.

Radical total hysterectomy and pelvic lymphadenectomy often are used as definitive treatment of cervical cancer if (1) the patient is pregnant, (2) large uterine or adnexal tumors are present, (3) the patient has chronic salpingitis, (4) there are small or large bowel adhesions in the pelvis or to the abdominal wall, (5) the patient is under age 35 and wishes to keep her ovaries, or (6) she refuses or abandons radiation therapy but is a good surgical risk.

Complications of Therapy

The mortality rate due to radiation is about 1% and that due to surgery is about 2%. The morbidity rates are approximately 2% and 5%, respectively.

Radiation therapy may cause early side effects, including nausea and vomiting, weight loss, dysuria, and urinary frequency. Such complications as tissue fibrosis, hemorrhagic cystitis, small or large bowel stenosis, or fistulas may develop later.

A serious complication of radical abdominal hysterectomy is

ureteric fistula. However, the incidence of this complication has been reduced to 3%–5% by better operative technique. Other serious problems include bowel injury, hemorrhage, wound infection or dehiscence, pulmonary embolism, atonic bladder with urinary retention, and cystic lymphangioma.

Prognosis

The earlier the stage at which cancer is diagnosed, the better the prognosis. Preinvasive cancer is commonly diagnosed in women <30 years, but most patients with invasive carcinoma are 40–50 years old at the time of diagnosis. Thus, it appears to take 5–10 years for carcinoma to penetrate the basement membrane and become invasive. Untreated patients usually die 3–5 years after invasion occurs.

Reported survival rates according to the stage at which the cancer is discovered vary widely. A composite of 5-year survival rates at major cancer centers worldwide where radiotherapy is the primary method of treatment is as follows: stage I 86%–89%, stage II 43%–70%, stage III 27%–43%, and stage IV 0–12%.

Chapter 20

Diseases of the Uterus

BENIGN UTERINE NEOPLASMS

LEIOMYOMA (MYOMAS, FIBROIDS, FIBROMYOMAS)

Leiomyomas are discrete, rounded, firm, white to pale pink, benign myometrial tumors composed mostly of smooth muscle with some connective tissue. Approximately 95% arise from the uterine corpus and ~5% from the cervix. Only occasionally do they arise from a fallopian tube or round ligament. *Leiomyomas are the most frequent pelvic tumors,* occurring in ~25% of white and ~50% of black women by age 50 years. Leiomyomas account for ~10% of gynecologic problems and have their peak incidence in the fifth decade. Although the cause is unknown, each tumor (98% are multiple) originates from a single muscle cell (whether an embryonic cell rest or blood vessel smooth muscle is unclear). They enlarge in response to estrogen. Thus, enlargement is marked with pregnancy. Premenarcheal leiomyomas are rare, and menopause or castration causes regression.

Uterine leiomyomas are classified by anatomic location (Fig. 20-1). Most commonly they are subserous (beneath the peritoneum), intramural (within the uterine wall), or submucous (only 5%–10% are beneath the endometrium). Leiomyomas may become pedunculated in either the subserous or submucous locations. A special variation of pedunculation is retroperitoneal extrusion between the leaves of the broad ligament (intraligamentous). Although adhesions to other organs are rare, in extreme cases pedunculated leiomyomas may derive their entire blood supply elsewhere, becoming parasitic.

Pathology

Only 2% of leiomyomas are solitary. They may grow to >45 kg. Each tumor is limited by a pseudocapsule, a potential cleavage

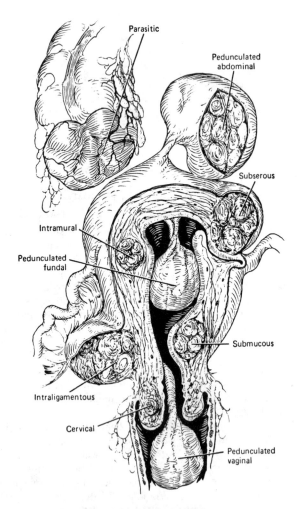

Figure 20-1. Myomas of the uterus.

plane useful for surgical enucleation. Leiomyomas may be multi-nodular and are generally lighter in color than normal myo-metrium. On typical *cut section,* leiomyomas exhibit a whorled or trabeculated pattern of smooth muscle and fibrous connective tissue in varying proportions. *Microscopically,* the myocytes are mature and of uniform size, with a characteristic benign appearance. The smooth muscle cells are arranged in bundles and have interspersed fibrous tissue in direct relation to the extent of atrophy and degeneration that has occurred. Telangiectasia or lymphectasia occasionally is present.

Blood supply is generally through one or two major arteries, and the tumors tend to outgrow their blood supply with subsequent degeneration. Of larger leiomyomas, two thirds demonstrate some degeneration. Acute leiomyoma degeneration is relatively uncommon, but this may be necrotic, hemorrhagic (red degeneration), or septic. Chronic degeneration may be atrophic, hyaline (65%), cystic, calcific (10%), myxomatous (15%), or fatty. Leiomyosarcomas occur in ~0.1%–0.5% of patients with leiomyomas. However, it is not known if they arise from the leiomyomas.

Clinical Findings

Symptoms and Signs

The majority (about two thirds) of women with leiomyomas are asymptomatic. When symptoms occur, they depend on the number, size, location, situation, and status (usually vascular supply) of the tumor(s). Gynecologic symptoms most commonly are abnormal uterine bleeding, pressure effects, pain, and infertility. Abnormal uterine bleeding is encountered in ~30% of patients with uterine leiomyomas. Menorrhagia is the most common abnormal uterine bleeding pattern, and although any pattern is possible, premenstrual spotting and prolonged light flow after menses often occur. Iron deficiency anemia commonly occurs as a result of the heavier menstrual blood loss. Rarely, a secondary polycythemia due to increased erythropoietin occurs with leiomyomas. The cause of this mechanism is uncertain.

The gynecologic symptoms resulting from leiomyomas exerting pressure are variable but most commonly include enlarging abdominal girth, pelvic fullness or heaviness, urinary frequency (from bladder impingement), and ureteral obstruction. Much less commonly encountered are large tumors causing pelvic congestion, with lower extremity edema or constipation. Parasitic tumors may cause intestinal obstruction. Cervical tumors may lead to leukorrhea, vaginal bleeding, dyspareunia, or infertility.

The most common pain (about one third of patients have pain) caused by leiomyomas is acquired dysmenorrhea. However, the most severe and characteristic pains with leiomyomas are associated with degeneration (especially, carneous or septic, in which there is a sudden onset of unremittent pain that may occur as an acute abdomen), torsion (usually recurrent acute pain), or uterine contractions while attempting to expel a pedunculated submucous tumor. Pelvic heaviness and a sensation of bearing down are common complaints with large tumors. Occasionally, pelvic impaction of a leiomyoma may create nerve impingement, with pain radiating to the back or lower extremities.

Uterine leiomyomas emerge as the sole abnormality in 2%–10% of infertility patients. The causal relationship remains unclear, but myomectomy may be indicated in long-standing infertility with no other demonstrable cause. Abortions probably occur two to three times more frequently in patients with leiomyomas. Thus, in recurrent pregnancy wastage with leiomyomas as the only abnormality, myomectomy is indicated. This results in term pregnancy rates of 40%–50%. Pregnancy complicated by leiomyoma may lead to abortion, premature labor, malpresentation, failure of engagement, unusual pain or tenderness, dystocia, desultory labor, and postpartum hemorrhage.

Physical examination (abdominal and pelvic) generally reveals firm, irregular but smooth, nodular masses attached to the uterus.

Laboratory Findings

Anemia is the most common laboratory finding with uterine leiomyomas (as a result of abnormal uterine bleeding and infection). Leukocytosis as well as elevated ESR may occur if leiomyomas are complicated by endometritis or carneous or septic degeneration.

Imaging

Ultrasound examination may be useful with leiomyomas to confirm the clinical diagnosis, measure the uterus and tumors, assist in diagnosis of difficult cases, and sequentially measure tumor size. X-ray is only diagnostic for calcific alterations or when there is urinary system impingement (IVP). MRI may be able to differentiate leiomyomas from leiomyosarcomas.

Differential Diagnosis

The uterine enlargement or irregularity caused by a leiomyoma also may be caused by pregnancy, adenomyosis, or mistaken ovarian neoplasm. Other conditions to be considered include subinvolution, congenital anomalies, adherent adnexa, omentum, or bowel, benign hypertrophy, and sarcoma or carcinoma.

Treatment

The treatment of leiomyomas obviously depends on a number of variables, including number, size, location, symptomatology, degeneration, reproductive desires (age, parity, wish to reproduce), general health, proximity to the menopause, and potential for malignancy. With small asymptomatic leiomyomas, conservative management (i.e., careful follow-up but no therapy) consists of examinations (and possibly ultrasonic imaging) every 4–6 months. Indeed, the majority may be managed this way, thus avoiding surgery.

The necessity for intervention generally is based on bleeding causing a falling HCT or Hgb despite adequate iron and nutritional therapy, a combined uterine–leiomyoma size such that the ovaries and masses cannot be assessed adequately on pelvic examination (about the size of a 12–14 week gestation), untoward leiomyoma location (e.g., cervical or leiomyoma causing ureteral obstruction), and pain or signs of symptomatic degeneration. Removal of leiomyomas during pregnancy is rarely warranted because of the extraordinary bleeding encountered. Even after delivery, surgical therapy should be delayed 3–6 months for tumor involution if at all possible.

When it is desirable to temporarily delay surgery (e.g., to correct a medical problem or to enhance hematologic status), cause the tumor to decrease in size preoperatively (e.g., to facilitate surgery), or circumvent surgery entirely (e.g., near the menopause), patients may be treated with an GnRH analog. These compounds cause pseudomenopause, with marked shrinking of the tumors.

Preoperatively, the usual gynecologic evaluations and a cytologic (Pap) smear. are required (Chapter 29). In patients with abnormal bleeding, a differential curettage is advisable to ascertain the endometrial status. In all women >35, in those >30 and anovulatory, and when the diagnosis is uncertain, the status of the endometrium must be known (i.e., rule out endometrial cancer). This may be established by hysteroscopy and directed biopsies or D & C. In the case of pedunculated submucous leiomyomas, excisional biopsy may be curative. Definitive surgery is usually myomectomy or hysterectomy. Myomectomy is employed for patients wishing to preserve fertility. However,

patients must be cautioned preoperatively that should myomectomy be impractical (e.g., due to tumor situation), hysterectomy will be necessary. Moreover, if the endometrial cavity is
entered during myomectomy, it may be prudent to deliver subsequent infants by elective cesarean section because of the hazard
of uterine rupture.

Occasionally, a pedunculated myoma can be removed vaginally if it is submucous, perhaps facilitated by uteroscopy.
Symptomatic, small leiomyomas may be removed by vaginal
myomectomy. Large leiomyomas or those with unusual placement will require abdominal myomectomy or hysterectomy.
The ovaries should be preserved if possible (especially in those
<40–45 years). However, if they are diseased or have a com-
promised blood supply or if the patient is postmenopausal, removal is warranted.

The *incidence of recurrence* following myomectomy is 15%–
40% even if all macroscopic leiomyomas are removed at the time
of surgery. At least one half of recurrent leiomyomas require
further surgical therapy. Hysterectomy is totally curative.

ADENOMYOSIS

See Chapter 26.

ENDOMETRIAL POLYP

Endometrial polyps are suggested by abnormal vaginal bleeding,
most commonly menometrorrhagia or postmenopausal light staining. Polyps occur from age 29 to 59, with the majority occurring
after age 50. *The incidence of asymptomatic polyps in postmenopausal women is ~10%.*

Endometrial polyps usually arise in the fundus and may be
attached by a slender stalk (pedunculated) or have a broad
base (sessile). Occasionally, polyps prolapse through the cervix. *Grossly,* endometrial polyps are velvety smooth, red to
brown, ovoid masses from a few millimeters to centimeters in
size. *Histologically,* endometrial polyps have stromal cores with
marked vascular channels and endometrial mucosal surfaces
that may cover glandular components. The distal polyp

may show stromal hemorrhage, inflammatory cells, ulceration, and engorged blood vessels. Occasionally, multiple polyposis occurs. Another uncommon variant is the pedunculated adenomyoma (differentiated by interlacing bands of smooth muscle).

The *differential diagnosis* includes submucous myomas, retained products of conception, endometrial cancer, and mixed sarcomas. Polyps are estrogen sensitive and may undergo malignant change, in which case a better prognosis is likely as compared with nonpolypoid endometrial cancer.

The *diagnosis* is made easily by hysteroscopy, and the treatment is excision. This may be accomplished easily by hysteroscopy followed by curettage of the stalk. A wire snare or scissors may be used to sever the base of a large polyp. It is wise to sample the endocervical canal by curettage when polyps are removed to rule out endometrial cancer. During D & C, explore the uterine cavity using an Overstreet or similar polyp forceps. Polyps tend to recur, and hysterectomy is definitive but rarely necessary for benign endometrial polyps.

ENDOMETRIAL HYPERPLASIA

Endometrial hyperplasia is an extremely important lesion because of its probable correlation with the majority of endometrial cancers. In occasional older patients, a less well differentiated endometrial cancer apparently can develop without intervening steps. Common agreement about the *terminology of endometrial hyperplasia* is awaited, but an attractive thesis is illustrated in Table 20-1. This hypothesis contends that first the endometrium responds to unopposed estrogenic stimulation with a very florid proliferative endometrium. Continued estrogenic stimulation causes the glands to dilate markedly, and the endometrium assumes a classic Swiss cheese appearance. With still further estrogenic stimulation, the glandular epithelium becomes more prominent. It is postulated that up to this point, with no atypia, the process is spontaneously reversible if estrogenic stimulation ceases or if progesterone is administered.

With continued stimulation, the adenomatous hyperplasia becomes progressively more atypical. In some cases, progestin therapy can reconvert the process to normal. Nonetheless, vigilance is required to be sure that the process does not progress to endometrial cancer. The alterations at this stage are based less

Table 20-1. Classification of endometrial hyperplasia and its relationship to endometrial carcinoma

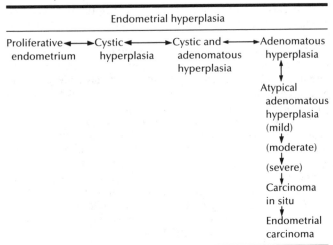

on the shape, crowding, budding, and glandular branching (architectural atypia) and more on the cytologic atypia—the major determinant of malignant potential. Progressive epithelial cellular atypia includes cellular abnormalities (e.g., piling up of cells), nuclear atypia, and the development of epithelial bridges. This is followed by irregular cell size, prominent nucleoli, occasional nuclear pleomorphism, mitosis, abnormal chromatin configuration and a high nuclear/cytoplasmic ratio. These alterations are further classified as mild, moderate, and severe. The *incidence* of endometrial hyperplasia is age related: 40–50 years (40%), 50–60 years (25%), <40 years (only 15%). The time required for conversion to malignancy may be 1–2 years. If untreated, at least 50% of patients with atypical adenomatous hyperplasia will develop endometrial cancer, whereas only 20%–25% of those with adenomatous hyperplasia will progress to cancer.

Therapy for endometrial hyperplasia is directly related to the degree of hyperplasia, the patient's age, and her desire for retention of reproductive capability. Moderate and severe atypical adenomatous hyperplasia in a woman past the reproductive age or one who does not want more children generally requires hysterectomy. If it is desirable to retain the uterus, and a careful D & C or preferably hysteroscopy with directed biopsies has been performed, therapy may consist of megestrol acetate (40–320 mg/day) for several months to totally suppress the endometrium. The endometrium must be thoroughly sampled at ≤6 month intervals to ascertain the success of therapy. Regardless of the severity of adenomatous hyperplasia, if abnormal bleeding recurs despite appropriate therapy, the endometrium must be promptly sampled.

Therapy for mild atypical adenomatous hyperplasia consists of D & C and perhaps a less potent progestin (e.g., medroxyprogesterone acetate 10 mg PO daily for 2 weeks to a month. The endometrium must be sampled again in 6–12 months. For continued atypical adenomatous hyperplasia in a woman not desiring reproduction, hysterectomy is justified. For adenomatous hyperplasia, a thorough D & C may be adequate primary therapy if progestin or induction of ovulation is then instituted. The latter is obviously undertaken only in those desiring reproduction. Endometrial sampling should be performed in 1 year to ascertain that the adenomatous hyperplasia has regressed.

The *prevention* of endometrial hyperplasia requires recognition of hyperestrogenic states (e.g., polycystic ovarian syndrome, feminizing tumors, postmenopausal estrogen replacement). These feature unopposed estrogen, and treatment includes appropriate progestin therapy.

ENDOMETRIAL CARCINOMA IN SITU

Carcinoma in situ of the endometrium is a very difficult diagnosis to make grossly or on frozen section at hysterectomy or at D & C. The primary difficulty is that microscopically the endometrial glands are not separated from stroma, myometrium, blood vessels, and lymphatics by a structure analogous to the basement membrane in squamous epithelial lesions. The usual criteria for diagnosis of endometrial carcinoma in situ include histologic staining qualities (endometrial carcinoma often has large, eosinophilic, pale-staining glandular cells whereas lesser lesions are more basophilic), loss of nuclear polarity (enhanced with endometrial carcinoma), and no vascular or lymphatic invasion (both occur with endometrial carcinoma). When the changes of severe atypical adenomatous hyperplasia are at a maximum and these criteria are met, the lesion is termed carcinoma in situ. Since endometrial carcinoma in situ cannot be distinguished from early invasive carcinoma on biopsy, both should be treated as endometrial carcinoma.

UTERINE MALIGNANCIES

ENDOMETRIAL CARCINOMA

Carcinoma of the endometrium *histologically* is usually adenocarcinoma (70%–80% in the United States), adenosquamous carcinoma (10%–20%), or adenoacanthoma (~5%). Other lesions are uncommon to rare. These include clear cell carcinoma, papillary serous carcinoma, secretory carcinoma, mucinous carcinoma, squamous cell carcinoma (from metaplasia or from cellular rests), carcinosarcoma (adenocarcinoma and sarcoma), and sarcoma from endometrial stroma (e.g., chondrosarcoma, leiomyosarcoma, myxosarcoma).

Although the *etiology of endometrial cancer remains unknown* and certainly numerous factors may be operative, unopposed estrogen is a primary associated factor. Moreover, the *incidence* of endometrial carcinoma is directly related to increased estrogen levels (endogenous and exogenous) and the duration of this stimulation. For example, endometrial carcinoma is four to eight times more common in women using unopposed estrogens for menopausal replacement and is more common in those with feminizing ovarian tumors and polycystic ovarian syndrome. Other known risk factors include obesity (20–50 pounds—3 times, >50 pounds—10 times), nulliparity (2–3 times), diabetes mellitus (2.8 times), and menopause >52 years (2.4 times).

Thus, women who have elevated levels of endogenous estrogen, those who are anovulatory, and those requiring estrogen replacement therapy should all receive close clinical follow-up (including periodic endometrial sampling) and consideration for cyclic progestin therapy.

Endometrial carcinoma is the most common female genital tract malignancy in developed countries. The chance of a woman in the United States developing endometrial carcinoma is ~1%. Overall, endometrial cancer is most prevalent in women between 50 and 70 years, and <5% of cases are diagnosed before 40 years of age. When the disease is revealed before age 35, it is almost always in association with a condition of unopposed estrogen. Just before menopause, about 10% of women with hypermenorrhea will have endometrial carcinoma. The incidence in nulliparas is 3 times that in multiparas. The occurrence of endometrial carcinoma is nearly 2 times that of ovarian cancer and >2.5 times that of cervical cancer, but it has a much better prognosis. Table 20-2 details the number of new cases and annual deaths from the most common genital tract cancers.

Table 20-2. Relative incidence and deaths from three most common genital tract tumors — 1988

Genital cancers	New cases	Deaths	Death/new case ratio
Endometrial	34,000	3,000	1/11.3
Ovarian	19,000	12,000	1/1.6
Cervical	12,900	7,000	1/1.8

Pathology

Endometrial adenocarcinoma is composed of malignant glands that vary from well differentiated (grade 1) to anaplastic (grade 3). Endometrial adenosquamous carcinoma consists of malignant glands and malignant squamous epithelium that are often poorly differentiated. Adenoacanthoma incorporates malignant glands and benign squamous metaplasia. It is usually well differentiated.

Endometrial carcinoma may spread in any of the following ways: within the endometrium as a surface growth (e.g., into the cervical canal), into the myometrium to the peritoneum and parametrium, via the uterine tube to the ovaries, to the uterine and cervical lymphatics, to the uterine arteries and veins, or to the pelvic and abdominal viscera by penetration through the serosa. Invasion of the myometrium and metastasis occur relatively late (Fig. 20-2). When invasion of the uterine wall does occur, the lymphatics are involved first and the venous and arterial channels later.

The uterine lymphatic drainage includes small lymphatic branches along the round ligament to the femoral nodes, infundibulopelvic ligament drainage to the paraaortic nodes from the tubal and ovarian pedicles, and broad ligament lymphatics to the pelvic nodes. The iliac, obturator, and sacral lymph nodes are commonly involved when there is endocervical involvement by an endometrial cancer. Reflux of cancer cells through the tubes results in dependent, lateral and posterior, peritoneal tumor implants. Vaginal metastases occur in 10%–15% of patients following hysterectomy. These are most commonly in the vaginal vault or along the urethra 1–2 cm from the urethral meatus. Spread may also occur via the uterosacral ligaments and presacral lymphatics to the iliac and periaortic nodes. Hematogenous metastases to the liver, lungs, and bones are not uncommon.

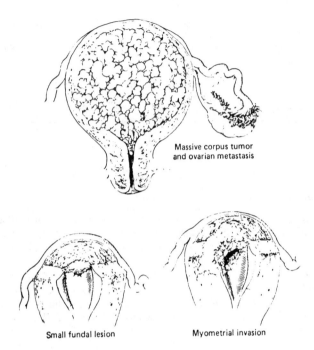

Massive corpus tumor
and ovarian metastasis

Small fundal lesion   Myometrial invasion

Figure 20-2. Adenocarcinoma of the endometrium.

Clinical Findings

Symptoms and Signs

The *peak incidence* of endometrial cancer is at 55–69 years of age. Endometrial cancer most commonly occurs in a woman who is infertile, nulliparous, diabetic, obese, and white. The classic symptom is perimenopausal or postmenopausal vaginal bleeding (in 80% of cases). In premenopausal women, the usual symptom is abnormal vaginal bleeding (the most frequent is menorrhagia). About 20% of postmenopausal bleeding is due to an underlying cancer, with 12%–15% being endometrial. Hemorrhage is rare, and pain is not usually a feature of this malignancy unless intrauterine infection or cervical obstruction occurs or the disease is far advanced. A watery, serous or sanguineous, malodorous vaginal discharge may occur occasionally.

In early cases, no alterations are detectable by physical examination, but as the cancer progresses, the uterus usually becomes larger, more globular, and irregularly softened. The cervix may soften, and the os may appear slightly patulous. In the older postmenopausal woman, cervical scarring or stenosis may obstruct external bleeding, and she may experience only uterine cramping. With cervical obstruction, diagnosis often is delayed, and pain, pyometra, or hematometra may slowly develop. If drainage is not accomplished, the uterus may rupture.

Laboratory Findings

Cytologic examination of cervical and vaginal smears must always be done in these cases, primarily to rule out cervical or vaginal neoplasia. Vaginal cytology reveals endometrial carcinoma cells in only 50% of cases, evidence of inadequate screening. Indeed, even intrauterine cytologic techniques are less effective than outpatient endometrial tissue sampling ($>90\%$) for diagnosis. Every suspected case of endometrial carcinoma must have the endocervix evaluated also before therapy is instituted. Hence, it is prudent to obtain endocervical curettage at the same time that the uterus is sounded and the endometrial tissue is sampled. However, most frequently a clinical staging examination with anesthesia is required, which includes examination under anesthesia, cystoscopy, proctoscopy, and fractional D & C (with accurate uterine measurement).

The usual laboratory workup of the endometrial cancer patient includes CBC, UA, liver function tests, BUN, creatinine, 2 h postprandial blood glucose, stool guaiac, and sigmoidoscopy.

Imaging

Obtain the following radiographs on all endometrial carcinoma patients: chest x-ray, IVP, and barium enema. Although hysterosalpingography has been used to detail the site and volume of tumor, it is not recommended because of the possibility of transtubal spread of cancer. The usefulness of ultrasonic scans appears to be limited to potential cases of hematometra or pyometra. CT scan is useful in evaluating local invasion as well as the abdomen and retroperitoneal nodes. MRI improves the accuracy of clinical staging and is very helpful in assessing myometrial invasion and lower uterine segment or cervical involvement.

Receptor Assay

Tumor receptor assays for estrogen and progesterone binding should be obtained to assist in planning adjuvant or subsequent hormone therapy. Generally, the better differentiated the tumor, the better the estrogen or progesterone receptor binding (e.g., stage I, grade 1, ~75%; grade 2, ~60%; grade 3, 25%)

Staging

Staging of endometrial carcinoma is based on the clinical extent of the disease, the histologic grade (differentiation of the neoplasm), and the presence or absence of cancer in the endocervical canal (Table 20-3). By using this staging at the time of diagnosis, the distribution of endometrial carcinomas is heavily weighted in the lesser categories: stage I 70%–75%, stage II 10%–15%, and the rest are stage III and stage IV. Current staging does not incorporate one other important prognostic indicator, the depth of myometrial invasion (hysterectomy required). This crucial detail, along with degree of anaplasia and cervical involvement, is directly related to nodal metastases, vaginal recurrence, and survival.

Differential Diagnosis

In the premenopausal female, a pregnancy must be ruled out. Other potentials in the diagnosis include uterine leiomyoma, endometrial hyperplasia, endometrial polyps, cervical polyps, other genital cancers (e.g., cervical, tubal, and ovarian), and metastatic cancers (e.g., bowel, breast, and bladder).

With increasing age, it is more likely that postmenopausal bleeding will be due to endometrial cancer, and by age 80, cancer is responsible in 50%–60% of cases.

Treatment

For optimal treatment results in endometrial cancer, therapy should be individualized by gynecologic oncologists in oncology centers. Surgery and radiation therapy are the two major therapeutic modalities for endometrial cancer. For stage I, grade 1 endometrial cancer, extrafascial total abdominal hysterectomy and bilateral salpingo-oophorectomy is the primary treatment of choice. Here, radiation therapy as a primary treatment averages a 20% lower cure rate. The *abdominal approach* to surgery is preferred because it allows the collection of peritoneal washings

Table 20-3. Clinical staging of carcinoma of the endometrium*

Stage 0	Carcinoma in situ. Histologic findings suggestive of malignant growth. (Cases of stage 0 should not be included in any therapeutic statistics.)
Stage I	Carcinoma is confined to the corpus.
Stage IA	Length of uterine cavity is ≤ 8 cm.
IB	Length of uterine cavity is > 8 cm. Stage I cases should be graded by histologic type as follows:
G1	Highly differentiated adenomatous carcinoma.
G2	Differentiated adenomatous carcinoma with partly solid areas.
G3	Predominantly solid or entirely undifferentiated carcinoma.
Stage II	Carcinoma has involved the corpus and the cervix.
Stage III	Carcinoma has extendeed outside the uterus but not outside the true pelvis.
Stage IV	Carcinoma has extended outside the true pelvis or has obviously involved the mucosa of the bladder or rectum. Bullous edema as such does not permit a case to be allotted to stage IV.

*Approved by the International Federation of Obstetricians and Gynecologists. Adopted by ACOG, 1976.
Note: On occasion, it may be difficult to decide whether the cancer involves the endocervix only or both the corpus and the endocervix. If a clear differentiation is not possible on examination of a specimen obtained by fractional curettage, adenocarcinoma should be classified as carcinoma of the corpus and epidermoid carcinoma as carcinoma of the cervix.

for cytology, permits evaluation of the peritoneal cavity for cancer spread, and allows survey of the retroperitoneal nodes. The cervix and tubes should be occluded to decrease the chance of cellular dissemination. If the tumor is grade 2 or 3 preoperatively, there is lymph node enlargement, or the surgical specimen (opened in the operating room) reveals deep myometrial penetration, lymph node dissection (aortic, iliac, and obturator) should be added if possible. Intraperitoneal radioactive colloids may be added postoperatively if positive washings are reported.

Adjuvant radiation therapy is recommended if there is one-third myometrial penetration by tumor, poor histologic differentiation, papillary serous or clear cell histology, lower uterine segment or cervical involvement, or extrauterine extension and for those at greater risk of metastasis. Adjuvant radiation therapy postoperatively in *stage I* reduces the rate of vaginal vault recurrence from 3%–8% to 1%–3% and is worthwhile for all other patients with resectable endometrial adenocarcinoma.

For *stage II,* the three options include radical hysterectomy and pelvic node dissection, primary radiation (intrauterine and vaginal implants plus external therapy) followed by extrafascial hysterectomy, and radiation without surgery. For *stage III,* therapy is usually total abdominal hysterectomy, bilateral salpingo-oophorectomy, and tumor debulking, followed by external radiation. However, other variations must be considered (e.g., individualized treatment of patients with vaginal extension). For *stage IV,* the uterus, tubes, and ovaries should be removed if possible, and the tumor should be debulked. This should be followed by radiation and hormone chemotherapy.

Endometrial carcinoma not amenable to surgery or radiation therapy may be treated with long-term (>3 months) *progesterone* (usually hydroxyprogesterone caproate or megestrol). The response rate is <35%, with a 20 month average response duration and 13% long-term remission of recurrent disease. Those responding survive 4 times longer than nonresponders, with ~30% of responders alive at 5 years. Indicators of good responsiveness include young patients, high levels of tumor receptors, well-differentiated tumors, and localized or late recurrence. Of the chemotherapy agents currently used for recurrent endometrial carcinoma, the most promising is tamoxifen, especially in the group with indicators of responsiveness.

Prognosis

Overall *5-year survival* of *stage I* endometrial carcinoma is 75%–95%. About 90% of recurrences occur <5 years. Those with *poorly differentiated tumors or deep myometrial invasion* have 5-year survivals of 50%–60%. In the latter group, there are 30%–40% positive pelvic nodes. Other overall 5-year survivals are *stage II* 50%–60%, *stage III* ~30%, and *stage IV* 5%–10%.

Sarcomas

Sarcomas of the uterus are heterogeneous, highly malignant tumors derived from mesodermal elements. They are uncommon, constituting only 2%–3% of all malignant tumors of the uterine corpus. The *etiology* of uterine sarcomas is unknown. However, there is a positive correlation between the mixed forms and prior pelvic radiation. Sarcomas usually occur after age 40 and spread by direct extension, lymphatic or hematogenous routes. Overall, sarcomas have a bad prognosis.

Classification and Staging

Several categories are necessary to classify uterine sarcomas: homologous (malignancies that histologically appear native to the uterus), heterologous (malignancies appearing foreign to the uterus), pure (composed of a single cell line), mixed (composed of ≥2 cell lines), and mesodermal, mullerian, or mesenchymal (depending on their differentiation). A summary of sarcoma classification is found in Table 20-4. Most clinicians apply the staging for endometrial carcinoma (Table 20-3) to sarcomas.

Pathology

About 55% of sarcomas (leiomyosarcoma) are derived from smooth muscle by heteroplasia, 40% are mixed mesenchymal or mesodermal tumors (probably related to endometrial stroma cells), <5% are carcinosarcoma, and the rest develop from blood vessels (angiosarcoma) or from connective tissue (reticulum cell sarcoma).

Sarcomas begin as localized silent tumors, gradually becoming diffuse and symptomatic on extension into and beyond the myometrium. Pain, obstruction, and inflammation do not occur until the tumor is moderately advanced. Extension into the uterine cavity or the formation of polypoid growths causes leukorrhea and abnormal bleeding. Metastases occur early via the bloodstream or lymphatics.

Leiomyosarcoma

A leiomyosarcoma rarely arises from a leiomyoma. Leiomyosarcomas usually occur in women in their 50s. The histologic features most correlated with outcome include the number of mitoses (per 10 hpf), vascular and lymphatic invasion, serosal extension, and degree of anaplasia. Mitoses per 10 hpf is closely associated with outcome: <5 usually is benign, ≥5 is diagnostic of leiomyosarcoma, 5–9 is low malignant potential, ≥10 has the worst prognosis. Premenopausal patients have a better prognosis than those who are postmenopausal. The overall 5-year survival

Table 20-4. Classification of uterine sarcomas*

Classification	Sarcoma
I. Pure sarcoma	
A. Homologous	
1. Smooth muscle tumors	Leiomyosarcoma
	Leiomyoblastoma
Metastasizing tumors with benign histology	Intravenous leiomyomatosis
	Metastasizing uterine leiomyoma
	Leiomyomatosis peritonealis disseminata
2. Endometrial stromal sarcoma	
a. Low grade	Endolymphatic stromal myosis
b. High grade	Endometrial stromal sarcoma
B. Heterologous	Rhabdomyosarcoma
	Chondrosarcoma
	Osteosarcoma
	Liposarcoma
C. Other sarcomas	
II. Malignant mullerian mixed tumors	
A. Homologous: Carcinoma and homologous sarcoma	Carcinosarcoma
B. Homologous: Carcinoma and heterologous sarcoma	
III. Mullerian adenosarcoma	Adenosarcoma
IV. Lymphoma	Lymphoma

*Modified from P. Clement and R.E. Scully. Pathology of uterine sarcomas. In: *Gynecologic Oncology.* M. Coppleson, ed. Churchill Livingstone, 1981, p 591.

is ~20%. However, when stage is considered (I and II), the survival is ~40%).

Leiomyoblastoma and Metastasizing Uterine Sarcomas with Benign Histology

Less common or unusual sarcomas, e.g., leiomyoblastoma, intravenous leiomyomatosis, metastasizing uterine leiomyoma, and leiomyomatosis peritonealis disseminata, must be differentiated from leiomyomas and leiomyosarcomas. Leiomyoblastomas are rare tumors made up of spindle-shaped, epithelial-like cells. They generally have <5 mitoses/hpf and are nearly always benign. Extrauterine intravenous extension of smooth muscle tissue (often described as wormlike) characterizes the rare intravenous leiomyomatosis. Metastasizing leiomyoma is characterized by extrapelvic smooth muscle nodules, found most frequently in the lymph nodes or lungs. Leiomyomatosis peritonealis disseminata is most frequently encountered during pregnancy. It may regress postpartum.

Endolymphatic Stromal Myosis

Endolymphatic stromal myosis occurs primarily in younger women (three fourths <50 years) and is frequently mistaken for leiomyomas because the primary clinical findings are abnormal uterine bleeding and an irregularly enlarged uterus. Histologically, these tumors consist of uterine stromal cells with a spindlelike appearance, having <10 mitoses/10 hpf. They are rare, being the least frequent among the uterine sarcomas, and are generally benign.

Endometrial Stromal Sarcoma

These uterine stromal cell sarcomas generally have >10 mitoses/ 10 hpf and carry a very poor prognosis. Endometrial stromal sarcoma is, like endolymphatic stromal myosis, usually found in women <50 years with abnormal bleeding and an irregularly enlarging uterus.

Malignant Mullerian Mixed Tumors (MMMT)

MMMTs occur in older women (generally >62 years) and generally occur clinically as postmenopausal bleeding with a large uterus. Prior pelvic radiation is a known etiologic association. Heterologous and homologous tumors occur with equal (albeit rare) frequency and have similar survival rates (overall 5-year survival ~20%) despite different histologic patterns.

Clinical Findings

Symptoms and Signs

A rapidly enlarging uterus or myoma may suggest sarcoma in a young girl or postmenopausal woman. Common complaints relative to sarcoma are abnormal uterine bleeding, abdominal enlargement, leukorrhea, urinary frequency, and pelvic discomfort. Protrusion of polyps through the cervix is ominous. Late manifestations are loss of weight, pain, orthopnea, jaundice, and edema of the legs.

Laboratory Findings

Anemia, increased ESR, and eosinophilia are reported in well-established sarcomas.

Imaging

Chest x-ray films should rule out pulmonary metastases. CT or MRI scans may be useful to detect abdominal or pelvic extension.

Cytologic Diagnosis and Biopsy

Vaginal cytologic examination may disclose malignant cells of endometrial sarcoma and mixed mesenchymal tumors, but they rarely indicate leiomyosarcoma or other sarcomas. Sarcomas arising from the endometrium can be diagnosed by biopsy or D & C, but leiomyosarcomas require more direct sampling.

Differential Diagnosis

A postmenopausal patient's leiomyoma that is rapidly enlarging, without large doses of estrogen, is a sarcoma until proven otherwise. In the premenopause, rapidly enlarging leiomyomas (particularly submucous) are usually benign. Metastatic carcinoma must also be considered.

Treatment

Therapy is largely surgical, with extrafascial total abdominal hysterectomy and bilateral salpingo-oophorectomy (TAH, BSO). In well-differentiated sarcomas, even more radical primary or secondary surgery may be justifiable. Radiation therapy may retard tumor growth and relieve distressing symptoms. However, radiation does not significantly increase life expectancy. Chemotherapy may be palliative and is most commonly used (multiple agent) to treat distant metastases.

Low-grade sarcomas (e.g., stromatosis) have a better prognosis than those of more malignant morphology or extent of growth. Well-encapsulated sarcomas incidentally discovered within leiomyomas metastasize infrequently, and cure is likely. Without treatment, invasive sarcoma of the uterus is fatal <18 months in 75% of patients. After therapy, 20%–30% survive 5 years.

GESTATIONAL TROPHOBLASTIC DISEASES

Gestational trophoblastic disease (GTD) is a general term for three tumors arising from fetal tissue containing both syncytiotrophoblastic and cytotrophoblastic cells: hydatidiform mole, chorioadenoma destruens (invasive mole), and choriocarcinoma. All three GTD tumors are the result of a genetic aberration whereby all of the tumor's chromosomal material is of paternal origin. Although the exact mechanism is not clear, there is inactivation or disappearance (perhaps via the polar body) of the ovum's chromosomal material, with subsequent ovum penetration by a diploid sperm or two sperms. *True* or *complete molar gestations* are usually euploid (46,XX), of paternal origin, and carry a 20% risk of malignancy. *Transitional molar gestations* are usually trisomic. *Partial moles* are triploid, of maternal and paternal origin, and are rarely malignant.

These tumors all have a characteristic tumor marker, human chorionic gonadotropin (hCG). The GTD tumors are currently the only disseminated solid tumors curable by chemotherapy alone.

HYDATIDIFORM MOLE

Hydatidiform mole occurs in 1/1500 in the United States and in 1/125 deliveries in Mexico. It is more commonly associated with previous molar gestation (increased over initial risk 20–40 times), low socioeconomic status, certain geographic locations (Southeast Asia and Mexico), poor diet (e.g., low protein, low folic acid, low carotene), and <20 years or >40 years. The overall recurrence is <5%.

Common *clinical findings* include uterine bleeding in the first trimester (90%), expulsion of vesicles (80%), rapid enlargement of the uterus (greater than expected by dates in 50%), multiple theca lutein cysts enlarging one or both ovaries (15%–30%), hyperemesis gravidarum (10%), onset of pregnancy-induced hypertension during the first trimester (10%–12%), and absent fetal heart tones.

Two tests (beta subunit hCG and ultrasonography) are invaluable in *diagnosis, management, and follow-up* of GTD tumors. Levels of hCG in urine or serum correspond to the number of viable tumor cells. Standard hCG levels are of value when high, but because most tests will not differentiate between LH and hCG, beta subunit hCG (β-hCG) levels are essential when hCG falls to the normal range of 20–30 mIU (the pituitary level of LH). Normal pregnancy is associated with β-hCG levels <60,000 mIU/ml, in contrast to levels of >100,000 mIU/ml seen in molar pregnancies.

Uterine *ultrasonography* demonstrates multiple echoes formed by the interface between the molar villi and surrounding tissue, with no gestational sac or fetus (or Swiss cheese pattern). Maternal hyperthyroidism occurs in 10% as a result of thyrotropin secretion by molar tissue.

Characteristic *gross pathologic findings* are multiple, 1–2 cm diameter, grapelike vesicles filling and distending the uterus. However, if small, hydatidiform moles may grossly resemble an abortus, and the diagnosis will only be made histologically. Edema of the villous stroma, avascular villi, and nests of proliferating syncytiotrophoblastic or cytotrophoblastic elements surrounding villi are characteristic *histopathologic findings*. Malignant sequelae occur more often if the trophoblastic cells are anaplastic or show proliferation.

Treatment consists of uterine evacuation as soon as the diagnosis has been confirmed. Suction curettage may be safely performed in uteri up to the size of 28 weeks gestation as long as precautions for emergency hysterectomy, hysterotomy, hypogastric artery ligation, and massive transfusion have been made. Oxytocin should be initiated intravenously once the uterine contents have been moderately decreased. Sharp curettage should follow suction curettage, and all specimens must be submitted for histopathology. If no further pregnancies are desired or in the older patient, hysterectomy may be the therapy of choice in the patient who is a good surgical risk.

CHORIOADENOMA DESTRUENS (INVASIVE MOLE)

Chorioadenoma destruens is simply a hydatidiform mole with myometrial invasion. Grossly, the tumor may penetrate the myometrium to such an extent that uterine rupture and hemoperitoneum occur. In addition to findings typical of a hydatidiform mole, the signs and symptoms in the cases of perforation are those of hemoperitoneum and may be life-threatening. The incidence of malignancy is ~10% in chorioadenoma destruens.

CHORIOCARCINOMA

Choriocarcinoma is an epithelial tumor composed of syncytiotrophoblastic and cytotrophoblastic cells that may accompany or follow any pregnancy, including ectopic. Microscopic examination of the tissue shows trophoblasts in sheets or isolated foci on a hemorrhagic or necrotic background. Choriocarcinomas occur in 1/40,000 normal pregnancies and 3%–5% of molar gestations.

The predilection for this disorder is increased 10 times in women of blood group A impregnated by a type O male (compared to a type A male). Women with blood type AB have a much poorer prognosis than any other blood group when malignancy occurs. Choriocarcinoma arising primarily has a worse prognosis than if it occurs after hydatidiform mole.

GENERAL PRINCIPLES OF GTD MALIGNANCY

Of those GTD patients developing malignancy, hydatidiform mole is responsible for 75% of those with nonmetastatic disease and for 50% of the metastatic disease. The rest occur after abortion, ectopic gestation, or term pregnancy. The presence of an excessively large uterus with multiple lutein cysts is associated with a malignancy risk of 57%.

If malignancy is diagnosed, the studies to be performed (in addition to those noted previously) include chest x-ray, CT scan and MRI of the brain, lungs, liver, and kidneys looking for metastatic disease. Liver and renal function tests should be performed. Establishing the ratio of hCG in CSF to that in serum will be helpful in follow-up of brain metastases. Fortunately, malignancy is most often confined to the uterus.

During the period of surveillance for malignant trophoblastic disease, be certain that pregnancy is avoided. This may be best accomplished using oral contraceptives. β-hCG levels should be obtained weekly until undetectable. Pelvic examination should be performed 1 week after evacuation, followed by examination every 4 weeks to evaluate the change in size of the uterus and the presence of theca lutein cysts. Evaluation of the cervix, vagina, urethra, and vulva for metastases is also important.

For *therapy,* patients are generally divided into two groups: those with a natural history suggesting good prognosis and those with a likely poor prognosis. The patients with GTD and a probable *good prognosis* include those who have nonmetastatic disease as well as those with metastatic disease outside the uterus with the following: disease of <4 months duration, metastases confined to lungs or pelvis, serum β-hCG <40,000 mIU/ml, and no prior chemotherapy. Failure of initial drug therapy occurs in ~6.5% of those with nonmetastatic malignant disease and in ~10% of the good prognosis patients with metastases.

Patients having metastatic disease with *poor prognosis* include the following: disease of >4 months duration, metastases to brain or liver, unsuccessful previous chemotherapy, and those with GTD following a term pregnancy. Even the poor prognosis patients may eventually achieve remission in >85% with proper therapy.

Dactinomycin and methotrexate are the most effective single *therapeutic agents* used. Radiation and combination chemotherapy are usually reserved for the poor prognosis patients. However, the details of chemotherapy for gestational trophoblastic disease should be sought from definitive sources.

Chapter 21

The Ovary and Oviducts

OVARY

Ovarian tumors are classified as benign (neoplastic and non-neoplastic) or premalignant/malignant. Benign nonneoplastic disease of the ovary is usually of an inflammatory or infectious nature and is discussed in Chapter 22 and Chapter 26. Table 21-1 details a classification of nonneoplastic ovarian lesions, Table 21-2 is the WHO classification of ovarian neoplasms, and Table 21-3 gives the characteristics of common ovarian neoplasms.

BENIGN OVARIAN NONNEOPLASTIC CYSTS

The *clinical assessment and therapy* of benign ovarian masses have been greatly aided by modern imaging techniques and the use of oral contraceptives to decrease pituitary gonadotropin stimulation. Ultrasonic scanning is the most frequently applied imaging technique for ovarian masses. Imaging modalities aid in the differentiation of ovarian enlargements from other masses or fullness in the pelvis, determine the structure of a tumor (solid or cystic, multilocular or unilocular), determine the size of a tumor (often difficult by physical examination in obese patients), and document the change in size of masses over time. In complex cases (e.g., cancer) more sophisticated imaging techniques (e.g., MRI) may assist in preoperative determinations.

Oral contraceptives administered daily for 4–8 weeks will resolve 80% of functional cystic ovarian masses not requiring surgery. Surgery for benign lesions in the premenopausal patient is removal of the lesion (cystectomy), not oophorectomy. The general indications for operative intervention are listed in Table 21-4.

Table 21-1. Classification of ovarian tumors

Nonneoplastic lesions
  Inflammatory diseases of the ovary
    Adhesive disease due to subacute or chronic infections
    Endometriosis
    Peritoneal inclusions
  Nonneoplastic cysts
    Follicle cysts
    Lutein cysts (corpus luteum, theca lutein cysts)
    Polycystic ovarian disease (Stein-Leventhal syndrome)
  Focal proliferation
    Thecosis
    Cortical granuloma
    Luteoma of pregnancy
Ovarian neoplasia (mesothelial)
  Mesothelial tumors (primarily epithelial)
    Serous
    Mucinous
    Endometroid
    Mesothelioid tumors
    Mesotheliomas
  Mesothelial tumors (primarily stromal)
    Fibroadenoma
    Cystadenofibroma
    Brenner tumor
    Granulosa-theca cell tumor
    Sertoli-Leydig cell tumor
    Gonadal stromal tumors
  Stromal (mesenchymal) tumors
    Fibroma
    Fibromyoma
    Gonadal stromal tumors
    Sarcoma
  Germ cell tumors
    Dysgerminoma
    Teratoma
      Embryonal
      Extraembryonal
        Endodermal sinus
        Polyvesicular vitelline (yolk sac)
        Choriocarcinoma
    Gonadoblastoma
Metastatic tumors and secondary malignant tumors

Table 21-2. World Health Organization
classification of ovarian neoplasms

Common epithelial tumors
Sex cord stromal tumors
Lipid (lipoid) cell tumors
Germ cell tumors
Gonadoblastoma
Soft-tissue tumors (not specific to ovary)
Unclassified tumors
Secondary (metastatic) tumors
Tumorlike conditions (not true neoplasm)

Table 21-3. Summary of characteristics of common ovarian neoplasms

| | Age* | % of all ovarian neoplasms | % of ovarian cancers | Benign % bilateral[†] | Malignant %[‡] | | |
					No	Yes	±
Epithelial							
Serous	30–50	20–50	35–40	10	70	20–25	5–10
Mucinous	30–60	15–25	6–10	8–10	85	5	10
Brenner tumor	40–50	1–2	<1	6	97	3	
Endometrioid	40–60	5	15–25				
Mesonephroid	>40	<5	5	Rare	70	30	
Germ cell							
Benign cystic teratoma	18–30	20–25	<1	12	>99	<0.5	
Dysgerminoma**	10–30	<1	0.1	5–30			

*The age given is for benign tumors, except where ** indicates malignant tumors. In the epithelial tumors, malignancy of each type generally occurs at an older age than the same benign tumor.
[†]Epithelial malignant tumors tend to have a higher incidence of bilaterality (serous cystadenocarcinoma 33%–66%, mucinous cystadenocarcinoma 10%–20%, malignant Brenner tumor up to 15%, endometroid carcinoma 13%–30%). This is not true of the germ cell tumors. Immature teratomas are 2%–5% bilateral, and other germ cell tumors are rarely bilateral, except dysgerminoma.
[‡]No, benign tumor %; Yes, malignant tumor %; ±, borderline.

Table 21-4. Indications for surgical exploration of patients with ovarian tumors

---

An ovarian cyst ≥5 cm persisting after 8 weeks of observation and/
  or oral contraceptive therapy
Any adnexal mass before menarche
An adnexal mass after the menopause
A solid mass at any age.
A cystic mass >8 cm in diameter.

Follicle Cyst

Follicle cysts are normal, transient, and often multiple, physiologic structures resulting from faulty resorption of the fluid from incompletely developed follicles. They occur most frequently in young, menstruating women and are the most common cysts found in normal ovaries. Their diameter may be microscopic to 8 cm (2 cm average). *Grossly,* they are translucent, thin walled, and filled with clear to slightly yellow fluid. *Histologically,* the wall of the cyst is formed by closely packed, round granulosa cells overlying a deeper layer of spindle-shaped theca cells.

Follicle cysts are usually asymptomatic and disappear spontaneously in <60 days. If symptoms occur, they usually involve an abnormally long or short intermenstrual interval. Intraperitoneal bleeding and torsion are rare complications. Any cyst that continues to enlarge or persist >60 days warrants further investigation. The usual investigation for cysts <4 cm is initial ultrasound examination, reexamination in 6 weeks and again in 8 weeks if the cyst persists. In follicle cysts ≥4 cm or if a small cyst is persistent, oral contraceptives for 4–8 weeks should cause resolution of the cyst.

Corpus Luteum Cyst

After ovulation, the granulosa cells becomes luteinized to form a corpus luteum. If blood leaks into the cavity during this process (which involves marked vascularization), a corpus hemorrhagicum is formed. Resolution involves resorption of the blood, and a corpus luteum cyst remains. A corpus luteum is termed a *corpus luteum cyst* if it is ≥3 cm. Occasionally, these cysts may be as large as 10 cm in diameter (average is 4 cm). Complications of this process may occur as a result of the original hemorrhage or as a result of the corpus luteum cyst.

A hemorrhagic corpus luteum usually causes local pain and tenderness (especially on pelvic examination). If the bleeding is so great that the ovarian capsule is ruptured, hemoperitoneum develops. Curiously, rupture is more frequent (two thirds) on the right. Bleeding usually causes a sudden, severe lower abdominal pain (but may have been preceded by aching discomfort). Pain most often occurs 14–60 days after the LMP. Not infrequently (about one fourth as frequent as bleeding ectopic pregnancy), the blood loss may be so severe that operative intervention (laparoscopy or laparotomy) is required to arrest the bleeding. The *usual operative intervention is ovarian cystectomy* with preservation of the ovary. The necessity for operation is established if the HCT of fluid obtained by culdocentesis is >15%.

If the hemorrhage is less severe, however, the pain and tenderness are associated with delayed menstruation or amenorrhea, and, thus, *corpus luteum cyst must be differentiated* from ectopic pregnancy as well as rupture of an endometrioma or adnexal torsion. This usually is accomplished by an hCG and an ultrasonic scan. In the absence of significant complications (hematoperitoneum or ovarian torsion), symptomatic expectant therapy (analgesia and observation) is advised.

In addition to spontaneously occurring corpus luteum cyst, *it is not uncommon for the corpus luteum of pregnancy to persist after a first trimester pregnancy loss.* All early corpus luteum cysts are purple to brown (depending on how long it has been since bleeding occurred) and smooth. In chronic cases, the wall may be gray-white. On cut surface, the cyst wall is usually yellow-orange, perhaps with a resolving blood clot, but in chronic cases, the cyst remnant may be gray-white to pale yellow. On *microscopic examination,* both the granulosa and theca cells are luteinized. In chronic cases, the cells may be atrophied due to pressure. The cyst is hormonally active, producing both estrogens and progesterone. Thus, *symptomatology* consists of menstrual abnormalities, unilateral pelvic pain, and a tender adnexal mass. Once ectopic pregnancy is excluded, conservative therapy (analgesics, observation, oral contraceptive therapy) may be instituted. Persistent cysts require 4–8 weeks of oral contraceptive therapy to resolve.

Theca Lutein Cyst

Theca lutein cysts usually are bilateral, small, and much less common than follicle or corpus luteum cysts. Theca lutein cysts are filled with straw-colored fluid. They are associated with gestational trophoblastic disease (i.e., hydatidiform mole, choriocarcinoma), multiple pregnancy or pregnancy complicated by diabetes mellitus or Rh sensitization, polycystic ovarian disease (Stein-Leventhal syndrome), and administration of ovulatory agents (e.g., clomiphene or hCG therapy).

Symptoms are usually minimal (e.g., pelvic fullness or pressure), even though the total ovarian size may be 10–20 cm. *Complications* are uncommon and include rupture (with intraperitoneal bleeding) and ovarian torsion. When theca lutein cysts are discovered, gestational trophoblastic disease must be ruled out. The cysts themselves require no therapy. Gestational trophoblastic disease is discussed elsewhere (p. 553).

Polycystic ovarian disease is seen in women 15–30 years old with bilateral enlarged polycystic ovaries, secondary amenorrhea, oligomenorrhea, and infertility. Obesity is common, and 50% are hirsute. The ovaries have a thick, whitish surface cortex with small fluid-filled follicle cysts below the surface (oyster ovaries).

The *diagnosis* is suggested from history and physical examination. The FSH is normal, and the LH is tonically elevated (without LH surge). The urinary 17-ketosteroid level may be elevated minimally. Diagnosis is confirmed by ultrasonography and laparoscopy.

Because these patients are anovulatory, the endometrium is stimulated by unopposed estrogen, thus increasing the risk for endometrial carcinoma.

The *treatment* is induction of ovulation, initially with cyclic clomiphene citrate, but hMG may be necessary (Chapter 27). Wedge resection has been successful in restoring fertility but should be used as a last resort because adhesive disease or ovarian insufficiency may result from surgery.

OVARIAN NEOPLASIA

Epithelial Tumors

Epithelial (mesothelial) tumors comprise 65% of all true ovarian neoplasms and ~85% of ovarian cancers. They arise from the original epithelial lining of the embryonic celomic cavity and are composed of both supporting connective tissue and ovarian stroma. Because ovarian stroma is present, all varieties of this tumor have a potential functional capacity. However, this group of tumors characteristically do not produce hormones. The several types of epithelial ovarian tumors include serous, mucinous, endometrioid, clear cell (mesonephroid), and Brenner tumors.

Serous Tumors

Serous tumors account for 20%–50% of all ovarian neoplasms and 35%–40% of ovarian cancers. About 70% of serous tumors are benign, 5%–10% have borderline malignant potential, and 20%–25% are malignant. Serous cystadenomas occur most frequently in women 30–50 years of age, and serous carcinomas occur in women >40 years. The tumor may enlarge to fill the abdominal cavity but usually weighs 4.5–9 kg. Few *symptoms* are reported. Serous tumors are generally discovered on routine pelvic examination. The tumor produces no hormones.

Originally, serous tumors are unilocular, contain a thin yellowish fluid, and have a smooth, fibrous capsule. Subsequently, they become multilocular, and papillary excrescences develop on both inner and outer surfaces. *Histologically,* serous tumors consist of fallopian tubelike, ciliated epithelial cells (cuboidal or low columnar cells). Small, sandlike, sharp, calcareous concretions (psammoma bodies) often are present within the tumor. They are well-differentiated (especially in younger women), whereas anaplastic lesions are more common in older patients.

Laboratory findings are not characteristically abnormal. Imaging is most helpful. X-ray studies may reveal the small calcifications of psammoma bodies. Ultrasonic scans or MRI are helpful in detailing the extent and configuration of the tumor. The *differential diagnosis* includes benign cystic teratomas, dysgerminomas, metastatic malignancy, and retroperitoneal tumors. *Complications* include malignancy, torsion, rupture, or intestinal obstruction.

Malignancy cannot be predicted by visual inspection. Serous tumors of low malignant potential are bilateral in 35%, with extraovarian extension in 30%. In contrast, 40%–60% of serous carcinomas are bilateral, with extraovarian extension in 85%. Over half are >15 cm, and malignant tumors may be unilocular or multilocular. Usually the more differentiated the tumor, the more likely it will be benign. Lesser differentiated serous carcinomas have a poor prognosis.

Malignant changes in cystadenomas are characterized by (1) excessive proliferation and extensive stratification of cells, (2) an intricate pattern with increased glandular elements, (3) spare stroma in proportion to epithelial cells, (4) anaplasia characterized by immature cells, variation in size and shape of cells and nuclei, numerous nucleoli, many undifferentiated cells, and numerous mitotic figures, and (5) invasion of the stroma or the capsule by glandular elements, with intralocular cyst formation.

Treatment of both benign and malignant tumors is surgical

removal individualized according to the operative findings. Pathology assessment is mandatory.

Cystadenofibroma and *fibrocystadenoma* are related, usually benign tumors, most commonly seen in the 40–60 year age group. There is a predominantly stromal component, with a variety of epithelial elements in the cystic areas. It is thought that cystadenofibroma and fibrocystadenoma are solid variations of serous cystadenomas.

Fibrocystic tumors are commonly unilateral (fibrocystadenoma is bilateral in 20%–25%), <3 cm in diameter (but up to 30 cm reported), and asymptomatic. On rare occasions, a hormone-producing tumor causes feminization. *Treatment* for cystadenofibroma and fibrocystadenoma is surgical removal, usually with hysterectomy and bilateral salpingo-oophorectomy in the postmenopausal woman. In premenopausal women, removal of the tumor (usually salpingo-oophorectomy) and inspection of the contralateral ovary probably is sufficient.

Mucinous Tumors

Mucinous tumors comprise 15%–25% of all ovarian neoplasms and account for 6%–10% of ovarian cancers. They are bilateral in 8%–10%. Mucinous tumors may be huge (>70 kg) but average 16–17 cm in diameter at diagnosis and are seen primarily in two age groups (10–30 years and >40 years). There are usually no *symptoms* other than fullness from an abdominal mass.

Mucinous tumors are smooth-walled with a tough parchmentlike capsule. They usually are multilocular, and contain brownish, thick, viscid liquid. *Histologically,* they are lined by endocervical-like or intestinal-like tall columnar epithelial and mucin-producing goblet cells. These tumors often develop a well-defined pedicle.

Mucinous tumors usually are of low malignant potential, but *mucinous carcinomas* account for 10%–20% of epithelial ovarian tumors. Stage I tumors are bilateral in only 10%. Extraovarian extension at diagnosis occurs in ~15% of the low malignant potential and in 40% of mucinous carcinomas.

The mucinous carcinoma has almost entirely intestinal-like cells. The tumor is composed of multiloculated cysts filled with viscous mucin. There may be solid areas of tumor, hemorrhage, or necrosis. These findings are not as predictive of malignant potential as in the serous tumors, however. The more differentiated the cells, the better the prognosis.

Peritoneal implantation of mucinous cells after extension or rupture of a mucinous ovarian tumor (usually of low malignant potential) or mucocele of the appendix results in propagation of tall columnar tumor cells and the accumulation of mucin within the abdomen known as *pseudomyxoma peritonei* (mucinous peritonitis). Although benign, this is a very serious complication leading to distention and multiple intestinal obstructions. It has a mortality rate of ~50%.

Treatment is unilateral salpingo-oophorectomy if the tumor is not bilateral and no malignancy is present. If malignancy is present, the primary therapy is surgical. Chemotherapy is less effective than for other ovarian epithelial cancers.

Endometrioid Tumors

Benign endometrioid neoplasms grossly resemble the far more common endometriosis (Chapter 26). Some pathologists believe the two must be differentiated from one another because ovarian endometrial neoplasms are composed of cells resembling the endometrial epithelium but do not have endometrial stroma and do not demonstrate the invasive characteristics of disseminated endometriosis. Moreover, it is believed that the endometrioid carcinomas arise from ovarian epithelium, as opposed to originating from endometriosis.

The *importance of endometrioid neoplasms is* not their frequency (~5%), but *their malignant potential* (~20% of all ovarian carcinomas). Endometrioid carcinoma usually occurs in women age 40–60 years. *Treatment* is similar to that of other ovarian cancers.

As in other ovarian cancers, the better differentiated the endometroid carcinoma, the better the *prognosis*. Recommended therapy is TAH, BSO, and omentectomy with removal of any affected pelvic tissues. The prognosis is improved if endometriosis is present. *Five-year survival* is ~80%. Adjunctive therapy includes radiation and chemotherapy, including progestational agents if progesterone receptors are present in tumor cells.

Brenner Tumor

The Brenner tumor (2%–3% of all primary ovarian tumors) is probably of epithelial origin. *Approximately 1%–2% are malignant,* and ~2% occur in association with a mucinous cystadenoma or benign cystic teratoma in the same or contralateral ovary. Brenner tumors occur in women 40–50 years of age. They are usually small (may reach 20 cm) and unilateral (5%–15%

bilateral). About 10%–15% are associated with endometrial hyperplasia.

Grossly, Brenner tumors are smooth, gray-white, solid neoplasms. On cut section, the tumor is homogeneous and gray to slightly yellowish with small cystic spaces. *Histologically,* the tumors have masses or nests of uniform epithelial cells surrounded by fibrous stroma. The epithelial cells have a coffee bean-appearing nucleus from a nuclear membrane indentation. *Therapy* is simple excision. Malignant tumors will require more extensive surgery and even adjuvant therapy.

It is rare for the Brenner tumor to undergo malignant transformation, but when this occurs, surgical therapy should be followed by radiation because chemotherapy is ineffective. If the tumor extends beyond the ovary at diagnosis, 5-year survival is extremely rare.

Mesonephroid Tumors (Clear Cell Carcinomas)

Mesonephroid tumors are a small group of ovarian neoplasms composed of scattered glycogen-rich pseudoglomerular cell groupings suggestive of the mesonephros. They commonly are multifocal and may involve the peritoneal surfaces from diaphragm to pelvis. Most mesonephroid tumors occur in women >40 years of age. *At least 30% of mesonephroid tumors are malignant.*

Grossly, mesonephroid tumors are unilateral, fairly well encapsulated, grayish brown, smooth, free, semisoft or cystic. Friable tissue and thin serous fluid fill the loculi and tissue spaces. Areas of cystic degeneration and even hemorrhagic extravasation may be seen. Most tumors are 10–20 cm in diameter. Two main *histologic types* are recognized: a semisolid clear cell variety and a more adenomatous papillary type with groups of prominent protruding hobnail epithelial cells studding the acinous spaces. The tumor cells may be mesothelial, ciliated, secretory, or a combination without mitotic activity. The *differential diagnosis* includes cystadenomas, metastatic clear cell carcinomas of renal origin, and other poorly differentiated tumors.

Mesonephroid carcinomas are rarely large and have both cystic and solid components. About 85% are diagnosed in women >40 years of age. The cell types may be either clear cell or pseudoglomerular, characteristic of the kidney tumor. Extraovarian extension occurs late and about two thirds are unilateral at presentation.

Hyperpyrexia and hypercalcemia are associated with mesonephroid carcinoma for obscure reasons. Otherwise, symptoms are similar to those of other ovarian cancers. The tumor must be differentiated from a renal tumor metastatic to the ovary. *Treatment* requires the elimination of as much of the tumor mass as possible: total abdominal hysterectomy, bilateral salpingo-oophorectomy, and tumor debulking. Radiation or chemotherapy is largely ineffective, and if the tumor has spread, the *prognosis* is guarded. Five-year survival is ~60% in stage I and almost zero in stage III or IV.

Germ Cell Tumors

Germ cell tumors are derived from ovarian germ cells and *comprise 20%–25% of all ovarian tumors*. Germ cell tumors may occur at any age, but they are more common in younger women, constituting ~60% of ovarian neoplasms occurring in infants and children. Although the vast majority are adnexal, they may be located anywhere from the base of the ovarian mesentery (in which the embryonic germ cells migrate to the gonad) to the ovary. The World Health Organization's classification of germ cell tumors is given in Table 21-5. Nearly all the tumors of this category are benign cystic teratomas.

Table 21-5. World Health Organization classification of germ cell tumors

Dysgerminoma
Endodermal sinus tumor
Embryonal carcinoma
Polyembryoma
Choriocarcinoma
Teratomas
 Immature
 Mature
  Solid
  Cystic
   Dermoid cyst (mature cystic teratoma)
   Dermoid cyst with malignant transformation
 Monodermal and highly specialized
  Struma ovarii
  Carcinoid
  Struma ovarii and carcinoid
  Others
Mixed forms

Teratomas

Generally, teratomas are tumors with one or more of the three embryologic layers, ectoderm, mesoderm, and endoderm. They may be benign (mature) or malignant (immature). They are also categorized by the predominant tissue type and their gross configuration (solid or cystic). Teratomas are usually found in the midline or unilateral in the ovary. Mature tissues (teeth, hair, skin, muscle, bone, cartilage) are easily recognized in the neoplasm. The extraembryonic tissues are of trophoblast or endodermal sinus origin. Teratoid tumors are usually asymptomatic unless *complications,* such as rupture, torsion, fistula formation, or peritonitis, occur. *Malignant teratomas are uncommon.* If there is a thyroid preponderance (struma ovarii) or carcinoid preponderance in the teratoma, *clinical symptoms* (hyperthyroidism, carcinoid syndrome) may become evident.

Benign Cystic Teratomas (Dermoid Tumors). Benign cystic teratomas are the most common ovarian tumors during the early reproductive years (18–30 years). Benign cystic teratomas are parthogenic in origin. Overall, *they comprise 20%–25% of primary ovarian tumors,* and about 10%–15% are bilateral. Benign cystic teratomas contain ectodermal (and often mesodermal) tissue in the form of macerated skin, hair, bone, and teeth. The cyst is filled with a heavy, greasy sebaceous material. A long pedicle is often present.

Benign cystic teratomas may be minute, but most weigh <0.5 kg, and they may be much larger. The tumor wall is smooth and tough. The neoplasm generally has a yellowish cast from sebaceous material within the tumor. On opening the tumor, striking amounts of grumous sebaceous material and hair are revealed. The various structures noted above may be apparent on *gross or histologic examination.* Most commonly, the cysts are lined by epidermal-like stratified squamous epithelium with sudoriparous and sebaceous glands as well as numerous hair follicles. Solid tumors are rare (<0.1% of all ovarian tumors).

Clinically, benign cystic teratomas float upward in the abdomen, elongating the ovarian pedicle and causing them to lie anterior and superior to the uterus (Kustner's sign). This is in contrast to other ovarian tumors, which are generally found posterior to the uterus. Few symptoms are related to this freely shifting, lower abdominal tumor unless it exceeds 10 cm (when it may exert nonspecific pressure symptoms). Thus, benign cystic teratomas are usually asymptomatic, although three major complications may cause striking symptoms. Torsion may occur with the usual abdominal pain. Rupture leads to peritonitis, and impaction in the pelvis during pregnancy can cause nonengagement of the fetus.

Imaging is very useful for diagnosis because calcified bone or teeth may be seen on ultrasonic scans or by radiography. *Laboratory studies* may reveal functional thyroid tissue (struma ovarii) in ~5% or the presence of carcinoid or choriocarcinoma revealed by their respective metabolites [T_4, 5-hydroxyindoleacetic acid (5-HIAA), and hCG]. *Never aspirate cystic tumors*, e.g., teratomas, through the cul-de-sac for diagnostic or therapeutic purposes because leakage may cause chemical peritonitis, adhesion formation, bowel obstruction, or spread of cancer.

Treatment is surgical removal of the tumor (cystectomy), leaving as much ovarian tissue as is identifiable to preserve fertility. Occasionally, it may be necessary to perform unilateral oophorectomy, but that is unusual. Care should be taken not to spill tumor contents into the pelvic cavity. At the time of surgery, the contralateral ovary should be inspected carefully. However, surgical incision (bivalving the ovary) for inspection is not only unnecessary, it is so inimical to future reproduction that it has been abandoned.

Malignant changes in mature teratomas occur very infrequently (<0.5%). Of these, squamous epithelial malignancies are the most common. When the tumor is confined to the ovary it is usually treated by excision. However, if the tumor has broken through the ovarian capsule, the prognosis is poor even with radiation or chemotherapy or both. Malignant struma ovarii may be treated effectively with ^{131}I.

Carcinoid elements in a teratoma may cause a *carcinoid syndrome* in ~30% of patients. Carcinoids occur in older women and tend to be unilateral and slow growing. If the patient is young and childbearing is desired, stage Ia tumors may be treated by unilateral salpingo-oophorectomy. More advanced cases and all of those who do not desire childbearing should be treated by bilateral salpingo-oophorectomy. Postoperatively, 5-HIAA may be used to monitor the success of treatment.

Malignant Teratomas.   Overall, immature (malignant) teratomas account for <1% of all ovarian tumors, but they are the second most common germ cell malignancy (after dysgerminoma). Moreover, since ~75% occur at <20 years of age, malignant teratomas comprise ~20% of malignant ovarian tumors in women under 20. Malignant teratomas are rarely bilateral, but ~5% of cases have a contralateral benign teratoma. Characteristically, these tumors grow rapidly and cause pain as an early feature. However, they do not produce hCG or AFP. At diagnosis, two thirds are confined to the ovary.

Malignant teratomas may be of three varieties: choriocarcinoma (tumor marker hCG), endodermal sinus tumor (tumor marker AFP), or polyvesicular vitelline. Dysgerminoma will be associated in ~30%.

Therapeutic decisions must incorporate tumor grade and the preservation of childbearing. Because the tumor is always unilateral, removal of the affected ovary is the only surgery required, but this must be followed by combined chemotherapy immediately thereafter. Preservation of the unaffected ovary maintains fertility in these young patients. If the tumor is confined to one ovary, there is no convincing evidence that bilateral salpingo-oophorectomy and hysterectomy will improve the outcome over unilateral salpingo-oophorectomy. However, for all ovarian tumors over grade 1 and those with metastasis, adjunctive chemotherapy is required. Additionally, if metastases exist, efforts should be made to sample as much of the tumor as possible. Following surgery, prolonged chemotherapy, e.g., VAC (vincristine, dactinomycin, and cyclophosphamide), has demonstrated effectiveness. Second-look surgery has documented the ability to convert immature to mature elements (which require no more therapy).

In the adult experiencing malignant degeneration of a benign teratoma, the tumor most often found is a squamous cell carcinoma. Nonetheless, mucinous cancers, malignant melanoma, mixed tumors, thyroid cancer, and others have been reported. The *prognosis* depends on the tumor type, grade, and extent of disease at diagnosis. The most common adjunctive therapy after surgery is total pelvic radiation, but this is not usually successful.

Dysgerminomas

Dysgerminomas are the most frequent malignant germ cell tumors and the most frequent ovarian malignancy in young women. Dysgerminomas account for 0.1% of ovarian malignancies and represent only 1% of germ cell tumors. Dysgerminomas are not hormonally active, being analogous to male seminomas. Dysgerminomas occur most commonly between 10 and 30 years of age (80% <30 years, 50% <20 years). They tend to grow rapidly and are bilateral in 10%–30% of cases. Clinically, dysgerminomas are most frequently identified because of abdominal enlargement (tumor growth and ascites). Acute pain may accompany capsular rupture.

These typically unilateral tumors are 3–5 cm in diameter in most cases. Dysgerminomas are grayish brown, smooth, rounded, thinly encapsulated, nonadherent, and semisolid (rubbery). On cut surface, the appearance is edematous and brainlike. Histologically, dysgerminomas are composed of primitive germ cell nests separated by lymphocytic infiltrated fibrous trabeculae. It is the tumor type occurring in dysgenetic gonads. Hemorrhage and cystic degeneration are common. Histologic grading cannot be applied to dysgerminomas. Giant cells representing trophoblastic elements may secrete hCG, which may cause a weakly positive pregnancy test in a rare patient. A teratoma may be associated with the dysgerminoma, but because of the high incidence of dysgenetic gonads in such patients, a karyotype should be performed.

If confined to one ovary, *treatment* by unilateral salpingo-oophorectomy is as effective (5-year survival >90%) as more extensive surgery. A 20% recurrence rate (particularly in tumors >15 cm) is likely, but since the tumors are radiosensitive (some cured after <3000 rad), radiotherapy is effective in elimination of recurrences. Close follow-up (CT scans, MRI) of patients is mandatory. Sampling the contralateral ovary at surgery is necessary because of the incidence of bilaterality. More advanced tumors should be treated with a combination of surgery and radiotherapy. Chemotherapy is useful in cases where radiotherapy fails or is not feasible.

Prognosis is related to tumor type (pure dysgerminomas have a better prognosis than mixed germ cell tumors), unilateral occurrence (better than bilateral), tumor size (better if <15 cm), encapsulation (better than spread beyond the capsule), lack of nodal metastasis, and absence of ascites. If the tumor is bilateral or if extraovarian extension has occurred, surgery should consist of TAH and BSO followed by chemotherapy or radiotherapy or both. The 5-year survival rate for unilateral disease (stage Ia) is ~95%. In more advanced disease, the 5-year survival rate is <70%.

Other Germ Cell Tumors

Endodermal sinus (yolk sac) *tumors* are rare (<1% of ovarian) malignancies. They occur primarily in young women (median 19 years) and may even affect small children. Endodermal sinus tumors produce AFP, which may be used for both identification and follow-up. *Treatment* for stage Ia is unilateral salpingo-oophorectomy. More advanced cases should receive chemotherapy (e.g., VAC). The *prognosis* must be guarded.

Embryonal carcinomas are rare malignant germ cell tumors that produce hCG and AFP. They occur primarily in young women and are treated similarly to endodermal sinus tumors.

Nongestational choriocarcinoma is a rare but highly malignant germ cell tumor occurring in young women (<20 years). Like gestational choriocarcinoma, these tumors produce hCG. Non-gestational choriocarcinoma must be treated with multiple-agent chemotherapy after surgical excision.

Combinations of the various germ cell tumors are called *mixed germ cell tumors*. Therapy must be individualized with consideration of the germ cell elements present.

Sex Cord Stromal Tumors

These tumors are derived from the sex cords and specialized stroma of the developing ovary. Cumulatively, *sex cord stromal tumors represent ~6% of ovarian neoplasms*. Although this tumor classification contains the majority of hormonally active ovarian tumors, some have no or low potential for hormone production (e.g., fibroadenoma, cystadenofibroma). Others have a high functional potential (e.g., granulosa-theca cell, Sertoli-Leydig, gonadal stromal tumors).

Tumors in this category may have a male or female differentiation based on their sex cord component (female is granulosa cell sex cord and theca cell or fibroblast stromal elements; male is Sertoli cell sex cord and Leydig cell stromal component).

Granulosa-Theca Cell Tumors

Granulosa-theca cell tumors may develop in any age group. They account for ~5% of patients with precocious puberty (<9 years). If granulosa-theca tumors occur during the menstrual years, ~5% will cause amenorrhea and signs of estrogen excess. Because of tonically elevated and unopposed estrogen levels, ovulation is inhibited, and the proliferative endometrium may become hyperplastic. Other symptomatology in the postmenopausal years is related to estrogen stimulation (breast soreness, fluid retention, nausea). In addition to endometrial hyperplasia, endometrial carcinoma may occur.

Granulosa-theca cell tumors are usually yellow-orange and <15 cm in diameter. Some may be microscopic. They usually are unilateral (3%–8% bilateral). Granulosa cell tumors are constituted primarily of granulosa cells with lesser thecal or fibrous elements. Characteristically, the granulosa cells surround Call-Exner bodies (eosinophilic areas) set in a follicular pattern. Luteinization may occur, and the primary hormone production is estrogen. Mitoses are normal in the proliferating granulosa of the normal developing follicle. Hence, mitotic figures are not abnor-

mal in these tumors. The *histologic pattern* is not directly correlated with clinical malignant potential. The very well differentiated tumors tend to be benign, but these tumors overall tend to be
low-grade malignancies, often with late (>5 years) recurrences
(some after 10–15 years).

Treatment is surgical excision of the ovary containing the tumor unless both ovaries are involved or no further children are
desired, in which case total hysterectomy and bilateral salpingo-
oophorectomy are advised. Both chemotherapy and radiation
therapy are useful adjuncts. *Prognosis* is adversely affected by
tumors >15 cm in diameter, advanced clinical stage, tumor rupture, or high incidence of mitoses in the tumor. The 10-year
survival rate is ~90%.

The luteoma of pregnancy is discussed elsewhere.

Sertoli-Leydig Cell Tumors

The Sertoli-Leydig cell tumor classicially is a gonadostromal lesion with tubular differentiation. *These tumors are rare* (<500
cases reported) and occur in women in the reproductive age.
Sertoli-Leydig cell tumors cause hirsutism and masculinization in
one third of patients. Rarely, they produce estrogens.

Grossly, Sertoli-Leydig cell tumors are unilateral, small, solid
tumors with a smooth capsule. The color varies, but most are
yellowish brown. They have *histologic components* that resemble
the testis (tubules of Sertoli cell surrounded by Leydig cells). A
karyotype should be performed to rule out the Y chromosome.

Therapy has generally been surgical, but insufficient data exist to detail adjunctive therapy. Since the tumors behave as low-
grade malignancies, the 5-year survival is high (70%–90%). *Prognosis* is adversely affected when tumors are poorly differentiated
or are in an advanced stage.

Fibromas and Thecomas

These tumors represent up to 4% of ovarian tumors and include
the fibroma, fibrothecoma, and thecoma. Fibroma is by far the
most frequently seen in this category, and fibroma tends to become larger than the others. Fibromas are not usually hormonally active and are usually found on routine pelvic examination as a firm adnexal mass. Tumors in this category arise from
the undifferentiated mesenchymal component. They are most
commonly seen in patients aged 40–60 years. When functioning

components are present (thecal cells), expect signs of estrogen stimulation.

Grossly, tumors of this group are typically unilateral, grayish white, encapsulated, round, lobulated tumors, which rarely are >10 cm diameter. Thecomas consist entirely of stromal (theca) cells, and fibromas are composed of fibrous (spindle-shaped) cells. Combinations of the two components occur.

Meigs-Demons syndrome (transudative hydrothorax and ascites associated with a *benign* ovarian tumor) may be present. Ovariectomy results in resolution of Meigs-Demons syndrome in <2 weeks.

In premenopausal patients, these usually benign tumors should be *treated* by unilateral salpingo-oophorectomy. If the patient is postmenopausal, hysterectomy and bilateral salpingo-oophorectomy are advised. The *prognosis* is good.

Gynandroblastomas

These rare sex cord stromal tumors consist of both female and male cell types.

Gonadal Stromal Tumors (With or Without Tubular Structures)

These tumors may be well-differentiated (Pick's adenoma), intermediate (poorly defined tubules with gonadal stromal cells with interstitial cell foci), or sarcomatoid (stromal) tumors (no tubular structures). Gonadal stromal tumors are usually feminizing. They are unilateral (bilateral in <5%) and infrequently progress to malignancy (<10%). The patient is usually a younger woman, although all ages have been reported. *Treatment* is aimed at preserving the uterus and one ovary unless the karyotype reveals a Y chromosome.

Hilus Cell Tumor

The hilus cell tumor is a virilizing ovarian neoplasm (hirsutism, alopecia, enlarged clitoris, sometimes deepening of voice) in perimenopausal or early postmenopausal women. Endometrial hyperplasia may develop in some patients, suggesting simultaneous androgenic and estrogenic effect. The tumor is brown to yellowish brown, typically unilateral, and <4–5 cm in diameter. An adrenal tumor and familial hirsutism must be ruled out. *Treatment* is surgical removal of the tumor. The prognosis is good.

Gonadoblastoma

Gonadoblastomas are rare tumors with germ cell (often dysgerminoma-like) and sex cord-stromal (often immature granulosa and Sertoli cell-like) elements. In pure form, these tumors do not metastasize. There is a higher occurrence of gonadoblastoma in phenotypic females with a Y chromosome. Such patients should be advised to have the gonads removed.

Like the germinoma, the gonadoblastoma is also common in dysgenetic gonads. Most patients will be phenotypic and genetic females, but a karyotype should be performed to rule out a Y component. The *pathologic features* of this tumor are the unencapsulated germ cell, an attempt at tubule formation, folliculoid pattern with nests of granulosa cells surrounding large eosinophilic bodies, and focal calcification. *Therapy* consists of bilateral salpingo-oophorectomy.

Lipoid Tumors

These very rare tumors (<100 cases) may cause virilization or excess cortisol production and are composed of cells that resemble cells of the adrenal cortex, Leydig cells, or luteinized ovarian cells. Occasionally, metastases have occurred. *Treatment* requires removal of the involved ovary, but data are insufficient to detail total therapy.

Unclassified Tumors

Multifocal neoplasia and ovarian neoplasia associated with other types of genital cancer are difficult to classify. Because the ovarian mesothelium and the endometrium have a common embryonic origin, tumors may arise in separate foci in the ovary and endometrium without representing metastatic disease. If the lesions are truly multifocal, the prognosis is much improved (80% 5-year survival) compared to metastatic disease (30%–35%).

Treatment of multifocal ovarian cancer is the same as for endometrial carcinoma, i.e., TAH and BSO. Because 25% of the ovarian tumors are not palpable at surgery, they may be an incidental finding during therapy for primary uterine cancer.

Secondary (Metastatic) Tumors

Metastatic Tumors from Genital Primary Malignancy

Metastatic disease to the ovary from the lower genital tract is rare (1%–2%) but may represent direct extension through the broad ligament rather than true metastatic disease.

Metastatic Ovarian Tumors from Extragenital Primary Malignancy

Metastases to the ovary are common, especially if the primary cancer is in the breast or gastrointestinal tract. *These represent 1% of all ovarian neoplasia.* They are commonly bilateral (75%) and may reach massive proportions. The cell pattern will vary depending on the primary malignancy. One recognizable tumor, Krukenberg tumor, is characterized by coarse, abundant, occasionally edematous stroma with islands of moderately large epithelial cells with mucin-laden or vacuolated cytoplasm and eccentrically placed, small hyperchromatic nuclei resembling signet rings. The *primary tumor* is usually stomach but may be intestinal, breast, or thyroid in origin. Slight estrogen production is not unusual. *Treatment* is surgical, with removal of as much tumor as possible, followed by adjunctive chemotherapy. The overall *prognosis* is most discouraging.

Malignant and Premalignant Ovarian Neoplasia

Approximately 15% of ovarian tumors are malignant, and ovarian cancer is the fifth leading cause of death in women. The incidence of malignancy increases with age, averaging 50–59 years. Over 80% of deaths from ovarian cancer occur between 35 and 75 years. The lifetime risk of developing ovarian cancer in the United States (unchanged in 30 years) is 1.4%. Because these tumors are difficult to diagnose and treat early, the *5-year sur-*

vival rate is only 35%–38%, despite improved chemotherapy and radiotherapy.

Staging

The most widely used staging for ovarian neoplasia is that of the International Federation of Gynecology and Obstetrics (FIGO) (Table 21-6). Recall that ovarian cancer staging includes all of the operative findings, in contrast to cancer of the cervix and vulva, where staging is based on the nonoperative clinical findings.

Pathophysiology

Although *ovarian cancer accounts for 15%–20% of female reproductive tract cancer,* it causes more deaths than the others combined. Ovarian cancer is usually silent until palpable or widely disseminated.

Ovarian cancer is more frequent in infertile women or in those who have had repeated spontaneous abortion, delayed childbearing, or breast cancer. In the United States, the incidence is 6–7/100,000, with about equal rates in blacks and whites.

Malignant ovarian tumors in children are most often of germ cell origin, whereas those of adult women are malignant epithelial tumors (>90%), of which 70% have metastasized outside the pelvis at the time of diagnosis. The site of metastatic disease is as follows: peritoneum (85%), pelvic and aortic lymph nodes (80%), omentum (70%), contralateral ovary (70%), mediastinal or supraclavicular lymph nodes (50%), liver (35%), pleura (33%), lung (25%), uterus (20%), vagina (15%), bone (15%), spleen (5%–10%), kidney (5%–10%), adrenal (5%–10%), skin (5%–10%), vulva (1%), and brain (1%).

The ovaries may become the site of metastases of other primary tumors or may be involved by simple extension.

Diagnosis

There is no routine screening test available for ovarian cancer. Symptoms of pain may occur with significant distention, inflammation, torsion, or traction. Pelvic pressure may be reported if the

Table 21-6. International Federation of Gynecology and Obstetrics (FIGO) staging of ovarian neoplasms (modified, 1985)

Stage		Characteristics
Stage	I	Growth limited to the ovaries.
	Ia	Growth limited to one ovary; no ascites. No tumor on the external surface; capsule intact.
	Ib	Growth limited to both ovaries; no ascites. No tumor on the external surface; capsule intact.
	Ic	Tumor either stage Ia or Ib but with tumor on surface of one or both ovaries; or with capsule ruptured; or with ascites present containing malignant cells or with positive peritoneal washings.
Stage	II	Growth involving one or both ovaries with pelvic extension.
	IIa	Extension and/or metastases to the uterus and/or tubes
	IIb	Extension to other pelvic tissues.
	IIc	Tumor either stage IIa or IIb, but with tumor on surface of one or both ovaries; or with capsule(s) ruptured; or with ascites present containing malignant cells or with positive peritoneal washings.
Stage	III	Tumor involving one or both ovaries with peritoneal implants outside the pelvis and/or positive retroperitoneal or inguinal nodes. Superficial liver metastasis equals stage II. Tumor is limited to the true pelvis but with histologically proven malignant extension to small bowel or omentum.
	IIIa	Tumor grossly limited to the true pelvis with negative nodes but with histologically confirmed microscopic seeding of abdominal peritoneal surfaces.
	IIIb	Tumor of one or both ovaries with histologically confirmed implants of abdominal peritoneal surfaces none >2 cm in diameter. Nodes are negative.
	IIIc	Abdominal implants >2 cm in diameter and/or positive retroperitoneal or inguinal nodes.
Stage	IV	Growth involving one or both ovaries with distant metastases. If pleural effusion is present, there must be positive cytology to allot a case to stage IV. Parenchymal liver metastasis equals stage IV.

tumor is large. Enlarging abdominal girth, weight gain or loss, and gastrointestinal symptoms ranging from indigestion to intestinal obstruction may occur with ovarian cancer. Diagnosis depends on appropriate clinical, laboratory, and surgical evaluation.

Clinical Evaluation

A careful history and complete physical examination are most important. The most common physical findings are adnexal masses, an abdominal mass, ascites, or nodulation. Any fixed mass in the posterior cul-de-sac must be considered as possibly malignant, as is any large, fixed mass.

Laboratory Evaluation

Preoperative evaluation for suspected ovarian cancer includes complete blood count and typing, blood chemistry, urinalysis, cervical and vaginal cytology, radiographs of the chest and abdomen, intravenous pyelography, barium enema, and possibly liver function tests, coagulation profile, GI series, proctosigmoidoscopy, liver and bone scans. Ultrasonography, CT scan, or MRI of the pelvis also may be helpful. Finally, Ca_{125} or CEA tumor antigens may assist in evaluation for malignancy.

Surgical Evaluation

Surgical exploration is necessary to obtain tissue for histologic study, to stage the tumor, and, hopefully, to effect cure. A midline incision of sufficient size to allow intact tumor removal and complete exploration is necessary. Peritoneal washing is performed if there is no peritoneal fluid available for cytologic sampling in unilateral disease. Lavage with 100 ml saline should be performed in four areas.

1. Undersurface of the diaphragm
2. Lateral to the ascending colon
3. Lateral to the descending colon
4. The pelvic peritoneal surfaces

Washings are less helpful if malignant extension to the peritoneal surfaces or omentum has occurred or if the entire tumor cannot be removed. Both visualization and palpation of all peritoneal surfaces and abdominal organs are mandatory to search for metastatic disease. Any suspicious area(s) should be biopsied.

The tumor should be removed after exploration unless it is so large that surgical elimination is impossible.

Treatment

Standard therapy consists of total abdominal hysterectomy (TAH), bilateral salpingo-oophorectomy (BSO), and omentectomy. Retroperitoneal nodes should be palpated and biopsied if suspicious. As much tumor as possible (debulking) should be removed to decrease overall tumor mass. However, more radical surgery has not been proven to be of added benefit. Frozen sections may be helpful, but permanent histologic sections must be reviewed carefully before prognosis is given. In the woman with an epithelial or germ cell neoplasm of low malignant potential who understands the risks for late recurrence (10 year survival ~95%) and who wishes to preserve childbearing potential, surgery may be more conservative.

In some cases, the disease is too extensive for total hysterectomy, adnexectomy, and omentectomy. In such cases, as much tumor as possible should be removed to improve the results of adjunctive therapy (chemotherapy and radiation therapy). Chemotherapy is the preferred initial adjunctive therapy, since radiation therapy has limitations (e.g., damage to the liver or kidneys). Reexploration (second-look surgery) may be of benefit if remarkable response to adjunctive therapy is documented in previously inoperable cases. Response rates of 40%–45% can be anticipated.

THE OVIDUCT

BENIGN TUMORS

These neoplasms are usually asymptomatic and are not palpable. They usually are discovered incidentally during surgery or investigative procedures.

Cysts of the uterine tube are fairly common, most often occurring near the fimbriated end as the result of occlusion of the accessory lumina of the tube during embryogenesis. On rare occasion, pregnancy may develop in the cyst or torsion may occur. Otherwise, they are asymptomatic.

Epithelial polyps may be located in the cornual portion of the tube. More distal tubal polyps are rare. *Mesotheliomas* are <1.5 cm in diameter. They are asymptomatic and found incidentally. *Leiomyomas* occur primarily in the cornual portion of the tube. *Tubal teratomas* have the same elements as ovarian teratomas but are located on the uterine tube.

MALIGNANT TUMORS

Primary Oviduct Carcinoma

Primary tubal carcinoma is the least common cancer of the female reproductive tract. It is associated with nulliparity in ~50% of the cases and usually becomes symptomatic in the early 50s. Like ovarian cancer, there are few complaints other than an intermittent serosanguineous discharge in ~30%. Occasionally, vaginal cytologic studies will be positive and lead to further investigation. Ascites is rare. Early in the disease, a slightly tender adnexal mass may be palpated during pelvic examination. Ultrasonography may demonstrate a partially cystic, partially solid mass separate from the ovary and uterus. Hysterosalpingography should be avoided, or dispersal of malignant cells into the peritoneal cavity may occur. Laparoscopy is of little value, since treatment is surgical excision. Barium enema and chest x-ray should be part of the workup, but liver and bone scans are rarely necessary. *Late manifestations* are lower abdominal discomfort or enlargement and intestinal obstruction.

The vast majority (95%) of primary tubal cancer is papillary adenocarcinoma. In 40%–50%, bilateral tumors are found, which may represent bilateral primary disease rather than metastases. With time, the papillary tumor progresses to papillary-alveolar, then to alveolar carcinoma. Extratubal extension does not necessarily portend poor prognosis.

Treatment is hysterectomy and bilateral salpingo-oophorectomy. Surgery is followed by chemotherapy or radiation therapy.

Other Malignant Tumors of the Oviduct

Other tumors of the oviduct include *mixed mesodermal tumors, choriocarcinoma,* and *mesonephroma. Therapy* is essentially the same as for the same tumor type located in the ovary or uterus.

ADNEXAL TORSION

Most commonly, torsion of the ovary and tube occur together, although the ovary alone may occasionally be twisted on its pedicle. *Adnexal torsion accounts for ~3% of gynecologic operative emergencies.* Adnexal torsion occurs more often in children. In adults (the average patient is in her mid-20s), 50%–60% of torsions occur with an ovarian mass (most common at ~8–12 cm), and the most common ovarian tumor involved is benign cystic teratoma. However, solid benign tumors, serous cysts, and even paraovarian cysts may have a predilection to cause torsion. Pregnancy is also a predisposition. The right ovary is involved more frequently than the left. Interestingly, if a woman has one episode, she has a 10% chance of contralateral involvement.

The usual *symptom* of adnexal torsion is abdominal pain. This pain is acute and unilateral. Associated nausea and vomiting occur in two thirds of patients. Intermittent pain may have preceded the final event, and a sudden change in position may be the precipitating factor. Expect tenderness to palpation, but rebound tenderness is uncommon. As the infarction progresses, there may be low-grade fever and leukocytosis.

Grossly, the involved adnexa is cyanotic to nearly black in color and edematous. On cut section and *histology,* hemorrhagic infarction is found. A twisted pedicle with vascular compromise must not be untwisted because untwisting may discharge an embolus. An oophorocystectomy should be performed by doubly ligating the pedicle slightly below the area of the twisting, taking care not to include adjacent structures (e.g., the ureter). Occasionally, it may be possible to salvage the ovary or tube with incomplete torsion (i.e., without vascular compromise) by carefully releasing the pedicle, performing a cystectomy, and stabilizing the ovary by shortening the ovarian ligament with sutures. However, risk of emboli must be recognized.

Chapter 22

Sexually Transmitted Diseases

A sexually transmitted disease (STD) is any infection acquired primarily through sexual contact. STD is a general term, and the causative organisms, which are harbored in the blood or body secretions, include viruses, mycoplasmas, bacteria, fungi, spirochetes, and minute parasites (e.g., crab lice, scabies). Some of the organisms involved are found exclusively in the genital (reproductive) tract, but others exist simultaneously in other systems. Additionally, various STDs often coexist, and when one is found, others should be suspected. There is a range of intimate bodily contact that may transmit STDs, including kissing, sexual intercourse, anal intercourse, cunnilingus, anilingus, fellatio, and mouth or genital to breast contact. Physicians are required to report most STDs to local public health departments.

The vast majority of female genital tract infections are acquired sexually. Female genital tract infections are divided into lower genital tract and upper genital tract (or pelvic) infections. The lower genital tract infections (including a number of STDs and their sequelae) are discussed in Chapters 17 and 18, and they include viral infections (herpes simplex, human papillomavirus, and molluscum contagiosum) and vulvar infestations (pedicularis pubis and scabies). Common types of vulvovaginitis (e.g., *Trichomonas, Gardnerella,* and *Candida*) and some of the sequelae of STDs (e.g., infections of Bartholin glands and cervicitis) also are discussed in Chapter 17. This chapter deals with upper genital tract infections, the most serious, most directly sexually transmitted diseases and their sequelae.

SEXUALLY TRANSMITTED DISEASES CAUSED BY ORGANISMS

HUMAN IMMUNODEFICIENCY VIRUS (HIV) INFECTIONS

The human immunodeficiency virus (HIV) was first reported to cause disease in 1981. In the US AIDS is now the fifth leading cause of death among women of childbearing age. Moreover, it is the leading cause of death in this age group in New York City. This is now a worldwide crisis, with millions affected, especially in developing countries. One of the problems in recognition of HIV infection is a long, asymptomatic latency of 2 months to 5 years. The mean age at diagnosis of HIV infection is 35 years.

The virus is present in blood and all body fluids and is transmitted by sexual contact (>70%), by parenteral exposure to infected blood or body fluids, or by transplacental passage of the virus from mother to fetus. The highest-risk groups for HIV infection are homosexuals, bisexual men, intravenous drug abusers, and hemophiliacs receiving blood transfusions. Others at high risk are prostitutes and heterosexual partners of men in the high-risk groups. All blood must be screened for HIV before transfusion to minimize transfusion risk. Women acquire the virus more easily from men rather than the reverse because the concentration of HIV in semen is high and mucosal breaks at the introitus or vagina with intercourse occur more commonly than do breaks in penile skin.

Although anti-HIV antibodies develop within 12 weeks of exposure, 45%–90% of persons infected with HIV will develop symptoms of an acute infection similar to mononucleosis within a few months. They experience weight loss, fever, night sweats, pharyngitis, lymphadenopathy, and an erythematous maculopapular rash. Most of these symptoms resolve within a few weeks, although the patients remain infectious despite being asymptomatic. Some will progress to develop symptoms of AIDS-related complex (ARC), with early immunosuppression (decreased CD4+ lymphocytes). ARC is usually marked by generalized lymphadenopathy, weight loss, diarrhea, malabsorption, and wasting. Some patients experience further immunosuppression and develop AIDS (any of the symptoms of acute sepsis, opportunistic infections, Kaposi's sarcoma, cognitive difficulties, or depression). *Once AIDS has been diagnosed, mortality exceeds 90%*. Immunologic abnormalities associated with AIDS include (but are not limited to) lymphopenia, decreased T helper cells, decreased T lymphocytes, hypergammaglobulinemia, and an inverted T4/T8 ratio.

Since there is no cure for HIV, current *therapy* only slows the progression of the disease. Hence, there is every reason to stress *prevention*. Other than abstinence or having a monogamous relationship with a known noninfected partner, using latex condoms lubricated with nonoxynol 9 is the most effective method of limiting the risk of infection. If a woman is HIV positive, she should be counseled (1) not to donate blood, plasma, tissue, or organs, (2) to avoid pregnancy, (3) to maintain a monogamous relationship, and (4) to assiduously use condoms lubricated with nonoxynol 9 during any sexual contact.

HIV antibody testing begins with the enzyme-linked immunosorbent assay (ELISA), which has a >95% sensitivity and a >99% specificity if repeatedly positive. If the ELISA is positive, a Western blot assay must be performed to confirm the diagnosis. False negative results are rare unless the patient is too early in the disease to have formed antibodies. HIV screening (after informed consent has been obtained and assurances of confidentiality provided) should be encouraged for women in the following categories: intravenous drug users, prostitutes, sex partner(s) of men who are HIV positive or at risk for HIV, those with other sexually transmitted disease, those who received blood transfusions between 1978 and 1985, those with clinical signs and symptoms of HIV infection, inhabitants of a country with high endemic heterosexual HIV infection, prison inmates, and one who considers herself at risk.

Pregnancy does not appear to alter the progression of HIV infection, but *the chance of the fetus acquiring the virus is 20%–50%*. The neonate may be infected during labor and delivery by maternal blood or body fluids or may be infected during breastfeeding. The mode of delivery does not influence the development of pediatric AIDS. The acute illness associated with HIV in pregnancy may be misdiagnosed if HIV serologic testing is not performed. When HIV infection is diagnosed during pregnancy, treatment should be delayed because of the teratogenic potential of the medications used. The pregnant HIV-infected woman should be screened for other STDs, along with evaluation for opportunistic infection. A baseline serologic study for CMV and toxoplasmosis, TB skin testing, and chest radiograph are recommended.

Care of the HIV-positive woman and her infant in the peripartum and postpartum interval includes protection of health care workers by using universal infection control guidelines (e.g., water-repellent gowns, gloves, masks, goggles for potential splash situations, wall or bulb suctioning). Scalp electrodes and fetal scalp blood samples should be avoided (potential entry site for HIV if fetus is not already infected). Circumcision should not be done if the neonate is HIV positive. Since anti-HIV IgG antibody passes through the placenta, the infant may be seropositive without being infected. Abnormal facial features have been described in some HIV-positive newborns, but this is not common. If neonatal/pediatric AIDS develops, the course of the disease is much more rapid than in adults, with death in months rather than years.

GONORRHEA

Neisseria gonorrhoeae (one of the most common causes of STD) is a gram-negative diplococcus that usually resides in the female in the urethra, cervix, pharynx, or anal canal. The infection primary involves the columnar and transitional epithelium of the genitourinary tract. The organism is very fastidious and sensitive to drying, sunlight, heat, and most disinfectants. Special media (e.g., Thayer-Martin) are required to achieve optimal recovery. Culture of the lower genital tract is usually obtained by rotating a cotton swab for 15–20 sec deep in the endocervical canal. If a rectal swab is taken, the incidence of recovery increases from 85% to >90%. In upper genital tract infections (salpingitis, peritonitis) proven by laparosocopically obtained culture, only ~50% of the lower genital tract cultures will reveal *N. gonorrhoeae.*

After exposure to an infected partner, 60%–90% of women and 20%–50% of men will become infected. Untreated, 10%–17% of women will develop pelvic inflammatory disease (PID). If a woman is positive for *N. gonorrhoeae,* she has a 20%–40% chance of also having chlamydial infection, syphilis, or hepatitis.

Early symptoms typically include vaginal discharge, urinary frequency, and rectal irritation. Some report burning, itching, or inflammation of the vulva, vagina, cervix, or urethra, although most women are asymptomatic. Bartholin duct(s) and gland(s) may be involved, as evidenced by swelling or abscess formation (Chapter 17). Acute pharyngitis and tonsillitis may occur, but this is uncommon. Rarely, the asymptomatic carrier will develop a disseminated infection with polyarthralgia, tenosynovitis, and dermatitis or meningitis or endocarditis. Although ophthalmic infection most commonly occurs in neonates born to an infected mother, adult ophthalmitis may result from autoinoculation.

The *diagnosis* may be presumed when a stained smear from the involved sites reveals intracellular gram-negative diplococci. However, confirmation after growth on selective medium is essential. The culture for gonorrhea must include penicillin resistance testing because 2%–3% of strains in the United States are penicillin resistant. Gonorrhea must be reported to the state public health authorities.

The patient and all sexual partners must be treated. Other concomitant diseases must be ruled out and treated if present. The preferred adult regimen for uncomplicated disease, according to the Centers for Disease Control (CDC), is ceftriaxone 250 mg IM, followed by doxycycline 100 mg PO bid for 7 days. Alternate regimens include (1) spectinomycin 2 g IM, followed by doxycycline (as above) for patients who cannot tolerate ceftriaxone (however, spectinomycin is not reliable therapy for pharyngeal infection), (2) ciprofloxacin 0.5 g or norfloxacin 0.8 mg orally once (for those nonpregnant only), plus doxycycline (as above), (3) cefotaxime 1 g or ceftizoxime 0.5 g IM, plus doxycycline (as above), and (4) cefuroxime axetil 1 g with probenecid 1 g PO once, plus doxycycline (as above) in cases acquired from a source proven not to be penicillinase producing. If tetracyclines are contraindicated or not tolerated, erythromycin base or stearate 500 mg or erythromycin ethylsuccinate 800 mg PO qid for 7 days is acceptable. Because of the emergence of resistant organisms, repeat cultures must be performed within 7 days of completion of therapy to ensure cure.

Disseminated disease requires hospitalization. Meningitis and endocarditis must be confirmed or ruled out. Recommended therapy is ceftriaxone 1 g IM or IV qd or cefotaxime or ceftrizoxime 1 g IV q8h. Patients with allergy to beta-lactamase drugs may be treated with spectromycin 2 g IM q12h. If sensitivity testing confirms that the organism is penicillin-sensitive, ampicillin 1 g q6h may be given. Whichever regimen is chosen, therapy should be continued for 7 days. Oral medications include cefuroxime axetil 0.5 g q12h, Augmentin 0.65 g q8h, or ciprofloxacin 0.5 g q12h (if not pregnant).

The *prognosis* for properly treated gonorrhea is good, but future fertility may be compromised.

CHLAMYDIAL INFECTIONS

Chlamydia trachomatis is an obligate intracellular microorganism with a cell wall similar to that of gram-negative bacteria. Although they are classified as bacteria, contain both DNA and RNA, and divide by binary fission, *Chlamydia* grow only intracellularly, as do viruses. Since most of the *C. trachomatis* serotypes attack only columnar epithelial cells (except the aggressive L serotypes), signs and symptoms tend to be localized to the infected area (e.g., eye or genital tract) without deep tissue invasion.

Cervicitis

C. trachomatis cervical and tubal infections occur in women of young age (2–3 times higher in women <20 years), with numerous sexual partners, of low socioeconomic status, with other STDs, and with oral contraceptive use. Barrier contraception tends to decrease the infection rate. Pregnant women have an incidence of 8%–12%.

Signs and Symptoms

Typically, a mucopurulent discharge develops with cervical chlamydial infection, and the cervix shows hypertrophic inflammation (mucopurulent cervicitis). The infection may be asymptomatic in 15% of nonpregnant, sexually active women.

Laboratory Findings

The most frequently used method of detection is a direct fluorescein-conjugated monoclonal antibody test (available in kit form). This is rapid, sensitive (85%–93%), and specific (~99%). Specimens are generally obtained as described for gonorrhea (p 586). Tissue culture is required for culture of *C. trachomatis,* and because of the high cost, limited availability, and 2–6 day delay, it is used infrequently. Although Giemsa staining of conjunctival specimens in neonates is fairly successful in identifying chlamydial inclusions, this technique is only 40% accurate in genital infections.

Differential Diagnosis

N. gonorrhoeae is the only other predominant organism causing a mucopurulent cervicitis. Thus, fluorescent antibody tests or cultures on selective medium are mandatory for differentiation. Both organisms may be present simultaneously.

Treatment

Cure rates of >95% can be achieved with the use of one of several regimens. The preferred regimen is tetracycline 500 mg PO qid for 7 days or doxycycline 100 mg bid for 7 days. If tetracyclines cannot be taken or are contraindicated, erythromycin base 500 mg qid for 7 days, or erythromycin ethylsuccinate 800 mg qid for 7 days may be prescribed.

Complications

The primary complication of *C. trachomatis* cervical infection is salpingitis. Unfortunately, if the patient is pregnant and untreated, the vaginally delivered neonate will develop chlamydial conjunctivitis in 50% of cases and late onset pneumonitis in 10%. Premature delivery and early postpartum endometritis are also associated problems.

Salpingitis

C. trachomatis salpingitis may be as prevalent as that caused by *N. gonorrhoeae*. However, there are marked differences in the pathophysiology and symptomatology. *C. trachomatis* salpingitis (which is also an ascending infection) has an insidious onset, it usually causes minimal symptoms, and the organism remains in the tube (primarily in the epithelium) for months. In contrast, *N. gonorrhoeae* infections have an acute onset, cause more acute symptoms, and remain in the tubes only 24–48 h. Gonorrheal infections appear to have a much greater cytotoxic effect on the tubal epithelium.

Although *C. trachomatis* salpingitis usually causes fewer symptoms, the gross appearance of the tubes suggests even more severe involvement. Salpingitis is a consequence of *C. trachomatis* cervicitis. *Treatment* of *C. trachomatis* salpingitis may be accomplished with tetracyclines or erythromycin. The sequelae of *C. trachomatis* salpingitis include ectopic pregnancy and infertility, although the exact incidence of these complications is unknown.

Lymphogranuloma Venereum

The L serotypes of *C. trachomatis* cause lymphogranuloma venereum, which usually occurs in tropical or subtropical areas (including the southern United States). The incubation period is

7–21 days, and men are affected 6 times more often than women. In the United States, <500 cases/year are reported, and most occur in men.

Lymphogranuloma venereum begins with a vesicopustular eruption that progresses to very painful inguinal and vulvar ulceration, lymphedema, and secondary bacterial invasion. *Clinically,* a depression between the groups of inguinal nodes and the genitocrural fold produces the appearance of a double genital crural fold (the groove sign). There is a reddish to purplish blue, hard induration that occurs 10–30 days after exposure. Anorectal lymphedema causes painful defecation and blood-streaked stools. Later in the disease, progressive rectal strictures form, which may even prevent defecation. Vaginal strictures may cause distortion and narrowing, with resultant dyspareunia. Headache, arthralgia, chills, and abdominal cramps may occur late in this disease. Late complications include vulvar elephantiasis.

The *diagnosis* is confirmed by tissue culture and serotype determination, but complement fixation for *Chlamydia* with titer ≥ 1:16 is presumptive, as is a rising titer (>1:64 is diagnostic). Immunofluorescent testing is available. The *differential diagnosis* for the cutaneous lesions includes granuloma inguinale, tuberculosis, syphilis, chancroid, vulvar cancer, genital herpes, and Hodgkin's disease. With systemic symptoms, meningitis, arthritis, peritonitis, and pleurisy must be considered.

Treatment for lymphogranuloma venereum includes doxycycline 100 mg PO bid for 21 days. *Persistent disease* requires a second course. Alternative drugs include tetracycline, erythromycin, or sulfisoxizole, each at 500 mg PO qid for 21 days. After the disease is under control, surgery may be necessary (e.g., partial vulvectomy). Abscesses should not be excised but treated by aspiration. Anal strictures should be dilated weekly. A diversionary colostomy may be required for severe anal stricture.

SYPHILIS

Syphilis is a disease caused by the spirochete *Treponema pallidum,* which is transmitted by direct contact with an infectious moist lesion. These organisms can pass through intact mucous membranes or abraded skin or may be acquired transplacentally. A single sexual encounter with an infected partner carries ~10% chance of acquiring syphilis. Untreated, the disease progresses from primary to secondary to latent and, finally, to tertiary syphilis. Congenital syphilis has its own course and symptoms. There are ~280,000 new cases of syphilis in the United States each year.

The *primary lesion* of syphilis is the hard chancre, an indurated, firm, painless papule or ulcer with raised borders, which appears 10 days to 3 months (average is 3 weeks) after the treponemes have entered the body. The chancre may be located on the external genitalia, cervix, or vagina or any area of skin or mucous membrane of the body but is often not noted in women. The primary lesion persists for 1–5 weeks and is followed in most by spontaneous healing. Any lesion suspected of being a chancre should be subjected to darkfield examination, seeking treponemes, because culture is not available. *Serologic tests for syphilis* should be performed weekly for 6 weeks or until positive (usually reactive 1–4 weeks after the chancre appears).

The generalized cutaneous eruption (macular, maculopapular, papular, or pustular) of *secondary syphilis* appears 2 weeks to 6 months after the primary lesion. The rash is a diffuse, bilateral, symmetric papulosquamous eruption that may involve the palms and soles. Perineal lesions (moist papules, condyloma latum) are present and positive for treponemes on darkfield examination or immunofluorescent studies. Other mucous patches may be present, as well as patchy alopecia, hepatitis, or nephritis. Generalized lymphadenopathy is typical. The secondary lesions last 2–6 weeks and heal spontaneously. Serologic tests are almost always positive at this stage.

Latent syphilis is untreated syphilis after secondary symptoms have subsided. These patients remain infectious for 1–2 years and may have relapses resembling the secondary stage. Latency may be lifelong or end with the development of tertiary syphilis, which occurs in one third of patients.

Tertiary syphilis is marked by the presence of destructive lesions of skin, bone (gummas), cardiovascular system (e.g., aortic aneurysm or insufficiency), or nervous system disorders (e.g., meningitis, tabes dorsalis, paresis). Tertiary syphilis is fatal in 25% of those affected.

Although the *maternal course of syphilis* is unaltered by pregnancy, it is frequently not recognized unless detected by serologic screening. The treponemes may pass transplacentally throughout pregnancy, but if the disease is discovered and treated <18 weeks gestation, the fetus appears to suffer few sequelae. After 18 weeks, the classic signs of congenital syphilis occur in the fetus. The risk of *fetal infection* is greater during the secondary stage than during the primary or latent stages. The incidence of stillbirth and premature delivery is increased with syphilis. Hydramnios may be present. The placenta is involved; it has a waxy, hydropic appearance. Infection late in pregnancy results in fetal or neonatal infection in 40%–50%.

Congenital syphilis occurs in the fetus or newborn whose mother has untreated syphilis. Depending on time of acquisition of infection, there may be signs of intrauterine infection (e.g., hepatosplenomegaly, radiographic changes in bone, anemia, jaundice, lymphadenitis, meningitis), or the baby may appear unaffected, only to develop signs and symptoms equivalent to secondary syphilis sometime after birth.

Classically, the newborn with congenital syphilis may be undergrown, with wrinkled facies because of reduced subcutaneous fat. The skin may have a brownish (café-au-lait) tint. The most common lesion of early congenital syphilis in the newborn is a bullous rash, so-called syphilitic pemphigus. Large blebs may appear over the palms and soles and, occasionally, in all other areas. Seropurulent fluid from the lesions swarms with treponemes. Mucositis identical with that of secondary syphilis in older patients may be noted in the mouth and upper respiratory passages of the newborn. The nasal discharge (syphilitic snuffles) is very infectious because it contains large numbers of *T. pallidum.*

The bones usually show signs of osteochrondtitis, and on x-ray, an irregular epiphyseal juncture (Guerin's line) is characteristic. Abnormalities of the eyes and other organs or the central nervous system may be apparent at birth, or defects may develop later in untreated cases. Any infant with the stigmata of syphilis should be placed in isolation until a definitive diagnosis can be made and appropriate treatment given.

Because serologic testing evaluates IgG antibodies that are transplacentally acquired, the baby will be positive if the mother is positive. Effective neonatal treatment is shown by progressively falling titers over weeks to months.

Laboratory Findings

Visualization of the treponemal organisms requires the presence of a moist cutaneous lesion for darkfield examination (fresh smear), immunofluorescent staining (dried smear), or silver staining for the treponemes in a biopsy specimen. Because the organisms are demonstrable for only a short time, *diagnosis* usually relies on history and serologic testing.

Screening for syphilis is accomplished primarily by nonspecific nontreponemal antibody testing (e.g., VDRL, RPR). All pregnant women should be tested at the first visit. High-risk patients should be screened at 28–32 weeks gestation and at delivery. These tests become positive 3–6 weeks after infection. The titers are high in secondary syphilis and fall to low titers or even become negative in late syphilis. Titers that have a fourfold drop or are falling in early syphilis indicate adequate treatment.

False positive tests may be associated with collagen disease, infectious mononucleosis, malaria, leprosy, febrile illnesses, vaccination, drug addiction, old age, and pregnancy itself. The titer seen with false positive tests usually is low. However, any positive test should be investigated by an antitreponemal antibody test. The most widely performed antitreponemal antibody test is the fluorescent treponemal antibody absorption (FTA-ABS) test. The test remains positive regardless of therapy. Thus, titers are not determined.

Differential Diagnosis

The differential diagnosis for primary syphilis includes chancroid, granuloma inguinale, lymphogranuloma venereum, herpes, carcinoma, scabies, trauma, lichen planus, psoriasis, drug eruption, aphthosis, mycotic infection, Reiter's syndrome, and Bowen's disease.

The differential diagnosis for secondary syphilis includes pityriasis rosea, psoriasis, lichen planus, tinea versicolor, drug eruption, "id" eruptions, perleche, parasitic infection, iritis, neuroretinitis, condylomata accuminata, acute exanthems, infectious mononucleosis, alopecia, and sarcoidosis.

Treatment

Treatment should be initiated if exposure has occurred even if evidence of disease is not present. During pregnancy, it is better to treat any suspicion of disease rather than risk congenital syphilis.

Contacts and patients with early syphilis (primary, secondary, and latent <1 year) should be treated with one of the following regimens: (1) benzathine penicillin G 2.4 million units IM, (2) tetracycline hydrochloride 500 mg PO qid or doxycycline 100 mg bid for 14 days (for penicillin allergy but not during pregnancy), or (3) erythromycin (stearate, ethylsuccinate, or base) 500 mg PO qid for 15 days (30 g total) for penicillin allergy and if unable to take tetracycline. A short-lived (<24 h) febrile reaction occurs in 50%–75% of those receiving penicillin therapy, presumably due to a release of toxic treponemal products. The fever, which occurs 4–12 h after injection, is a *Jarisch-Herxheimer reaction*.

Congenital syphilis is treated with benzathine penicillin G 50,000 units/kg IM if the infant is asymptomatic and there is no evidence of neurosyphilis. Symptomatic congenital syphilis or neurosyphilis is treated with aqueous crystalline penicillin G 50,000 units/kg/day IV, divided in two doses for 10 days or aqueous procaine penicillin G 50,000 units/kg daily for 10 days.

Chancroid

Chancroid (soft chancre) is caused by the gram-negative rod *Haemophilus ducreyi* and is uncommon in the United States (<1500 cases/year). This infection begins in females as a papule or vesicopustular lesion on the perineum, cervix, or vagina 3–5 days after exposure. The lesion progresses over 48–72 h to a very tender saucer-shaped ragged ulcer. Several ulcers may develop in a cluster. The heavy discharge produced by the ulcer(s) is foul-smelling and infectious. Over 50% of patients develop painful inguinal lymphadenitis that may become necrotic and drain spontaneously. Aspiration of pus from a bubo may yield the organism. Syphilis must be ruled out, although the *differential diagnosis* also includes herpes simplex, lymphogranuloma venereum, and granuloma inguinale.

Treatment includes sitz baths, soap and water plus antibiotics. The therapeutic regimen will vary depending on sensitivity of the pathogen. Ceftriaxone 250 mg IM qd, erythromycin 500 mg PO qid, and trimethoprim (160 mg)/sulfamethoxazole (800 mg) PO bid have been effective. Treatment should continue for a minimum of 10 days until the ulcer(s) and lymph nodes are healed. Abscessed nodes should be aspirated rather than incised and drained.

Granuloma Inguinale

Granuloma inguinale is caused by *Calymmatobacterium granulomatis*. A characteristic finding in the lesions is the Donovan body (bacteria encapsulated in mononuclear leukocytes). It is almost never seen in the United States (~100 cases/year) but is common in India, Brazil, and the West Indies. The incubation period is 1–

12 weeks. Granuloma inguinale may be spread by repeated sexual or nonsexual contact.

The disease usually is localized to the vulva and inguinal area but may involve the cervix, uterus, ovary, or mouth. It begins as an asymptomatic papule or nodule that ulcerates to form a red, granular area with sharp borders. The ulcer drains a foul-smelling discharge. Healing is extremely slow, but there are few local or systemic manifestations. Satellite ulcers may coalesce into one large ulcer. Buboes may occur late in the disease. Pain may be present if the urethra or anus is involved.

Late complications include dyspareunia if the introitus constricts from chronic disease. The *differential diagnosis* includes carcinoma, chancroid, lymphogranuloma venereum, and syphilis. The *diagnosis* is confirmed by finding Donovan bodies in a biopsy specimen or smear using Wright, Giemsa, or a silver stain.

The drug of choice for *treatment* of granuloma inguinale is tetracycline 500 mg qid for a minimum 21 days. Other choices include erythromycin 500 mg qid for 14–21 days, doxycycline 100 mg bid for 21 days, or sulfamethoxazole 1 g bid for 21 days.

PELVIC INFECTIONS

Infections may occur in any or all portions of the upper genital tract: endometrium (endometritis), uterine wall (myositis), oviducts (salpingitis), ovary (oophoritis), uterine serosa and broad ligaments (parametritis), and pelvic peritoneum (peritonitis). A functional classification of pelvic infections is shown in Table 22-1.

Organisms may disseminate to and throughout the pelvis in any of five ways.

1. *Intraluminal.* Nonpuerperal acute pelvic inflammatory disease nearly always (~99%) follows a progression of entrance of pathogens through the cervix into the uterine cavity. Infection then spreads to the uterine tubes, with pus eventually entering the peritoneal cavity from the ostia. Organisms known to spread by this mechanism include *N. gonorrhoeae, C. trachomatis, Streptococcus agalactiae,* cytomegalovirus, and herpes simplex virus. Three fourths of women with acute PID have concomitant endometritis, whereas ~40% of those with mucopurulent cervicitis and 50% of those with positive *C. trachomatis* or *N. gonorrhoeae* endocervical cultures have concomitant endometritis. The endometritis phase is generally asymptomatic, often brief, and occurs at the end of a menses.

2. *Lymphatic.* Puerperal infections (including abortion) and

Table 22-1. Functional classification of pelvic infections

Pelvic inflammatory disease (PID)
  Limited (salpingitis)
  Pelvic abscess (cul-de-sac or tuboovarian)
Puerperal infections
  Cesarean section (common)
  Vaginal (uncommon)
Postgynecologic procedure infection
  Acute PID after diagnostic instrumentation
  Abortion-related infections
    Postabortal cellulitis
    Incomplete septic abortion
  Cuff cellulitis and parametritis
  Vaginal cuff abscess
  Tuboovarian abscess
Pelvic infection secondary to other infections
  or intraabdominal accidents
    Appendicitis
    Diverticulitis
    Tuberculosis
    Traumatic viscus rupture

IUD-related infections are disseminated through the lymphatic system, as are nonpuerperal *Mycoplasma* infections.

3. *Hematogenous.* Hematogenous dissemination of pelvic disease is limited to certain diseases (e.g., tuberculosis) and is uncommon in the United States.

4. *Intraperitoneal.* Intraabdominal infections (e.g., appendicitis, diverticulitis) as well as intraabdominal accidents (e.g., perforated viscus or ulcer) may lead to an infectious process involving the internal genital system.

5. *Contiguous.* The postgynecologic surgical infections are the result of local spread of infection from areas of tissue necrosis and infection.

Pelvic Inflammatory Disease (PID)

Although PID is an inexact term including infection of any portion of the upper genital tract, the designation is useful because these infections are so interrelated. PID is an extraordinary health problem. There are about 1 million cases of acute PID a year in the United States, and the total cost is estimated to exceed $3.5 billion per year. PID affects 1%–2% of sexually active females yearly and is more frequent in young women (75% of those affected are <25 years). In the United States, PID annually results in 2.5 million physician visits, nearly 270,000 inpatient admissions, about 120,000 operative procedures, and 0.29 deaths/100,000 women age 15–44.

Spontaneous PID (usually arising after a menstrual period) in sexually active females accounts for 85% of cases, but 15% occur after procedures in which the mucosal surface is injured (e.g., IUD insertion, endometrial biopsy, curettage, hysterosalpingogram). In <1% of PID, transperitoneal spread to the upper genital tract occurs from appendicitis, diverticulitis, or traumatic rupture of a viscus.

Approximately two thirds of acute pelvic infections are polymicrobial. *N. gonorrhoeae* is responsible for one third of acute PID, *N. gonorrhoeae* with a mixed endogenous anaerobic and aerobic flora is responsible for another one third, and mixed anaerobes and aerobes are responsible for the remaining third. In combination with other organisms, *C. trachomatis* is found in up to 30% of cases. The aerobes and anaerobes found in PID usually are normal vaginal and gastrointestinal flora. The anaerobes (e.g., *Bacteroides, Peptostreptococcus, Peptococcus*) predominate in abscesses. Common aerobes include *Escherichia coli,* group B *Streptococcus, Streptococcus faecalis,* and coagulase-negative *Staphlococcus. Mycoplasma hominis* and *Ureaplasma urealyticum* do not appear to be pathogenic in PID.

The *signs and symptoms* of acute PID are generally nonspecific but are related to both the extent of the infection and the organisms involved. Lower abdominal pain of <7 days duration occurs in >90% of patients with acute PID. The pain is usually characterized as constant and dull but is enhanced by movement or sexual activity. Endocervical infection is present in 75% of patients with PID. Abnormal vaginal bleeding occurs in 40% of patients. Other symptoms are nonspecific, including fever (30%), malaise, and headache.

The white blood cell count may be normal, increased, or decreased and should not be relied on to rule out PID. Abdominal x-ray films (KUB and upright) may demonstrate adynamic ileus or free peritoneal gas or both. Abdominal ultrasound is very useful. Culdocentesis is simple, relatively painless, and may be diagnostic. Pus suggests a ruptured tuboovarian abscess, ruptured appendix, ruptured viscus, ruptured diverticular abscess, or a uterine abscess involving a myoma. Cloudy fluid suggests pelvic peritonitis (as seen with acute gonococcal salpingitis), twisted adnexal cyst, or other causes of peritonitis (e.g., appendicitis, pancreatitis, cholecystitis, perforated ulcer, carcinomatosis, echinococcosis). Blood may be found with ruptured ectopic pregnancy, hemorrhage from corpus luteum cyst, retrograde menstruation, ruptured spleen or liver, gastrointestinal bleeding, or acute salpingitis. Laparoscopy should be performed if there is any doubt about the diagnosis.

The infection may be so widespread that in 5%–10% of acute PID, perihepatic inflammation develops. Here, the symptoms are right upper quadrant distress, pleuritic pain, and right upper quadrant tenderness. This condition is called the Curtis-Fitzhugh syndrome and often results in perihepatic adhesions.

Early diagnosis and prompt effective treatment may decrease the sequelae (e.g., pelvic adhesions, tissue necrosis, abscess formation, intestinal obstruction, infertility, tubal pregnancy), but 25% of women with acute PID develop significant complications. There is a 6–10 times increase in ectopic pregnancy and a 4 times increase in chronic pelvic pain. Infertility is enhanced, depending on the number and severity of attacks.

PID may be decreased or prevented by limiting the number of sexual contacts, determining if sexual contacts have STDs, using condoms, spermicides, diaphragms and spermicides, and employing postcoital toilet (urination, washing or douching with antiseptic solution).

Acute Salpingitis

As noted previously, the most common organism initiating acute salpingitis-peritonitis is *N. gonorrhoeae*. Approximately 15% of asymptomatic infections will result in acute salpingitis.

Symptoms and Signs

Typically, salpingitis occurs in young (often teenage) women who have multiple sexual partners and are not using vaginal contraception. *Symptoms* typically begin shortly after cessation of menstrual flow or following instrumentation. The onset of lower abdominal and pelvic pain (frequently bilateral) is usually acute but may be insidious. Pain may radiate from the back down the leg(s). There may be a purulent vaginal discharge. Systemic symptoms include fever (30%), headache, malaise, nausea, and vomiting.

Physical examination reveals abdominal tenderness, usually of the lower quadrants. Rebound tenderness is noted in the presence of peritonitis. Bowel sounds may be decreased or absent. The paraurethral and Bartholin glands may be inflamed and discharging purulent material. The cervix often exudes a purulent discharge. Movement of the cervix or uterus is exquisitely painful. The adnexa are tender to palpation. The criteria for diagnosis of salpingitis are summarized in Table 22-2.

Laboratory Findings

A smear of the cervical discharge nearly always reveals infection and may suggest the etiology (e.g., gram-negative diplococci of *N. gonorrhoeae*), but culture confirmation is essential, using selective media. The WBC may be elevated or normal. Women with suspected PID should have a sensitive hCG test because 3%–4% of them will have ectopic gestation. Culdocentesis usually produces cloudy fluid, which should be sent for cell count

Table 22-2. Criteria for diagnosis of salpingitis

Criteria	
Abdominal direct tenderness, with or without rebound tenderness	
Tenderness with motion of cervix and uterus	All 3 necessary for diagnosis
Adnexal tenderness	
	plus
Gram stain of endocervix positive for gram-negative, intracellular diplococci	
Fever (>38°C)	
Leukocytosis (>10,000)	One or more necessary for diagnosis
Purulent material (WBCs present) from peritoneal cavity by culdocentesis or laparoscopy	
Pelvic abscess or inflammatory complex on bimanual examination or on sonography	

Modified from W.E. Hager, D.A. Eschenbach, M.R. Spence, et al. Criteria for diagnosis and grading of salpingitis. *Obstet Gynecol* 61:114, 1983.

(>30,000 WBC/ml is associated with PID), gram stain, culture, and sensitivity.

If abdominal x-ray films show evidence of free air under the diaphragm, laparotomy is mandatory. Ultrasonic scanning is useful in the patient who is too tender to examine properly to rule out ectopic gestation or to reveal abscesses.

Differential Diagnosis

Included in the differential diagnosis are appendicitis, ectopic pregnancy, ruptured corpus luteum cyst with hemorrhage, diverticulitis, infected septic abortion, degeneration of a uterine leiomyoma, torsion of an adnexal mass, endometriosis, acute urinary tract infection, ulcerative colitis, and regional enteritis.

Treatment

Free peritoneal air is a surgical emergency, but the decision to hospitalize for treatment is most frequently based on the following findings: peritonitis in upper quadrants (nonpelvic peritonitis), gastrointestinal symptoms (including ileus), tuboovarian abscess, pregnancy, uncertain diagnosis, presence of an intrauterine device, history of instrumentation, inadequate response to outpatient therapy, or nulliparity.

Patients requiring hospitalization should be put at bedrest, initially kept NPO, given IV fluids, and placed on nasogastric suction for abdominal distention or ileus. Antibiotic therapy should be IV until the patient has shown clinical improvement for 48 h. Drug regimens include

1. *Doxycycline* 100 mg IV bid plus *cefoxitin* 2 g IV qid, followed by *doxycycline* 100 mg PO bid to complete 10–14 day therapy

2. *Clindamycin* 900 mg IV tid plus *gentamicin or tobramicin* 2 mg/kg IV initially, 1.5 mg/kg thereafter q8h, followed by *doxycycline* 100 mg PO bid for 10–14 days or *clindamycin* 450 mg qid for 10–14 days

If the organism is *N. gonorrhoeae* and is penicillin resistant, *spectinomycin* 2 g IM should be administered. An IUD should be removed once therapy has been begun. Analgesics with or without codeine may provide relief.

Surgical exploration is reserved for those in whom life is threatened, the condition deteriorates, a tuboovarian abscess ruptures, a pelvic abscess is pointing into the cul-de-sac, the abdominal symptoms persist despite intensive therapy, and there are persistent masses. In women not desiring future childbearing, the tuboovarian masses may be removed. However, in the majority, every effort should be made to preserve ovarian function, especially in those who may want in vitro fertilization, when the uterus should remain.

Treatment is reasonable on an outpatient basis for the majority of mild PID (~75% of cases). The patient must not be pregnant and must not appear acutely ill, and the diagnosis must be certain. Outpatient regimens include (1) cefoxitin 2 g IM plus probenecid 1 g PO, (2) ceftriaxone 250 mg IM plus probenecid 1 g PO. Both should be followed by doxycycline 100 mg PO bid for 14 days or tetracycline 500 mg PO qid for 14 days. Erythromycin 500 mg PO qid for 14 days may be used if the patient cannot take tetracyclines. The patient should be reevaluated in 48–72 h after starting therapy. If she fails to improve, she should be hospitalized for treatment. Follow-up examination, including cervical cultures, should be performed 2 weeks after therapy to assure a cure.

Prognosis

The prognosis depends on prompt therapy with broad-spectrum antibiotics and rest. *Complications* include hydrosalpinx, pyosalpinx, tuboovarian abscess, infertility, ectopic pregnancy (at least 2 times increased), and chronic pelvic pain (20% after just one episode). The prognosis for fertility decreases substantially with each infection. Infertility is present in 12%–18% with the first (or only) episode of acute salpingitis, 25% with two episodes, and 60% with three episodes of salpingitis. Recurrent infections are so common (25%) that in the past a designation of *chronic infection* was given to cases in which therapy was appropriate but the patient returned with another infection.

Pelvic Abscess

Cul-de-Sac Abscess

Pelvic abscesses may be tuboovarian or in the cul-de-sac. Most often, pelvic abscesses follow acute pelvic infection or septic abortion, although they may follow appendicitis, perforated viscus, or recurrent pelvic infection. *Bacteroides* (either *fragilis* or *bovis*) is the most commonly cultured organism. The symptoms may be those of acute pelvic infection plus a fluctuant mass in the adnexa or cul-de-sac. Pain usually is more severe than with acute PID or salpingitis, especially to the rectum and back and during defecation.

The *differential diagnosis* includes tuboovarian abscess, periappendiceal abscess, ectopic pregnancy, retroflexed and incarcerated uterus, endometriosis, diverticulitis with perforation, and carcinomatosis.

Antibiotic *treatment* must be effective against both aerobic and anaerobic bacteria. Recommended regimens include (1) penicillin G 20–30 million units IV per day, plus chloramphenicol 4–6 g IV per day (monitor for idiosyncratic aplastic anemia), (2) penicillin G 20–30 million units IV per day, clindamycin 600–1200 mg IV qid, and gentamicin 5 mg/kg per day, (3) cefoxitin 8–12 g IV per day and gentamicin or tobramycin 5 mg/kg/day, and (4) cefotaxime 6–8 g IV per day.

The patient should be reevaluated frequently (and gently) for signs of peritoneal involvement or dissection into the rectovaginal septum with fixation. If any of these occur, surgical intervention is necessary. If extension downward occurs, vaginal drainage with a large Pezar-type catheter should be accomplished. This should be followed by low-pressure irrigation with sterile saline q6h until the space is obliterated. If fever persists despite antibiotic therapy, percutaneous drainage and irrigation of the cul-de-sac may be performed.

If peritoneal signs develop or if the patient's condition deteriorates despite therapy, an exploratory laparotomy is indicated. When the patient has no further desire for children, total abdominal hysterectomy (TAH), bilateral salpingo-oophorectomy (BSO), and lysis of adhesions should be performed. More conservative surgery may be dictated by age, parity, condition of the tubes and ovaries, and desire for childbearing. In some cases, salvage of even an ovary may be desirable.

Although the *prognosis for fertility* is guarded, the overall *prognosis* is good if the abscess is localized and is treated early. If rupture into the peritoneum occurs, the prognosis is serious.

Tuboovarian Abscess (TOA)

Although tuboovarian abscess may occur after an initial episode of acute salpingitis, it most often is associated with recurrent adnexal infections (Fig. 22-1). The ovarian site of ovulation is thought to be a portal of infection for abscess formation. TOA is bilateral in 60%–80%.

Fulminant peritonitis with a 5%–10% mortality rate results

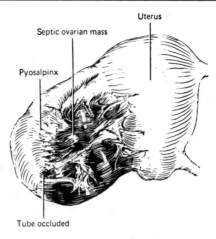

Figure 22-1. Tuboovarian abscess.

from sudden rupture of an abscess, whereas a slow leak may result in signs and symptoms of a cul-de-sac abscess. Granulomatous disease (e.g., tuberculosis, actinomycosis) and use of IUDs are associated with TOA.

Patients may be asymptomatic or clearly be in septic shock. The typical patient has a history of previous pelvic infection, is young, with low parity, and has had symptoms for <1 week. The onset is usually 2 weeks after menses, with pelvic and abdominal pain (of varying degrees), nausea, vomiting, fever, and tachycardia. The entire abdomen is tender, and guarding may be present. Because of extreme tenderness of the adnexa, pelvic examination may be difficult. Culdocentesis may rupture the abscess, thus ultrasonography is preferred for diagnosis. The WBC count may be low, normal, or greatly elevated. The abdominal x-ray may show adynamic ileus or free air under the diaphragm if rupture has occurred.

The *differential diagnosis* in the asymptomatic patient may be ovarian cyst, ovarian neoplasm, unruptured ectopic pregnancy, uterine leiomyoma, hydrosalpinx, or periappendiceal abscess. In the symptomatic patient whose tuboovarian abscess remains unruptured, the differential diagnosis includes appendiceal abscess, appendiceal rupture, diverticular abscess, perforated diverticulum, perforated peptic ulcer, porphyria, and diabetes mellitus. *Complications* include septic shock, septic emboli, peritonitis, bowel obstruction, recurrent infection, ectopic pregnancy, and infertility.

Treatment depends on whether or not the abscess is symptomatic and whether or not it has ruptured. If the tuboovarian abscess is unruptured and asymptomatic, it may be treated by antibiotics (see below). If the mass does not shrink within 2–3 weeks of antibiotic therapy or increases in size, surgery is indicated. Usually TAH and BSO are performed, although a more conservative approach (unilateral adnexectomy) is reasonable in select patients. If the abscess is unruptured but symptomatic, the patient should be hospitalized, placed at bedrest in semi-Fowler position, and maintained NPO, with nasogastric suction applied, and she should receive IV fluids, with close monitoring of electrolytes. Antibiotics should be administered IV in one of the following combinations.

1. Penicillin G (or Ampicillin) and chloramphenicol
2. Penicillin G (or Ampicillin) plus metronidazole
3. Clindamycin plus an aminoglycoside (gentamicin, amikacin, tobramycin)
4. Cefoxitin or cefamandole plus either clindamycin, metronidazole, or choramphenicol
5. Moxalactam or cefotaxime with or without clindamycin, metronidazole, chloramphenicol, or an aminoglycoside

If the initial therapy results in improvement, continue oral antibiotics (tetracycline, doxycycline) for 10–14 days. If rupture or leakage is suspected or if the patient does not respond to antibiotic therapy, perform an exploratory laparotomy. *About 50% of patients with unruptured symptomatic tuboovarian abscess will require surgery.*

A ruptured tuboovarian abscess is a life-threatening emergency and must be treated as such. Admit the patient to an intensive care unit (or its equivalent) in preparation for surgery. Monitor urine output hourly, and monitor the central venous pressure, administer oxygen, and correct hypovolemia. Corticosteroids (e.g., methylprednisolone succinate 15–30 mg/kg IV q4–6h for 4 doses) may be advisable. Surgery must be performed as soon as the patient has stabilized sufficiently to tolerate a major operation.

The abdomen should be entered through a midline incision. The pus encountered should be sent for aerobic and anaerobic culture. The entire abdomen should be explored, and all abscesses should be drained. Thorough irrigation with suction is necessary. Normally, TAH and BSO are performed, but therapy must be individualized. Supracervical hysterectomy may be necessary to shorten operative time in the unstable patient. Drains should be inserted through the open vaginal cuff or cul-de-sac.

Leave drains in place as long as there is purulent discharge. Close the fascia but leave the subcutaneous space open.

The *prognosis* for survival with an unruptured tuboovarian abscess is excellent, although fertility is markedly diminished. *Mortality* from ruptured tuboovarian abscess is 5%–10%, with sterility a consequence of hysterectomy/oophorectomy.

POSTOPERATIVE PELVIC INFECTIONS

Hysterectomy carries a high rate of infection presumably because the vaginal flora cannot be eliminated from the operative site. The common infectious sequelae of hysterectomy includes cuff induration (cellulitis), infected cuff hematoma (cuff abscess), salpingitis, pelvic cellulitis, suppurative pelvic thrombophlebitis, and tuboovarian abscess. These infections are usually polymicrobial. The incidence of posthysterectomy infection may be lowered to 5% by a single dose of prophylactic antibiotic therapy.

Postoperative infection usually begins as cuff cellulitis that spreads from the vaginal apex to the parametrial tissues. If there is a hematoma present, an abscess forms. Antibiotic therapy and adequate drainage may halt further progression to salpingitis, diffuse pelvic cellulitis, and tuboovarian abscess. If the pelvic veins become involved (as is common with anaerobic infection), suppurative pelvic thrombophlebitis results, and septic emboli may occur to lungs, brain, spleen, and other sites.

Clinical Findings

Postoperative pelvic infection causes fever (>38°C or >100.8°F) within 24–36 h in 50% of patients. Alternatively, temperature elevation may be due to atelectasis, urinary tract infection, or phlebitis. Early onset of fever without symptoms may resolve spontaneously, whereas fever by 72 h may require antibiotic therapy.

Examination of the vaginal cuff after hysterectomy may disclose hyperemia, edema, and purulent or seropurulent exudate whether the wound is infected or not. If the host immune system cannot control the inoculum of vaginal flora, the parametrium will usually become indurated, causing pain and tenderness. Infection may then spread to the tubes and ovaries, followed by paralytic ileus. Spiking diurnal fever after the sixth postoperative day is suggestive of suppurative pelvic thrombophlebitis. The patient may not appear toxic (despite a high temperature) unless septic embolization has occurred.

Palpation is difficult, but ultrasonography may detect an infected pelvic hematoma. Typically, there may be no abnormality other than fever. An unexpectedly low HCT and fever are suggestive of an infected hematoma.

Because *laboratory and x-ray findings* are not often helpful in making the diagnosis of postoperative pelvic infection, the *diagnosis* must be made clinically. If the next step is a workup for postoperative fever, it is useful to recall the clinical mnemonic *3 Ws* (wound, wind, and water). Include in the *differential diagnosis* atelectasis, which causes fever within 12–36 h and is suggested by auscultation and demonstrated by chest x-ray films. Dehydration may cause mild fever within 24–48 h of surgery and usually can be suspected by the patient's clinical appearance, fluid losses, urine output, and HCT. The abdominal incision may become infected and should be probed carefully if the pelvic examination is unremarkable. Except for extremely virulent infections (e.g., clostridia), it is uncommon for the abdominal wound to cause marked fever before the third postoperative day.

Other causes of postoperative fever to be ruled out include phlebitis and urinary tract infection. Phlebitis of a superficial vein at an IV site may cause fever, especially if antibiotics are being infused. Urinary tract infection is common after gynecologic surgery because of the use of indwelling catheters. However, fever usually occurs principally when pyelonephritis is present.

Complications

Complications of postoperative infections include wound abscess, tuboovarian abscess, pelvic or intraabdominal abscess, metastatic septic emboli, and septicemia.

Prevention

Conscientious attempts should be made to prevent or decrease sepsis because of the severity of postoperative pelvic infection. Helpful measures include

1. *Preoperative vaginal douches* with topical antibacterial agents (e.g., povidone-iodine, hexochlorophene) for several days

2. *Preoperative insertion of antibacterial vaginal creams* or suppositories (especially if vaginitis or cervicitis is present)

3. *Meticulous operative hemostasis* without strangulation of tissues

4. *Use of nonreactive suture material*

5. *Suction drainage* at sites of suboptimal hemostasis (with vaginal surgical margin left open or closed)

6. *Prophylactic antibiotics* preoperatively with two optional additional doses 6 and 12 h postoperatively (*Note:* usual drugs for single-dose prophylaxis are cefonicid, ceforanide, cefotaxime, cefotetan, ceftriaxone, and cefuroxime)

7. *Treatment of a mild infection* before it becomes severe

Treatment

Treatment depends on diagnosis. A cuff hematoma or abscess must be adequately drained and antibiotics must be initiated. Single-agent therapy with one of the newer cephalosporins usually eliminates fever within 48–72 h. Large hematomas will require suction drainage and more prolonged antibiotic therapy. Tuboovarian abscess therapy has been described previously. Diagnosis of suppurative pelvic thrombophlebitis is made by exclusion when fever persists after 7–10 days of antibiotic administration. Heparin 5000 units q4h IV should be administered. If fever persists despite heparin and antibiotic therapy, addition of another antibiotic effective against anaerobic organisms (e.g., clindamycin, chloramphenicol, metronidazole) is recommended. Surgical intervention is usually necessary only if heparin therapy is contraindicated, if embolization continues despite adequate therapy, or if the patient fails to respond to therapy.

Pelvic Tuberculosis

Pelvic tuberculosis (TB), often resulting from lymphatic spread of pulmonary TB, is rare in the United States and complicates pulmonary tuberculosis in about 5%. Direct extension to other abdominal organs from the pelvic organs is common. The pelvic organs primarily involved are oviducts and the endometrium.

Clinical findings may be minimal. Presentation may be for infertility, although pelvic pain, dysmenorrhea, or signs of tuberculous peritonitis may be present. Patients with abdominal symptoms may complain of low-grade fever and weight loss. Tuberculous peritonitis is usually accompanied by ascites. If the pelvic TB is found incidentally during pelvic surgery, it may be mistaken for chronic pelvic inflammation. However, the adhesions are much more dense, with loss of cleavage planes, the tubes are segmentally dilated, and the tubal ostia are usually not occluded with TB.

The *diagnosis* may be suspected given a history of TB, positive TB skin test, or chest x-ray consistent with TB. Hysterosalpingography during infertility workup may be suggestive when films reveal an irregular tubal lining, segmental areas of tubal dilatation, and saccular diverticula extending from the ampulla (characteristic of granulomatous disease). Abdominal x-ray may show calcified inguinal and periaortic lymph nodes. The diagnosis is confirmed when acid-fast bacteria are found on Ziehl-Neelsen stain and mycobacteria are cultured on Lowenstein-Jensen medium from samples obtained from menstrual discharge, curettage, or peritoneal biopsy.

The *differential diagnosis* includes schistosomiasis, enterobiasis, lipoid salpingitis, carcinoma, chronic pelvic inflammation, and mycotic infections. *Complications* are sterility and TB peritonitis.

Treatment consists of a 24–36 month course of standard TB drugs using a combination of several of the following drugs: isoniazid (INH), streptomycin, ethambutol, cycloserine, and rifampin. The reader is referred to medical texts describing specific TB therapeutic regimens.

The *prognosis* is good if diagnosis is made early and treatment is instituted, but the incidence of fertility remains low.

Chapter 23

Menstrual Abnormalities and Complications

ABNORMAL UTERINE BLEEDING

Abnormal uterine bleeding may be caused by hormonal factors, complications of pregnancy, systemic diseases, endometrial abnormalities (polyps), uterine or cervical problems (leiomyomas), or cancer. However, the pattern of abnormal bleeding is often very helpful in individualizing diagnosis.

Menorrhagia (hypermenorrhea) is prolonged or heavy menstrual flow that may be further complicated by clots. Menorrhagia may be caused by leiomyomas (often submucous), pregnancy complications, endometrial hyperplasia, adenomyosis, malignancy, or coagulopathies.

Metrorrhagia (intermenstrual bleeding) is defined as bleeding at any time between menstrual periods. The causes of metrorrhagia include midcycle (ovulatory) bleeding, endometrial polyps, endometrial or cervical cancer, endogenous estrogen production, and exogenous estrogen administration.

Menometrorrhagia is bleeding occurring at irregular intervals. Generally, the amount and duration of bleeding vary. The causes of menometrorrhagia are the same as those of metrorrhagia.

Polymenorrhea is menstrual-like bleeding that occurs too frequently. The usual cause of polymenorrhea is anovulation, but occasionally a shortened luteal phase may be the fault.

Postcoital (contact) *bleeding* must be investigated to rule out cervical cancer, although the most common causes are benign and include cervical eversion, cervical polyps, and cervical or vaginal infections.

Hypomenorrhea (cryptomenorrhea or spotting) is unusually light menstrual bleeding. Possible causes are obstructions (e.g., hymenal or cervical), uterine synechiae (Asherman's syndrome), and inappropriate oral contraceptive dosage (correctable).

Oligomenorrhea is defined as menstruation occurring at an interval >35 days.

DIFFERENTIAL DIAGNOSIS

The differential diagnosis of abnormal uterine bleeding must include the possibility of gynecologic but nonuterine bleeding. The most common causes of vulvar and vaginal bleeding are atrophic vulvovaginitis, infectious vulvovaginitis, local trauma, and genital cancer. Cervical causes of bleeding include eversion, erosion, cervical polyps, pedunculated leiomyomas, and cancer. With the exception of tubal ectopic gestation, other causes of bleeding from the uterine tube are unusual (e.g., salpingitis or tumors). The ovarian causes of vaginal bleeding include functional ovarian cysts, estrogen-producing tumors, and ovarian neoplasms.

Uterine causes of abnormal bleeding are endometritis, endometrial hyperplasia, endometrial cancer, endometrial polyps, adenomyosis, submucous leiomyomas, IUD pressure, or reaction to oral contraceptives or exogenous steroids. Systemic conditions that may cause abnormal uterine bleeding include hypothyroidism, hepatic dysfunction (abnormal estrogen metabolism), coagulopathies, blood dyscrasias, and extreme weight loss (e.g., eating disorders or excessive exercise leading to anovulation). The use of anticoagulants or adrenal steroids may lead to abnormal uterine bleeding also.

Nongynecologic causes of bleeding that may be confused with abnormal uterine bleeding include anorectal or urologic problems.

DIAGNOSIS

The history of abnormal uterine bleeding must detail the intervals between bleeding, the duration and amount of the bleeding, the character of the blood loss (e.g., color, consistency, clots), and when the abnormal pattern began. Seek additional information to properly evaluate the bleeding, including obstetric history, contraceptive history, postcoital bleeding, LMP, LNMP, menarche (or menopause), and alteration in general health. The patient-generated contemporaneous menstrual record is invaluable.

To evaluate abnormal uterine bleeding, perform a careful general physical examination, noting systemic health and conducting a pelvic evaluation. Obtain a cytologic smear to screen for uterine or cervical malignancy. An enlarged or irregular uterus suggests leiomyomas, and a symmetrically enlarged uterus is more commonly noted with endometrial cancer or adenomyosis. Pelvic examination should reveal vulvar, vaginal, and cervical lesions (e.g., atrophic, inflammatory, neoplastic), and bimanual examination should reveal uterine, tubal, or ovarian masses.

If pregnancy is not a factor (a pregnancy test may be required), sample the endometrium by endometrial aspiration (using a suction curette or Vabra-type aspirator), endometrial and endocervical biopsy, hysteroscopy with directed biopsies, or D & C. The exact modality for diagnosis depends on the patient's age, parity, and anatomy.

TREATMENT

Treatment of abnormal uterine bleeding must be individualized depending on the diagnosis.

DYSFUNCTIONAL UTERINE BLEEDING (DUB)

DUB is abnormal uterine bleeding occurring when all pathologic causes have been excluded. DUB is most common at the extremes of reproductive age (20% of cases are in adolescents, 40% are in patients >40 years). DUB may be caused by a persistent corpus luteum cyst or a short luteal phase, but most patients are anovulatory. Anovulation results in continuous estrogen stimulation of the endometrium, with resultant hyperplasia, periodic partial endometrial breakdown, and irregular bleeding.

At menarche, anovulation with subsequent irregular menses is common. Usually, only pelvic examination and exclusion of pregnancy are necessary before therapy is begun. The therapeutic goals are control of bleeding, stabilization of the endometrium, and induction of controlled menstruation. The endometrium may be stabilized and the bleeding checked (usually in 12–14 h) by the administration of high-dose estrogen-progestin oral contraceptives. After the oral contraceptives are withdrawn, expect 5–7 days of heavy bleeding followed by renewal of more normal endometrium. An alternative is administration of progesterone (e.g., medroxyprogesterone acetate 10 mg/day for 10 days). Occasionally, it may be necessary to give high doses of conjugated estrogens first to control very heavy bleeding. Finally, prescribe cyclic therapy (either oral contraceptives or estrogen and estrogen-progesterone, e.g., conjugated equine estrogens 1.25 mg/day for 1–25 days, medroxyprogesterone acetate 10 mg/day for 10–25 days) for three to six cycles. Often after 2–3 months of cyclic therapy, spontaneous ovulation and normal menstruation will occur.

Endometrial sampling before initiating therapy as outlined becomes more important with increasing age, especially in the premenopausal woman, when hysteroscopically guided biopsies and endocervical curettage are especially revealing. Hormone therapy may be accomplished, but the patient should be continued on cyclic estrogen-progesterone therapy. In later years, if this is unsuccessful (or if hormones are contraindicated), consider abdominal or vaginal hysterectomy.

POSTMENOPAUSAL BLEEDING (PMB)

PMB is defined as bleeding occurring after >12 months of amenorrhea in a woman of menopausal age (>45 years). PMB is far more likely to be of pathologic origin than is abnormal uterine bleeding during the reproductive years. Therefore, it is mandatory that PMB be thoroughly investigated. Although nongynecologic bleeding is more common in this age group, it is always wise to exclude gynecologic causes. The *differential diagnosis* of pathologic causes of PMB includes atrophic endometrial bleeding, endometrial hyperplasias (cystic, adenomatous, and atypical), endometrial polyps, submucous leiomyomas, sarcoma, endometrial carcinoma, cervical carcinoma, endocervical carcinoma, fallopian tube carcinoma, an estrogen-producing ovarian tumor, and ovarian carcinoma.

AMENORRHEA

Amenorrhea is the absence of menses during the reproductive years. It is a symptom not a diagnosis. The most common cause of amenorrhea is physiologic, i.e., pregnancy, nursing, or the puerperium. When pathologic, amenorrhea may be caused by genetic, anatomic, or endocrine disorders and is classified as primary or secondary.

PRIMARY AMENORRHEA

Primary amenorrhea is failure of menses to occur by age 16.5 years or within 2 years of full secondary sexual characteristic development. It is infrequent (0.1%–2.5%), and the etiologies causing primary amenorrhea may be pathophysiologically classified by physical examination, with emphasis on breast development (secondary sexual characteristics), the external genitalia, and whether or not a uterus is present. Most commonly, the external genitalia are normal.

Ambiguous Genitalia

Those patients with ambiguous genitalia usually have been exposed to excessive androgens in utero. Ambiguous genitalia usually are encountered at a much earlier age and are discussed on page 682.

Breast Development and Uterus Present (Group A, Table 23-1)

Primary amenorrhea with normal breast development and a uterus occurs in one third of cases. Of these, one quarter are caused by hyperprolactinemia. Others are due to exogenous estrogens. The rest of these patients have diagnoses similar to those with secondary amenorrhea (Table 23-1). Thus, testing and therapy should proceed as is discussed for secondary amenorrhea.

Breast Development Absent and Uterus Present (Group B, Table 23-1)

This category is the most commonly encountered situation (one half) in patients with primary amenorrhea.

Gonadal Failure

The *causes* of gonadal failure are mainly chromosomal or genetic: partial or total absence of an X chromosome (eg, 45,X, 46,XX, p-, or q-), mosaicism (e.g., X/XX), pure XX and XY gonadal dysgenesis, and 17α-hydroxylase deficiency (with 46,XX karyotype).

Two or more normal X chromosomes are necessary for normal ovarian development. Without them, fibrous bands (gonadal

Table 23-1. Differential diagnosis of primary amenorrhea with normal external genitalia based on breast development and uterine presence or absence.

	Uterus present	Uterus absent
Breast development present	**Group A** Hypothalamic Pituitary Ovarian Uterine	**Group C** Congenital uterovaginal agenesis Androgen insensitivity (testicular feminization)
Breast development absent	**Group B** Gonadal failure CNS-hypothalamic-pituitary disorders	**Group D** 17,20-Desmolase deficiency Agonadism 17α-Hydroxylase deficiency (46,XY)

streaks) often replace normal ovarian development, and there is no ovarian hormonal production and no secondary sexual characteristics. Gonadotropin levels in such cases are high, as with ovarian failure. Other stigmata of X chromosome abnormality include short stature (<63 inches) and major cardiovascular or renal anomalies in one third of these patients.

The most common X chromosome abnormality is *Turner's syndrome* (45,X), which occurs in 1 in 2000 live births. Individuals with Turner's syndrome or Turner's mosaicism (45,X/XX) have normal migration of the oogonia to the genital ridge. Although some fetal ovarian development may occur, it soon undergoes accelerated degeneration, resulting in streak ovaries. Individuals with mosaicism have been reported to menstruate briefly, but conception is very rare. Females with deletion of the short arm of an X chromosome phenotypically resemble those with 45,X.

Gonadal dysgenesis is considered pure if the primitive oogonia do not migrate to the genital ridge, resulting in streak gonads that cannot produce hormones. This probable genetic disorder includes normal stature and phenotype in both 46,XX and 46,XY. If this maldevelopment occurs with 46,XX there will be no ovarian hormones produced. However, development of both internal and external genitalia is not dependent on estrogen. Primary amenorrhea is the usual result. When the syndrome is incomplete, a few such individuals may have some follicles and occasional menstruation. In 46,XY karyotypes, failure of primitive germ cells to migrate to the genital ridge results in a streak gonad that produces neither testosterone nor mullerian-inhibiting hormone (MIH). The resulting internal and external genitalia are female. Since estrogen is not produced, breast development does not occur, and the doctor usually is consulted because of delayed onset of puberty rather than primary amenorrhea.

Patients with 17α-hydroxylase deficiency are very rare. They lack the enzyme necessary to convert progesterone to cortisol and, thus, have high progesterone levels and low cortisol levels. They also may have hypernatremia (with hypertension) and hypokalemia, as well as elevated ACTH and mineralocorticoid levels. These patients require sex steroids and cortisol replacement.

CNS-Hypothalamic-Pituitary Abnormalities

Patients with these lesions have low gonadotropin and estrogen levels.

Hypothalamic Disorders. Normal hypothalamic function requires pulsed release of GnRH from the arcuate nucleus into the hypophyseal portal system about every hour. GnRH causes release of LH and FSH from the pituitary, which stimulate ovarian follicular growth and ovulation. Absence of GnRH, abnormal transport of GnRH, or abnormal pulsation of GnRH will result in *hypogonadotropic hypogonadism.*

Defective GnRH Transport. Conditions that will interfere with GnRH transport include those that destroy the arcuate nucleus or compress or disrupt the pituitary stalk. These problems include trauma, tumors (e.g., craniopharyngioma, germinoma, glioma, teratoma, or endodermal sinus tumor), Hand-Schuller-Christian disease, sarcoidosis, tuberculosis, and radiation.

Defective GnRH Pulse Production. If the GnRH pulse frequency or amplitude is severely reduced, little or no FSH and LH will be released, no ovarian follicles will develop, and estradiol will not be secreted. Although this may be idiopathic, it is seen also in prepubertal girls and in those with anorexia nervosa, severe stress, starvation, prolonged vigorous exercise, and hyperprolactinemia. If GnRH pulsation amplitude or frequency is less severely reduced, there may be diminished LH and FSH production that may result in follicular stimulation insufficient for full development and ovulation, but estradiol will be secreted. This too may be idiopathic, or the condition may occur as the result of stress, hyperprolactinemia, marked athletic activity, or early eating disorders.

Congenital Absence of GnRH. Congenital absence of GnRH (Kallmann's syndrome) is associated with anosmia. LH and FSH are not released from the pituitary so that follicular development and ovulation cannot occur.

Pituitary Disorders. Pituitary lesions (excluding chromophobe adenomas) are rarely the primary cause of amenorrhea. Congenital absence of the pituitary is exceptional and lethal. On rare occasion, isolated congenital abnormalities of LH or FSH occur, resulting in anovulation and amenorrhea. Acquired pituitary dysfunction may occur as the result of Sheehan's syndrome (postpartum necrosis of the pituitary secondary to severe hypotension from hemorrhage), hemosiderosis (destruction of the cells producing FSH and LH by iron deposits), and pituitary hyperplasia or pituitary adenomas (both cause high prolactin levels).

Breast Development Present and Uterus Absent (Group C, Table 23-1)

Congenital Uterovaginal Agenesis (Rokitansky-Kuster-Hauser Syndrome)

Congenital absence of the uterus is usually an isolated developmental defect occurring in 1 in 4000–5000 female births. This contributes about 15% of individuals with primary amenorrhea. The ovaries function normally. Therefore, these individuals generally have normal secondary sexual development and no endocrinopathies. However, the uterus and upper (or total) vagina are absent. Associated abnormalities include renal (one third), skeletal (one eighth), and an enhanced rate of cardiac and other abnormalities.

Androgen Insensitivity

Primary amenorrhea is often the reason individuals seek medical assistance who have 46,XY karyotype but are phenotypically female. The fetus does not develop male genitalia unless testosterone and its active metabolite dihydrotestosterone (DHT) are present. Thus, any disorder of fetal testosterone production, metabolism, or its receptors will result in a phenotypic female. In addition, the fetal testis produces mullerian-inhibiting factor (MIF), which is responsible for regression of the mullerian structures (i.e., uterus, uterine tubes, and upper two thirds of the vagina).

Androgen insensitivity (testicular feminization) occurs with normal fetal testosterone production as the result of either absent or defective androgen receptors in the genital anlagen and mesonephric ducts. Because MIF production is normal, the mullerian structures regress, and there are no uterine tubes, uterus, or upper vagina. Since these patients produce some estrogen, breast development may be normal, and the abnormality may not be diagnosed until they are investigated for primary amenorrhea.

Breast Development Absent and Uterus Absent (Group D, Table 23-1)

Any enzymatic defect in the biosynthesis of testosterone that occurs before the production of androstenedione will result in an individual with female external genitalia but no mullerian structures (i.e., MIF is produced). If the enzymatic defect occurs after androstenedione is formed but there is no testosterone production, the patient will have ambiguous external genitalia and no mullerian structures.

This group includes <1% of all primary amenorrhea patients and comprises *17,20-desmolase deficiency, agonadism, and 17α-hydroxylase deficiency (46,XY)*. Generally, they are male in karyotype, have elevated gonadotropin levels, and have testosterone in the normal or below-normal female range. With both 17,20-desmolase deficiency and 17α-hydroxylase deficiency, individuals have an enzymatic defect in the path of testosterone synthesization. As a result, they develop female, not male, external genitalia. MIF is produced by the testes, causing female internal genitalia regression.

Regression of the fetal testis at <7 weeks results in a clinical picture indistinguishable from pure gonadal dysgenesis. If regression of the testis occurs between 7 and 13 weeks, MIF and testosterone production have had time to affect genital differentiation sufficiently to result in ambiguous genitalia.

SECONDARY AMENORRHEA

Secondary amenorrhea is the lack of menses for >6 months in a woman who has previously had normal menstruation or lack of menses for three typical intervals in the oligomenorrheic woman. Secondary amenorrhea occurs in 0.7%–3% of women. It is predisposed by age (<25 years), by previously having menstrual irregularities, by extraordinary emotional stress, or by marked physical stress.

Ovarian Dysfunction

The most common cause of ovarian dysfunction is *polycystic ovaries* (*Stein-Leventhal syndrome*). Pathologic findings consist of ovaries with multiple small antral follicles, well-developed stromal tissue, and a thick pseudocapsule. The abnormality is believed to be the result of increased androgen (from either the ovary or adrenal gland), with subsequent conversion to estrogen in the adipose tissue. Because levels of sex steroid-binding globulin are low, free estrogen levels are increased. Elevated estrogen stimulates the pituitary to increase the LH/FSH ratio, which results in aberrant follicular development, anovulation, and increased ovarian androgen production. That androgen is, in turn, converted to more estrogen: a vicious cycle. Amenorrhea may be primary or secondary.

Ovarian Failure

Primary ovarian failure is demonstrated by the presence of elevated gonadotropins and low estradiol (*hypergonadotropic hypogonadism*). Secondary ovarian failure is demonstrated by normal or low gonadotropins and low estradiol (*hypogonadotropic hypogonadism*) and usually is secondary to hypothalamic dysfunction. If ova are depleted <35 years, ovarian failure is considered premature, and premature menopause is the result.

Causes of primary gonadal failure include idiopathic premature ovarian failure, steroidogenic enzyme defects, true hermaphroditism, gonadal dysgenesis, ovarian resistance syndrome, postoophorectomy injury (after wedge resection or bivalve operations), autoimmune oophoritis, postinfection, postradiation, and postchemotherapy. Many of these become evident by careful history and examination.

Ovarian resistance (Savage's syndrome) is characterized by ovaries containing primordial germ cells and elevated levels of circulating FSH and LH. Receptor resistance is postulated.

Systemic Causes

In addition to previously listed processes, obesity may result in amenorrhea, presumably by the same hormone imbalance mechanism as that found in polycystic ovarian syndrome. Other endocrinopathies causative of obesity include hypothyroidism, Addison's disease, Cushing's syndrome, and chronic renal failure.

DIAGNOSIS OF AMENORRHEA

The diagnostic goal is to determine which organ is primarily responsible for amenorrhea so that appropriate therapy, if any, can be initiated. A careful history and physical examination are mandatory.

Rule Out Anatomic Abnormalities

There are five common anatomic disorders in 46,XX individuals that may lead to amenorrhea.

1. Mullerian dysgenesis (congenital absence of the uterus and upper vagina)
2. Vaginal agenesis (congenital absence of the vagina)
3. Transverse vaginal septum (from the failure of fusion of the mullerian and urogenital sinus-derived portions of the vagina)
4. Imperforate hymen (does not allow menstrual blood egress from the vagina)
5. Asherman's syndrome amenorrhea secondary to intrauterine synechiae. Asherman's syndrome may occur as the result of such procedures as myomectomy and cesarean section but most often follows complicated D&C (e.g., vigorous elimination of endometrium, infected products of conception), or it may result from tuberculous endometritis.

Imperforate hymen, transverse vaginal septum, and vaginal agenesis can be identified or ruled out by examination.

Of prime importance in evaluating primary amenorrhea is to determine whether or not the patient has a uterus (by examination, ultrasound). If the uterus is absent, a karyotype and testosterone level should be obtained because 46,XY is highly likely.

Rule Out Pregnancy

If a uterus and patent vagina are present, pregnancy should be ruled out before extensive testing is begun, whether amenorrhea is primary or secondary.

Perform a Progestin Challenge Test

The diagnostic workup for the patient who has secondary amenorrhea with normal prolactin levels and absence of galactorrhea begins with a progestin challenge test to determine whether or not the ovary is producing estrogen. Either medroxyprogesterone acetate 10 mg PO daily for 5 days or progesterone 100–200 mg IM as a single dose is given. The exogenous progestin administered will produce menses if the endometrium has been normally primed with estrogen. If bleeding does not follow, either there is no (or inadequate) estrogen or the patient has Asherman's syndrome.

Asherman's syndrome can be diagnosed by hysterosalpingography, by hysteroscopy, or by obtaining weekly progesterone levels and demonstrating any in the ovulatory range (>3 ng/ml) not associated with menses. In these patients, providing estradiol 2.5 mg PO for 25 days with medroxyprogesterone acetate 10 mg PO on days 16–25 will be diagnostic of Asherman's syndrome if menses do not occur.

If the progestin challenge is positive (menses occurred) and the patient has evidence of hirsutism, *polycystic ovary syndrome, ovarian tumor,* or *adrenal tumor* should be suspected. If the patient with a positive challenge test is not hirsute, *mild hypothalamic dysfunction* is likely, possibly the result of such factors as emotional or physical stress, weight loss, obesity, or psychologic disorder, or the problem may be idiopathic.

Evaluate the Hypothalamic-Pituitary Axis

If Asherman's syndrome has been ruled out, yet menstrual bleeding did not occur with progestin challenge, serum FSH levels should be obtained. If FSH is >40 mIU/ml, *gonadal failure* is the diagnosis, and a karyotype should be performed to identify the genetic etiology for the premature menopause. Autoimmune causes should be investigated also, since they may be treatable. If the FSH level is <40 mIU/ml, severe *hypothalamic dysfunction* is present (hypogonadotropic hypogonadism).

If a uterus and patent vagina are present, serum TSH and

prolactin levels should be obtained to aid in evaluation of the hypothalamic-pituitary axis.

If breast development is present, the patient with primary amenorrhea should undergo the same workup as for secondary amenorrhea. If breast development is absent, workup should progress as for progestin challenge-negative secondary amenorrhea.

Galactorrhea-Hyperprolactinemia Syndrome

Consideration of the differential diagnoses of galactorrhea-hyperprolactinemia should begin when galactorrhea is noted on physical examination in a patient with elevated prolactin levels. The *differential diagnosis* includes pituitary tumor, hypothyroidism, idiopathic hyperprolactinemia, drug-induced hyperprolactinemia (dopamine antagonists, e.g., phenothiazines, thioxanthines, butyrophenone, diphenylbutylpiperidine, dibenzoxazepine, dihydroindolone, and procainamide derivatives, catecholamine-depleting agents, and false transmitters, e.g., alpha-methyldopa), interruption of the normal hypothalamic-pituitary relationship, and peripheral neuronal stimulation varying from chest wall stimulation (e.g., thoracotomy, mastectomy, thoracoplasty, burns, herpes zoster, bronchogenic tumors, bronchiectasis, chronic bronchitis), nipple stimulation, spinal cord lesions (e.g., tabes dorsalis, syringomyelia) to CNS disease (e.g., encephalitis, craniopharyngioma, pineal tumors, hypothalamic tumors, pseudotumor cerebri).

The *workup* for amenorrhea associated with galactorrhea-hyperprolactinemia begins with obtaining serum level of TSH. If the TSH is elevated, treat the hypothyroidism. If TSH is normal, obtain a CT or MRI scan of the sella turcica. If the sella appears normal and prolactin levels are <50–100 ng/ml, repeat the prolactin level every 6 months and sella turcica scans every 1–2 years. If the sella is abnormal or the prolactin level is >50–100 ng/ml or if visual fields are restricted, an *adenoma* or *hyperplasia* may be present.

TREATMENT OF AMENORRHEA

Management of the amenorrheic patient depends on the individual's desire to ovulate (menstruation, pregnancy) and the etiology of the amenorrhea. If amenorrhea is secondary to hypothyroidism, thyroid hormone replacement may be the only therapy required. If the patient has amenorrhea-galactorrhea with pituitary macroadenoma, surgical removal of the adenoma should be considered. However, postoperatively, ~50% will require bromocriptine to induce ovulation. If the patient has amenorrhea-galactorrhea without adenoma or with microadenoma, therapy with bromocriptine alone (2.5 mg PO bid) probably will induce ovulation. The dosage can be titrated until the serum prolactin level falls to normal. The drug may be discontinued once an ovulatory pattern is established or continued until pregnancy occurs.

If the patient has primary ovarian failure, the likelihood for ovulation is practically nonexistent unless the cause is autoimmune oophoritis, which may respond to corticosteroid therapy. If the karyotype reveals a Y chromosome, the ovaries should be removed to decrease the risk of tumor formation.

Progestin challenge-negative patients (hypoestrogenic hypothalamic amenorrhea) are treated using hMG, often in combination with clomiphene citrate to induce ovulation. Care must be taken to avoid overstimulation of the ovaries. Because the primary problem is a deficiency or abnormal pulse frequency of GnRH, pulsatile GnRH can be administered SC or IV to induce ovulation, although GnRH therapy is expensive.

Progestin challenge-positive patients almost always respond to clomiphene citrate. The initial dosage is 50 mg PO daily for 5 days. Ovulation usually occurs 5–10 days after the fifth dose. If the starting daily dose is insufficient, increase it gradually to a maximum of 250 mg/day. If there is still no response and androgens are elevated, adding corticosteroids may be effective. If combination therapy is ineffective, hMG may be added to the regimen.

If polycystic ovaries are present, the drug of choice is clomiphene citrate, followed by hMG if unsuccessful. Although surgical wedge resection may lead to ovulation, it may also lead to adhesions and mechanical infertility and, thus, should be reserved until other therapy has been tried and proven to be unsuccessful.

Progestin challenge-negative patients who desire menses without ovulation are best treated with oral contraceptives combining estrogen 0.625–1.25 mg on days 1–25 plus 5–10 mg medroxyprogesterone on days 16–25 to maintain bone density and prevent genital atrophy. Adequate daily calcium intake should be assured.

Progestin challenge-positive patients should be given progestins to avoid endometrial hyperplasia and the increased risk of endometrial carcinoma. This can be accomplished easily using oral contraceptives in patients <35 years. Otherwise, give medroxyprogesterone acetate 10 mg PO daily for 10–13 days every 1–2 months.

Prognosis of Amenorrhea

Because amenorrhea is amenable to therapy in almost all cases, the prognosis is good. The exceptions are premature ovarian failure and reproductive organ absence. With the use of either one or a combination of hormones (e.g., hMG, GnRH, corticosteroids) and medications (e.g., bromocriptine, clomiphene citrate), almost all other amenorrheic patients with ovaries may be induced to ovulate.

COMPLICATIONS OF MENSTRUATION

Dysmenorrhea

The definition of dysmenorrhea is severe, painful cramping in the lower abdomen just before or during the menses. Other *symptoms* may include sweating, tachycardia, headaches, nausea, vomiting, diarrhea, and tremulousness. Dysmenorrhea is probably the most common complaint of gynecologic patients, *affecting 75% of all women*. Of those affected, 50% report mild symptoms (i.e., no systemic symptoms, medications not often required, and work rarely affected), 30% have moderate symptoms (i.e., few systemic symptoms, medication required, work moderately affected), and 20% have severe symptoms (i.e., multiple symptoms, poor medication response, and work inhibited). Dysmenorrhea is more likely to occur in women who have first-degree relatives with dysmenorrhea and is less likely to occur in those who have delivered a child or take birth control pills.

Primary dysmenorrhea denotes women without pathologic indications or conditions potentially causative of the symptomatology. Primary dysmenorrhea begins near menarche (<20 years). It is likely that elevated prostaglandin $F_{2\alpha}$ in the secretory endometrium leads to painful uterine contractions and other symptoms of primary dysmenorrhea. Indeed, prostaglandin-synthetase inhibitors (PGSIs) alleviate symptoms in nearly three fourths of sufferers. A special rare form of dysmenorrhea is *membranous dysmenorrhea*. It is the painful passage of the intact endometrial lining through the cervix.

Relief of mild primary dysmenorrhea is usually possible with aspirin or acetaminophen. For some mild cases, nearly all moderate cases, and some severe cases, PGSIs (ibuprofen 400–800 mg q6h, naproxen 250–500 mg q6h, naproxen sodium 275–550 mg q6h, and mefenamic acid 250–500 mg q6h) generally afford relief of acute pain. Cyclic administration of oral contraceptives, usually low dose but with a higher estrogen content, will prevent dysmenorrhea. Cervical dilation rarely helps. Very occasionally, medication will not help, and surgical therapy becomes necessary. Procedures that have been used include uterosacral ligament division, presacral neurectomy, and hysterectomy. Obviously, such choices must be weighed carefully, and all options must be discussed with the patient.

Secondary dysmenorrhea includes conditions or pelvic pathology that cause the pain. Secondary dysmenorrhea is usually acquired later in life (>30 years). Conditions capable of causing dysmenorrhea include endometriosis (Chapter 26), adenomyosis (p 660), pelvic infection and adhesions (p. 596), pelvic congestion, cervical stenosis, endometrial polyps causing a cervical outflow obstruction, conditioned behavior, stress, and tension.

Pelvic congestion syndrome is caused by engorgement of the pelvic vessels and is characterized by burning or throbbing pelvic pain, worse on standing and at night. The vagina and cervix may reveal vasocongestion, and there may be uterine enlargement, with tenderness. *Laparoscopy* reveals uterine congestion as well as engorgement or varicosities of the broad ligament and pelvic veins. The pathophysiology is not understood, and the condition appears to be related to tension and psychosomatic problems. *Therapy* (usually counseling) is directed toward relief of tension and psychosomatic problems, but occasionally even medical pain management fails, and hysterectomy is a last resort.

During menses, *cervical stenosis* (either external or internal os) may impede menstrual flow. This increases intrauterine pressure and leads to retrograde menstrual flow through the fallopian tubes. Cervical stenosis may be congenital, secondary to cervical injury (e.g., childbirth), caused by infections, or due to operative injury (e.g., electrocoagulation, conization). Clues to *diagnosis* include scant menstrual flow with severe cramping throughout menses, scarring of the cervix, and difficulty passing a uterine sound. The diagnosis may be confirmed by hysterosalpingogram. *Therapy* consists of progressive cervical dilation using laminaria or dilators of progressive size. Pregnancy and delivery (cervical dilation) are usually curative.

Very occasionally, an *endometrial polyp* or *polypoid leiomyoma* will act as a ball-valve during menses. This too may be confirmed by hysteroscopy or hysterosalpingography. *Treatment* consists of hysteroscopic resection of the lesion.

Conditioned behavior as an etiology for dysmenorrhea requires that a reward or control results from the symptoms and that no other cause can be found. Confirmation of this as an etiology may be accomplished by use of a personality profile test (e.g., Minnesota Multiphasic Personality Index). *Treatment* involves sensitive reeducation or reconditioning. *Stress* and *tension* as a cause for dysmenorrhea are usually characterized by a history of gradual onset, with the symptoms worsening at times of stress. *Therapy* is directed to stress reduction.

MASTODYNIA

Mastodynia (or mastalgia) is the pain and breast enlargement caused by edema and engorgement of the vascular and ductal system, generally in response to the luteal phase of the menstrual cycle. It is a diagnosis of exclusion and is reserved for cases of nearly intolerable symptoms with no palpable abnormalities save tenderness and generalized tissue thickening. *It must be differentiated from neoplasms* (usually painless except for fibrocystic breast disease) and *mastitis* (rare except in postpartum patients).

General *therapy* usually consists of breast support, avoidance of methylxanthines (in case of some fibrocystic breast disease component), avoidance of excessive salt, occasional diuretics, and perhaps vitamin E (1200–1800 U/day). Specific therapy may be low-dose testosterone (5 mg every other day when symptoms are present) or danocrine 100–400 mg/day for up to 6 months. Should virilization begin to appear with use of testosterone, discontinue the therapy immediately.

PREMENSTRUAL SYNDROME (PMS)

Although PMS is variably defined and probably is a symptom complex once referred to as premenstrual molimina, Dalton has indicated that to be defined as PMS, sufferers must exhibit (at the minimum) edema, weight gain, restlessness, irritability, and increased tension. Symptomatology must occur in the second half of three consecutive menstrual cycles, and there must be a symptom-free interval of at least 7 days in the first half of the cycle. PMS must be severe enough to require medical intervention. *PMS oc-*

curs to some degree in up to 90% of women; 20%–40% are mentally or physically limited, and 2%–3% have severe distress with true incapacitation. PMS rarely occurs in adolescents, and the peak incidence is in the late 20s to early 30s.

There is disagreement concerning symptoms and criteria for *diagnosis.* More than 150 symptoms have been related to PMS (e.g., fluid retention, mastodynia, headaches, bloating, irritability, tension, anxiety, accident proneness, sleep alterations, mood swings, social withdrawal, antisocial behavior, increased crying, and changes in sexual desire). The *etiology* of PMS also is unknown, but estrogen-progesterone imbalance, excess aldosterone, hypoglycemia, hyperprolactinemia, abnormal prostaglandin activity, premenstrual fall in endogenous endorphins, and psychogenic factors have been proposed. If there is associated psychiatric illness, it is most likely depression. Most authorities recommend keeping a daily symptom diary with relation to the menstrual cycle.

Treat the symptomatology. Therapy is extremely controversial and has included (all of undocumented efficacy) progesterone (400 mg/day vaginal suppositories in the second half of the menstrual cycle), oral contraceptives, vitamins (B_6 50–200 mg/day), diuretics (spironolactone is most frequently used), PGSIs, bromocriptine (only for those with hyperprolactinemia, mastodynia, and breast engorgement), minerals, natural substances for sedation, and laxatives. Other therapeutic suggestions include high-protein well-balanced diet, more regimented daily life (especially exercise and rest), restriction of salt, sugar, caffeine, alcohol, and smoking, use of relaxation techniques (including biofeedback), and behavioral techniques. Group support, empathy, and a special interest in the problem are essential to successful management.

Chapter 24

Contraception

Contraception (pregnancy avoidance) is practiced for many reasons, such as pregnancy planning, limiting the number of children, avoiding medical risks of pregnancy (especially with heart disease, diabetes mellitus, or tuberculosis), and controlling the world population. The use of contraception is increasing in developed countries, but some forms are economically out of reach for those in developing countries.

Of the US female population age 15–44, it is estimated that 30% are not sexually active, 5% are not using contraception, and 60% are using a contraceptive. Table 24-1 shows an approximate distribution of the different contraceptives used in the United States and their relative effectiveness. Contraceptives usually fail when they are unacceptable (and therefore not often used) or when pregnancy inadvertently occurs. This is difficult to quantify, but the latter is termed the *failure rate* and is expressed as pregnancies per 100 women at 1 year, or per 100 woman-years. Pearl's index is another way of expressing the pregnancy rate.

$$\text{Pregnancy rate} = \frac{\text{Pregnancies X 1200}}{\text{Woman-months of use}}$$

The life table method is an actuarial expression of pregnancy or discontinuation at various intervals and may be a superior method for quantifying contraceptive information. Whatever type of assessment is used, it is important to differentiate between method effectiveness and use effectiveness. *Method effectiveness* is the rate of contraceptive effectiveness when always used correctly, whereas *use effectiveness* is the overall effectiveness in actual use. Effectiveness is materially enhanced by women wishing to prevent (as opposed to delay) pregnancy, those >30 years, those having higher education, and women of higher socioeconomic status.

Laws regarding the prescription and sale of contraceptives vary from state to state and country to country. In the United States, regulations may vary also with regard to the prescription of contraceptives to patients <18 years.

Table 24-1. Types of contraceptives used in the United States and failure rates

	% using method*	First year failure†
Sterilization	35	<0.2
Female	(20)	
Male	(15)	
Oral contraceptive	30	1–3
Condom	13	1–10
IUD	6	2–5
Diaphragm	6	6–14
Spermicide	4	6–18
Withdrawal	3	4–12
Rhythm	2	8–19
Douche and other	<0.5	4–12

*% of women using contraception.
†Pregnancy per woman-years.

There is no perfect contraceptive when one considers both side effects and effectiveness. All contraceptives have advantages and disadvantages, which must be integrated carefully with the patient's status. Therefore, careful individualization is necessary to avoid undesirable side effects and to optimize patient acceptance. Informed consent regarding the benefits, risks, and alternatives of contraceptives should be documented.

METHODS OF CONTRACEPTION

COITUS INTERRUPTUS

Withdrawing the penis before ejaculation is moderately effective in preventing pregnancy. It has the disadvantages of requiring male self-control and the occurrence of pregnancy from semen escaping before ejaculation or semen deposition at the vaginal introitus.

DOUCHING AFTER COITUS

The intent of this method is to wash semen out of the vagina before sperm can enter the cervix. Since sperm are found in the cervical mucus within 90 sec of ejaculation, the effectiveness of this method of contraception is marginal.

CONTRACEPTIVE SPONGE

A polyurethane sponge containing the spermicide nonoxynol 9 is available without prescription for insertion before intercourse. It is effective for 24 h after wetting, and a loop to the sponge facilitates removal. It is less effective than diaphragm and spermicide. Occasional cases of toxic shock syndrome (TSS) have been reported in association with the use of the sponge.

SPERMICIDAL PREPARATIONS

A variety of spermicidal creams, jellies, foams, gels, and suppositories are available without prescription and are effective as spermicides as well as barriers to contraception. All of these agents require insertion into the vagina before each coitus. Failure may occur with improper insertion or if inadequate time is allowed for vaginal dispersal of the agent. Some women or men will experience chemical irritation requiring discontinuance or change to a different product or method. Some of the available preparations also provide a good prophylactic effect against sexually transmitted diseases (STD) caused by, e.g., *Neisseria gonorrhoeae*, *Treponema pallidum*, *Candida albicans*, and *Trichomonas vaginalis*.

VAGINAL DIAPHRAGM

This simple rubber device acts as a mechanical barrier between the cervix and penis, and it holds contraceptive cream or jelly to the cervix and upper vagina. The diaphragm must be fitted properly during a pelvic examination using fitting rings.

The *disadvantages* of this method are the need for fitting, the need for insertion in anticipation of intercourse, and the possibility of the diaphragm becoming dislodged during coitus.

Diaphragms are less effective in the first few months of use (presumably because the patient is less familiar with usage). The *failure rate* for the diaphragm is 2–3 pregnancies/100 woman-years.

CERVICAL CAP

The cervical cap is a barrier device covering the cervical portio. The latest cap has a one-way valve allowing uterine and cervical fluids to escape while preventing entrance of sperm. Cervical caps probably should not be left in place for >72 h to avoid infection. The *disadvantage* of this method is that each cap must be individually molded for every patient because cervical anatomy varies greatly. The first-year failure in motivated patients is ~9%.

CONDOM

The condom is a penile sheath made of latex, rubber, plastic, or animal membrane that serves as a barrier. The addition of a vaginal spermicide makes this method very effective if used properly. The additional advantage of protection against STD is lost if the animal membrane variety is used or if petroleum jelly is used with the latex product. Among the *disadvantages,* manufacturing defects occur in ~3/1000. Moreover, if withdrawal of the penis occurs after detumescence, semen may leak into the vagina. Both partners may complain of decreased sensation during intercourse. However, the widespread availability, low cost, and effectiveness in prevention of STDs make it the most commonly used barrier contraceptive in the world. The *pregnancy rate* with condoms is ~0.9–3.5/100 woman-years.

PERIODIC ABSTINENCE (RHYTHM METHOD)

Since women are fertile for only ~24 h after ovulation, conscientious avoidance of intercourse for the 2 days before ovulation and 2–3 days after ovulation should provide effective contraception. The difficulty is to determine prospectively, with reasonable certainty, when ovulation will occur. Thus, several adjuncts may be used to increase precision in identifying the time of ovulation.

Three methods are commonly available to predict the day of ovulation. The *calendar method* predicts ovulation 14 days before the next menstrual period as determined by months of careful documentation of the length of the woman's menstrual cycles. Basal body temperature (BBT) is recorded immediately on awakening, before any activity is performed. The BBT rises abruptly 0.3–0.4°C (0.5–0.7°F) with ovulation (Fig. 24-1).

Checking the cervical mucus for consistency may assist in determination of ovulation. This has been used as an aid to the rhythm method. The *laboratory determination of the abrupt surge of LH with ovulation* (*LH peak*) is the most reliable method of determining ovulation. However, one must obtain serial serum LH levels, which is expensive and impractical for the avoidance of pregnancy. All in all, the BBT determination and cervical mucus assessment are the most reliable, practical methods to determine the infertile periods of the cycle. Nevertheless, ~20% of fertile women have such menstrual cycle variability that accurate prediction of ovulation is difficult, if not impossible. As a consequence, the *failure rate* of the rhythm method is high.

Prolongation of Lactation

Prolonged nursing (1–2 years, without supplementation) provides some contraceptive benefit (i.e., pregnancy is delayed 5–10 months on average compared with those who do not nurse). However, since about 6% of women will ovulate before the first postpartum menstrual period, relying on lactation alone for contraception is questionable.

Oral Contraceptives

Combined Hormonal Contraceptives

The oral contraceptive formulations currently available in the United States are all *19-nortestosterone derivatives.* They all share an ethinyl group in the 17 position that enhances their oral activity. There are only two with predominant estrogenic activity, whereas five have actual *progestogenic effect.* The estrogens are ethinyl estradiol and mestranol, its 3-methyl ether derivative. The progestins are norethindrone, norethynodrel, norethindrone acetate, ethynodiol diacetate, and norgestrel (Table 24-2).

Synthetic estrogens and progestins given to prevent ovulation

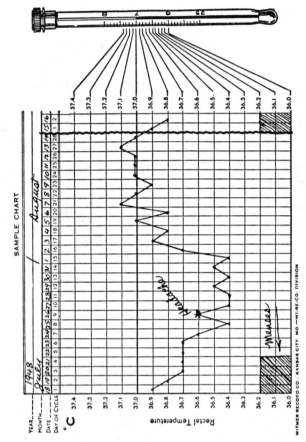

Figure 24-1. Basal body temperature recording. The temperature (vaginal or rectal) must be taken immediately on awakening every morning, before any activity whatsoever. The thermometer is allowed to remain in place for at least 5 min, and the recording is made immediately. This procedure must be continued over a period of at least 3 cycles to obtain an accurate chart. (Courtesy of Witmer Record Co.)

Table 24-2. The 19-nortestosterone oral
contraceptives available in the United States

Estrogenic	Progestogenic
Ethinyl estradiol	Norethynodrel
Mestranol	Norethindrone
	Norethindrone acetate
	Ethynodiol diacetate
	Norgestrel

are almost 100% effective in preventing pregnancy when taken as directed (*pregnancy rate of ~0.2%/year*). Combination pills containing both estrogen and progestin (often in different combinations) are taken daily for 20–21 days, with no pill or inert pills taken for 7–8 days to maintain a 28 day cycle. Withdrawal bleeding usually occurs 3–5 days after completing a 20–21 day regimen of two hormones.

Method of Action

With the combined contraceptive regimen, FSH and LH levels remain constantly low. Thus, the follicle is not stimulated to develop, and ovulation does not occur. They also cause scant, viscid cervical mucus, alter the endometrium, and reduce ovarian responsiveness to gonadotropin stimulation.

Benefits and Risks

In addition to extremely effective contraception, the *advantages* of combination oral contraceptives are decreased incidence of heavy menstrual bleeding, menstrual irregularities, ovarian cysts, iron deficiency anemia, benign breast disease, ectopic pregnancy, endometrial cancer (<50%), osteoporosis, TSS, breast fibroadenomas (reduced 85%), chronic cystic breast disease (50%), rheumatoid arthritis, and PID (50% decrease). Ovarian cancer is decreased 50% by the use of oral contraceptives. Moreover, oral contraceptives are helpful in conditions of unopposed estrogen and perhaps in endometriosis.

There are two major *disadvantages* of oral contraceptives. First is an increased incidence of thromboembolic disease, especially in smokers (4–5 times nonusers). The death rate from thrombo-embolic disease in users is 3/100,000. Although certainly less than the death rate from pregnancy and delivery (9/100,000, excluding illegal abortions), it is a risk. Second is the increased incidence of coronary artery disease (2.7 times nonusers age 30–39 and 5.7 times nonusers age 40–44) in women who smoke. This association is so strong that oral contraceptives are contraindicated in women >35 who smoke.

All *side effects* are reduced with lower-dose products. Even so, the estrogenic components occasionally cause depression, mood changes, sleepiness, nausea, breast tenderness, fluid retention (usually <3–4 pounds), hypercoagulability (ethinyl estradiol), and hypertension (transient). Progestogens may cause weight gain, acne, nervousness, or failure of withdrawal bleeding. Both act to cause irregular bleeding or chloasma. There is lowered effectiveness if oral contraceptives are taken with rifampicin (often used to treat tuberculosis). Additionally, barbiturates, sulfonamides, cyclophosphamide, ampicillin, and penicillin may exert a similar effect. Thus, the use or barrier contraceptives is recommended when oral contraceptive users must take these medications.

Oral contraceptive use does not cause atherosclerosis and is not associated with increased incidence of breast, endometrial, or cervical cancer. The occurrence of liver cancer (rare) may be slightly increased. Oral contraceptive use does not, overall, appear to impede future pregnancies.

Contraindications

Oral contraceptives are *contraindicated* in pregnancy (virilization of female fetus), nursing mothers (decreased milk production), those with vascular disease (thrombophlebitis, thromboembolism, atherosclerosis, stroke), lupus, diabetes mellitus, severe heart disease, SS hemoglobinopathies, hypertension, hyperlipidemia, smoking habit and age >35 years, and cancer of the breast or endometrium. *Relative contraindications* include migraine headaches, depression, and heavy smoking at age <35 years. Women with oligomenorrhea, amenorrhea (except for polycystic ovarian syndrome), or galactorrhea should have a definitive diagnosis before starting oral contraceptives.

Prescribing Oral Contraceptives

A complete history and physical examination should identify contraindications to oral contraception. A CBC, UA, and cervical cytology are obtained. Obtain documented (written) informed consent. In patients ≥35 years or those with a family history of diabetes, vascular diseases, or liver disease, the following should be determined: a 2 h postprandial blood glucose, HDL and LDL cholesterol, total cholesterol, triglycerides, and liver function studies. Follow-up of any abnormality is mandatory.

Products containing 30–35 μg of ethinyl estradiol are often used as a trial oral contraceptive. Oral contraceptives may be given to sexually active adolescents who have had a minimum of three regular (ovulatory) menses without fear of causing epiphyseal closure. After a first trimester abortion, oral contraceptives may be started immediately. In contrast, they should be started 1 week after second trimester abortions. In nonnursing mothers, oral contraceptives may be started 2–3 weeks after delivery.

The patient should be seen after 3 months for a nondirected history and blood pressure recording. Thereafter, the patient should be seen annually for history, blood pressure, weight, physical examination, and cervical cytology.

Nonstop Progestin Minipill

Taking low doses of progestin daily is a reasonably reliable method of contraception (2–7 pregnancies per 100 woman-years). Ovulation is not prevented however. The exact mechanism of action is unknown, but the *advantages* include no estrogen side effects and no sequencing of pills, with the daily administration. The *disadvantages* are irregularity of the ovulatory cycle, occasional abnormal bleeding patterns, and an increased incidence of ectopic pregnancy. There is probably no enhancement of thromboembolism, hypertension, nausea, and breast tenderness. Ideal patients for this method may be those with estrogen intolerance or lactating women (although long-term effects on the offspring from the small amount of progestin in the milk are unknown).

Postcoital Pill

If coitus occurs 2–6 days before ovulation, ovulation usually will be suppressed and pregnancy avoided by the use of oral contraceptives. The failure rate is 0–2.4%. The prevention of pregnancy after coitus is most often used in women who have been raped.

Two tablets of ethinyl estradiol 0.05 mg and dl-norgestrel

0.5 mg q12h for two doses, or the equivalent, is effective (1.6% pregnancy rate), as is progestin alone (norgestrel 1 mg) 1–8 h after unprotected intercourse. In the past, large doses of estrogenic compounds were used postcoitally to prevent pregnancy, but since they cause severe nausea and vomiting, they have largely been abandoned.

PARENTERAL HORMONAL CONTRACEPTION

Injectable Progestogens

Hormones injected in depot form may effectively prevent pregnancy for up to 1 year. This method prevents ovulation by suppressing anterior pituitary function. The most commonly used preparation is a 21-carbon progesterone, depomedroxyprogesterone acetate (DepoProvera) 150 mg every 90 days. With this agent, the resultant hormonal imbalance may cause atrophy of the endometrium and irregular or absent menstrual bleeding for months. The *disadvantage* is delay in reestablishing ovulation after discontinuation of the injections (6–12 months).

Implantable Progestin Capsules

Slender implantation capsules of progestin have become available in the United States. Six capsules are inserted through a 2 mm skin incision beneath the skin of the nondominant upper inner arm in a fan-shaped pattern under local anesthesia. The skin, about four fingerbreadths from the medial epicondyle, is cleansed with three applications of an antiseptic solution (e.g., providone-iodine), a sterile fenestrated drape is applied, and an intradermal wheal is created with a local anesthetic through a 25 gauge needle. Using an 18–22 gauge 1.5 inch needle, 1 ml of local anesthetic (e.g., 1% lidocaine with 1:4000 epinephrine) is injected along each anticipated site for the capsule. The proximal ends of the capsules are 15 degrees apart (and close enough to be removed by a single small incision) in a splayed pattern extending over 75–90 degrees. Using a sharp trocar or a No. 11 scalpel blade, an incision is made and the capsules are inserted from the most medial to the most lateral. The incision, which does not require suturing, is covered with a compression dressing (to prevent bruising) for 24 h.

Intrauterine Contraceptive Devices (IUD)

Of the many intrauterine contraceptive devices that have been on the market over the years, only two types are available in the United States, Progestasert and Copper TCu 380A. IUDs are inserted into the endometrial cavity and prevent implantation through a variety of local mechanisms.

The device usually is inserted during the menses to ensure the avoidance of pregnancy and better patency of the cervical canal. The device can be inserted at any time during the menstrual cycle, however (Fig. 24-2).

The cervix is cleansed using a topical antiseptic, the anterior lip is grasped with a single-toothed tenaculum, and with gentle

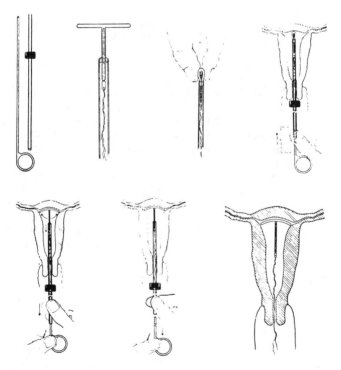

Figure 24-2. Insertion of the Tatum-Zipper Copper T. (From H.J. Tatum. In: R.C. Benson, ed., *Current Obstetric & Gynecologic Diagnosis & Treatment,* 4th ed. Lange, 1982.)

traction, the uterine cavity length and direction are determined using a sound. This is followed by insertion of the IUD using its accompanying insertion tube. The monofilament plastic tail is allowed to protrude from the cervix to aid later removal and to allow periodic digital palpation by the patient as a check (usually after each menses) for its presence. Complications of insertion include pain and, occasionally, syncope (especially in nulligravidas). Care and appropriate insertion technique should avoid perforation of the uterus (rare).

The *advantages* of the IUD include long-term protection without active participation by the patient except for occasional digital checking for expulsion. Fertility returns promptly after the device is removed. The *disadvantages* of the IUD include continued cramping in some, expulsion during menses (especially in the first few months after insertion), abnormal bleeding (less frequent if the device is the proper size), and ectopic pregnancy (3.8%). If the patient cannot feel the IUD string and did not notice expulsion, she should be examined and radiographs should be taken to locate the device. The string may have separated, but the device may also have perforated the uterus (<1/1000 insertions). If the patient becomes pregnant with a device in place, she must be warned of the enhanced rate of septic abortion, and pregnancy termination should be offered.

Contraindications to IUD include pregnancy, severe cervicitis, malignancy of the genital tract, recent class III or IV cytologic (Pap) smear without definitive diagnosis and treatment, uterine bleeding of unknown etiology, abnormal uterine cavity, acute or subacute salpingitis, cervical canal stenosis, and previous ectopic pregnancy.

An *IUD should be removed* when uterine cramps are severe, when bleeding is excessive or prolonged (increased bleeding during the first three or four menses after insertion are to be expected), when perforation has occurred (IUD removal by laparoscopy or colpotomy may be possible), if the device is displaced into the cervix, if pregnancy occurs (spontaneous abortion risk is 50% if not removed), and if bacterial salpingitis occurs (most frequently <4 weeks after insertion).

Chapter 25

The Nonreproductive Years

CLIMACTERIC

The climacteric is that phase of the aging process in which a woman passes from reproductive to nonreproductive capability. Menopause is life after the last menstruation. Thus, premenopause is that phase of a woman's life before menopause, and postmenopause is the phase of life after menopause.

To understand the physiology of the climacteric requires a brief review of ovarian physiology. Primordial germ cells migrate to the genital ridge by 5 weeks gestation. Successive mitotic cellular divisions form oogonia, which in turn give rise to oocytes. Although there are approximately 7 million oogonia present in the fetus at 20 weeks gestation, their numbers gradually decline, leaving 2 million at birth and only 300,000 at puberty. This reduction continues until menopause. The oogonia are reduced by atresia (the primary cause of loss) and ovulation (400–500 per lifetime).

Menopause occurs when oocytes responsive to gonadotropins disappear. The average age of menopause in the United States is 49–50, and it relates to health and genetic background. The age of menopause is not correlated with age at menarche, height, weight, parity, or prolonged use of oral contraceptives.

Early menopause has been associated with smoking, infection, chemotherapy (especially alkylating agents), radiation, surgical procedures that impair ovarian blood supply, tumors, or surgical removal of the ovaries (usually for treatment of endometriosis or estrogen-sensitive neoplasia). Early menopause has even been related to left-handedness, although menopause is not classified as being premature unless menses cease at <35 years of age.

PREMENOPAUSE

The length of the menstrual cycle shortens from 35 days at age 15 to 30 days at age 25 to 28 days at age 35. This is due to shortening of the follicular phase of the cycle. The luteal phase is unaffected by aging. The transition from premenopause to menopause may be marked by wide variations in menstrual cycle length. This transition period tends to be shorter when menopause occurs at an early age. Because the maturation of follicles in the premenopausal period is irregular, ovulation may or may not occur. The likelihood of conception occurring during this transition period is minimal. Hormone secretion by these follicles is variable but diminished.

Progesterone levels remain similar to those in younger women, but premenopausal women have lower estradiol levels. Although LH levels are similar to those in younger women, FSH levels are elevated, especially during the early follicular phase. The elevated FSH levels may stimulate the release of bursts of estradiol from the residual follicles, causing estrogen stimulation of the endometrium, which in the absence of regular progesterone secretion results in irregular bleeding.

HORMONAL CHANGES WITH MENOPAUSE

With the cessation of follicular activity, major changes in estrogen, progesterone, androgen, and gonadotropin secretion occur within 6 months (Table 25-1).

Estrogen

With menopause, estrogen production, especially estradiol, declines even further from the levels in the premenopause. The residual estradiol is produced indirectly by the adrenal glands. Both estrone (the major contributor) and testosterone are converted to estradiol in peripheral tissues. Estrone has a diurnal variation with a peak level in the morning and a nadir in early evening. Peripheral aromatization of adrenal androstenedione to estrone accounts for most of the estrone production.

Progesterone

Since progesterone is produced by the corpus luteum, postmenopausal progesterone levels are only 30% of those seen in

Table 25-1. Mean serum concentrations of hormones in premenopausal and postmenopausal women

Hormone	Premenopausal (ng/ml)	Postmenopausal (ng/ml)
Androstenedione	1.5	0.6
Dehydroepiandrosterone	4.2	1.8
Dehydroepiandrosterone-S	1600	300
Estradiol	0.05	0.013
Estrone	0.08	0.029
Progesterone	0.47	0.17
Testosterone	0.32	0.25

ovulating women during the follicular phase. The adrenal gland is presumed to be the source of the small amount of progesterone in postmenopausal women.

Androgens

Androstenedione is the predominant androgen secreted by developing follicles. With cessation of follicular development in postmenopausal women, androstenedione levels fall by 50%. Diurnal variation of androstenedione can be shown to follow adrenal gland activity after menopause. Only 20% of androstenedione is secreted by the ovary after menopause. Overall, testosterone production postmenopausally is decreased by less than a third. Diurnal variation is notable. A relatively large portion of testosterone is secreted by the postmenopausal ovary. This continued testosterone production combined with relatively low estrogen levels may result in slight virilism. Dehydroepiandrosterone (DHEA) and dehydroepiandrosterone sulfate (DHEAS) are produced primarily by the adrenal gland (<25% by the ovary). With aging, DHEA production falls by 60% and DHEAS falls by 80%.

Gonadotropins

After menopause, LH and FSH increase substantially. FSH and LH levels are both 4–30 mIU/ml during reproductive life, except briefly during the preovulatory surge, when they increase

to >50 mIU/ml and >100 mIU/ml, respectively. After menopause, the levels of both are >100 mIU/ml. FSH rises sooner
and at a more rapid rate than does LH. Both FSH and LH
show pulsatile bursts every 1–2 h, thought to be secondary to
pituitary response to hypothalamic release of gonadotropin-
releasing hormone (GnRH). Low estrogen levels increase pituitary sensitivity to GnRH.

CLINICAL FINDINGS

Reproductive Tract

Both the duration and flow of menstrual blood gradually diminish prior to the menopause until only spotting is followed by
cessation. On rare occasion, abrupt cessation occurs. In some
women, vaginal bleeding will be heavier or more frequent, occasionally with intermenstrual bleeding. Menopause cannot be diagnosed until cessation of menses has exceeded 6–12 months.

Decreased estrogen levels are responsible for atrophic changes
in the entire reproductive tract. The vaginal epithelium thins, and
the capillary bed is closer to the surface, making the vagina appear
hyperemic. Minimal trauma may result in mild vaginal bleeding.
Bacterial invasion may occur. The vaginal rugae gradually disappear. As time passes, the capillary bed decreases, and the vagina
becomes pale, shiny, and smooth.

Vaginal cytologic smears may be obtained to assess estrogenic
activity. Either the maturation index (a differential count of the
parabasal, intermediate, and superficial squamous cells) or the
cornification count (the percentage of precornified vs cornified
cells) may be used. Because there can be great variation in the
findings, the vaginal smear should be used only as a gross estimate of estrogenic status of the woman. It cannot diagnose the
climacteric state, although cytology may be helpful in determining the dosage of replacement estrogen required to reverse vaginal atrophy and may help to diagnose genital tract malignancy or
infection.

The cervix contracts in size, and cervical mucus production
decreases. The uterus and tubes atrophy as the myometrium and
endometrium shrink. This change is of benefit to women with
leiomyomas or adenomyomas because these lesions tend to atrophy as well. Endometrial biopsy may show tissue changes ranging from a scanty basal atrophic pattern to a moderately proliferative pattern. However, if glandular hyperplasia is present, this

indicates excessive estrogenic stimulation, and further investigation is necessary.

Because the decrease in ovarian size is substantial after menopause, a palpable ovary in a postmenopausal woman (the palpable ovary syndrome) should be considered neoplastic until otherwise explained. Progressive loss of pelvic tissue tone accompanies estrogen deficiency and contributes to the increased incidence of enterocele, rectocele, cystourethrocele, and uterine prolapse often seen in postmenopausal women.

Urinary Tract

Estrogen maintains the epithelium of the bladder and urethra. Hence estrogen deficiency causes atrophic cystitis and urethritis, characterized by urgency and frequency without dysuria or pyuria. Urethral tone decreases, occasionally allowing the meatus to protrude (a reddened caruncle).

Breasts

Breast size decreases progressively during the climacteric.

Hot Flushes

Hot flushes, or flashes, will occur in 75% of women who lose ovarian function, either through menopause or by bilateral oophorectomy. The episodic sudden flushing causes perspiration even in a cool environment. The vasomotor episodes are described as starting with a sensation of pressure in the chest or head that increases until a feeling of heat or burning is experienced in the face, neck, and chest, immediately followed by sweating especially involving the head, neck, chest, and back. Some report palpitations, vertigo, weakness, fatigue, or a feeling of faintness. The frequency may be from one to two per hour to one to two per week. The durations of the episodes vary from momentary to 10 min, with an average duration of 4 min. If flushes occur, 80% can expect them to recur for 1 year, and at least 25% will experience flushes for 5 years.

Only slight changes in blood pressure or heart rhythm have been demonstrated, but cutaneous vasodilatation, decreased core temperature, sweating, and increased pulse rate are documented. The symptoms may relate to a malfunction of the central thermoregulatory system. Despite a falling core temperature, the patient feels hot and attempts cooling by fanning or moving to an open door or window. Apparently at climacteric, the set point for temperature in the hypothalamus is reset temporarily at a lower point. Withdrawal of estrogen rather than lack of estrogen appears to be responsible, since young girls do not have hot flushes nor do those with gonadal dysgenesis (unless estrogen is given, then withdrawn). There appears to be a correlation of hot flushes with the pulsatile release of gonadotropins. If the flushes occur at night, frequent awakening may lead to sleep deprivation (e.g., fatigue, irritability, anxiety, memory loss). The most effective treatment is estrogens. Progestins also have been shown to be effective in treatment of hot flushes.

Cardiovascular System

Heart disease in women <55 years is less common and less severe than in men of the same age. However, for each decade >55, the death rate from heart attack increases 2 times in men and 3 times in women. Smoking increases the risk in both groups. The risk of heart disease increases the younger the age at menopause.

Estrogen replacement therapy decreases the risk of heart disease and decreases the death rate as well. Cholesterol levels increase about 16 mg/dl with menopause, but this increase is not lowered by replacement estrogens. Estrogens increase the high-density lipoproteins by 10% and decrease the low-density fraction. Triglyceride levels are increased by replacement estrogens. This effect on lipid metabolism may be profound in cases of familial hyperlipidemia.

Although menopause has no consistent effect on blood pressure, replacement estrogens increase both systolic and diastolic blood pressure. The change in blood pressure associated with estrogen therapy occurs via the renin-angiotensin-aldosterone system, thus resulting in vasoconstriction and fluid retention. The increase is usually mild, and no increased incidence of stroke has been documented because of this shift. Menopause does not affect carbohydrate metabolism. Replacement estrogen either has no effect on carbohydrate metabolism or may decrease glucose tolerance slightly without increasing insulin secretion.

In the United States, the decrease in the female death rate from heart disease has coincided with the increased use of replacement estrogen therapy. The female death rate has declined by >30%, whereas male deaths from heart disease declined only 20% during the same time.

Osteoporosis

Osteoporosis is the loss of bone density without change in its chemical composition. It may be the most significant health hazard associated with the climacteric because of the resulting fractures, disability, and invalidism. Death within 6 months of hip fracture occurs in 15%–20%, with substantial morbidity in the survivors. Trabecular bone loss is greater than cortical bone loss (50% and 5%, respectively). Osteoporosis occurs in both sexes, more in women and earlier than in men (beginning as early as age 30 and 45–50, respectively). There are racial differences in the incidence of osteoporosis, with the highest incidence in Caucasians, followed by Orientals, and lowest in blacks. Smoking increases osteoporosis. Thin women and those who do not exercise are more susceptible.

The bone loss is the result of bone resorption exceeding bone formation, with a calcium loss of approximately 15 mg/day between 50 and 70 years of age (net loss 100 g). The exact mechanism is unclear, but estrogen replacement therapy results in decreased bone resorption and decreased bone calcium loss. However, new bone formation does not occur with this therapy. Effects of estrogen on parathyroid hormone receptors and calcitonin are being studied. Osteoporosis in itself is not painful, but fractures are. Vertebral body fractures are most common, leading to a hunched posture (dowager's hump). Hip and arm fractures are increased substantially, as well as rib fracture, often after seemingly trivial accidents.

Early *diagnosis* is important, and *therapy* must be initiated early enough to decrease the risk of pathologic fractures. Bone densitometry studies are an excellent means of measuring trabecular bone mass. If presentation is atypical, other bone diseases must be considered, such as osteomalacia, multiple myeloma, osteitis deformans (Paget's disease of bone), metastatic cancer, or hyperparathyroidism. These may be differentiated by evaluating the results of serum calcium and phosphate levels, 24-h urinary calcium, parathyroid hormone, or serum protein electrophoresis.

Low-dose estrogen begun shortly after menopause can retard or arrest bone loss. Conjugated estrogens, 0.625 mg, or its equivalent demonstrate benefits for at least 10 years. Elemental calcium supplementation (1000–1500 mg) is also of benefit. If the patient is vitamin D deficient, vitamin D should be given. Low-dose calcitonin plus calcium has been shown to increase body calcium stores for up to 2 years. High-dose sodium fluoride will increase trabecular bone but has toxic side effects. Etidronate disodium (Didronel), a sulfone successfully used to treat Paget's disease of bone, may be useful in the prevention or treatment of postmenopausal osteoporosis, especially in women who cannot take estrogens (e.g., after treatment for breast cancer).

Skin

Estrogen receptors are present in skin, especially of the face, thigh, and breasts. With aging, the skin becomes thinner, with a loss of elasticity leading to wrinkling. These changes are most pronounced in areas exposed to sunlight (e.g., face, neck, hands). In animal studies, estrogen increases skin cell growth, changes dermal collagen content, alters skin vascularization, and enhances dermal water. However, estrogen in skin creams or lotions may cause systemic problems and should only be used under physician direction, if at all.

Hair

Changes in hair (thinning) may be in part the result of low estrogen with sustained testosterone levels. The fine hair decreases on the face with the growth of coarse hair, especially on the upper lip (moustache) and chin. Pubic and axillary hair decrease, and slight baldness may appear. Body and extremity hair may increase or decrease.

Psychologic Aspects

Psychologic disturbances increase during the climacteric. Hot flushes, sleep disturbance, and vaginal atrophy may play a significant role. Many family changes may be occurring concomitantly, with slight alterations in the woman's appearance. The incidence of severe psychiatric illness is not increased by menopause, but estrogen therapy may improve the emotional state by relieving hot flushes, insomnia, or vaginal atrophy.

Excess Endogenous Estrogens

Occasionally, women will show signs of estrogen excess, with uterine bleeding, mastodynia, edema, leiomyoma growth, and increased endometriosis. When such symptomatology of estrogen excess develop in postmenopausal women, one of three mechanisms is likely: (1) increased androgen production, (2) increased aromatization of androgens, or (3) excess estrogen production. Increased androgen production is usually associated with an ovarian or adrenal neoplasm. Increased aromatization of androgen is associated with hyperthyroidism, obesity, or liver disease. Increased androgenic estrogen may be associated with obesity, likely due to the increased conversion of androstenedione to estrone in adipose tissue.

TREATMENT

When a woman seeks relief of symptoms of the climacteric, a discussion of the physiologic changes she is experiencing may be helpful to understand the therapeutic goals. She should be made aware of the benefits of and alternatives to estrogen replacement therapy.

Absolute *contraindications* to estrogen replacement are undiagnosed vaginal bleeding, acute liver disease, chronic hepatic dysfunction, acute vascular thrombosis, neuroophthalmologic vascular disease, and endometrial or breast carcinoma (estrogen may stimulate the growth of malignant cells). Estrogens are not contraindicated in treated cervical carcinoma. Undesirable side effects may be seen in patients given estrogens with hypertension, seizure disorder, uterine leiomyomas, fibrocystic disease of the breast, familial hyperlipidemia, some collagen diseases, chronic thrombophlebitis, diabetes mellitus, migraine headaches, or gallbladder disease.

The use of replacement estrogen without progestins in the postmenopausal woman increases her risk of developing endometrial carcinoma. Although the incidence of endometrial cancer is increased, the risk of death from this is not increased if careful observation of these patients allows diagnosis of cancer in the early stages.

There may be a slightly increased risk of breast carcinoma with the use of replacement estrogens. However, studies have not shown consistent results relative to those at greatest risk. Nonetheless, high estrogen doses have been implicated in breast cancer development.

Thromboembolic disease may be worsened due to the estrogen effect on the clotting mechanism. Estrogen increases the coagulability of blood via platelet changes, the coagulation system itself, and the fibrinolytic sequence. Estrogen also increases vascular endothelial proliferation and decreases venous blood flow slightly. However, the low doses of estrogen used in replacement therapy usually do not significantly increase the risk of thromboembolic disease. This must be considered, however, in certain women.

Gallbladder disease increases with estrogen replacement, presumably due to the increase in cholesterol and triglycerides. However, heart disease is decreased with the use of low-dose estrogens. Since the age-adjusted mortality rate of death from heart disease is 4 times that of death from breast cancer or endometrial cancer combined, this benefit should be stressed.

Progestin-Estrogen Therapy

Current recommendations include progestin therapy with estrogen therapy because studies have shown that the risk of endometrial carcinoma is decreased if endometrial tissue exposed to estrogen is periodically opposed by progestin. The duration of progestin therapy is critical for this effect, since 7 days/month is ineffective, whereas 13 days is protective. Long-term estrogen replacement is necessary to prevent osteoporosis (e.g., 4 years is insufficient). The effects of long-term progestin therapy are unknown but seem to be limited to periodic vaginal bleeding. If the patient has no uterus, progestins are not indicated.

Although the hormones may be replaced orally or by injection, certainly the oral method is more convenient. The starting dosage of estrogen is 0.625 mg/day of oral conjugated equine estrogens or estropinate for 25 days, with no therapy for the rest of the month. If the lower dose does not prevent hot flushes, a higher dose may be given and tapered as soon as possible. Norethindrone (Norlutate) should be avoided, since this preparation blocks the beneficial effects of estrogen on lipid metabolism. If the uterus is present, medroxyprogesterone acetate 10 mg/day should be given during the last 13–15 days of estrogen replacement each month.

If estrogen replacement is contraindicated or refused, hot flushes may be reduced in 90% by medroxyprogesterone 150 mg/month IM or 10–40 mg/day PO. Less effective than estrogen is norgestrel 250 μg/day PO. Conjugated estrogen vaginal cream 1 g every other day may relieve symptoms of vaginal atrophy.

Chapter 26

Endometriosis and Adenomyosis

ENDOMETRIOSIS

Endometriosis is the extrauterine occurrence of endometrial glands and stroma, most often involving the ovaries or dependent visceral peritoneal surfaces. Although benign, endometriosis is progressive, tends to recur, may be locally invasive, may have widespread disseminated foci (rare), and may exist in pelvic lymph nodes (30%). The etiology is unknown, but several mechanisms may be important in pathogenesis. Endometriosis represents a very significant problem in gynecology, with *10%–20% of menstruating women affected*. Endometriosis is found in 30%–45% of infertile women. Endometriosis is responsible for 20% of all gynecologic operations and is the single leading nonobstetric cause (>5%) of hospitalization for women age 15–44.

PATHOLOGY

Although some contend that it may be entirely a microscopic diagnosis, with no grossly visible alterations, most authorities maintain that grossly visible changes are necessary for a clinical diagnosis. Early lesions appear as red petechiae on the pelvic peritoneal surfaces. With accumulation of menstrual-like detritus, these multifocal lesions develop into small (1–10 mm), flat to cystic, dark (blue, brown, or black) lesions with hemorrhage into adjacent tissues. Collectively, these changes are often described as a powder-burn appearance. They also cause thickening and scarring of the contiguous peritoneal surfaces. As the disease progresses, the size and number of these lesions increase, and extensive adhesions form. The largest cysts occur in the ovary, where they are termed endometriomas and are filled with thick, chocolate-colored blood.

Pelvic endometriosis is characteristically multifocal, involving (in order of decreasing frequency) the ovary (50%), cul-de-sac, uterosacral ligaments, posterior uterine surface and broad ligaments, and the remaining pelvic peritoneum. The bladder (10%–15%), ureters (<1%), and bowel (rectosigmoid 10%–15%, appendix 14%–30%) may be affected by implants leading to scarring, obstruction, or blood in the urine or stool. Distant sites of endometriosis are rare but have been reported in the lung, brain, and kidney.

The most characteristic histology (endometrial glands, stroma, and hemorrhage into adjacent tissues) is found in early lesions. With progression, the wall of the implant may be lined by a monolayer of connective tissue cells, or no lining may be identifiable. Indeed, viable endometrial glands and stroma may not be found in about 25% of cases. Characteristically, the fibrotic cyst wall contains hemosiderin-laden macrophages. In part, these progressive alterations may explain the 8% incidence of disagreement between the operative and pathologic diagnoses.

Pathologic Physiology

Although a single etiology for endometriosis has not emerged, several observations and potential mechanisms seem to generally explain pathogenesis. Endometriosis has a multifactorial inherited predisposition. The risk of endometriosis in first-degree female relatives of an afflicted woman is increased 7 times. Women with a family history of endometriosis develop the disease earlier in life, and it is more likely to be advanced when compared to those without first-degree relatives with endometriosis.

Retrograde menstruation (which probably occurs in the majority of women) with direct implantation of fragments of viable endometrium was a cause of endometriosis advocated by Sampson. This readily explains the usual distribution of lesions. However, retrograde menstruation does not explain why distant metastases occur or why the majority of women do not develop endometriosis. Another theory is that multipotential cells of the celomic epithelium may undergo metaplasia. This induction phenomenon as a cause for endometriosis was advocated by Meyers and subsequently modified by others as either a spontaneous or induced alteration (perhaps by factors within the menstrual discharge). The metaplasia theory assists in answering some (e.g., deep rectovaginal septal) cases but fails to provide a complete answer. Women with endometriosis may have a defect in local cell-mediated immunity. Finally, lymphatic and vascular metastasis may explain the rare remote endometrial implants, to the lung, for example.

How endometriosis causes pelvic pain and infertility is only partially understood. However, pain and infertility may be related mechanically by direct extension of the process. On the other hand, patients with endometriosis have an increased number of anovulatory cycles, luteal phase defects, luteinized but unruptured follicles, and galactorrhea. These problems all seem related to a relative hyperprolactinemia. In addition, there are increased amounts of prostaglandin precursors, prostaglandins (Pg), and prostaglandin metabolites in the peritoneal fluid and peritoneal washings from infertile patients with endometriosis. Notably increased are thromboxane B_2, 6-ketoprostacycline $F_{1\alpha}$, $PgF_{2\alpha}$, and PgE. Enhanced amounts of peritoneal fluid also roughly parallel the severity of endometriosis.

Endometriosis may enhance spontaneous abortion. In support, several studies have detailed a decrease in the rate of spontaneous abortion (44%–82%) after therapy eliminating endometriosis.

DIAGNOSIS

Typical patients with endometriosis are in their mid-30s, nulliparous, and involuntarily infertile and have secondary dysmenorrhea and pelvic pain. However, the diagnosis of endometriosis may be difficult because one third of endometriosis cases are asymptomatic, there is no correlation between extent of the disease and symptomatology (i.e., minimal disease may cause severe pain, whereas large endometriomas may be asymptomatic), endometriosis frequently appears in atypical fashions (e.g., teenagers, multigravidas, asymptomatic ovarian tumors), and the symptomatology varies with the anatomic site of endometriosis.

Symptoms and Signs

The usual symptomatology includes pelvic pain, infertility, and abnormal bleeding.

Pelvic Pain

Pelvic pain is the cardinal symptom of endometriosis. Characteristically the pain is chronic and recurrent and presents as acquired or secondary dysmenorrhea. The pain usually occurs 24–48 h premenstrually and subsides sometime after the onset of menstruation. However, discomfort may include the entire menstrual interval. The pain is characterized as constant, usually in the pelvis or low back (sacral), However, pain may be unilateral or bilateral and may radiate to the legs or groin. When compared to primary dysmenorrhea, the pain is more constant and less often in the midline. Other pelvic symptoms include severe cramping, pelvic heaviness, and pelvic pressure.

Gastrointestinal symptoms may occur, whether or not the bowel is actually involved, e.g., cyclic abdominal pain, intermittent constipation, diarrhea, dyschezia, and blood in the stool. Urinary symptoms include urinary frequency, dysuria, perimenstrual hematuria, or hydronephrosis. Deep penetration with intercourse may evoke severe pain (dyspareunia) which may last for 1–2 h. Unusual symptoms about the time of menses have been reported: seizures (CNS implants) and hemothorax or hematemesis (pulmonary implants).

Infertility

Endometriosis is diagnosed nearly twice as often in infertile women as in those who are fertile. Thus, it must be suspected in every case of infertility (Chapter 27).

Abnormal Bleeding

Abnormal bleeding, not associated with anovulation, occurs in 15%–20% of women with endometriosis. The characteristic patterns are premenstrual spotting or menorrhagia or both.

Physical Examination

External endometriosis usually occurs on the cervix and is associated with an enhanced frequency of *internal endometriosis*. Other external endometriosis is usually iatrogenic, occurring in surgical incisions. On physical examination, endometriosis classically causes tender nodularity of the uterosacral ligaments. With progression, the uterus becomes retroverted and fixed, usually with posterior cul-de-sac scarring and tenderness. The ovaries may be enlarged (rarely symmetrically), tender, and fixed to adjacent structures (e.g., broad ligament or lateral pelvic sidewall). In advanced cases, the pelvic structures become rigid and unyielding.

Laparoscopy

Laparoscopy is generally used to confirm the diagnosis of endometriosis. Biopsy of selected implants may reveal the characteristic pathology. Although this is not necessary to complete the diagnosis, it is useful for subsequent therapy and overall prognosis. The American Fertility Society's classification (Table 26-1) quantifies severity based on the characteristic of the lesions, resultant adhesions, ovarian cysts, scarring and retraction, fixation of pelvic structures, and obliteration of the cul-de-sac. Occasionally, confirmation of the diagnosis and staging are accomplished during a laparotomy, e.g., for ruptured ectopic pregnancy.

ENDOMETRIOSIS DURING ADOLESCENCE AND AFTER MENOPAUSE

Endometriosis is present in two thirds of adolescents who have significant morbidity associated with their menses. Adolescents account for 8% of women with endometriosis. Of the teenagers with endometriosis, 10% have congenital obstruction to menstrual outflow. The symptoms in this age group most indicative of endometriosis are increasing acquired dysmenorrhea, chronic pelvic pain, bowel changes with menses, and abnormal vaginal bleeding. Thus, diagnostic laparoscopy should be considered in truly symptomatic adolescents. Rarely, postmenopausal endometriosis is due to the use of unopposed exogenous estrogens.

DIFFERENTIAL DIAGNOSIS

The differential diagnosis of endometriosis most commonly includes primary dysmenorrhea, chronic pelvic inflammatory disease, leiomyoma with degeneration, pelvic adhesions, adenomyosis, ovarian malignancy, and functional bowel disease. Less commonly, the following conditions should be considered in the

Table 26-1. American Fertility Society revised classification of endometriosis

THE AMERICAN FERTILITY SOCIETY
REVISED CLASSIFICATION OF ENDOMETRIOSIS

Patient's Name _____ Date _____

Stage I (Minimal) · 1-5
Stage II (Mild) · 6-15
Stage III (Moderate) · 16-40
Stage IV (Severe) · >40
Total _____

Laparoscopy _____ Laparotomy _____ Photography _____
Recommended Treatment _____
_____
Prognosis _____

PERITONEUM	**ENDOMETRIOSIS**	<1cm	1-3cm	>3cm
	Superficial	1	2	4
	Deep	2	4	6
OVARY	R Superficial	1	2	4
	Deep	4	16	20
	L Superficial	1	2	4
	Deep	4	16	20

	POSTERIOR CULDESAC OBLITERATION	Partial		Complete	
		4		40	

	ADHESIONS	<1/3 Enclosure	1/3-2/3 Enclosure	>2/3 Enclosure
OVARY	R Filmy	1	2	4
	Dense	4	8	16
	L Filmy	1	2	4
	Dense	4	8	16
TUBE	R Filmy	1	2	4
	Dense	4*	8*	16
	L Filmy	1	2	4
	Dense	4*	8*	16

*If the fimbriated end of the fallopian tube is completely enclosed, change the point assignment to 16.

Additional Endometriosis: _____

Associated Pathology: _____

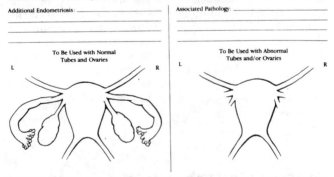

To Be Used with Normal Tubes and Ovaries

To Be Used with Abnormal Tubes and/or Ovaries

Courtesy of the American Fertility Society.

differential diagnosis: salpingitis isthmica nodosa, chronic ectopic gestation, carcinoma of the colon or rectum, and diverticulitis. Rupture of an endometrioma appears as an acute abdomen and must be differentiated from bleeding corpus luteum, ectopic gestation, appendicitis, and diverticulitis.

MINIMAL DIAGNOSTIC CRITERIA

In some cases, the symptomatology and physical examination are so classic that the diagnosis seems obvious, and it is tempting to base the diagnosis entirely on the history and physical examination. However, the diagnosis must exclude other conditions because of the serious lifelong implications for the patient. It is strongly recommended that laparoscopy with documented visualization of gross lesions and pathologic demonstration of characteristic glands and stroma be the minimal diagnostic criteria. Additionally, laparoscopic visualization allows staging of the disease.

THERAPY

One must individualize therapy for endometriosis to include the patient's desire for fertility, her age, severity of symptoms, location of the lesions, stage of the disease, and other concurrent significant abnormalities. Various therapeutic options are outlined in Table 26-2.

Observation and Palliation

Observation is warranted in some patients (e.g., those with minimal disease or near the menopause) but should be undertaken with the knowledge that physical examination alone is not likely to detect any save the very gross disease. Analgesic therapy is purely palliative, regardless of the agent used, but may be useful in combination with other therapy.

Pregnancy was once described as curative for endometriosis, but this is untrue. Indeed, endometriomas may increase rapidly in size during the first trimester of pregnancy but generally decrease in size during the third trimester. Rupture of endometriomas has been reported at any time during pregnancy. Once menses return after the puerperium, endometriosis will continue to progress.

Table 26-2. Therapy options for endometriosis

A.	Observation	
B.	Palliation	
	1.	Analgesics
	2.	Nonsteroidal anti-inflammatory agents
	3.	Prostaglandin synthetase inhibitors
	4.	Pregnancy
	5.	Infertility studies
C.	Endocrine therapy	
	1.	Danazol
	2.	GnRH agonists
	3.	Estrogen-progestogens
	4.	Progestogens
	5.	Androgens
D.	Surgical therapy	
	1.	Conservative surgery
	2.	Procedures for pain relief
	3.	Definitive surgery

Endocrine Therapy

Danazol

The most common medical treatment of endometriosis is danazol (17-alpha-ethinyltestosterone). However, this may change with the availability of GnRH. Danazol is mildly androgenic and anabolic, but it also binds to androgen receptors, progesterone receptors, and sex hormone-binding globulin. This results in a threefold increase of free testosterone. The result is marked endometrial atrophy (both within the uterus and within the lesions). Amenorrhea and inhibition of ovulation occur within 4–6 weeks of therapy. Unfortunately, because of these clinical alterations, the overall effect was erroneously termed pseudomenopause. The clinical state induced by danazol, although it is hypoestrogenic and hypoprogestational, more closely resembles that induced by androgens. It lacks most of the physiologic alterations of the menopause.

The dosage of danazol for suppression of endometriosis is 400–800 mg/day for 6–9 months. For therapy >6 months, serum liver enzymes should be determined. Danazol may be started on the fifth day after menses. For the first month, barrier contraceptives should be used because danazol may masculinize a female fetus should pregnancy occur. Success is most marked when treating endometriomas <2 cm in diameter. After a full course of therapy, 90% of patients will be objectively improved and 75% will report symptomatic improvement. However, 15%–30% will have recurrence of symptoms in <2 years. The fertility rate is improved to 40% (uncorrected).

Danazol is expensive, and 80% of patients have side effects (10%–20% severe enough to discontinue the medication). The most common side effects in a representative series include acne (>15%), hot flashes (15%), uterine spotting (10%), gastrointestinal disturbances (8%), weakness and dizziness (8%), hirsutism (6%), edema (6%), decreased breast size (5%), weight gain (8–10 pounds in 5%), and change in libido (3%–5%). Less common side effects include muscle cramps (4%), voice changes (3%), atrophic vaginitis (3%), and migraine headaches (2%). Although more difficult to quantify, emotional lability and depression also may occur.

Gonadotropin-Releasing Hormone (GnRH) Agonists

By relatively long-term binding to LHRH receptors, the GnRH analogs suppress the pituitary-ovarian axis, creating low levels of FSH and LH as well as estrogen and progesterone levels in the menopause range. This causes endometrial atrophy. Administration of GnRH agonists is usually subcutaneous or intranasal. This is effective (85%) in objectively decreasing endometriosis. Ovulation resumes relatively quickly (45 days) after discontinuation of the medication. Although general usage has just begun, there appear to be fewer side effects and better tolerance than with danazol.

Estrogen-Progestogen and Progestogen Therapies

Whereas cyclic hormones may induce endometrial growth, continuous estrogen-progestogen or progestogen alone suppresses the growth pattern. Thus, constant (daily) regimens of estrogen and progestin, oral contraceptives, or progestogen all cause endometrial atrophy. Low estrogen combination oral contraceptives with high progestin activity are most commonly used in the treatment of endometriosis as 1 tablet per day starting on the third day of menses until breakthrough bleeding occurs. When this develops, doubling the dosage generally will relieve the breakthrough bleeding, and after 5 days of elevated amounts, the dosage may be returned to 1–2 pills per day. This may be continued for 6–9 months.

There may be an initial (first 6 weeks) slight exacerbation of clinical symptoms and even a slight risk of endometrioma rupture. Side effects include nausea, breast tenderness, weight gain, chloasma, depression, irritability, edema, and rarely hypertension. Alternatively, medroxyprogesterone may be used (100 mg IM every 2 weeks for four doses, then 200 mg monthly for four doses). Medroxyprogesterone may be used by the older woman after completed childbearing, but this program should be avoided in those who want to conceive because of the extremely variable and often long interval before ovulation resumes (1 year is not uncommon). Breakthrough bleeding is the most frequent side effect, but unpleasant mood alterations may cause patient discontinuance. These therapies currently are reserved for those with mild endometriosis who do not desire immediate fertility and are not candidates for other treatments. These regimens are less effective (both objectively and subjectively) than danazol and have a greater patient discontinuance (one third) because of side effects. Uncorrected pregnancy rates are 30%.

Currently, androgens (methyltestosterone), estradiol, and gastrinone are used rarely to treat endometriosis.

Surgical Therapy

The indications for surgery for endometriosis are summarized in Table 26-3. Increasingly, endocrine therapy is being applied before and after surgery. Conservative surgery is performed to retain and enhance the patient's reproductive capability. The goals are removal of all macroscopic endometriosis, division of adhesions (especially ovarian and tubal), preservation of reproductive function, and restoration of normal anatomy. All this may be accomplished by laparoscopy using the argon laser for photocoagulation and the Nd:YAG or CO_2 laser for vaporization of endometriotic foci. With conservative surgery, a D&C may be a wise addition to ascertain that no obstruction exists to menstrual outflow, as the latter may enhance retrograde bleeding, a predisposition of endometriosis.

At laparotomy, microsurgical techniques should be used, e.g., operative site magnification, minimal tissue trauma, fine polyglycolic suture, careful reperitonealization, intraperitoneal dextran, corticosteroids, and prophylactic antibiotics. With laparotomy, it is good practice to do a round ligament uterine suspension to prevent the uterus and adnexa from adhering in the cul-de-sac.

Table 26-3. Indications for surgical therapy

Rupture of endometrioma (a surgical emergency)
Ureteral or bowel obstruction
Tuboovarian masses (>5 cm)
Endometriomas (>8 cm)
Severe, incapacitating symptoms
Pain worsening with medical therapy
Infertility for >1 year despite conventional therapy

Elective appendectomy is not recommended because of the slightly enhanced risk of infection.

Pregnancy rates following conservative surgery are inversely related to the stage of the disease, i.e., 75% with mild endometriosis, 50%–60% for moderate disease, and 30%–40% for severe disease. Recurrence necessitating further surgery occurs in >10% of patients within 3 years and in 35% of patients within 5 years. The initial severity of endometriosis does not predict recurrence. Pregnancy delays but otherwise does not influence recurrence rates.

Indications for surgery to relieve pain are severe midline dysmenorrhea or dyspareunia or both. For the former, a presacral neurectomy is most often accomplished, whereas uterosacral ligament resection is the most common operation for treatment of the latter. These procedures often are performed through the laparoscope.

In patients who do not desire future reproduction or who have debilitating disease despite medical and conservative surgical therapy, ablative surgery may be the best alternative. In the younger woman (generally to the mid-30s), ovarian preservation with total abdominal hysterectomy may be indicated. Only 10% of patients thus treated will suffer progression of their endometriosis.

Definitive surgical therapy involves removal of all sites of endometriosis, abdominal hysterectomy, bilateral salpingo-oophorectomy, lysis of adhesions, and appendectomy. The last is recommended because of a 14%–30% finding of microscopic endometriosis in the appendix. It is prudent to place the patient who has had definitive surgical therapy on medroxyprogesterone or continuous oral contraceptive therapy for 1 year even though the risk of recurrence after definitive surgical therapy is 3%.

Endometriosis of the bowel most commonly involves the appendix or rectosigmoid and is usually only a small serosal involvement. Occasionally, more extensive involvement may be clinically signaled by large bowel cramping, lower abdominal pain, dyschezia, perimenstrual blood in the stool, palpation of a rectal shelf, or palpation of a pelvic mass. Endocrine therapy is not effective in advanced cases. Surgical therapy must be individualized and may vary from superficial excision to bowel resection.

Most urinary tract endometriosis is an incidental finding of peritoneal involvement over the bladder and responds well to medical or surgical therapy. However, ureteral obstruction may occur without the usual symptoms (hematuria, flank pain) in one third of patients. The obstruction is nearly always in the distal third of the ureter and responds poorly to medical therapy. The usual surgical therapy is ureterolysis or ureteroneocystostomy.

PREVENTION

The only currently effective preventive measure for endometriosis is to ensure adequate menstrual outflow. Other suggestions remain unproven, including early marriage, early pregnancy, avoidance of partial salpingectomy, irrigation or isolation of operative sites, and annual pelvic examinations.

ADENOMYOSIS

Adenomyosis is the presence of endometrial glands and stroma within the myometrium. It may be a diffuse process, with many areas demonstrating continuity between the endometrium and the glands and stroma within the myometrium, or the adenomyotic foci may be isolated in the myometrium. Expect hypertrophy of the smooth muscle adjacent to the ectopic endometrial glands and fibrosis. In large isolated areas of adenomyosis, the process resembles a leiomyoma and is termed *adenomyoma.* Adenomyosis regresses after menopause. It is a pathologic diagnosis of unknown etiology.

The usual *symptoms of adenomyosis* include hypermenorrhea (50%) and often severe acquired premenstrual and menstrual dysmenorrhea (30%). However, 30% of patients are asymptomatic. Classically, physical examination reveals the uterine fundus to be diffusely enlarged. Occasionally, softened areas of adenomyosis may be noted just before or during early menstruation. The condition is more likely to occur in parous women >30, and it is uncommon in nulliparas. Adenomyosis is found in 20% of hysterectomy specimens, but the correct diagnosis is made preoperatively in less than one third of cases. MRI is useful in the detection of adenomyosis but is seldom used for this purpose. Adenomyosis frequently is complicated by chronic anemia (common), primary adenocarcinoma (rare), and endolymphatic stromal myosis (stromatosis) (also rare).

The *differential diagnosis* includes pregnancy, submucous leiomyoma (leiomyomas are associated in 50%–60% of cases of adenomyosis), pelvic endometriosis (complicates 15% of adenomyosis), pelvic congestion syndrome, idiopathic uterine hypertrophy, and endometrial cancer.

Treatment of adenomyosis is symptomatic if childbearing potential is retained. Hormone therapy is not beneficial. Occasionally, an isolated adenomyoma can be removed surgically, but the usual curative therapy is hysterectomy.

Chapter 27

Infertility and Related Issues (Special Fertility Procedures, Hyperandrogenism)

INFERTILITY

Infertility is a defined as the failure to conceive after 1 year of attempting pregnancy. *Primary infertility* denotes those patients who have never conceived. *Secondary infertility* applies to patients who have conceived previously. Approximately 15% of couples experience infertility, which may result from subfertility or sterility (the innate inability to conceive) in either partner or both. The female is responsible in 40%–50% of cases. The male is responsible in 30% and is contributory in another 20%–30% of couples. However, it is crucial to recall that multiple etiologies are found in 40% of infertile couples.

The *incidence* of infertility has increased (perhaps 100% over the past 20 years) in developed countries because of increasing sexually transmitted disease (especially gonorrhea and *Chlamydia,* causing subsequent tubal damage), an increased number of sexual partners (increasing the potential for acquiring STDs), intentionally delaying pregnancy, the contraceptive(s) used, and smoking (>1 pack/day decreases the chance of pregnancy by >20%). Infertility accounts for 10%–20% of all gynecologic office visits.

Fertility rates are established using *fecundibility* (the chance of pregnancy per month of exposure). Only 25% of young healthy couples having frequent intercourse will conceive per month (60% by 6 months, 75% by 9 months, and 90% by 18 months). Fecundibility declines with age, and the effect is more pronounced in women than in men. By 36–37 years, the chance of pregnancy is less than half that at 25–27 years.

Careful evaluation should detect probable cause(s) for infertility in 85%–90%. Happily, even without therapy, 15%–20% of infertile couples may be expected to achieve pregnancy over time. Therapy, excluding in vitro fertilization, will result in pregnancy in 50%–60%.

ETIOLOGY

The causes of infertility may be classified as male-coital factors (40%), cervical (5%–10%), uterine-tubal (30%), ovulatory factors (15%–20%), and peritoneal or pelvic factors (40%). A few genetic causes (e.g., primary amenorrhea) are recognized.

Male-Coital Factors

Male factors include abnormal spermatogenesis, abnormal motility, anatomic disorders, endocrine disorders, and sexual dysfunction. The anatomic abnormalities possibly responsible are congenital absence of the vas deferens, obstruction of the vas deferens, and congenital abnormalities of the ejaculatory system.

Abnormal spermatogenesis may occur as the result of mumps orchitis, chromosomal abnormalities, cryptorchidism, chemical or radiation exposure, or varicocele. Abnormal motility is seen with absent cilia (Kartagener's syndrome), varicocele, and antibody formation.

The male factor *endocrine disorders* include thyroid disorders, adrenal hyperplasia, exogenous androgens, hypothalamic dysfunction (Kallmann's syndrome), pituitary failure (tumor, radiation, surgery), and hyperprolactinemia (tumor, drug-induced). An elevated FSH commonly indicates parenchymal testicular damage, since inhibin, produced by the Sertoli cells, is the primary feedback control of FSH secretion.

Cervical Factors

Cervical factors of female infertility may be congenital (DES exposure, mullerian duct abnormality) or acquired (infection, surgical treatment).

Uterine-Tubal Factors

Uterine-tubal factors are most commonly structural abnormalities (e.g., DES exposure, myoma, failure of normal fusion of the reproductive tract, previous ectopic pregnancy).

Ovulatory Factors

Ovulatory factors involve CNS function, metabolic disease, or peripheral defects. CNS defects include chronic hyperandrogenemic anovulation, hyperprolactinemia (empty sella, tumor, drug-induced), hypothalamic insufficiency, and pituitary insufficiency (trauma, tumor, congenital). Metabolic diseases causing ovulatory factor defects are thyroid disease, liver disease, renal disease, obesity, and androgen excess (adrenal or neoplastic). Peripheral defects may be gonadal dysgenesis, premature ovarian failure, ovarian tumor, or ovarian resistance.

Peritoneal or Pelvic Factors

The two most common pelvic or peritoneal factors are endometriosis and sequelae or infection (e.g., appendicitis, pelvic inflammatory disease). Laparoscopy in women with unexplained infertility will reveal previously unsuspected pathology in at least 30% of patients. Endometriosis exerts a greater pejorative effect on fertility than can be explained on the basis of physical alterations (p 651).

DIAGNOSIS

Infertility evaluations should follow a progression of testing and procedures that takes into account probability (including individualization for the couple), invasiveness, risks, and expense. The basic evaluation usually requires 6–8 weeks to complete. Even if the history suggests a probable cause of infertility, completion of the evaluation of all major factors should be accomplished to avoid overlooking a secondary or contributory factor.

The *initial assessment* should include medical history for female infertility factors, including pubertal development, present menstrual cycle characteristics, contraceptive history, prior pregnancy and outcome, previous surgery (especially pelvic), prior infection, abnormal Pap smears and therapy, drugs and therapy, diet, weight stability, exercise, and history of in utero DES exposure (now rare).

Evaluation of Male Factors

The *initial test* for male infertility is the semen analysis because a normal semen analysis usually excludes a significant male factor (Table 27-1). The specimen should be obtained after 2–3 days abstinence and evaluated in the laboratory within 30–60 min of ejaculation.

The frequency of male factors, as well as risk and cost effectiveness, mandates male diagnosis in the initial phase of infertility investigation. The *medical history* for male factor infertility should include frequency of intercourse, difficulty with erection or ejaculation, prior paternity, past history of genital tract infections (e.g., mumps orchitis or chronic prostatitis), congenital anomalies, surgery or trauma (e.g., hernia repair, direct testicular trauma), exposure to toxins (medications, lead, cadmium, or radiation), diet, exercise, alcohol consumption, smoking >1 pack/day), illicit drug use, in utero exposure to DES, and unusual exposure to high environmental heat.

The *physical examination* should consider habitus and hair distribution (e.g., testosterone effect). The urethral meatus should be in the normal location. Testicular size may be compared to standard ovoids. Eliciting a Valsalva maneuver in the standing position should aid in the detection of a varicocele. Transrectal prostatic massage generally will produce sufficient secretions for microscopic examination. Excessive leukocytes in this or the semen analysis indicate infection.

Table 27-1. Normal semen analysis values

Parameter	Normal value
Volume	2–5 ml
Viscosity	Full liquefication <60 min
Count	40–250 M/ml (previously, down to 20 M/ml)
Motility	1st h ≥60%; 2–3 h ≥50%
Normal morphology	>60%
Dead sperm	<35%
White blood cells	<10/hpf

If the semen analysis is abnormal or borderline, the man's medical history over the past 2–3 months should be reviewed, recalling that spermogenesis requires 74 days. A repeat semen analysis should be performed 1–2 weeks later for comparison. Consider referral to a urologist specializing in infertility if a significant abnormality persists.

Because sperm must reach the ovum before fertilization can occur, infertility in the presence of normal semen values suggests that there may be an abnormally high attrition of sperm. *Cervical mucus studies* may clarify this problem.

Evaluation of Cervical Factors

Cervical factors are evaluated by physical examination and an appropriately timed postcoital mucus test. History of in utero DES exposure, abnormal Pap smears, cryotherapy, postcoital bleeding, or conization is suggestive of persistent cervical problems.

Normal cervical mucus in the preovulatory phase is thin, watery and acellular and dries in a ferning pattern. Mucus in this state acts as a facilitative reservoir for sperm. Cervical mucus is best evaluated on days 12–14 of a 28 day cycle. The amount and clarity of the mucus are recorded, and the pH should be ≥6.5. *Spinnbarkeit* (the stretchability of a strand of mucus) is ascertained by drawing out the mucus vertically (it should stretch to ≥6 cm).

The *Sims-Huhner test* evaluates the initial interaction of the sperm with cervical mucus. The test should be conducted in the periovular interval. Timing of the test may be enhanced using vaginal ultrasound to determine the presence or absence of a dominant follicle. Mucus is collected 2–4 h after intercourse. The mucus is placed on a clean glass slide under a coverslip and observed.

There should be >20 sperm/hpf, and large numbers of active sperm will be seen in the thin, acellular mucus. Lower numbers (<20/hpf) of motile sperm in favorable mucus may be present in normally fertile couples due to the stress of coitus at a prescribed time. The absence of sperm suggests *aspermia* or improper coital technique or specimen collection. Finding an adequate number of immobile sperm in favorable mucus requires an investigation for autoantibodies in the male or serum antibodies in the female. If a sufficient number of sperm are present but poorly motile, further assessment of the mucus and timing of the test is indicated. If the mucus tests are repeatedly abnormal despite apparently favorable mucus, a crosscheck using donor mucus and donor sperm is reasonable. *Antibody studies* may determine the antigenic site (sperm head, midpiece, or tail) and are more likely to be positive in men who have a history of trauma, infection, or previous surgery.

In vitro fertilization is the ultimate test for male factor infertility. A sperm penetration test may be useful. This uses a hamster egg to demonstrate the ability of the sperm to penetrate a zona-free oocyte using a known fertile donor as control. Abnormality is indicated by <10% penetration. Negative penetration of healthy appearing, mature ova by partner sperm with simultaneous positive penetration by donor sperm may provide the diagnosis.

Diagnosis of Uterine-Tubal Factors

Both *history* and careful *pelvic examination* are essential initial steps in detection of uterine-tubal factors. Key details of the history include menstrual problems, pelvic infections (pelvic pain), STD, appendicitis, and abdominal trauma or surgery. Suggestive findings on pelvic examination include uterine irregularities, pelvic masses, and uterine deviation or fixation.

It is uncommon for submucous myomata, endometrial polyps, or bicornuate uterus to cause infertility, although each of these is associated with an enhanced rate of abortion. Tubal *fimbrial occlusion* is the most common of the three usual locations, followed by *midsegment and isthmus-cornual occlusion.* Midsegment occlusion is nearly always due to tubal sterilization but may be secondary to tuberculosis. The major causes of isthmic-cornual occlusions are infection, maldevelopment, endometriosis, adenomyosis, or salpingitis isthmica nodosum.

Hysterosalpingography (HSG) (Fig. 27-1), hysteroscopy, laparoscopy, or a combination of these is required to determine patency of the tubes. HSG is performed as an outpatient procedure using a radiopaque dye (first water-soluble and, after patency is assured, an oil-based contrast medium) instilled into the uterine cavity via a small transcervical catheter. Radiographs should document the fluoroscopically observed findings. Uterine contour, tubal patency, and ability of the dye to freely transit the tubes to enter the pelvis are evaluated. The oil-based dye provides a better image but has a greater risk of retention and granuloma formation. The water-based dye causes less cramping and allows better definition of the rugae. Abnormal findings include intrauterine synechiae (Asherman's syndrome), congenital malformations of the uterus, polyps, submucous leiomyomas, proximal or distal tubal occlusion, and salpingitis isthmica nodosa.

The major risk of HSG is infection. Thus, HSG should not be

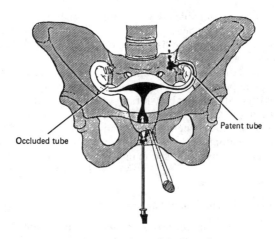

Figure 27-1. Hysterosalpingography.

performed during even suspected active inflammation or when there is an adnexal mass. Broad-spectrum antibiotic therapy (e.g., doxycyline) may be prudent if recent STD screening has not been performed. The test is also contraindicated if there is allergy to the dye.

Laparoscopy may demonstrate tubal abnormalities (e.g., agglutinated fimbria, endometriosis) that probably would not be seen on HSG. Hysteroscopy performed concomitantly with laparoscopy may give further information regarding uterine contour or polyps. Endometriosis (Chapter 26) is an important cause of infertility and is suggested by a history of worsening dysmenorrhea or dyspareunia but usually cannot be diagnosed short of visual inspection. Some endometriosis may be eliminated during laparoscopic diagnosis if informed consent has been obtained and preparations have been made for laser surgery or operative pelviscopy.

Laparoscopy may be indicated relatively early in the investigation of infertility if pelvic factors are suggestive or in older patients, whereas it may be the last test performed in a young woman when all other studies are negative. It may be considered together with ovarian stimulation and ovum collection in longstanding infertility using in vitro fertilization or by placing sperm and ovum directly into the tube to allow a trial of normal transport to the uterus.

Evaluation of Ovulatory Factors

Ovulating women usually have regular cycles (22–35 days). Substantiating symptoms may be useful, especially premenstrual (breast changes, bloating, and mood change). The physical examination and proper timing, coupled with cervical mucus evaluation, may determine ovulation. The usual screening test to confirm ovulation are basal body temperature (BBT) (see Fig. 24-1) and the midluteal serum progesterone.

BBT is taken on awakening before any other activity. After ovulation, a temperature elevation of 0.4°F occurs due to the thermogenic effect of progesterone. Progesterone levels as low as 5 ng/ml may indicate ovulation, but midluteal levels usually are >10 ng/ml.

Irregular menses, absence of premenstrual molimina, continued ferning of dried cervical mucus, low midluteal progesterone levels, and absence of midcycle BBT elevation all indicate probable failure of ovulation. Treatment of ovulation failure is discussed under therapy. Abnormal BBTs, spontaneous abortion(s), endometriosis, and poor cervical mucus may indicate a *luteal phase defect.* Confirmation of this diagnosis is accomplished by endometrial histologic study, including dating of endometrial biopsies (best taken from the superior, anterior uterine fundus) in relation to menses. Dating of the endometrium is accomplished by the criteria illustrated in Figure 27-2. Should the histologic date of the biopsy lag by more than 2 days in two cycles, this diagnosis is confirmed. An additional ovulatory abnormality is the luteinized unruptured follicle (LUF) syndrome. In LUF, the oocyte is trapped or not released from the follicle (as determined by laparoscopy) despite indirect signs of ovulation.

Evaluation of Peritoneal and Pelvic Factors

In women with unexplained infertility, laparoscopy can identify previously unsuspected pathology in 30%–50% of patients. The most common condition diagnosed is endometriosis. Other conditions (e.g., unexpected adhesions) also may be encountered.

TREATMENT

Male and Coital Factors

Smoking, alcohol, and drug use should be stopped. Eliminate sources of increased scrotal temperature (e.g., saunas, hot tubs,

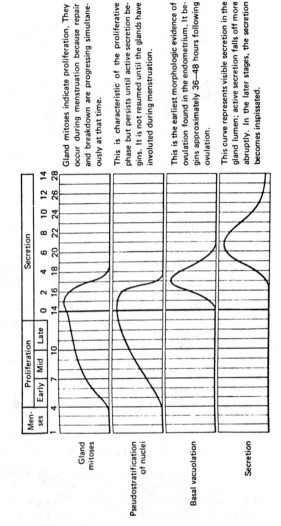

Men-	Proliferation			Secretion								
ses	Early	Mid	Late									
1	4	7	10	14 16	0 2	4 18	6 20	8 22	10 24	12 26	14 28	

Gland mitoses

Pseudostratification of nuclei

Basal vacuolation

Secretion

Gland mitoses indicate proliferation. They occur during menstruation because repair and breakdown are progressing simultaneously at that time.

This is characteristic of the proliferative phase but persists until active secretion begins. It is not resumed until the glands have involuted during menstruation.

This is the earliest morphologic evidence of ovulation found in the endometrium. It begins approximately 36—48 hours following ovulation.

This curve represents visible secretion in the gland lumen; active secretion falls off more abruptly. In the later stages, the secretion becomes inspissated.

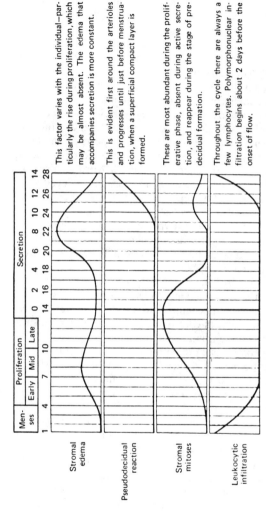

This factor varies with the individual—particularly the rise during proliferation, which may be almost absent. The edema that accompanies secretion is more constant.

This is evident first around the arterioles and progresses until just before menstruation, when a superficial compact layer is formed.

These are most abundant during the proliferative phase, absent during active secretion, and reappear during the stage of predecidual formation.

Throughout the cycle there are always a few lymphocytes. Polymorphonuclear infiltration begins about 2 days before the onset of flow.

Figure 27-2. Dating the endometrium. Approximate relationship of useful morphologic factors. (Modified after J.P.A. Latour. From Noyes, Hertig, and Rock, Dating the endometrial biopsy. *Fertil Steril* 1:3, 1950.)

or jockey shorts underwear) with their adverse effect on spermatogenesis. Lubricants and douching should be eliminated. The woman should lie on her back for at least 15 min following coitus (to facilitate semen retention and progression). Infrequent or poorly timed intercourse is a common cause of infertility. Hence, coitus every 2 days during the periovulatory interval (e.g., days 12–16 of a 28 day cycle) should be advised.

Azoospermia because of chromosomal abnormalities, congenital abnormalities (other than congenital absence of the vas deferens), and elevated FSH cannot be reversed. Therefore, artificial insemination with donor sperm or adoption are the only alternatives. There have been occasional reports of successful pregnancy in congenital absence of the vas deferens by using sperm aspirated from the epididymis and in vitro fertilization. Hypothalamic or pituitary hormone insufficiency-induced azoospermia may be treated by replacement hormone therapy, with varying results. Successful reversal of azoospermia secondary to vasectomy by performance of a vasovasostomy is influenced by the duration of occlusion and whether or not autoantibodies have formed. Patency can be achieved in 75%–90%, with resultant pregnancy rates of 33%–70%.

Varicoceles are present in approximately one third of men evaluated for infertility, and varicocelectomy has been shown to improve sperm parameters in up to two thirds. However, postoperative pregnancy rates in controlled studies reveal no statistical difference between the treated and untreated.

Low semen volume is a problem notoriously difficult to treat. This is usually treated by artificial insemination with husband's semen (AIH). Here, 0.1 ml of liquefied semen is placed in the endocervical canal and the rest in a cervical cup. When *high semen volume* is accompanied by *low sperm count,* a split ejaculate technique may be useful. In this technique, the first portion of the ejaculate, which has a much higher sperm count, is collected and used for AIH. If necessary, several first ejaculates may be pooled and saved by freezing, to be used later for AIH.

Oligospermia (low sperm count) or *asthenospermia* (low sperm motility) if due to an endocrinopathy may respond to specific hormonal therapy (e.g., human menopausal gonadotropin—hMG)—for hypothalamic-pituitary failure, bromocriptine for hyperprolactinemia, or thyroid replacement for hypothyroidism). In idiopathic oligoasthenospermia, clomiphene (not FDA approved for this purpose) may be useful. When specimen quality cannot be improved by other means, the semen may be washed and the sperm concentrated into a smaller volume by slow centrifugation. The resultant semen then is only used for intrauterine insemination accurately timed by daily LH levels or ovulatory stimulation.

If *sperm autoantibodies* are present, suppression of the immune response by steroids may be initiated. However, in vitro fertilization may be necessary in some of these cases to achieve pregnancy.

Intrauterine insemination with washed semen (to eliminate prostaglandins) has been shown to be effective in cases where the sperm parameters are normal and the postcoital examinations are abnormal. This is not true in the reverse instance. If postcoital tests are normal but the sperm characteristics are not, artificial insemination offers little benefit.

In vitro fertilization and gamete intrafallopian transfer (GIFT) offer therapy most likely to be successful in male factor infertility with abnormal sperm factors. Both are invasive and expensive procedures. Moreover, several attempts may be necessary to achieve pregnancy (reported pregnancy rate per cycle is 15%–20%).

Cervical Factors

If the cervix is abnormal as a result of treatment (e.g., coagulation, cryotherapy) or congenital malformation, intrauterine insemination with washed sperm over three cycles should achieve pregnancy in 30%–40%. If cervical mucus is not adequate at midcycle, low-dose estrogen administered during the mid- to late follicular phase of the cycle may be effective. Human menopausal gonadotropins may be necessary to improve the cervical mucus when low-dose estrogen is ineffective. Nonetheless, close monitoring is recommended to avoid multiple gestation or hyperstimulation syndrome. If these are ineffective, intrauterine insemination may be performed. When the cervical mucus is altered by inflammation or infection, empiric tetracycline therapy (doxycycline 100 mg bid for both partners) is advocated.

Uterine-Tubal Factors

Microsurgical tuboplasty is 60%–80% effective in achieving pregnancy with tubal occlusion. However, correction of isthmic occlusions and neosalpingostomy are significantly less successful. Ectopic gestation occurs in 10% of conceptions after surgical tubal repair. Fibroids significantly distorting the endometrial cavity or submucous myomas may warrant removal in the treatment of infertility. Periadnexal adhesions may be lysed by operative laparoscopy.

Ovulatory Factors

When anovulation is the etiology of female factor infertility, successful induction of ovulation will result in pregnancy <1 year in 80%. If pregnancy does not occur despite documented ovulation, other factors must be investigated. Ovulation can be induced in 90%–95% of anovulatory patients, except those with an elevated FSH. An elevated FSH is pathognomonic of ovarian failure or ovarian resistance, and no further testing is warranted. The only hope for pregnancy is embryo or ovum donation. A pregnancy rate of up to 20% per transfer is likely, but the ethical, psychologic, and legal issues of this procedure must be considered.

The initial drug used to induce ovulation is *clomiphene citrate*. Of anovulatory women whose ovaries are producing estrogen, 70% will ovulate with this drug. Ideally, it is given for 5 days in the early follicular phase, since it acts as an antiestrogen. Ultrasound and hormonal testing may be required to evaluate patient response. Dosage or timing adjustment or additional hormone therapy (e.g., steroids, estrogen, midcycle hCG) may be necessary to achieve success.

Stimulation with *human menopausal gonadotropins (hMG)* generally is reserved for those who do not respond to clomiphene, those who respond but no pregnancy results, in cases of hypothalamic insufficiency, or in unexplained infertility. Monitoring of estrogen levels and ultrasonic determination of the number of follicles stimulated as well as the degree of maturity of ova are requisites. Most often, administration of hCG is necessary to trigger ovulation. Although ovulation can be achieved in 85%–90% using hMG, the risk of multiple births is 20%.

If investigation reveals an elevated prolactin level, a TSH determination is necessary to rule out hypothyroidism. If present, hypothyroidism should be treated. Many drugs can elevate prolactin levels, and these should be terminated. After pituitary adenoma and hypothyroidism have been eliminated in the etiology of elevated prolactin, *bromocriptine therapy* may be initiated and continued until pregnancy is confirmed. Despite its use in early pregnancy, there is no documented increase in the incidence of malformation or spontaneous abortion over that seen in the general population.

If the infertility is secondary to an inadequate luteal phase, *clomiphene* may be used successfully in the early follicular phase to recruit additional follicles (thus enhancing progesterone levels in the luteal phase). Other methods of therapy to be considered for an inadequate luteal phase are progesterone supplementation during the luteal phase and hCG injections.

Peritoneal and Pelvic Factors

Endometriosis and the residual of salpingitis are two of the most common causes of infertility. If medication or conservative surgery is ineffective in treating endometriosis or adhesive problems (regardless of cause), IVF or GIFT may be offered.

Combined Factors

When combined factors are documented, therapy can be performed sequentially or simultaneously depending on individual circumstances.

Unexplained Infertility

When no etiology for infertility can be found, no specific therapy is likely to be successful. Even without therapy, the couple can be given the statistical chance of pregnancy of 60% within 3–5 years. If age is a factor or infertility has been long-standing, advanced reproductive technologies warrant discussion with the involved couple. The option of giving hMG (Pergonal) combined with timed inseminations offers some hope short of IVF. If the former is unsuccessful, IVF should be offered.

PSYCHOLOGIC ASPECTS OF INFERTILITY

Infertile couples need considerable psychologic support. Infertility may engender feelings of inadequacy, loss of self-image, or fears regarding their own sexuality. This is particularly true if one is found to be at fault. Anger, accusations, or depression may predominate as frustration and disappointment recur on a monthly basis when pregnancy is not achieved. Some may become so obsessed with basal body temperatures, timed intercourse, and other aspects of therapy that the couple's interpersonal relationship suffers. An additional burden or stress may be the expense of investigation and therapy. Many insurance carriers pay little or nothing toward the expense involved.

Infertility can engender the progression through all of the phases of the *grief reaction:* denial, anger, bargaining, depression, and acceptance. Many couples become willing to try any technique that they may read or hear about, especially from well-meaning friends or relatives. Support groups may be of help—the national organization RESOLVE can provide informal support and referral for professional counseling.

Emphasize the fact that unlike many disorders (e.g., appendicitis), infertility can rarely be reversed overnight and that the couple should accept a process that may take months rather than days or weeks to diagnose and treat. Pregnancy usually occurs in 6–9 cycles if a true cause can be found. A time limit must be set for the expected resolution of the problem to avoid endless procedures or regimens delaying acceptance of failure and initiation of alternatives (e.g., acceptance of childlessness or adoption).

SPECIAL FERTILITY PROCEDURES

In Vitro Fertilization

In vitro fertilization-embryo transfer (IVF-ET) is the technique of removing the ovum (egg) from the ovary, fertilizing it in the laboratory, then placing the resulting embryo into the uterus. Since the first IVF-ET success in 1978, it has become invaluable in the treatment of otherwise untreatable infertility. Success in achieving pregnancy after ovum retrieval is 15%–20% per cycle, and 70%–80% of those carry the pregnancy to term. The usual *indications* for IVF-ET are bilateral tube abnormality (e.g., postsalpingectomy, postsevere salpingitis), antisperm antibodies, extensive endometriosis, oligospermia, and long-standing unexplained infertility.

Technique

Superovulation. Several methods may be used, including (alone or in combination) clomiphene citrate, hMG, hFSH, and GnRH.

Ultrasound scans. Determining the number and growth of

ovarian follicles is necessary, since at least two or three follicles should be developing simultaneously to enhance the possibility of successful ovum retrieval.

Hormonal monitoring. Serum estradiol levels are useful in predicting which cycle is most likely to result in pregnancy. LH levels are closely followed because an unexpected LH peak may result in ovulation before a scheduled ovum aspiration.

Ova retrieval. Ova are aspirated 24 h after injection of hCG or the onset of a spontaneous LH surge. Aspiration may be accomplished via laparoscopy or under indirect visualization using ultrasound and a percutaneous-transvesical or transvaginal approach. The advantage of the ultrasonographic technique is that this program may be outpatient oriented and there is no need for anesthesia. After the ovary is identified, each preovulatory follicle is punctured, and the contents are aspirated. The aspirate is immediately transferred to the laboratory.

Ova identification and classification. The ova are identified microscopically and classified as mature (expanded cumulus oophorus) or immature (compact cumulus). Mature ova have undergone the first meiotic division and are fertilized 5 h after aspiration. Immature ova may be incubated for up to 36 h before fertilization.

Sperm capacitation. Since freshly ejaculated sperm cannot fertilize an ovum, the sperm must be capacitated by a short incubation in culture medium.

Fertilization. With each ovum are mixed 10,000–50,000 motile sperm, and incubation is initiated.

Incubation. An atmosphere of 5%–20% O_2 and 5% CO_2 and culture medium supplemented by maternal serum or human cord serum are used for incubation. During incubation, the preparation is examined for the presence of pronuclei (fertilization has occurred) or blastomeres (cleavage has occurred).

Embryo transfer. The fertilized ova are replaced in the uterus after 48–72 h incubation, usually at the 2-cell to 8-cell stage. This is accomplished by aspiration of the ova into a small catheter, which is then passed transcervically. The ova are injected into the uterine cavity to complete the process.

Potential complications of the procedure are those associated with anesthesia and laparoscopy and those of any pregnancy. For example, ectopic pregnancy may occur. Because of the increased risk of multiple gestation with subsequent fetal wastage, most centers implant only three to four embryos a cycle. If there are excess fertilized ova, the options include freezing (for later use or donation to another infertility patient), discarding them (unwise), or experimentation (controversial).

Ovum Transfer

Ovum transfer is removal of an ovum from a fertile woman after insemination (usually by an infertile woman's husband) at the time of ovulation (LH peak). The ovum donor and the recipient must ovulate within 2 days of each other. Three to 4 days after insemination, the uterus of the donor is lavaged to attempt ovum retrieval (hopefully fertilized). The term pregnancy rate is 3%. Because the process is patented, the technique may be performed only in clinics licensed to do so. The major complication is failure to lavage a fertilized ovum from the donor, resulting in undesired pregnancy.

Gamete Intrafallopian Tube Transfer

Gamete intrafallopian tube transfer (GIFT) is similar to IVF-ET and is used in patients with patent uterine tubes. After superovulation and collection of the ova, ova and sperm are mixed, then immediately placed into the uterine tube, where natural fertilization can occur. The reported pregnancy rate for this technique is 20%–30% per cycle.

HYPERANDROGENISM

The primary androgen produced by the ovaries is *testosterone,* and the primary androgen from adrenal glands is *dehydroepiandrostene sulfate (DHEAS).* Androgen production in the ovary is stimulated by pituitary LH and in the adrenal is stimulated by pituitary ACTH. Most androgens are bound to specific proteins in the circulation and, while bound, are largely biologically inactive. On reaching the target tissue, androgens are further metabolized, often regaining biologic activity. For example, testosterone is 99% bound while in the circulation but, on reaching the skin, is converted to dihydrotestosterone (by 5α-reductase), an even more potent androgen than testosterone. The sebaceous glands are very sensitive to androgens, and oily skin and acne are early signs of hyperandrogenism. The hair follicle is moderately responsive to androgens, and hirsutism is a further response to increasing androgenicity. Finally, with marked androgenicity, signs of masculinization appear in the woman (virilization).

These include temporal balding, deepening of the voice, breast atrophy, increased muscle mass, and cliteromegaly.

The total testosterone produced by a mature female is 0.35 mg/day. Ovarian secretion accounts for 0.1 mg, 0.2 mg comes from peripheral conversion of androstenedione, and 0.05 mg is from peripheral conversion of DHEAS. The ovary and adrenal gland secrete about equal amounts of androstenedione and DHEA. Thus, about two thirds of a woman's daily testosterone comes from the ovaries. Therefore, increased levels of testosterone suggest an ovarian origin.

POLYCYSTIC OVARY SYNDROME (PCOS)

Polycystic ovary syndrome is the most common cause of female hyperandrogenism. The *etiology* of PCOS is unknown, but heredity, central catecholamine abnormalities, obesity, and stress are associated factors. The most common *symptom* is infertility, which occurs in 75% of patients. Other manifestations of PCOS include hirsutism (70%), menstrual irregularities (amenorrhea 50%, functional bleeding 30%, dysmenorrhea 25%), obesity (40%), and virilization (20%). Only 15% of those with PCOS will have biphasic body temperature, and even less will have cyclic menses. A feature of PCOS is enlarged ovaries (often 5 cm) that have a smooth, white, thickened pseudocapsule, immediately beneath which are numerous follicular cysts surrounded by hyperplastic luteinized theca interna cells.

PCOS is marked by increased gonadotropin-releasing hormone (GnRH) pulse frequency and tonically elevated levels of LH (generally >20 mIU/dl). Estradiol not bound to sex hormone-binding globulin (SHBG) is increased (total estradiol is not) because of a decreased SHBG (due to increased androgen levels and obesity), which stimulates GnRH pulsatility. This results in androgen excess (from both ovaries and adrenals) and anovulation. However, the hyperandrogenism is mild (if elevated, testosterone 70–120 ng/dl and androstenedione 3–5 ng/dl; about one half have elevated levels of DHEAS).

Because the FSH levels are usually low, an LH/FSH ratio >3 may be useful in *diagnosis* of PCOS (when LH is >8 mIU/dl). Ovaries of PCOS patients do not produce more estradiol from androstenedione (in fact, because of less FSH, the ovaries have lower aromatase levels). However, the increased circulating androstenedione is peripherally converted to estrone, resulting in elevated estrone levels. The important interrelationships in PCOS are graphically demonstrated in Table 27-2.

Mild hyperprolactinemia is found in 20% of women with PCOS.

STROMAL HYPERTHECOSIS

The peak age of of women with stromal hyperthecosis is 50–70 years, in keeping with the gradual onset of this uncommon disorder. Like PCOS, stromal hyperplasia is associated with enlarged ovaries (5–7 cm in diameter). Stromal hyperthecosis is usually bilateral and is characterized by stromal proliferation with foci of luteinization. There are no subcapsular cysts like those found in PCOS. The theca cells produce gradual but ever increasing amounts of testosterone (usually >2 ng/dl). Again, in contrast to PCOS, stromal hyperthecosis patients tend to have advancing virilization over a course of years.

ANDROGEN-PRODUCING OVARIAN NEOPLASMS

Neoplastic androgen-secreting ovarian disorders typically have a rapid onset of hirsutism, amenorrhea, and virilization. These neo-

Table 27-2. Probable interrelationships in PCOS*

Hypothalamus	Pituitary	Ovaries/ adrenals	Circulation	Result
GnRH pulsatility	↑ LH	↓ E_2 ↑ T	↓ Unbound E_2 ↓ SHBG	
		↑ A_2	↑ Unbound T + A_2	Excess androgen Anovulation LH/FSH ratio >2–3

*GnRH, gonadotropin-releasing hormone; LH, luteinizing hormone; FSH, follicle-stimulating hormone; E_2, estradiol; T, testosterone; A_2, androstenediol; SHBG, sex hormone-binding globulin.

plasms are usually unilateral and palpable on *pelvic examination*. Testosterone is the most commonly secreted androgen (usually >200 ng/dl) in these disorders. The most common of the tumors causing hyperandrogenism are the *Sertoli-Leydig cell* and *hilus cell tumors*. The neoplasms produce testosterone and almost always lead to virilization. The less common ovarian neoplasms leading to hyperandrogenism include *lipoid cell* (adrenal rest) *tumors* (produce testosterone or DHEAS or both), *granulosa-theca cell tumors* (can produce testosterone in addition to increased estradiol), *Brenner tumors,* and *Krukenberg tumors* (unusual, rarely produce testosterone). Also to be considered are *ovarian tumors*, whether benign or malignant, primary or metastatic in origin. They do not secrete androgens but stimulate the ovarian stroma to do so.

Sertoli-Leydig cell tumors are uncommon (<1% of solid ovarian tumors). They are most often diagnosed in menstruating women (20s–40s) and are associated with hirsutism, virilization, and a palpable ovarian mass (85%). Hilar (Leydig) cell tumors are most frequent after the menopause. They are not usually palpable but cause rapid development of virilization. Testosterone levels are high, but DHEAS levels are normal. Gonadoblastomas are a very rare cause of hyperandrogenism, most often occurring in phenotypic females with gonadal dysgenesis and a Y chromosome.

Hyperandrogenism during pregnancy may be caused by a luteoma of pregnancy or by hyperreactio luteinalis. Hyperreactio luteinalis is defined as bilateral cystic ovarian enlargement. The ovaries may be 20–30 cm in diameter and consist of innumerable thin-walled cysts. These give the mass a bluish to gray ovarian color and a honeycombed appearance. The cysts are lined by luteinized thecal lutein cells from the ovarian connective tissue.

A luteoma of pregnancy is a unilateral or occasionally bilateral (30%) benign solid ovarian tumor (50%) caused by a hyperplastic reaction of ovarian theca lutein cells. They are discrete and brown to reddish brown and may have a cystic component. Luteomas are more common in black multiparas.

Both luteoma and hyperreactio luteinalis are benign and hCG-dependent. They regress after pregnancy and should not be removed unless other problems intervene (e.g., torsion). The majority of cases are asymptomatic and are found incidentally. Should *symptoms* occur, they are usually nonspecific, i.e., a sense of pressure, ascites, or increasing abdominal girth. Although the majority are not hyperandrogenic, some produce high levels of testosterone and androstenedione. Thus, the mother is virilized in 30%, and a female fetus is at risk of virilization.

HYPERANDROGENISM OF ADRENAL ORIGIN

Excess androgens from the adrenal glands may be the result of neoplasia, inborn errors of biosynthesis of adrenal hormones, or inappropriate stimulation of the adrenal gland. Adrenal neoplasias typically produce DHEA with blood levels >7000 ng/ml. On rare occasions, testosterone will be secreted (blood levels >200 ng/ml). Androgens are intermediates in the biosynthetic pathway for cortisol. Consequently, a disorder that causes an increase in cortisol production (e.g., Cushing's syndrome) may concomitantly increase androgen levels.

Cushing's Snydrome

Cushing's syndrome may have three *etiologies:* adrenal tumors, ectopic production of adrenocorticotropic hormone (ACTH) by a nonpituitary tumor, or excess production of ACTH by the pituitary (Cushing's disease). All result in excessive production of glucocorticoids. The *classic findings* include centripetal obesity, dorsal neck fatpads, abdominal striae, muscle wasting, weakness, hirsutism, and menstrual irregularity. Cushing's syndrome is *diagnosed* by the dexamethasone suppression test.

Androgen-producing adrenal tumors are usually adenomas or carcinomas. Characteristically, symptoms have a rapid onset. The tumors produce DHEA, DHEAS (>8 μg/dl), and androstenedione. CT scan of the adrenals facilitates diagnosis.

Congenital Adrenal Hyperplasia (CAH)

CAH results from enzymatic deficiencies (21-hydroxylase or 11B-hydroxylase) inherited as autosomal recessive traits. The 21-hydroxylase deficiency is the most common form. Because both conditions result in diminished cortisol biosynthesis, ACTH is increased. ACTH leads to enhanced intermediate compounds before the enzymatic defect. Thus, elevations of 17-hydroxypregnenolone and 17-hydroxyprogesterone (17-OHP) occur and are subsequently converted to DHEA and androstenedione. The latter compounds are in turn peripherally converted into testosterone. Female infants with this disorder are often diagnosed shortly after birth due to ambiguous genitalia. *CAH is the most common cause of ambiguous genitalia in the newborn.*

Milder deficiencies also occur and may not be diagnosed until puberty or later. CAH may account for 5% of women with hirsutism. Characteristically, these women have a history of prepubertal accelerated growth but overall reveal short ultimate height and postpubertal hirsutism. They may exhibit mild virilization and DHEAS levels >5 μg/dl. Measurement of 17-OHP >8 ng/dl facilitates *diagnosis*. However, when 17-OHP is 3–8 ng/dl, an ACTH stimulation test may be diagnostic.

DIAGNOSIS

A complete medical history is essential. This must include the menstrual and family history. Onset of symptoms should be noted as well as drug ingestion, whether current or in the recent past. Use of body building programs and food supplements should not be overlooked. *Physical examination* should include vital signs, body habitus, hair pattern, and presence or absence of skin and fat changes consistent with Cushing's syndrome, as well as signs of virilization in addition to hirsutism. The pelvic examination should consider ovarian size or masses.

Initial *laboratory testing* should include serum testosterone and DHEAS levels. Serum testosterone <200 ng/dl rules out testosterone-secreting neoplasms, whereas serum DHEAS <7000 ng/ml eliminates significant adrenal pathology. A testosterone level >200 ng/dl is indicative of ovarian tumor until proven otherwise (i.e., study of the adrenals is essential only if no ovarian mass is present). If the patient is anovulatory or oligoovulatory, FSH, LH, and prolactin levels may be helpful. Elevated LH levels (especially LH/FSH ratio >3) suggest polycystic ovary disease. Prolactinoma may cause elevated prolactin levels.

Screening for hypercortisolemia requires a 24 h urine for urinary-free cortisol or 17-hydroxycorticosteroids (17-OHCS). More definitive testing includes an overnight dexamethasone suppression test. Obtain an outpatient baseline plasma cortisol determination. Administer dexamethasone 1 mg PO at 11 PM the same day. Obtain a plasma cortisol level again at 8 AM the next day. The cortisol level will be suppressed (<5 ng/dl) in normal patients but not in Cushing's syndrome. False positives may occur in obesity, chronic illness, or with phenytoin use.

If cortisol suppression does not occur, a 2 day low-dose dexamethasone test is in order. This is performed after two baseline 24 h urine collections for free cortisol and 17-OHCS levels have been obtained. Dexamethasone 0.5 mg is given q6h PO for 2 days. A 24 h urine is collected during the second day for free cortisol and 17-OHCS. Normal patients' 17-OHCS will be suppressed to <2 mg/g of creatinine. Moreover, free cortisol levels will be below normal values. In contrast, in Cushing's syndrome, the 17-OHCS will be >2.5 mg/g of creatinine.

Cushing's disease may be distinguished from Cushing's syndrome by using higher doses of dexamethasone over a 2 day test (disease shows suppression from baseline levels). Then, ACTH levels should be elevated.

Late-onset congenital adrenal hyperplasia is uncommon in adult women. It may be diagnosed by documenting increased serum 17-OHP. Mild deficiency may be detected only by ACTH stimulation to demonstrate the partial block of 21-hydroxylase activity.

Differential Diagnosis

The differential diagnosis of hyperandrogenism must include idiopathic hirsutism, polycystic ovary syndrome, stromal hyperthecosis, androgen-producing ovarian tumors, Cushing's syndrome or disease, congenital adrenal hyperplasia (adult manifestations), androgen-producing adrenal tumors, androgen excess in pregnancy (luteoma or hyperreactio luteinalis), exogenous or iatrogenic androgen administration (testosterone, danazol, anabolic steroids, or synthetic progestins), and abnormal gonadal or sexual development (idiopathic hirsutism, polycystic ovarian syndrome, and stromal thecosis are the most frequent).

Treatment

Therapy depends on the etiology of the hyperandrogenism as well as the desire for childbearing. Ovarian and adrenal tumors must be treated surgically. Congenital or acquired adrenal hyperplasia should be treated with hydrocortisone. Cushing's disease (tumor) is treated by transsphenoidal pituitary surgery. If unsuccessful, pituitary radiation or bilateral adrenalectomy is indicated. Acromegaly is treated by transsphenoidal hypophysectomy.

After serious disease and neoplasm are ruled out and a decision is made regarding further childbearing, medical therapy is indicated. This entails ovarian or adrenal suppression or the blocking of peripheral androgen effects. If infertility is a problem, ovulation induction is advisable after complete evaluation using appropriate drugs (clomiphene, bromocriptine, hMG, GnRH).

GnRH inhibits the secretion of gonadotropins from the pituitary to inhibit the secretion of androgens and estrogens from the ovary. Although reported to be effective in >60%, long-term effects are unknown. Further studies are warranted before general use of GnRH is advocated. Wedge resection of the ovary is not recommended as treatment for hyperandrogenism. Although it may induce ovulation, androgen levels decrease only transiently, and its success rate to decrease hirsutism is only 15%.

PROGNOSIS

Although the underlying cause may be corrected, the signs of hyperandrogenism may be difficult or impossible to reverse. Therefore, therapeutic efforts focus primarily on hirsutism.

HIRSUTISM

Androgen-Dependent Hirsutism

Hirsutism, the excessive growth of androgen-dependent sexual hair, is the most common sign of female hyperandrogenism. However, hirsutism is but one manifestation of hyperandrogenism. Hirsutism generally has a gradual onset and, in milder forms, occurs primarily on the upper lip and chin. With increasing severity, hair growth progresses to the cheeks, intermammary chest, abdomen, inner thighs, lower back, and intergluteal areas. Hirsutism may result from excessive production of androgens by the ovary, adrenal gland, or both. However, medications, e.g., exogenous androgen administration, must be considered also. Whereas the testosterone levels in virilization are usually >2 ng/ml, with hirsutism, the levels are <1.5 ng/ml. Rarely, the hair follicles themselves may have an increased sensitivity to androgen without an excess of circulating androgen.

The *disorders to be differentiated* from hirsutism are virilism (as noted earlier and characterized by more extensive androgen-stimulated changes), idiopathic hirsutism, and hypertrichosis. Hypertrichosis denotes excessive growth of the nonsexual hair (e.g., forehead, distal extremities). Hypertrichosis may result from starvation, traumatic skin irritation, drugs (e.g., phenytoin, diazoxide, minoxidil), and such disorders as acromegaly, porphyria, dermatomyositis, hypothyroidism, Hurler's syndrome, trisomy E, and Cornelia de Lange syndrome.

Most women with hirsutism will have no specific cause identified. For them, medical *therapy* is only moderately successful. The most common drugs used to treat hirsutism are oral contraceptives, medroxyprogesterone, dexamethasone, and spironolactone. Dexamethasone is effective in many whose hirsutism is of adrenal origin. The dose is 0.5–1 mg orally at night. Morning cortisol levels must be monitored to prevent oversuppression of the adrenals, however.

Combination oral contraceptives (estrogen + progestins) are effective in decreasing hair growth in 50%–60%, although to normalize testosterone levels may require 3 months. The effect of therapy is the inhibition of LH secretion by progestins and increased testosterone binding by SHBG (estrogen elevates SHBG). SHBG-bound testosterone will not be bound by receptors. In addition, combination oral contraceptives decrease DHEAS levels, possibly by suppressing ACTH release. This, in turn, decreases adrenal androgens. Progestins alone may be given in regular form (Provera, 30–40 mg/day) or in depot form (Depo-Provera, 150–400 mg IM every 3 months). Because the depot form may cause long-term suppression of the ovary, it should not be used if pregnancy is desired in the near future. In addition to the LH suppression, medroxyprogesterone acetate acts by increasing metabolic clearance of testosterone.

The growth cycle of hair is long (6–24 months), and once stimulated, much lower levels of androgen are necessary to sustain that growth. Therefore, patients should be cautioned not to expect a therapeutic response for 6–12 months. However, some decrease in hair diameter and lightening of hair color may be noted during that time. If adequate suppression of testosterone and DHEAS for 6–12 months has been documented without a decrease in hirsutism, the dose may be increased and another medication may be added or substituted. If the androgen levels do not decrease as expected with therapy or if hirsutism is progressive despite therapy, further evaluation for a slow-growing neoplasm should be initiated.

Idiopathic Hirsutism (Familial or Constitutional Hirsutism)

When hirsutism is present without ovarian or adrenal dysfunction and exogenous sources of androgens are absent, it is termed idiopathic. Idiopathic hirsutism is particularly common in those of Mediterranean or Near East descent. This condition is caused by abnormal peripheral androgen metabolism, i.e., increased 5_α-reductase activity converting normal levels of testosterone into higher than normal levels of DHT and adiol-G. Spironolactone, cimetidine, and cyproterone acetate afford effective *therapy* by blocking peripheral testosterone activity or interfering with 5_α-reductase activity.

Spironolactone lowers testosterone levels by inhibiting the biosynthesis of androgens and by competing for androgenic receptors in the hair follicle itself. The dosage is 50–200 mg/day. Cimetidine reduces hirsutism by peripheral inhibition of binding of dihydrotestosterone to androgen receptors. The dose is 300 mg PO 5 times per day.

Cosmetic therapy consists of bleaching, waxing, or depilatory use. Shaving and plucking may cause infection or scarring and are not recommended. Because permanent hair removal via electrolysis is expensive and painful, its use should be recommended only after 6–12 months of medical therapy.

Chapter 28

Other Gynecologic Problems

UTERINE POSITION AND MALPOSITION

UTERINE POSITION

Uterine position and axis are described by both the relationship to an imaginary line, equidistant from all bony structures through the true pelvis, and the relationship of the uterine axis to the cervical axis. The term *version,* with the appropriate prefix, ante- or retro- designates the uterine axis vis-a-vis the central pelvis. *Flexion* is the angulation of the axis of the uterus in relation to the axis of the cervix (Figs. 28-1 and 28-2).

The uterine axis usually deviates from that of the cervix by being anterior or posterior, and this is termed *anteflexion* or *retroflexion.* The corpus of the uterus is anteflexed in nearly 80% of women, and in the remaining 20% the corpus is retroflexed. Thus, *retroversion* implies that the axis of the body of the uterus is directed toward the hollow of the sacrum, but the cervix remains in its normal axis (Fig. 28-3). *Retrocession* implies that both uterus and cervix (to a lesser degree) are displaced backward toward the sacrum—away from the midpoint of the pelvis (Fig. 28-4).

Normally, because of the flexibility of the uterine supports, the position of the uterus may vary transiently as a result of pelvic inclination during sitting, standing, or lying down. In nulliparas and multiparas with good pelvic support, the cervical axis is usually directed posteriorly in the vaginal vault, almost at a right angle to the vaginal axis. Enlargement of the uterus by pregnancy or tumor may alter the relative fundal position. The uterus and cervix are often aligned with the vaginal axis following parturition or with relaxation of the pelvic floor because of laxity of the transverse cervical and round ligaments.

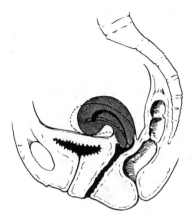

Figure 28-1. Anteflexion of uterus.

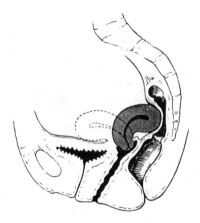

Figure 28-2. Retroflexion in an anteverted uterus.

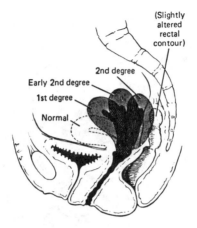

Figure 28-3. Degrees of retroversion of uterus without retroflexion.

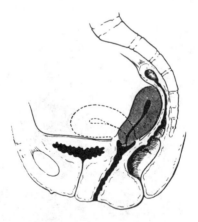

Figure 28-4. Retrocession of uterus.

UTERINE MALPOSITION

Uterine prolapse (even moderate) is nearly always associated with uterine retroversion or retrocession. *Nonfixed lateral uterine displacement* generally indicates displacement by tumors or shortening of the supports. *Fixed* (adherent) *lateral uterine version* may indicate endometriosis, adhesions, a tuboovarian mass, or tumor. Pelvic infections or endometriosis may obliterate the cul-de-sac and result in fixed uterine retroversion. A pyosalpinx or hydrosalpinx may draw the corpus backward and downward by its weight, whereupon adhesions add restriction to cause immobility. Speculum examination of the patient with retroflexion and retroversion of the uterus will reveal the cervix to be anterior, higher in the vagina than normally encountered, and pointing toward the symphysis pubis (as opposed to its normal posterior vaginal inclination). Bimanual examination ordinarily confirms this finding.

Differential diagnosis of unusual uterine positions includes a fundal fibroid, an ovarian tumor resting in the cul-de-sac, adherent retroposition of the uterus, salpingitis, or endometriosis. The *diagnosis* is most frequently clarified by a pelvic ultrasound examination.

Of women with retroposed uteri, <5% will have a complaint referable to posterior flexion or version of the uterus. When *symptoms* occur, they are most frequently backache, dysmenorrhea, or dyspareunia. These symptoms usually respond to correction of the retroposition of the uterus, which may be accomplished by manual replacement (rectovaginal manipulation of the corpus) (Fig. 28-5) and support using a vaginal pessary (Hodge type) (Fig. 28-6).

During early pregnancy, a retroflexed uterus may become incarcerated, often because of adhesions, and lead to acute urinary retention. In addition, because adherence interferes with normal fetal growth and development, abortion may result. This has been simply treated by catheterizing the bladder and using a vaginal mercury-filled balloon to gently displace the uterus anteriorly.

Adherent uterine fixations rarely cause uterine symptomatology. However, evaluation and appropriate therapy may be indicated for the underlying process creating the deviation. There are few indications for uterine suspension as a primary surgical therapy, although uterine suspension may assist in preventing uterine adherence to other pelvic structures in cases of pelvic endometriosis (p 659).

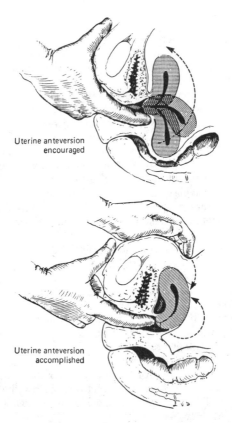

Uterine anteversion
encouraged

Uterine anteversion
accomplished

Figure 28-5. Bimanual replacement of uterus.

RELAXATION OF PELVIC SUPPORT

NORMAL SUPPORT OF PELVIC STRUCTURES

The cervix is normally relatively fixed in place by the dense fibrous and smooth muscle cardinal ligaments, which extend laterally to the pelvic sidewalls. At or just above the cervicouterine juncture, the relatively strong, primarily fibrous uterosacral ligaments attach posterior-lateral and extend to the sacrum to further support the uterus and cervix. The broad ligaments, a far weaker superior extension of the cardinal ligaments, are composed primarily of peritoneum and blood vessels.

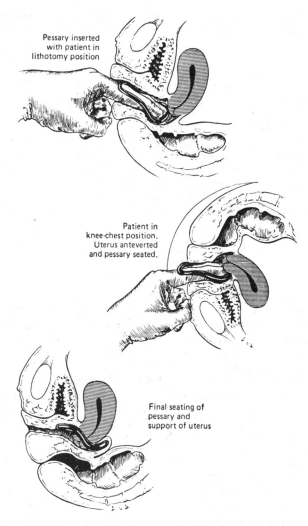

Pessary inserted
with patient in
lithotomy position

Patient in
knee-chest position.
Uterus anteverted
and pessary seated.

Final seating of
pessary and
support of uterus

Figure 28-6. Insertion of Hodge pessary if bimanual replacement of uterus is not successful.

The broad ligaments support the uterus laterally, and the round ligaments attach to the superior-lateral aspects of the corpus. Thus, the ligamentous support to the uterus is movable, in contrast to that of the cervix, which is not. The vagina is supported in part by the strong lower extension of the cardinal ligaments but pierces and is partly elevated by the muscles of the pelvic diaphragm (levator ani) and the perineum (perineal body, bulbocavernous muscle). Support of the lower vagina is intimately involved with that of the bladder and rectum.

With failure of support, the uterus, vagina, bladder, or rectum may first prolapse into, and finally protrude from, the vagina. It is so common for multiple problems to occur as a result of the basic defect that many authorities prefer the term *symptomatic pelvic relaxation* as the primary diagnosis, with a secondary description of the specific defects (e.g., cystocele) and their extent.

Vaginal Hernias

At least half of all parous women develop some degree of vaginal hernia (the most common are cystocele and rectocele), usually after the menopause. Approximately 10% of these are symptomatic and require treatment.

Vaginal herniations are caused by defects of the endopelvic connective tissue, fascia, or pelvic floor musculature. Such defects may occur as a result of congenital weaknesses, childbirth trauma, excessive strain on normal structures (e.g., straining with constipation), or musculofascial lacerations. Vaginal herniations rarely occur early in life, even after a traumatic delivery. The defects usually become evident only months or years later. The long delay in childbirth trauma becoming manifest is thought to be related to both intrinsic damage at the time and conversion of fibroelastic supports to fibrous (scar) tissue. The latter is much more prone to attenuation later. Thus, the climacteric and persistent stress of increased intraabdominal pressure cause gradual stretching of the damaged supports of the pelvic floor, bladder, or rectum.

Other contributing factors to prolapse are those that increase intraabdominal pressure and enhance strain on the pelvic structures. The following processes are associated with enhanced rates of vaginal herniation: congenitally deficient or relaxed pelvic support, obesity, chronic respiratory problems (asthma, chronic bronchitis, bronchiectasis), ascites, and sacral nerve disorders (injury to S1–4, the most common is diabetic neuropathy).

Types of Vaginal Hernias

Uterine (and Cervical) Prolapse

Prolapse of the uterus occurs most commonly in postmenopausal multiparous Caucasians. When the uterus prolapses, it carries the upper vagina with it. Figure 28-7 illustrates this condition.

Clinically, patients complain of a pelvic heaviness or dragging sensation. Other complaints may include low back pain, a sense of "something falling out," or a mass coming from the vagina. On physical examination, the descensus is apparent when the patient strains (i.e., increases intraabdominal pressure) or is demonstrated by gentle traction on the cervix (by grasping it with an Allis clamp or tenaculum).

The extent of uterine prolapse parallels the seriousness of separation or attenuation of its supporting structures. The degree of prolapse is graded by the extent of the cervical prolapse. A *first-degree prolapse* occurs when the cervix remains within the vagina, a *second-degree prolapse* exists when the cervix protrudes beyond the introitus, and a *third-degree prolapse* (com-

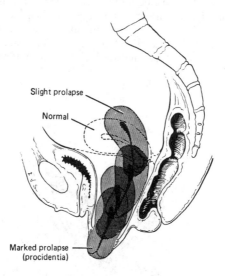

Slight prolapse

Normal

Marked prolapse
(procidentia)

Figure 28-7. Prolapsed uterus.

plete procidentia) implies that the entire uterus is outside the vulva. Often, the same grading is applied to other vaginal hernias to detail their extent.

The *differential diagnosis* of cervical or uterine prolapse includes only a nonprolapsed, hypertrophied, elongated, and often engorged, cervix. Rarely do cervical or uterine tumors have similar symptomatology.

Cystocele and Urethrocele

A cystocele is the prolapse of the bladder from its normal position into the vagina (Fig. 28-8). This hernia represents loss or a weakness of the pubocervical fascia. A urethrocele is defined as protrusion (a sagging) of the urethra into the vagina and is caused by loss of urethral attachments beneath the symphysis pubis. The urethra may assume a funnellike configuration. Frequently, the two defects occur together (*cystourethrocele*). The usual *symptomatology* of a cystocele includes a sensation of vaginal fullness, pressure, or falling out. On *examination,* a cystocele is marked by a soft, reducible mass bulging into the anterior vagina. With perineal depression and straining, the mass descends. Frequently, with a cystocele there is increased residual urine, which leads to urinary tract infection.

If there is an associated urethrocele, a downward and forward rotation of the urethra may be noted. Damage to the pubococcygeus portion of the levator musculature and the endopelvic fascia, often associated with a large cystocele, weakens and displaces the bladder neck and urethra. With a urethrocele if the

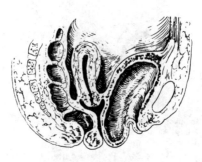

Figure 28-8. Cystocele.

bladder is even partially filled and the patient strains (e.g., cough), there may be stress incontinence of urine.

Rectocele

Loss of the rectovaginal septum and posterior vaginal wall support results in hernial protrusion of the rectum into the vagina, a rectocele (Fig. 28-9). The *symptomatology* of a rectocele includes a bearing-down sensation and vaginal fullness or heaviness. Additionally, patients with a rectocele may complain of constipation or the feeling of incomplete emptying of the rectum with bowel movement. In the most severe cases, the patient must place one or two fingers in the vagina (reducing the rectocele) to have a bowel movement.

On *physical examination,* a rectocele is revealed by retracting the anterior vaginal wall upward while having the patient perform a Valsalva maneuver. The rectum bulges into or through the vagina. Confirmation of the defect is afforded by placing one finger in the rectum and one in the vagina to detail the hernia and confirm loss of the rectovaginal septum. Most patients with rectocele also have hemorrhoids. In extreme forms, rectocele may lead to obstipation or fecal impaction.

Enterocele

Herniation of the cul-de-sac (pouch of Douglas) is defined as an enterocele. This hernia often contains loops of small bowel or

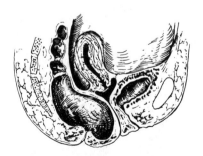

Figure 28-9. Rectocele.

omentum (Fig. 28-10). The bowel and omentum may be adherent to the peritoneum or freely movable. Enterocele may occur between the uterosacral ligaments into the rectovaginal septum with the uterus in place but is much more common following vaginal or abdominal hysterectomy.

Enteroceles are difficult to diagnose. *Symptomatology* is usually minimal (heaviness or internal weakness) or the same as with a rectocele. It is occasionally possible to differentiate the enterocele from a rectocele on physical examination by defining two hernias. This may be accomplished by seeking the bulge of the enterocele just above that of a rectocele as a bivalve speculum is slowly withdrawn from the vagina of the supine patient. The *diagnosis* can be confirmed by performing rectovaginal examination and asking the patient to cough. An impulse is felt against the fingertip opposing an enterocele (upper bulge) but not a rectocele (lower bulge). Also, if the enterocele is large enough to prolapse through the vaginal vault, transillumination may reveal bowel shadows. However, rectocele and enterocele are often only differentiated at the time of surgery. Enterocele is rarely a cause of intestinal obstruction.

Differential Diagnosis

Cysts of vestigial (wolffian) origin, semisolid tumors of the vaginal septa, and large inclusion cysts may be mistaken for cystocele or rectocele. A sizable cystocele may conceal a urethrocele. A

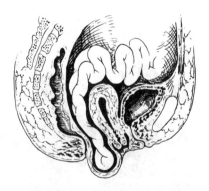

Figure 28-10. Enterocele and prolapsed uterus.

bladder or urethral diverticulum may be mistaken for a cystocele or urethrocele. The fullness of a high rectocele, prolapsed and adherent adnexa, a markedly retroflexed uterus, a soft cervical or uterine myoma, or retained fecal material may be confused with enterocele.

Diagnosis

There are no specific tests of value for detailing or diagnosing vaginal hernias. The workup generally is related to ascertaining fitness for surgery and excluding malignancy and other defects of the genital system. The diagnosis of urinary stress incontinence is reviewed on page 706. With complete procedentia any ulceration must be shown to be benign and resolved preoperatively.

Treatment

Treatment of vaginal hernias in postmenopausal patients usually involves the local or systemic administration of estrogen to enhance the vaginal mucosa, increase the blood supply to the region, and promote muscular tone. Kegel exercises (isometric contraction of the pubococcygeus muscles) may strengthen the musculature of the pelvic floor. In young women (who desire more children), it is common to defer surgical repair until after childbearing is complete or, when repair must be performed, to deliver subsequent pregnancies by cesarean section. In the woman who wishes to preserve her childbearing capability or in the medically compromised, pessary support (p 743) is palliative.

Therapy of uterine/cervical descensus most commonly is vaginal hysterectomy and resupport of the vagina using the uterosacral and cardinal ligaments. It is uncommon for cystocele to occur without some degree of rectocele, and vice versa. Until recently, the usual primary procedure for a cystocele and urethrocele was an anterior colporrhaphy. However, recurrence of stress urinary incontinence was high. Currently, urodynamic testing is performed before surgery so that the procedure most likely to effect cure may be determined. Many authorities recommend that even minor rectoceles be corrected at the time of urinary surgery to obviate the need for additional surgery at a later date.

Patients with recurrent cystourethroceles, those with severe stress incontinence of urine, and those in whom an abdominal procedure is necessary for other reasons may be treated with a Marshall-Marchetti-Krantz, Burch, or similar cystourethropexy (suspension) procedure (p 708). Posterior colporrhaphy is used to treat rectoceles. Repair of enteroceles is challenging (p 763), and the recurrence rate is >15% in all types of vaginal hernias after surgical repair.

GYNECOLOGIC UROLOGY

Because the female reproductive tract and lower urinary tract are so intimately related, consideration must be given to the lower urinary tract in evaluation of many gynecologic diseases.

ANATOMY AND PHYSIOLOGY

The urinary bladder is composed of three tightly woven muscle layers. Two of these layers extend into the urethra, forming longitudinal and circular muscle layers. Controversy exists as to whether or not a true striated muscle sphincter of the urethra exists because the pubococcygeus muscle acts as the sphincter of the urethra.

Innervation of the bladder is complex, with both autonomic and somatic nerves controlling the storage and expulsion of urine. Parasympathetic nerves from S2–4 stimulate bladder contractions. Beta-adrenergic fibers predominate in the bladder, and alpha-adrenergic fibers are dominant in the urethra. The smooth muscle of the urethra is contracted by the alpha-adrenergic system, and relaxation of the bladder and urethra are stimulated by the beta-adrenergic component. The pudenal nerve innervates the striated muscle present in the urethra.

The detrusor muscle relaxes as the bladder fills, thus allowing the intraluminal pressure to remain low. Although a smooth muscle, normally there is voluntary control, allowing micturition only when desired. When injury or disease is present, the intrinsic function of this muscle may be lost, resulting in incontinence.

Control of micturition involves the complex interplay of several systems. The urethra has two muscular layers (circular and longitudinal). Functionally, the pubococcygeus muscle acts as a striated muscle sphincter of the urethra. Urination is controlled by parasympathetic nerves from S2–4 (cholinergic nerve fibers), which stimulate bladder contractions, preganglionic sympathetic fibers from T10–L2, which are also cholinergic, postganglionic fibers from T10–L2 (adrenergic nerves) with beta fibers terminating mainly in the bladder and alpha fibers in the urethra.

Alpha-adrenergic stimulation contracts the ureteral smooth muscle. Beta-adrenergic stimulation relaxes both bladder and urethra. The detrusor muscle is composed of three muscular layers. It relaxes (within normal limits of volume) in response to increasing bladder volume, thus maintaining the same pressure.

Basic Evaluation of Urinary Problems

History

A careful history of medical and surgical treatment is important. Record the number and method of obstetric deliveries, as well as medications taken, pelvic or back surgery, neurologic disorders, and systemic disease processes. A history of tobacco use is also important because this may predispose to stress incontinence of urine.

Common Symptoms of Urinary Disorders

Dysuria

Dysuria is painful urination, often described as a burning sensation as urine flows through the urethra. Dysuria is a symptom of cystitis or urethritis but may result from chemical irritation, trauma, or atrophy (from estrogen deficiency). Dysuria must be differentiated from the burning associated with urine flowing over inflamed vulvar or vaginal tissues.

Frequency

Urinary frequency is a relative term, being defined as an increase in the number of voidings per 24 h for a given individual. Normal frequency varies from two to seven times per waking day. Urinary tract infection (UTI) is most often responsible for frequency, although interstitial cystitis, diabetes mellitus, emotional problems, or diuretics must be considered.

Urgency

Urgency is a sudden sensation of a need to void (often described as overwhelming). It is common in urinary tract disorders, especially with infection and interstitial cystitis.

Nocturia

Women who awaken more than once per night to void have nocturia. It may be the result of infection, a sleep disorder, or a neurologic problem. However, voiding more than once per night is common for the elderly. Recall that pregnancy, peripheral edema, and congestive heart failure cause diuresis in the recumbent position,

Enuresis

Enuresis is bedwetting. Although common in younger children, in an adult it is caused by either a neurologic or a psychogenic disorder or unrelieved urgency incontinence.

Stress Incontinence

Stress incontinence of urine is the involuntary loss of urine associated with increased intraabdominal pressure. Activites that increase intraabdominal pressure include sneezing, coughing, laughing, and stepping up or down. It is useful to ascertain the frequency of occurrence of stress incontinence and the amount of urine lost.

Urge Incontinence

Leakage of urine associated with the desire to void is termed urge incontinence, whether the urge is sudden or gradual in onset. Urge incontinence and stress incontinence may be concomitant.

Hesitancy

Hesitancy is the inability to start readily or maintain a stream of urine. This may be the result of poor urethral relaxation, inadequate detrusor contraction, partial urethral obstruction (from severe relaxation of pelvic supports), or overcorrection by cystourethropexy.

Postvoiding Fullness

A feeling of bladder fullness immediately after voiding is rarely a result of elevated residual urine volumes. Instead, it is often due to irritation (e.g., infection, trauma, inflammation, or foreign body), vaginal atrophy, or relaxation of pelvic supports. Residual urine volumes are generally low in postvoiding fullness.

Physical Examination

In the evaluation of urinary problems, a general physical examination and a complete pelvic examination should be performed. Evaluation for the relaxation of pelvic supports is important. The vagina should be inspected for evidence of inflammation, discharge, atrophy, scarring, stricture, abscess, or neoplasia. Urethral epithelial atrophy resulting from lack of estrogen stimulation is commonly associated with lower urinary tract symptoms in postmenopausal women.

The bladder and urethra should be palpated for tenderness or mass. Milking the urethra (stripping from proximal to distal) may disclose a discharge indicative of infection or diverticulum. To evaluate perineal neurologic integrity, assess the sensation of the perineum, the reflexes evaluated, and muscle strength. Evaluate the ability to contract and relax the pubococcygeus muscles and anal sphincter voluntarily.

Descent of the bladder or urethra is assessed during straining, with the patient in the dorsal lithotomy position. A lubricated cotton applicator is placed in the urethra to the urethrovesical junction The angle formed by the applicator stick and a line parallel to the floor is measured at rest and during a Valsalva (straining) maneuver. If the angle is <15 degrees both during rest and straining, good pelvic support is likely. If the angle is >30 degrees during straining, there is poor pelvic support. An angle of 15–30 degrees is inconclusive.

A urinary stress test should be performed to evaluate incontinence. The bladder is filled with a known volume of fluid (e.g., 300 ml) until it feels full but not uncomfortable. The patient is asked to stand with the feet a shoulder-width apart and to either cough eight or ten times or perform the Valsalva maneuver. The perineum is observed for leakage of urine. If incontinence occurs during the stress maneuver and ends shortly after straining is discontinued, the most likely cause is poor anatomic support. If the leakage is continuous or delayed, inadequate detrusor muscle control is likely. If the test is negative, mild incontinence may still be present, and further testing is necessary. Stress tests that include elevation of the vaginal wall during the test are not valid for predicting the effectiveness of surgery because they only show the effect of mechanical obstruction of the urethra.

EVALUATION AND THERAPY OF COMMON URINARY PROBLEMS

Urinary Tract Infection (UTI)

Because of the shorter urethra in females, UTI is more prevalent in women than in men, with an increasing incidence from adolescence to old age of 2%–20%. The organisms causing UTI are usually from the vagina or rectum and may ascend from the urethra (urethritis) to the bladder (cystitis) to the kidney (pyelonephritis). If urine contains >100,000 bacteria/dl in two clean-catch or one catheterized specimen, it is considered infected. Persons with poor hygiene, who void infrequently, or who have chronic urinary residual volume are most likely to develop UTI, as are those with renal stones, urinary tract anomalies, urinary reflux, or prolonged bladder catheterization.

The *signs and symptoms* of UTI may be minimal to severe, with dysuria, frequency, and urgency common in urethritis. Cystitis may be accompanied by suprapubic discomfort as well as urgency incontinence. Fever is usually present only with pyelonephritis. Back pain and anorexia are often associated findings in pyelonephritis, but asymptomatic renal infection does occur.

The *laboratory findings* suggesting UTI include pyuria (>6–8 WBC/hpf) in centrifuged urine sediment. Epithelial cells are usually of vaginal origin. A positive urine culture is diagnostic for many bacteria but will be negative in *Chlamydia* infection. Cystitis is often accompanied by hematuria. If WBC casts are present, pyelonephritis is likely. The WBC count on CBC may be elevated with pyelonephritis but may be normal in urethritis or cystitis.

The *differential diagnosis* includes vaginitis, especially from *Trichomonas* and herpes simplex. Pressure on the bladder from a pelvic mass may suggest cystitis.

Treatment for UTI is usually directed toward *Escherichia coli*, the most common offending organism. If it is the first episode of

UTI and is uncomplicated, the drugs of choice are ampicillin, trimethoprim-sulfamethoxazole, and nitrofurantoin. Once culture and sensitivity patterns are known, the drug dose or choice may be changed. Chronic or recurrent infections frequently are associated with resistant organisms requiring cephalosporins or aminoglycosides.

Dysuria may be relieved by urinary anesthetics (e.g., phenazopyridine hydrochloride). Administration of a single dose of antibiotic may cure simple cystitis. Pyelonephritis may require prolonged, even IV antibiotics. If bacteriuria persists after appropriate therapy, cystoscopy and intravenous pyelography (IVP) are indicated to rule out structural defects, stone, or tumor. Some recurrent UTIs result from contamination of the urethra during sexual intercourse and may be prevented by voiding immediately after intercourse, urinary antibiotics after intercourse, or nightly antibiotic prophylaxis.

Patients experiencing the symptoms of recurrent urethritis with negative bacterial cultures have *urethral syndrome.* Their symptomatology may be caused by organisms such as herpes simplex, *Chlamydia,* anaerobic bacteria, *Ureaplasma,* or *Mycoplasma.* Patients with urethral syndrome should be investigated for evidence of chemical or mechanical irritation of the urethra, as well as diverticula, stenosis, or a meatus opening into the vagina.

Approximately 20% of women >75 years are incontinent daily. Incontinence causes social and emotional distress as well as perineal irritation, vaginal discharge, dyspareunia, and unpleasant odors.

True Stress Incontinence

True stress incontinence (also termed *anatomic urinary stress incontinence*) is the involuntary loss of urine through the urethra simultaneously with an increase in intraabdominal pressure in the absence of detrusor muscle contraction. Because intraabdominal pressure is also transmitted (incompletely) to the proximal urethra, such activities as exercise or coughing may result in the loss of the pressure gradient and allow urine to escape.

Several mechanisms may be responsible for true stress incontinence: (1) anatomic descent of the proximal urethra below its normal intraabdominal position during stress-causing activities, (2) altered anatomic relationships between the urethra and bladder, resulting in vector forces directed from the bladder along the axis of the urethra, and (3) failure of the neuromuscular components that reflexly increase intraurethral pressure in response to increased intraabdominal pressure.

The *diagnosis* of true stress incontinence does not hinge on one test. The criteria include normal urinalysis, negative urine culture, poor anatomic support (as evidenced by the cotton-tipped applicator test, x-ray, or urethroscopy), demonstrable leakage with stress, and normal cystometrogram or urethrocystometry. Figure 28-11 details the common normal and abnormal bladder and urethral configurations.

The *signs and symptoms* of true stress incontinence are predominantly stress incontinence, although frequency, urgency, urge incontinence, and postvoiding fullness are common complaints. Dysuria and hematuria are uncommon unless there is a concomitant UTI. Approximately 75% of patients will have cystocele or urethrocele.

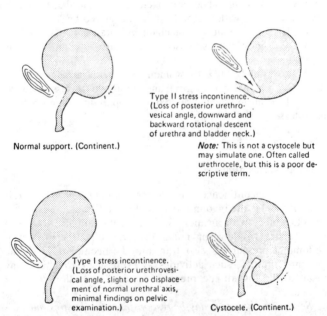

Normal support. (Continent.)

Type II stress incontinence. (Loss of posterior urethrovesical angle, downward and backward rotational descent of urethra and bladder neck.)

Note: This is not a cystocele but may simulate one. Often called urethrocele, but this is a poor descriptive term.

Type I stress incontinence. (Loss of posterior urethrovesical angle, slight or no displacement of normal urethral axis, minimal findings on pelvic examination.)

Cystocele. (Continent.)

Figure 28-11. Anatomic configuration of the bladder in normal (continent) women and women with stress incontinence. Drawn from cystourethrograms. (From T.H. Green, Jr, *Gynecology: Essentials of Clinical Practice,* 3rd ed. Little, Brown, 1977.)

Because treatment is based on correction of the anatomic abnormality, studies demonstrating poor support of the urethra are necessary before surgical correction. In 95%, the cotton-tipped applicator test will be abnormal. In the 5% with normal results, incontinence is the result of funneling of proximal urethra, severe scarring of the urethra, or atony of the urethral sphincteric mechanism. Urethral scarring will prevent movement of the applicator despite poor pelvic support. Therefore, a normal test should be followed by a straining cystogram or voiding cystourethrogram.

If the urinary stress test is negative, a pad test may be performed to document incontinence. A preweighed sanitary napkin is used to measure the volume of urine lost during exercise or whatever activity that precipitates stress incontinence in that woman. Colored fluid may be instilled into the bladder to visually demonstrate loss of urine.

A cystometrogram must be performed to rule out unstable bladder, overflow incontinence, reduced bladder capacity, or abnormal bladder sensation. If the bladder capacity is <300 ml or >800 ml, surgery is contraindicated.

Urethroscopy and cystoscopy may show diverticula, fistulas, neoplasia, calculi, or inflammation. Dynamic urethroscopy observes the urethrovesical junction during bladder filling and straining. If pelvic support is adequate during increased intraabdominal pressure maneuvers, the urethrovesical junction will close proximal to the tip located in the proximal urethra. If anatomic support is poor, the urethrovesical junction closes over the tip of the urethroscope.

Obtaining a urethral pressure profile can show weakness of the urethral sphincteric mechanism at rest, although this may not be exclusive to patients with true stress incontinence. It is most helpful in determining which patients with true stress incontinence will not benefit from surgical correction (i.e., when urethral closing pressures are very low at rest).

Treatment

Treatment may be either surgical, medical, or a combination of both. Severe incontinence is rarely cured by medical management. Surgical techniques that are successful initially may be followed by recurrence over the years due to the effects of aging and other disease processes that affect the continence mechanisms.

Medical Measures. Kegel isotonic exercises consist of repeated contractions of the pubococcygeus muscles to strengthen a weak pelvic floor musculature. The patient is instructed to squeeze the muscles used to stop urination 150–200 times per day. Good improvement is seen in 15%–30% with true stress incontinence, with some improvement in another 30%–40%. If the exercises are repeated less frequently, improvement may be marginal.

If the cause of incontinence is atrophic change from estrogen deficiency, estrogen replacement will result in resolution of stress incontinence in 10%–30% of postmenopausal women. Vaginal estrogen provides the most rapid response, but oral preparations maintain the patient's status as well as do vaginal preparations.

If the patient is taking medications that stimulate ganglionic or alpha-adrenergic blocking activity (e.g., guanethidine, methyldopa, prazosin), discontinuing their use may result in improved urethral tone and improved continence. Alpha-adrenergic agonists (e.g., phenylpropanolamine, pseudoephedrine) also may improve stress incontinence.

Other methods, such as electrical stimulation of the pelvic floor to increase urethral closure pressure or Teflon injected periurethrally to compress the urethral mucosa and cause a mild obstruction to urinary flow, have been performed with some success.

Surgical Measures. The goal of surgical procedures for incontinence is to elevate and support the urethrovesical junction to improve pressure transmission to the urethra during stress maneuvers. The procedures may be accomplished vaginally or abdominally. The cure rate depends on patient selection, accuracy of preoperative diagnosis, skill of the surgeon, and length of follow-up. Cure rates for the abdominal procedures are 85%–90% and for vaginal procedures 75%–85%.

The predominant *abdominal procedures* are the Marshall-Marchetti-Krantz (MMK) procedure, the Burch procedure, the paravaginal procedure, or various modifications. These procedures consist of placing sutures in the periurethral, vaginal, or perivaginal tissue to elevate the urethrovesical junction and attaching these sutures to relatively strong and permanent structures. The MMK uses the periosteum of the pubic symphysis for suture fixation, whereas the Burch procedure uses Cooper's ligaments. The obturator fascia, arcus tendineus of the pelvic fascia, insertion of the rectus fascia, and the periosteum of the pubic ramus have all been employed in various modifications.

Vaginal procedures for stress incontinence are based on the assumption that weakening of or damage to the endopelvic fascia between the vagina and bladder is responsible for the poor support. The initial procedure (Kelly plication) involves an anterior colporrhaphy with plication at the urethrovesical angle through a midline vaginal incision. Because long-term success is limited using the endopelvic fascia, employing stronger structures (e.g., pubourethral ligaments, periosteum of the pubic ramus, pubo-coccygeus muscles) has met with better results.

Combined vaginal-abdominal procedures resembling retro-pubic procedures performed primarily through the vagina have success rates almost as high as standard abdominal procedures.

Patients with urethral scarring or atony not amenable to stan-dard surgical therapy may benefit from placement of an artificial urethral sphincter that obstructs the urethra until the patient desires to void, at which time the artificial sphincter is emptied by an internal pumping system to relieve the urethral obstruction and allow the urine to flow.

A sling procedure using autogenous fascia (e.g., rectus fas-cia, fascia lata, round ligaments) or synthetic material that is passed under the urethra to support the urethrovesical junction and partially obstruct the urethra may be used if standard surgi-cal techniques are unlikely to succeed. The partial urethral ob-struction can be overcome sufficiently by some patients to allow voluntary voiding, whereas others will require intermittent self-catheterization or performance of the Credé maneuver (exter-nal abdominal pressure on the bladder).

Surgical complications include UTI, delayed postoperative voiding, dyspareunia, frequency-urgency syndrome, and surgi-cally induced unstable bladder, in addition to iatrogenic damage to the urinary tract, postoperative fistula, and bladder calculi from sutures perforating the bladder mucosa.

The *prognosis* for medical management is usually an improve-ment in symptoms but not cure. Surgical management is the only definitive cure for true stress incontinence. A poorer prognosis is likely for patients who have had a previous surgical failure, low urethral closing pressure at rest, concomitant local disease, com-bined urinary incontinence (true stress incontinence plus motor urge incontinence), or systemic diseases that make healing or technical performance of surgery difficult (e.g., diabetes melli-tus, obesity).

Motor Urge Incontinence

Motor urge incontinence, also termed *unstable bladder* or *de-trusor instability,* results from involuntary uninhibited detrusor muscle contractions. If the cause is neurologic, it is termed *hyperreflexic bladder.* Most cases are idiopathic, although infec-tion and obstruction may contribute.

Because the urine loss is unpredictable and large volumes may be lost, this condition causes considerably more distress than does true stress incontinence. About 1%–2% of adult females suffer from motor urge incontinence, with the highest incidence occurring in the geriatric population.

Normal micturition sequence is relaxation of the urethral sphincteric mechanism, followed by contraction of the detrusor muscle 1–3 sec later. The sequence is unchanged in motor urge incontinence, but the patient cannot voluntarily inhibit the action. It may occur at any bladder volume and may be spontaneous or provoked by physical, psychologic, tactile, or auditory stimuli. Approximately 25%–50% of patients with motor urge incontinence are incontinent only with provocation. About one third have concomitant true stress incontinence, making the distinction difficult. Most feel an urge to void immediately preceding the episode, but patients with neurologic disease may have no warning.

The *symptoms* include urgency, frequency, stress incontinence, and urge incontinence. Physical examination is usually normal unless detrusor hyperreflexia is present with associated neurologic abnormalities.

The *diagnosis* of motor urge incontinence is suggested by a several second delay in urine loss during a urinary stress test. The diagnosis is confirmed by cystometric evidence of involuntary detrusor contractions at rest, during bladder filling, or after provocative maneuvers. A smooth rise in pressure occurring simultaneously with visible urine leakage is typical. Urethrocystometry confirms that the involuntary contractions are preceded by a fall in urethral pressure. Urethroscopy and cystoscopy may reveal bladder trabeculation from hypertrophy of the detrusor muscle fascicles.

The *differential diagnosis* includes true stress incontinence and sensory urge incontinence. In the latter, the patient can inhibit the leakage with strong encouragement, whereas motor urge incontinence cannot be inhibited. True stress incontinence can be distinguished using provocative cystometry or simultaneous urethrocystometry.

Treatment

Behavior modification techniques using hypnosis, biofeedback, bladder retraining drills, and psychotherapy may be effective if neurologic disease is not responsible for the unstable bladder. Bladder retraining consists of having the patient void on schedule at intervals that are gradually lengthened in an attempt to regain cortical control over the voiding reflex. This may be effective in up to 80% but requires compulsive patient cooperation, and recurrence rates are high.

Medication will help in 50%–80% of patients. The most effective drugs are anticholinergic agents, but bladder analgesics, smooth muscle antispasmodics, calcium channel blockers, and prostaglandin synthetase inhibitors have been effective.

Surgery consisting of such procedures as denervation, cystoplasty, and urinary diversion usually are reserved for patients with severe permanent bladder instability from neurologic disease and when all other therapy fails.

Occasionally, indwelling catheters are used for patients who are severely incapacitated, but this adds the risk of chronic infection.

Prognosis

Recurrence rates are high, bladder retraining techniques require much time and effort, and medications have troublesome side effects. Hence, motor urge incontinence is likely to be a long-term problem not easily resolved. Theoretically, bladder retraining is ideal, since there are no side effects or surgery involved. If the patient responds initially, she is likely to respond to retraining should a recurrence develop.

Sensory Urge Incontinence

Sensory urge incontinence is diagnosed when incontinence occurs with a feeling of urgency in a stable bladder without marked descent of the urethra and bladder. The most common causes are infection, diverticula, neoplasia, foreign body, and psychologic and neurologic factors.

It is caused by either urethral relaxation or voluntary detrusor contraction. Normally as the bladder fills, there is a reflex urge to urinate that is subconsciously inhibited until the bladder is full. Conditions that irritate the bladder or urethra (e.g., infection, trauma) overstimulate this reflex, resulting in intermittent urethral relaxation. This allows the dribbling of small amounts of urine, which further stimulates the bladder. If the patient fails to concentrate on maintaining continence, the detrusor may contract after urethral relaxation, resulting in a larger volume of urine lost.

Clinical findings typically include a small bladder capacity on cystometry that normalizes under anesthesia unless scarring is present. Urethral pressure profiles or simultaneous urethrocystometry reveals urethral relaxation or marked variations in urethral pressure. Cystometrograms show no detrusor activity as long as the patient concentrates on not voiding. Urethroscopy and cystoscopy are essential to avoid missing local treatable problems.

Treatment

Therapy is directed toward the direct cause if one is present. Treat infection (urinary or vaginal) with antibiotics. Chronic infection may have prolonged symptomatology due to the residual inflammation and edema long after bacteria have been destroyed. Urethral dilatation and instillation of anti-inflammatory agents into the bladder may provide relief. Neoplasia, diverticula, and calculi require surgery or lithotripsy. Estrogen deficiency may be responsible for sensory urge incontinence and is treated by estrogen replacement vaginally or orally.

The *prognosis* is good with cure of the underlying disorder. Chronic causes may result in recurrence or only partial relief.

Overflow Incontinence

Overflow incontinence is the result of urinary retention with subsequent overflow. Causes of retention are multiple. Neurogenic retention may be a result of a denervated bladder with diminished or absent detrusor contractions or from detrusor-sphincter dyssynergia, in which the urethra fails to relax with voiding attempts. Diabetes and lower motor neuron disorders are most commonly responsible. Also, obstruction of the urethra may occur postoperatively, with severe relaxation of pelvic supports, or from pelvic masses. Medications (e.g., ganglionic blockers, anticholinergic agents, alpha-adrenergic agonists, and spinal or epidural anesthesia) may cause overflow incontinence. Acute or chronic overdistention of the bladder results in myotonic decompensation and subsequent inability to contract. This may be idiopathic or psychogenic in origin.

Cystometric findings typically reveal a large bladder capacity (as much as 1200 dl) with decreased sensation of the bladder and poor to absent detrusor contractility.

Treatment

Treatment in cases of acute retention is directed toward drainage to prevent myotonic decompensation, chronic retention, infection, and obstructive uropathy. To reduce urethral closing pressure and increase detrusor contractility, alpha-adrenolytic agents (e.g., prazosin, phenoxybenzamine), striated muscle relaxants (e.g., diazepam, dantrolene), and cholinergic agents (e.g., bethanecol) are used. If the patient has chronic urinary retention, intermittent self-catheterization is helpful.

Bypass Incontinence

Urinary leakage will occur whenever the urethral sphincteric mechanism is bypassed. Abnormalities, such as fistulas, ectopic ureters, and urethral diverticula, are the most common causes of bypass incontinence. Both fistulas and diverticula may mimic true stress incontinence, with exacerbation during stressful activity. The urinary diverticula may retain urine until the patient stands upright to walk or increases intraabdominal pressure, although the volume lost is usually less than with true stress incontinence.

Treatment

Treatment is surgical with a good prognosis if successful. However, damage to the urethral sphincteric mechanism during surgery will result in incontinence.

Psychogenic Incontinence

Stress incontinence, sensory urge incontinence, motor urge incontinence, and overflow incontinence may all have psychogenic origins. *Surgery* is usually unsuccessful in relieving psychogenic incontinence and should be avoided if possible. *Psychiatric and medical therapy* have the best chance of success as long as the patient's underlying psychologic conflicts are resolved.

Interstitial Cystitis

Interstitial cystitis is a chronic inflammatory condition almost exclusively of women, most of whom are perimenopausal. It may represent a defect in the protective glycosaminoglycan layer of the transitional epithelium (of uncertain origin) or an autoimmune disease.

Urinary frequency, urgency, suprapubic pain, discomfort with voiding, and dyspareunia strongly suggest urinary infection. However, when the symptomatology persists despite treatment for minimal urinary findings (including negative cultures), suspect interstitial cystitis. Interstitial cystitis is associated with stress or urge incontinence, which must be confirmed by urodynamic studies. Urethral syndrome is commonly a misdiagnosis for interstitial cystitis, but the latter may be noted in patients with hypersensitive bladders.

Chronicity of the urinary symptoms with suprapubic pain strongly suggests interstitial cystitis. Cystoscopy typically reveals a pancystitis and, occasionally, a localized fibrotic scar(s) or ulceration (Hunner's ulcer). Biopsies disclose chronic inflammation (including numerous mast cells) in the submucosa and muscularis, without evidence of cancer.

There is no cure for interstitial cystitis. Analgesics, bladder drill, or other feedback programs should relieve patients with slight to moderate interstitial cystitis. In severe cases, bladder distention under anesthesia or instillation of dimethyl sulfoxide or oxycholoresene sodium (Chlorpactin WCS-90) may give more lasting relief. Resection or laser therapy of a Hunner ulcer may be helpful. Cystectomy or urinary diversion may be warranted in severe recalcitrant cases.

Urethral Caruncle

A small, reddened, sensitive, fleshy excrescence at the urethral meatus is called a caruncle. Most caruncles represent eversion (ectropion of the urethra) or infection at the urinary meatus or both. However, vascular anomalies or benign or malignant tumors also may cause caruncle formation. The vast majority of caruncles are benign, persistent lesions. Caruncles may occur at any age, but postmenopausal women are most commonly affected.

Caruncles appear as small, vividly red, sessile or flattened masses protruding from the urethral meatus. They may bleed, exude, or cause pain depending on the cause, size, and integrity. Dysuria, frequency, and urgency are uncommon. Laboratory tests are not diagnostic. If cancer is suspected, biopsy must be performed.

Estrogen *therapy* for postmenopausal women and avoidance of local irritation will probably prevent and even heal caruncle formation. Infections, including STDs, must be treated with appropriate antibiotics. Estrogen (vaginal suppositories of estradiol

0.5 mg every other night for 3 weeks) may be given before specific therapy in postmenopausal patients who have not been receiving estrogen.

If the caruncle is not markedly infected or malignant, light fulguration under local anesthesia, cryosurgery laser vaporization, or excision may be performed. If stenosis develops, the urethral meatus must be dilated. The *prognosis* is excellent in benign cases but guarded when malignant change has occurred.

Urethral Diverticulum

Urethral diverticulum is a sacculation caused by (1) congenital cystic dilatation of paraurethral (wolffian) remnants, (2) infection of the paraurethral glands, with rupture to the urethra, or (3) urinary, obstetric, or gynecologic injury. Most patients are 40–50 years of age and multiparous.

The mid- or distal third of the urethra is the usual site. With congenital malformation, the cystic structure, usually 1–4 cm in diameter, may be an angled or multiloculated cavity. Calculi are present in the diverticulum in 10%–20% of patients.

Clinical Findings

Urinary urgency, frequency, nocturia, dribbling after urination, discharge of urinous or bloody, purulent fluid following stripping of the urethra, vaginal pain, dyspareunia, urethral tenderness, pelvic discomfort, and vaginal fullness occur. There may be indefinite anterior vaginal fullness that is periodically painful.

Radiopaque contrast fluid studies generally will outline the diverticulum. Ultrasonography is not diagnostic. Insertion of a small urethral sound will demonstrate a slight stricture of the urethra and the diverticulum just beyond. Air cystoscopy or panendoscopy will reveal the diverticular opening in most cases.

Complications

Urethrovaginal fistula may follow unsuccessful diverticulectomy or spontaneous rupture (often during labor), erosion by stone, incisional drainage, or fulguration of the cystic abnormality. Transitional cell carcinoma or adenocarcinoma may develop in urethral diverticula. Stricture of the urethra may be a consequence of extensive or complicated surgery.

Differential Diagnosis

Urethritis is unassociated with postvoiding discharge or local fullness. Urethral abscess is a phase of diverticulum development. Urethrocele is not a swelling or herniation but a disengagement of the urethra from the points of attachment. Tumors may be primary or secondary and are firm, semifixed, and nontender.

Treatment

Transvaginal diverticulectomy with urethral catheter drainage for 10 days for patients with a symptomatic urethral cyst usually is curative.

URINARY TRACT INJURIES FOLLOWING OBSTETRIC AND GYNECOLOGIC SURGERY

Iatrogenic fistulas may occur in any part of the urinary tract and result from direct or indirect injury. Occlusions usually involve the ureter and occur as a result of angulation or obstruction by a suture, scarring after injury, endometriosis or infection or as a complication of the treatment of pelvic cancer. The kidney is rarely damaged directly during gynecologic surgery. The incidence of urinary tract injury in medical centers in the United States is about 0.8% following major gynecologic surgery and 0.08% following obstetric surgery.

Postpartum fistulas of the bladder or urethra generally are caused by continued pressure of the presenting part or by instrumentation. There is usually a history of prolonged labor (especially of the second stage) or complicated operative delivery.

Clinical Findings

Symptoms and Signs

Unilateral ureteral injury usually causes flank pain, tenderness, and fever but does not alter the urinary volume. Ureteral injury may result in constriction of the ureter, fistula, or infection. Escape of urine from the abdominal or vaginal incision indicates ureteral or bladder fistulas or both. Ileus often follows urinary obstruction or extravasation. Urinary infection, especially with partial obstruction of the ureter, results in chills, fever, renal pain, and costovertebral and loin tenderness. In the absence of preexisting bacteriuria, complete obstruction of one ureter usually is asymptomatic. If urine leaks into the peritoneal cavity, there will be signs of free peritoneal fluid and peritoneal irritation. If leakage is retroperitoneal, regional pain and a fluid collection will develop.

Signs of perirenal or psoas inflammation are secondary to retroperitoneal extravasation or urine. Anuria and uremia follow complete bilateral ureteral occlusion. In acute cases, rule out dehydration, shock, lower nephron nephrosis, and congestive heart failure.

Laboratory Findings

1. Passage of a urethral catheter should reveal obstruction.
2. Urethroscopy will often expose blockage, perforating suture, or fistula.
3. Cystoscopy will disclose large vesical fistulas, but small fistulas may escape detection.
4. Retrograde studies of the urinary tract are especially useful to rule out ureteral injury. If the ureteral catheters pass readily to both renal pelves and clear urine is returned, ureteral injury is excluded, except perhaps in a case of a crushing injury or small perforation. If one of these complications seems likely, the catheter should be secured in the ureter for splinting and drainage for the 10–14 days necessary for healing.

Ureteral Constriction

Obtain blood creatine and BUN tests to identify renal impairment. Ultrasonographic or x-ray findings may disclose ureteral obstruction, fistula, or urinary extravasation. CT is the best radiographic modality for evaluating ureteral obstruction. It can also assess the degree of renal compromise, determine the site of a fistula or an obstruction, and determine the presence of extravasated urine.

Even the freshly occluded kidney will not excrete the contrast agent on excretory urography. Although the urogram can be used as a screening test, it is not as sensitive as CT for detecting extravasated urine. Moreover, the presence of intestinal gas will reduce the clarity of the roentgenogram.

Retrograde urography may be useful when a ureteral catheter is blocked by an occlusion. A radiopaque catheter should be used so that the level of the obstruction can be observed on the film. Injection of a contrast medium into a Braach bulb catheter may reveal a fistula above the bulb fixed in the most distal portion of the ureter.

Bladder Fistula and Extravasation

Obtain an anteroposterior scout film of the pelvis. Fill the bladder with 50 ml of suitable radiopaque medium in 200 dl of water, and take a second film. Drain the bladder, and obtain a third film at once. Slight extravasation, not visible in the second film, may be clearly seen in the third.

Complications

Peritonitis is the most serious complication of urinary tract injury. Anuria or oliguria may be associated with fatal uremia after bilateral ureteral occlusion. Other complications are psoas or perirenal abscess or thrombophlebitis. Urinary tract infection usually follows partial ureteral obstruction.

Differential Diagnosis

Clear, yellowish, odorless drainage from the abdominal wound may represent ascites or exudative peritoneal fluid, an antecedent of wound dehiscence. Thin, brownish discharge from an abdominal or vaginal suture line may be serum from a seroma or hematoma. In ureteral obstruction, oliguria or anuria may be due to shock, dehydration, or lower nephron nephrosis, abdominal distention may indicate dynamic ileus caused by intestinal obstruction or adynamic ileus due to peritonitis, fever may be due to an infected wound, peritonitis, or thrombophlebitis, and kidney pain and costovertebral or flank tenderness may be due to nephrolithiasis, ureterolithiasis, or pyelonephritis.

Prevention

Adequate preliminary studies of the urinary tract and full knowledge of the anatomy and pathologic processes involved are essential before surgery. The ureters should be catheterized and identified initially in all difficult cases, and the wire stylet should be left in the ureteral catheter for identification—to prevent the ureter from being cut or clamped by mistake.

All structures must be identified before clamping, incision, and ligation, and care must be taken to prevent undue traction and needless denudation of the ureter and base of the bladder. Only fine absorbable sutures should be used in or around the urinary tract. Multiple ligatures should not be used for hemorrhage. Instead, pressure should be applied and a single bleeding point secured. The integrity of the bladder and the course of the ureters must be traced at the completion of each abdominal operation if surgery was near the ureter.

The surgeon should personally remove ureteral catheters after surgery if it is decided not to leave them in place. A hang-up may indicate ureteral constriction.

Treatment

Emergency Measures

Treat shock, blood loss, and dehydration as indicated and catheterize the bladder. If oliguria or anuria is present, obtain creatine and BUN. Check the specific gravity of the urine.

Surgical Measures

1. *Bilateral ureteral obstruction.* If both ureters are obstructed and the patient is a poor surgical risk, nephrostomy or unilateral tube ureterostomy is preferred. Use the largest urethral catheter that will enter the ureter. The other kidney should not be left obstructed for more than a few days. As soon as the patient becomes a satisfactory operative risk, relieve the second blocked kidney by nephrostomy or tube ureterostomy. Deligation alone is not satisfactory unless it can be performed easily. If deligation is done, insert a splinting catheter through a longitudinal incision several centimeters above the point of obstruction, pass it to the kidney, bring it out from the urethra, and fix it to a Foley retention catheter for 10–14 days. Then remove both catheters. The retroperitoneal area must always be drained through a separate lower quadrant or flank stab wound.

A gallbladder T tube can be used in lieu of a catheter when (1) the crossarm of the T is notched at the vertical segment, (2) the ureter is incised longitudinally several centimeters about the defect, (3) the tube is inserted so that its lower arm splints the point of injury, (4) the upper arm of the tube is fixed in the proximal ureter, and the long arm is carried out retroperitoneally through a stab wound in the flank, (5) a drain is placed in the retroperitoneal space underlying the T tube and allowed to remain until drainage ceases (about 1 week after removal of the tube).

2. *Vesicoperitoneal fistula.* Perform laparotomy as soon as the diagnosis is established. With closure of the fistula in two layers using fine catgut, avoid the mucosa in suturing. Drain the bladder by cystostomy or with a Foley retention catheter, and use pelvic suction drainage for about 7 days.

3. *Vesicovaginal fistula.* Treat local infection by removing old sutures and concretions and by giving systemic antibiotics. Repair is indicated as outlined for vesicoperitoneal fistula. In general, attempts at closure should be delayed until 4 months or more after injury, although the use of steroids and intensive antibiotics may allow more immediate repair. All but large, inaccessible, immobile vesicovaginal fistulas (85%–90% of the total) should be closed transvaginally.

4. *Ureterovesicovaginal fistula.* Close the fistula abdominally using relatively few fine, absorbable, interrupted mattress sutures and avoiding the mucosa. Pursestring sutures should not be used.

Reimplantation of the severely damaged or severed ureter into the bladder (ureteroneocystostomy) is preferable to ureteroenterostomy on the same side. The bladder should be drained by cystostomy or with a Foley retention catheter, and suction drainage should be used for about 7 days.

Ligation of the damaged ureter and sacrifice of the kidney on the involved side are almost always contraindicated. The opposite kidney may be deficient or it may fail.

Prognosis

Most ureteral repairs are successful if performed carefully and if urinary and extraperitoneal drainage is ensured.

Very small vesicovaginal fistulas often close spontaneously if the bladder can be kept collapsed and infection prevented.

Urethral fistulas are notoriously resistant to spontaneous closure if a urethral catheter is used. Many heal well, however, when simply repaired and when a cystostomy is used instead of a urethral catheter.

ANORECTAL PROBLEMS

Common lesions of the anal canal are shown in Figure 28-12.

PROCTALGIA FUGAX

Proctalgia fugax, so-called rectal spasm or rectal neuralgia, is a
sudden cramping rectal pain of short duration. It is uncommon,

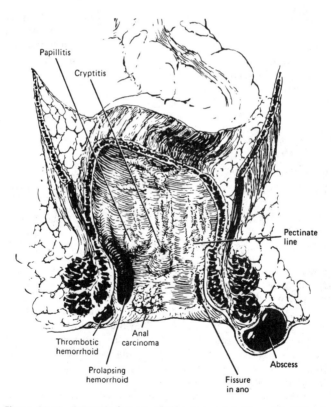

**Figure 28-12. Common lesions of the anal canal. (From J.L. Wilson,
Handbook of Surgery, 5th ed. Lange, 1973.)**

and its cause is not known. However, partial intussusception of redundant rectal mucosa is suspected.

Cramping rectal pain begins without warning, ranges in intensity from marked to agonizing, and tends to recur. The discomfort starts low in the rectum and moves higher (perhaps combined with the urge to defecate). Pain is associated with sweating, agitation, and even collapse. It subsides gradually, leaving the patient weak and shaken.

Rectal examination readily differentiates proctalgia fugax from thrombosed hemorrhoids, fissure in ano, or abscess. The pain of factitial proctitis, which may follow intravaginal radium therapy or local treatment of acute rectal disease, is constant and is accompanied by rectal bleeding and ulceration. Sigmoidorectal obstruction causes extreme, unrelenting, progressive pain and is not likely to recur.

Ample sedation and filling of the rectum with 200–300 ml of air or warm fluid may give dramatic relief. Recurrent attacks may be treated by submucosal injections of a solution containing 4% phenol, 50% glycerine, and water. Injections of 1 ml each at four points 1 cm apart just below the rectosigmoid junction may be curative.

ANAL CONDYLOMAS
(See Condylomata Acuminata, p. 496)

HEMORRHOIDS

Hemorrhoids (piles) are anorectal varicosities caused by lax pelvic veins and venous stasis. Internal hemorrhoids lie above the anorectal or mucocutaneous dentate line and are derived from the superior and middle hemorrhoidal veins. They usually are located in the right anterior and both posterior quadrants of the rectum. Internal hemorrhoids are covered by a thin rectal mucosa and are innervated by autonomic nerves.

External hemorrhoids develop below the mucocutaneous line and may appear in any quadrant. They are covered by skin, are supplied by the inferior hemorrhoidal vein, and are innervated by cutaneous nerves. Combined external and internal hemorrhoids are uncommon, but they may be serious if they involve at least a third of the anorectal margin.

Hemorrhoids cause itching, pain (the most severe occurs with thrombosis), protrusion, and bleeding. Most women with hemorrhoids develop them during pregnancy or delivery. Never assume that hemorrhoids are the cause of bleeding from the bowel until careful and complete physical, proctologic, and laboratory studies have failed to reveal cancer, a benign tumor, or other local or systemic disease.

Prevention includes good bowel habits, avoidance of straining, and prompt treatment of diarrhea and anorectal disorders. No therapy is required for asymptomatic hemorrhoids. Stool softeners, laxatives, and fiber-rich foods together with ample fluids should be given. Hemorrhoids causing mild or infrequent symptoms are treated with warm sitz baths, astringent ointments, or suppositories and oral analgesics. Avoid using sensitizing local anesthetics or antibiotics. Take measures to correct faulty bowel function.

Hemorrhoids with moderate symptoms (large or prolapsed hemorrhoids) should be treated as for mild symptoms. One hemorrhoid a week may be injected with 1 ml of 5% quinine and urea solution or 5% sodium morrhuate solution using a 22-gauge needle. Hemorrhoids with severe symptoms (large or strangulated hemorrhoids) are acutely painful. These and thrombosed external hemorrhoids should be incised under local anesthesia and the clot removed. For the first 24 h after clot formation, treat as for mild symptoms. Later, consider hemorrhoidectomy.

Symptomatic hemorrhoids during pregnancy should be treated for mild symptoms if possible. Hemorrhoidectomy should be deferred until after the puerperium.

Open radial hemorrhoidectomy (vascular ligation and excision) is the preferred *surgical* method. A cleansing enema should be administered before hemorrhoidectomy. Avoid packs or drains after surgery. Cover the incision with moist gel sponge. The patient should receive daily sitz baths, mild laxatives, and parenteral analgesics. Antibiotics may be given if needed. Perform gentle digital rectal dilation 5–7 days postoperatively and repeat two or three times every 5–7 days to prevent bridging and fistula formation.

Complications of hemorrhoidectomy include postoperative bleeding, perianal hematoma, infection, fecal impaction, delayed healing (with granulation tissue), rectal stenosis, and recurrence of hemorrhoids. Hemorrhoids are never precancerous, but cancer may coexist. Hemorrhoidectomy is curative. Hemorrhoids are unlikely to be permanently cured by injection therapy, but complications are uncommon.

FISSURE IN ANO

Anorectal mucosal lacerations occur frequently as a result of sudden or marked distention during a difficult bowel movement.

Acute fissures, although temporarily painful and perhaps associated with scant bleeding, generally heal rapidly. Chronic fissures may be persistent: either they fail to heal, or they heal and break down. Recurrent fissures may be associated with the eventual development of a sentinel pile, hypertrophic papillae, and anal spasm (especially painful on rectal examination).

Treatment of acute fissures is the same as that for hemorrhoids with mild symptoms. A single application of a mild styptic, such as 1% silver nitrate solution, may be beneficial.

For chronic or recurrent fissures, surgical excision of the sentinel pile or papilla and the fissure, preferably without suture closure, may be required. Postoperative care is similar to that after hemorrhoidectomy.

FISTULA IN ANO

Anal fistula (Fig. 28-13) is a chronically suppurating rectoperineal tract usually caused by pyogenic bacteria, often after obstetric trauma. A complete fistula has an internal (rectal) opening

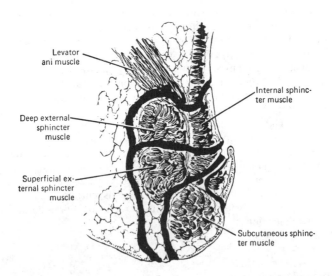

Figure 28-13. Cross-section of muscles of anal wall showing usual paths of anal fistulas. (From J.L. Wilson, *Handbook of Surgery*, 5th ed. Lange, 1973.)

and one of more external (perianal) openings. An incomplete or blind fistula has an internal opening only.

Many others are associated with repair of a third-degree or fourth-degree perineal laceration. Anal fistulas develop from an anal crypt, usually preceded by anal abscess.

Pain is reported when the fistula closes temporarily, suppuration develops, and drainage brings relief. Periodic soiling by fecal discharge is a common complaint. If the internal opening of a complete fistula is above the sphincter, involuntary passage of flatus is reported commonly.

Devious sinus tracts cause difficulty in identification of the internal opening. Injection of 1 part hydrogen peroxide and 2 parts methylene blue into the external openings releases oxygen by contact with the discharges. The blue dye is carried through the tract, and on anoscopic examination, the colored solution can be seen to bubble from the opening. For x-ray studies, injection of iodized oil (Lipiodol) may outline the fistulous tract.

Intestinal parasites should be identified by means of scrapings. Proper closure of an episiotomy or a complete perineal laceration usually will prevent fistula in ano. Prompt and adequate treatment of proctitis should prevent fistula in ano.

Chemotherapy should be used if parasites, e.g., *Eilistlytica,* are present. Incision of the entire fistula with excision of all portions of the tract is the only curative treatment. Do not close with sutures, since healing should occur by granulation. If the fistula is not totally exposed and removed, recurrence is likely.

ANAL INCONTINENCE

Anal incontinence follows obstetric lacerations, anorectal operations (especially fistulectomy), and neurologic disorders involving spinal nerves S2–4. When incontinence is the result of trauma or a complication of surgery, operative correction is indicated after the inflammation has subsided and initial healing is complete. Most serious lacerations due to childbirth injury should not be repaired until about 6 months after delivery.

ANAL CANCER

Anal cancer—almost always squamous cell type—represents only 1%–2% of all cancers of the colon, rectum, and anus. The cause is not known, but chronic granulomatous anal lesions are suspected.

Anal cancer appears as a slightly raised, firm, ulcerative, and slightly tender area. Anal cancer is frequently confused with chronic fissures in ano or bleeding hemorrhoids and is treated palliatively. It may be difficult to cure if the cancer extends upward into the sphincter and around the anus and metastasizes to the inguinal glands.

Biopsy of suspected or frankly tumorous anal lesions should be done under local anesthesia. Ample excision of very small anal cancers is feasible. However, most lesions are large when they are first diagnosed accurately and require abdominoperineal resection and radical groin resection. Radiation treatment, even for palliation, is unsatisfactory.

The *5-year survival rate* is only about 50%.

PSYCHOGENIC (ATYPICAL) PELVIC PAIN

Psychogenic (functional) pelvic pain is discomfort for which no organic cause can be found. It is usually chronic or recurrent. Women 25–45 years of age are most susceptible. The reported incidence in gynecologic patients in the United States is 5%–25%, depending on the interests and skills of the reporting physician.

Pain not attributable to physical causes may result from exaggeration of normal physiologic impulses, ignorance, fear, or tension, or from a lowered perceptual threshold to disturbing stimuli. Pain is associated with past or present environmental factors. The patient's complaint is often fixed on one anatomic area or organ system.

Before the pain is labeled psychogenic, there are four other alternatives to consider: the pain is from a disease process that is not yet detectable, the pain may be associated with vascular disorders where no disease process can be observed, the pain may be due to nongynecologic causes (e.g., gastrointestinal, genitourinary, or skeletal), and the psychogenic overlay is the result of chronic pain. To be classified as chronic the pain must be at least of 6 months duration.

A reasonable approach is to determine what organic problems are present and what psychologic factors are present and to treat both.

Clinical Findings

Symptoms and Signs

Complaints are almost invariably multiple. In addition to pelvic pain, most patients also report dyspareunia, dysmenorrhea, abnormal menses, and other pelvic complaints. There may be numerous abdominal scars, indicating polysurgery.

The patient insists that she is in great pain, but in at least 25% of cases no physical abnormality can be found. In the rest, insignificant physical variations or minimal lesions may be present.

The *historical investigation* should include a description and timing of the pain (when, where, why, what relation to menses, relation to stress, degree, and character). It should be determined if the patient has pain in other parts of the body (e.g., headache, backache, genitourinary tract). A careful menstrual and sexual history should be taken. Her work and leisure habits should be discussed. Inquiry should be made about pelvic and abdominal infections, previous operative procedures, and other gynecologic disorders (e.g., endometriosis, adenomyosis). A thoughtful social history should be obtained, including marital status, children, stresses in life (childhood, adolescent, adult), and history of physical or sexual abuse. Patients with chronic pelvic pain are more likely to experience depression, substance abuse, sexual dysfunction, and somatization disorders. They are more likely to have been sexually abused as a child or as an adult.

The *laboratory evaluations* include CBC, ESR, VDRL, UA and culture, and cervical cytology.

Special Examinations

Ruling Out Organic Disease. After appropriate initial evaluation, it may be necessary to rule out organic disease by laparoscopy, ultrasound, CT scan, MRI, gastrointestinal endoscopy, and genitourinary studies. Psychologic testing should be performed by those expert in the field.

Complications

Psychoneurosis may progress to psychosis. A despondent patient may commit suicide. If unaffected uterus or ovaries are removed, the symptoms may be transferred to the gastrointestinal or urinary tract.

Differential Diagnosis

Psychogenic disease can be differentiated from organic disease by ruling out the latter or by recognition of psychoneurosis or psychosis while investigating organic pathology. Most patients with psychogenic pelvic pain have many characteristic features that make a direct diagnosis possible without extensive studies.

Chronic salpingitis or urinary tract infection, spastic and other types of colitis, and endometriosis must be ruled out, perhaps by laparoscopy. A comparison of organic and psychogenic pelvic pain may be helpful in diagnosis (Table 28-1).

Prevention

Sex education, counseling, and early recognition and treatment of emotional illness are the best preventive measures.

Treatment

After examination and observation, the patient should be reassured and given simple symptomatic therapy. The physician must be empathetic, unhurried, and a good listener.

Once the diagnosis is established, the disorder must be explained to the patient in direct, convincing terms. The patient should be given an acceptable escape. A useful analogy may be that of tension headache. The physicians must gain the patient's cooperation, perhaps via reorientation and reeducation.

Table 28-1. Differentiation of organic and psychogenic pain

	Organic	Psychogenic
Type	Sharp, cramping, intermittent	Dull, continuous
Time of onset	Any time; may awaken patient	Usually begins well after waking, when social obligations are pressing
Localization	Localizes with typical point tenderness	Variable, shifting, generalized
Progress	Soon becomes either better or worse	Remains the same for weeks, months, or years
Provocative tests	Often reproduced or augmented by tests or manipulation, not mood	Not triggered or accentuated by examination but by interpersonal relationships

Simple analgesics are useful. Do not give sedatives, tranquilizers, amphetamines, or narcotics because these patients tend to be prone to addiction. Sedatives may lead to depression and suicide. Be prepared to spend a great deal of time talking to the patient. Do not perform operative procedures except on definite surgical indications. Psychotherapy or referral to a psychiatrist may be required. Every effort must be made to assist her to adjust socially.

Prognosis

These patients often refuse psychotherapy, withdraw early from a treatment program, and change physicians frequently. The medical future is bleak unless the patient confronts the real problem. Reassurance and symptomatic therapy result in temporary improvement in about three fourths of patients. Psychiatric treatment results in lasting improvement in many patients.

DYSPAREUNIA

Dyspareunia (painful coitus) may be functional (psychogenic), organic, or both. Functional dyspareunia occurs most frequently and is more difficult to treat. Either type may occur early (primary) or late (secondary) in the sexually active interval of life. The site of discomfort may be external (at the introitus) or internal (deep within the vagina or beyond), and some women describe both types of pain. Functional dyspareunia may be caused by psychosexual problems, a previous extremely negative experience (e.g., sexual molestation), fear of genital damage, fear of sexually transmittable disease, or fear of pregnancy.

Vaginismus, an involuntary spasm of the muscles of the introitus and levators when the thighs are abducted, is an indication of extreme anxiety. It may be due to psychologic factors or personal emotional problems, or it may occur in anticipation of or in response to pain.

External organic dyspareunia may be due to an occlusive or rigid hymen, vaginal contracture due to any cause, or inflammatory disorders. Traumatic or infectious processes are seen in younger patients and atrophic vulvovaginitis in postmenopausal women.

Organic causes of internal dyspareunia include vaginal disorders, severe cervicitis, marked fundal retroposition, uterine prolapse or neoplasm, tuboovarian disease, pelvic endometriosis, and severe disorders of the lower urinary tract or colon.

Psychiatric evaluation is indicated if complex psychosexual problems seem to be present. Specialized techniques of physical examination, e.g., cystoscopy, may be required to rule out organic disease.

Functional dyspareunia can be treated only by counseling and psychotherapy. Both partners should be interviewed. Information on contraception is often helpful. The importance of foreplay before sexual intercourse must be emphasized. An appropriate water-soluble vaginal gel may be useful. Adequate estrogen treatment often is required for postmenopausal women. The treatment of organic dyspareunia varies and depends on the basic underlying cause.

For functional dyspareunia, hymenal-vaginal dilations by the patient with a conical (Kelly) dilator or test tubes of graduated sizes may give confidence. Lubricants or anesthetic ointment applied to the introitus gives some relief but is of no permanent value. Organic dyspareunia due to vaginal dryness may be treated with a water-soluble lubricant. Estrogen therapy is indicated for senile vulvovaginitis.

Hymenotomy, hymenectomy, perineotomy, and similar procedures should be performed only on clear indications. Obstructive lesions should be corrected. Treat symptomatic vaginitis or cervicitis appropriately.

Few patients with functional dyspareunia are quickly and easily cured, even with psychotherapy. Organic dyspareunia subsides promptly after elimination of the cause.

Chapter 29

Gynecologic Procedures and Surgery

GYNECOLOGIC PROCEDURES

EXFOLIATIVE CERVICAL CYTOLOGIC STUDY (PAPANICOLAOU SMEAR)

Exfoliative cytologic examination of specimens from the lower genital tract (Pap smear) has been so valuable in the detection of premalignant and malignant lesions that it has been almost universally adopted as the primary cancer screening method for cervical cancer, an integral part of the health care of women. This has resulted in a >50% reduction of invasive cancers of the cervix alone. Although cervical cytology may detect endometrial cancer (in 15%–50%), it does not carry the same reliability as a screening tool for endometrial neoplasia.

Screening Guidelines

A. Initial gynecologic screening at age 18, or when the individual becomes sexually active.

B. Women whose initial smear is negative (without significant atypia) should have a second smear within 1 year to rule out a false-negative smear.

C. High-risk women should be screened annually, i.e., those with a history of early sexual activity or those with multiple sexual partners.

D. Low-risk women may be screened every 1–3 years at the discretion of the physician. These are women with late exposure to coitus, those with only one sexual partner, and women after two successive negative annual smears. (Some authorities contend it is too difficult to ascertain low risk and simply recommend annual screening.)

E. Postmenopausal women should receive annual screening.

F. Women after hysterectomy should have an initial smear following surgery; if this is negative, cytology should be repeated every 3 years.

Technique

Materials necessary for a Pap smear include a cervical spatula, shaped tongue depressor or cotton swab, glass slides and a means to identify the slide and patient, a speculum (warm, without lubricant), a jar of fixative (97% ethanol) or spray fixative (e.g., Pro-Fixx or AquaNet) (Fig. 29-1).

The objective is to sample secretions from the endocervical canal, the transitional zone, and the vaginal pool. The last site is less productive and, therefore, of lesser priority. Sampling is accomplished by gently wiping away excess mucus and obtaining endocervical canal samples using the moist cotton swab or cervical spatula. This is smeared onto a glass slide and fixed. An Ayers spatula or similar device is used to lightly scrape the entire transformation zone. In those with a small external os, a brush device may be helpful in guaranteeing that endocervical cells are sampled. This sample is spread on a slide and fixed immediately. Finally, the vaginal pool may be sampled by using the same Ayers spatula (again, fixing immediately).

Cervical *cytologic results* are reported as normal, atypical (inflammation, possible dysplasia), metaplasia, mild dysplasia, moderate dysplasia, severe dysplasia–carcinoma in situ, probable invasive cancer. Most reports also include additional information (e.g., when to come for the next visit).

COLPOSCOPY

The colposcope is a binocular microscope of low magnification (10–40×) used for direct visualization of the cervix. Although colposcopy does not replace other methods of diagnosing cervical abnormalities, it is an important additional tool. The patients who most benefit from colposcopy are those with abnormal Pap smears. Colposcopy is also used to evaluate women who were exposed to DES in utero and in gyncecologic cancer therapy follow-up.

Occult neoplasms in the upper cervical canal, where 10%–15% of cervical cancers develop, cannot be detected by colpos-

Materials Needed:
One cervical spatula, cut tongue depressor, or cotton swab.
One glass slide (one end frosted). Identify by writing the patient's name on the frosted end with a lead pencil.
One speculum (warm but without lubricant).
One bottle of fixative (97% ethanol) or spray-on fixative, eg, Pro-Fixx or Aqua-Net.

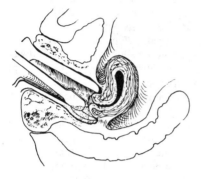

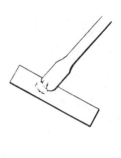

1. Obtain vaginal pool material from the posterior fornix.

2. Place adequate drop 1 inch from end of slide, smear, fix, and dry.

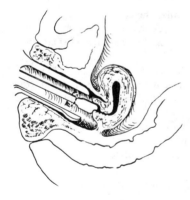

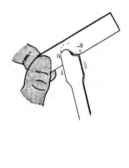

3. Obtain cervical scraping from complete squamocolumnar junction by rotating spatula 360° around external os, high up in the endocervical canal.

4. Place the material 1 inch from end of slide, smear, fix, and dry.

Figure 29-1. Preparation of a Papanicolaou cytosmear.

copy. Therefore, endocervical curettage should be performed in women who are being evaluated for abnormal cervical cytology.

Normally, columnar epithelium covers the ectocervix until adolescence, when it gradually changes to a squamous surface. The transformation zone can be inspected easily with the colposcope, and dysplastic surface changes can be identified. These include white epithelium (e.g., sheet of layered metaplastic cells), a mosaic pattern (e.g., sharply outlined cells and cell groups), punctation (e.g., vascular tufts between cell clusters), and leukoplakia (e.g., abnormal pale cell plaques).

Colposcopy allows recognition of cellular dysplasia, and vascular or tissue abnormalities not otherwise visible. Colposcopy allows selection of cancer-suspicious areas for biopsy. A green filter accentuates the vascular changes (which frequently accompany pathologic alteration). Dilute (3%) acetic acid solution is used to remove mucus and to facilitate visualization. Other chemical agents and stains may also be used to improve visualization. A camera attached to the colposcope facilitates follow-up. Colposcope-directed biopsy decreases the number of false-negative reports and may eliminate the need for conization of the cervix, a cause of morbidity.

To perform colposcopy, proceed as follows.

1. Insert a speculum and visualize the cervix.
2. Cleanse the cervix with 3% acetic acid. This removes excess mucus, blanches the surface, and accentuates normal epithelium.
3. Focus the colposcope on the cervix, beginning with low power (usually 13.5×). Inspect the squamocolumnar junction (transformation zone) carefully. A significantly abnormal area usually can be fully outlined.
4. Take biopsy specimens with a Kevorkian or similar biopsy forceps, and record the sites most suggestive of cancer.
5. Consider whether endocervical curettage should be performed.

Effective use of the colposcope requires thorough training and extensive experience.

EVALUATION OF PATIENT WITH ABNORMAL CERVICAL CYTOLOGY

In summary, a *normal* smear requires follow-up as noted previously. An *atypical* smear (inflammation, possible dysplasia) requires treatment against the offending agent and repeat cytology

6–8 weeks after the infection is eliminated and the tissue has healed. If the report on repeat cytology is possible dysplasia, colposcopy is warranted. Pap smears indicating *metaplasia, mild, moderate, or severe dysplasia–carcinoma in situ,* all require prompt repeat cytology and colposcopy. Any abnormal areas must be biopsied, and endocervical curettage must be performed. *Possible invasive cancer* requires immediate colposcopy and biopsy (including conization if necessary).

CULDOCENTESIS
(See Ectopic pregnancy, p 299)

SOUNDING THE UTERUS

The uterus may be sounded to determine the patency of the cervical canal, the presence of cervical or uterine lesions that will bleed on contact, the size of the uterus, the position of the uterine fundus, and the direction of the uterine canal (before endometrial biopsy or other instrumentation). Intrauterine pregnancy must be ruled out before uterine sounding. Use a sterile, malleable, calibrated (in centimeters) instrument, e.g., Sims or Simpson uterine sound (7 mm diameter).

Visualize the external cervix with a speculum, and carefully apply an antiseptic solution (e.g., povidone-iodine). Bend the sound to the estimated curvature of the cervicouterine axis. After warning the patient of possible slight pain, grasp the cervix (on either anterior or posterior lip) by a double-toothed Braun or Allis clamp and exert gentle traction toward the introitus, using the nondominant hand. This immobilizes the cervix and straightens the endocervical canal.

Use the index finger and thumb of the dominant hand to gently insert the sound in the cervicouterine axis while pressing the third and fourth fingers against the vulva to brace the hand. A slight, transient resistance may be encountered at the level of the internal os. An obvious obstruction is encountered at the vault of the uterine cavity. Exert special care to avoid perforation of the uterus at the level of the cervicouterine junction (particularly in marked flexion) and at the top of the fundus. Note the length of the cervical canal, the direction of the axis, the depth of the uterine cavity, and any obstruction, distortion, or free bleeding.

In the absence of cervical stenosis and extreme flexion of the corpus, gentle traction and sounding of the uterus cause only a few slightly menstruallike cramps. Careful patient preparation and analgesics if necessary make the procedure tolerable.

If sounding of the uterus is impossible with the usual instruments, try a fine, soft wire probe. Then use Hegar dilators (No. 5–10) to dilate a stenotic cervix. The diagnosis of an abnormally wide internal cervical os (notably incompetent) is confirmed if a No. 8 Hegar dilator passes without resistance.

BIOPSIES

Vulvar (see p 503)
Cervical

Multiple cervical biopsies may be performed in the office with little or no discomfort or danger, using Tischler, Schubert, Kevorkian, or similar punch biopsy forceps. Polypoid lesions may be removed by torsion or excision (Figs. 29-2 and 29-3). For microscopic analysis, do not crush the tissue. Anesthetics are not required because the cervix is relatively insensitive to this type of pain.

After detailing the areas to be biopsied by colcoscopy, immobilize the cervix using a tenaculum. First biopsy the posterior lip (so bleeding from more anterior biopsies will not obscure the field). The most frequent biopsy sites are at or near the squamocolumnar junction. Place the tissue in fixative (e.g., 10% formalin) immediately. Bleeding is variable and unpredictable. If necessary, control bleeding by pressure, Negatol, acetone, 5% silver nitrate solution, or fine catgut sutures.

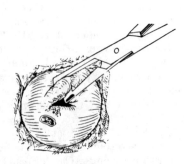

Figure 29-2. Multiple punch biopsy of cervix with Tischler forceps.

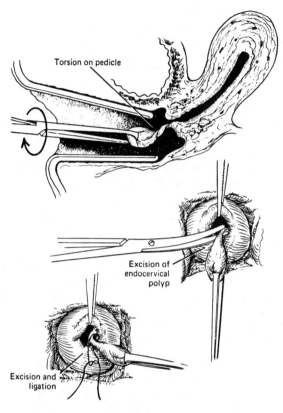

Figure 29-3. Three methods of cervical polypectomy.

Endocervical Curettage

This procedure is commonly used as an adjunct to colposcopy in an effort to guarantee sampling of the entire endocervix. Stabilize the cervix using a tenaculum or Allis clamp, and curette the endocervix throughout its circumference by taking downward strokes from the internal to the external os with a Kevorkian or other small curet. Fix these strips of tissue immediately and submit them for pathology diagnosis. Anesthesia is rarely required, the procedure generally is very short (<2 min), and bleeding is minimal. The principal complication is uterine perforation (usually at the cervicouterine junction).

Endometrial Biopsy

For endometrial biopsy, no anesthesia or only mild analgesia or paracervical block is required. *Contraindications* to endometrial biopsy include pregnancy, marked cervical stenosis, acute cervicitis, friable, bleeding cervical abnormalities, and profuse bleeding at the initiation of endometrial curettage.

The most common endometrial biopsy instrument currently used is a tubular plastic device for aspiration of strips of endometrium. After antiseptic preparation, sound the uterus. Next, direct the curet to the fundus and gently stroke downward against the uterine wall to the cervix while exerting gentle suction. Perform on both anterior and posterior uterine walls. Place the tissue obtained in fixative immediately.

INDUCED ABORTION

Induced abortion is the artificial termination of a previable pregnancy. In the United States, elective abortion is persistently controversial. Our purpose is to provide timely information, not to debate issues or enter into controversy. Therefore, in this summary, there is no attempt to influence patients or health care providers for or against abortion, and none should be inferred.

In the United States, about 25% (>1.5 million) of all pregnancies are terminated by induced legal abortion. Approximately 3% of women of childbearing age have an abortion annually. Nevertheless, the distribution is heavily weighted toward those of younger age (one third age <20, one third age 20–24) and the unmarried (75%). The vast majority of abortions (90%) are performed ≤8 weeks gestation, and 85% are accomplished by suction curettage, 10% by surgical curettage, and the rest by stimulation of uterine contractions. At the time of writing, trials are about to begin on an oral abortifacient.

Indications

The most controversial abortions are totally elective (patient demand). Social indications for interruption of pregnancy are probably the next most debated indications and cover a broad spectrum: preservation of mental health, excessive family size, poverty, incest, and rape.

Perhaps the least controversial are those termed "medically indicated." Examples of medical diseases said to require interruption of pregnancy to preserve maternal life or vital functions include neuropsychiatric disorders (authorities disagree regarding qualifications), bilateral renal insufficiency, chronic resistant pyelonephritis, class III or IV cardiac disease, e.g., intractable atrial fibrillation, coronary occlusion, marked impairment of pulmonary ventilation (vital capacity of <1400 ml in the average-size person), progressive loss of vision or Kimmelstiel-Wilson syndrome in patients with diabetes mellitus, thromboembolic disorders, severe hemoglobinopathies, gammaglobulinopathies, clotting defects, severe ulcerative colitis, invasive cervical cancer, and stage II breast carcinoma.

Obstetric complications that seriously affect the fetus when abortion should be considered include rubella before 12–14 weeks gestation, severe isoimmunization, fetuses with known morphologic defects (e.g., anencephaly, acardius), and fetuses with known congenital disorders (e.g., Tay-Sachs disease, osteogenesis imperfecta, trisomy 13).

Laboratory Studies

Ultrasound scanning is performed both to confirm the pregnancy and to determine the gestational age. If no fetal sac or fetal heartbeat is present, a qualitative hCG is performed.

Counseling

The physician has the responsibility to explain the reputed advantages, disadvantages, and alternatives of elective abortion, just as with other procedures. Additionally, the patient should be assured of continued empathetic quality care whatever her decision.

The patient must be informed about the nature of the procedure and its risks, including possible infertility or even continuation of pregnancy. All reasonable alternatives must be explored. The rights of the spouse, parents, or guardian vary considerably from state to state but must be considered. Permission must be obtained. State or provincial laws must be obeyed, with special reference to residence, indications for abortion, duration of pregnancy, consent, and consultations required or advisable.

Protracted guilt feelings for the loss of the fetus and remorse may result from induced abotion, particularly when religious and social conflicts complicate the decision to abort. The reported incidence of serious emotional sequelae following induced abortion is <5%. Follow-up and special care for those adversely affected should be afforded the patient.

Methods

Early Medical Abortion

An experimental (in the United States) medication (RU486), which appears generally safe and effective ≤7 weeks gestation, is being used for early pregnancy termination elsewhere in the world. Whereas the future of the compound in the United States is in doubt (clinical trials are just beginning), its use is very likely to increase elsewhere.

Vaginal Evacuation

Two main techniques are used for vaginal evacuation of pregnancy, suction curettage and D & C. The stated *advantages* of suction curettage (compared to D & C using standard curets) are that suction curettage is more rapid (3 min average), less cervical dilation is necessary (thus, less likelihood of cervical tears and an incompetent cervix), fewer failed abortions result, less anesthesia and analgesia are required, blood loss is less, infection is less common, and there is less trauma to the uterus (protection of the basalis and muscularis layers makes traumatic amenorrhea and intrauterine adhesions less likely).

Very early abortion (first 3–4 weeks of gestation) by low-pressure suction curettage is accomplished using a 4–5 mm flexible plastic cannula without cervical dilatation or anesthesia. This is termed menstrual extraction or menstrual regulation. This procedure has a relatively high rate of failed abortion and is contraindicated in women with acute cervicitis or possible salpingitis.

Suction curettage requires cervical dilatation as well as some form of anesthesia (e.g., paracervical block) when performed at 6–12 weeks gestation (Fig. 29-4). However, cervical dilatation can be accomplished using osmotic dilators (e.g., segments of Laminaria). When dry, osmotic dilators are small (2–3 mm diameter), but the material is very hygroscopic and capable of expanding to 2–3 times its original diameter. The dilators must remain in the cervix for at least 6–8 h to reach full size. Now synthetic osmotic dilators also are available. The stated *advantages* of this method are less pain (compared to mechanical dilatation) and fewer cervical lacerations. A *disdvantage* is that

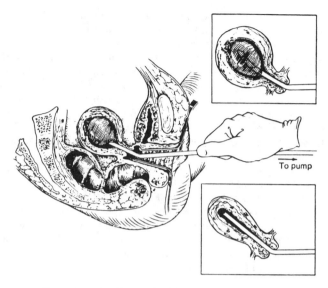

Figure 29-4. Suction method for therapeutic abortion.

the dilators must be placed in the cervix some hours before the procedure.

After 12–13 weeks of pregnancy, suction curettage is usually performed on an outpatient basis in an operating suite. These later terminations (generally up to 20 weeks—called dilatation and evacuation, D & E) require several osmotic dilators or graduated mechanical dilators, a larger suction cannula, and forceps to complete evacuation. Currently, this technique has fewer complications than the various methods for induction of uterine contraction, but it carries a higher incidence of uterine perforation and bowel damage. This technique is more rapid than induction of contractions but requires greater technical expertise. The long-term effects (primarily of possible cervical trauma) remain unknown. It is less expensive than prostaglandin-oxytocin-induced abortion.

Induction of Uterine Contractions

With Live Fetus. The various *techniques* of second trimester abortion by induction of contractions include intraamniotic saline infusion (100–200 ml 20% solution), intraamniotic infusion of prostaglandin ($PGF_{2\alpha}$, 40 mg), intravaginal prostaglandin vaginal suppositories (E_2, 20 mg), and intramuscular 15-methyl $PGF_{2\alpha}$. The coagulation system is altered temporarily by injection of hypertonic saline (decreased fibrinogen and platelets, increased fibrin degradation products), and the patient's fluids and electrolytes must be monitored carefully.

The *noninvasive techniques* (using prostaglandins) require less technical expertise and have a lower morbidity. However, prostaglandins should not be used in patients with asthma or in those who have had prior uterine surgery. The prostaglandins usually cause marked gastrointestinal side effects (nausea, vomiting, diarrhea), which require appropriate premedication. However, the success rate is >95%.

With Dead Fetus in Second or Third Trimester. PGE_2 suppositories are most successful for use after spontaneous fetal death when it occurs in the second or third trimester. As with the other prostaglandins, PGE_2 suppositories must be repeated, result in a rapid abortion (8–12 h), and induce all the side effects noted above, plus chills and fever.

Hysterotomy and Hysterectomy

Abdominal or vaginal hysterotomy, major surgery, has the disadvantage of much higher morbidity and should be avoided if possible. Hysterectomy, feasible up to 23 weeks gestation, is rarely warranted in the first trimester. Hysterectomy may be justified for patients requiring hysterectomy for other reasons or for those who desire the ultimate sterilization.

Follow-Up of Patients After Induced Abortion

Rh_o immune globulin (e.g., RhoGAM) should be administered ≤72 h after abortion if the patient is Rh negative (except when the father is Rh negative). For the first trimester abortion, the recommended dose of Rh immune globulin is 50 μg IM, and for second trimester abortion, the dose is 300 μg IM. As with term gestations, if there is evidence of fetal–maternal hemorrhage, additional Rh immune globulin should be given.

The patient should take her temperature daily and avoid coitus, douching, and use of vaginal tampons until her follow-up visit (>2 weeks). Effective contraception should be made available according to the patient's needs and desires. She should report fever, unusual bleeding, or flulike symptoms at once. She should be offered counseling and support similar to that following term pregnancy and delivery. Follow-up care should include pelvic examination to rule out continued pregnancy, endometritis, parametritis, salpingitis, or failure of involution.

Complications

The major complications of induced abortion include uterine perforation, pelvic infection, hemorrhage, and embolism. The mortality rate for legal abortions in the United States is 3/100,000 (vs 9/100,000 for pregnancy). The longer the duration of gestation, the greater the threat to the mother's life. A 5% morbidity rate is common in the first trimester. The morbidity rate is >15% in second trimester abortions.

USE OF VAGINAL PESSARIES

The vaginal pessary is a rubber or plastic prosthesis, often with a metal band or spring frame. The usual widely accepted *indications* for pessaries include poor-risk patients or those who refuse surgery for uterine prolapse or other vaginal hernias, aiding preoperative healing of cervical stasis ulcerations associated with cervical prolapse, nonoperative reduction of cystocele or rectocele, and to facilitate the evaluation and performance of hysteropexy (by holding the uterus in position). A vaginal pessary is probably most useful for the support of a prolapsed uterus or cervical stump.

Pessaries are *contraindicated* in patients with acute genital tract infections and in those with adherent uterine retroposition. In most cases, adequate anterior support and a reasonably good perineal body are required. Otherwise, the pessary may slip from behind the symphysis to be extruded from the vagina.

The various useful *types of pessaries* are shown in Figures 29-5 and 29-6. The Hodge pessary (Smith-Hodge, or Smith and other variations) is an elongated curved ovoid that supports the uterus after repositioning. The Gellhorn and Menge pessaries are for correction of marked prolapse when the perineal body is adequate. The Gehrung pessary rests in the vagina, cradling the cervix between the long arms, while it arches to the anterior vaginal wall to reduce a cystocele. Hard or soft ring pessaries (as well as the hollow plastic ball or sponge rubber bee cell) distend the vagina, elevate the cervix, and reduce cystocele and rectocele by direct pressure. Inflatable pessaries function similarly. If the

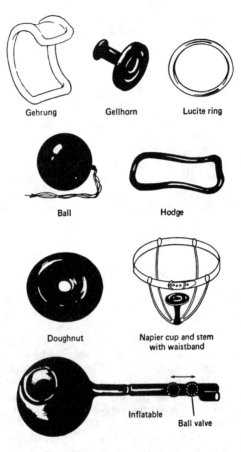

Figure 29-5. Types of pessaries.

perineum is inadequate, these pessaries may require a perineal belt and pad for support. The Napier pessary has a cup-stem arrangement supported by a belt and affords uterine support for a prolapsed cervix or uterus when the perineum is incompetent.

Pessaries are never curative, but they may be useful for months or years of *palliation*. Nonetheless, their use should be properly supervised. A neglected pessary may encourage genital infection(s) and may even cause fistulas. If the pessary is displaced, becomes uncomfortable, or requires cleaning, it must be

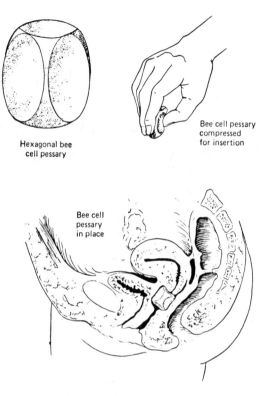

Hexagonal bee
cell pessary

Bee cell pessary
compressed
for insertion

Bee cell
pessary
in place

Figure 29-6. Bee cell pessary.

removed. The frequency of removal varies dpending on the pessary and the patient's status. To preserve the vaginal mucosa, a bee cell or inflatable pessary should be removed and cleaned nightly. Other pessaries may be left in longer. Acetic acid douches help to maintain hygiene while wearing a vaginal pessary.

When pessaries are fitted, the patient should be shown how to insert, remove, and clean it. Patients should be warned of difficulties, e.g., pessaries may cause infection, pressure necrosis, and ulceration or fistulas. Patients should be closely supervised. If not contraindicated, estrogen cream will assist in preserving the vaginal mucosa.

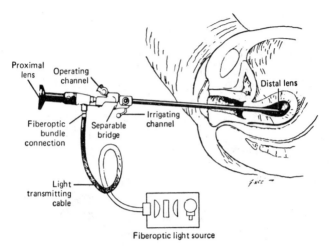

Figure 29-7. Diagrammatic representation of hysteroscope in use. (From R.F. Valle and J.J. Sciarra, *Minn Med* 1974;57:892.)

HYSTEROSCOPY

Hysteroscopy is visual examination of the uterine cavity with a small fiberoptic endoscope (Fig. 29-7). Paracervical anesthesia or analgesia is generally required, although general anesthesia may be necessary. After appropriate preparation with an antiseptic solution, the uterus is gently sounded and the cervix is dilated sightly to accept the hysteroscope. Intrauterine instillation of 35% dextran, dextran and saline, or CO_2 is used to slightly distend the uterus.

This technique is useful for removal of a foreign body (e.g., a intrauterine device), diagnosis of abnormal uterine bleeding (a polyp or other small tumor not discovered by other techniques), biopsy of specific sites (e.g., D & C may miss areas of endometrial cancer), lysis of intrauterine synechiae (i.e., Asherman's syndrome), some infertility investigations, removal of polypoid leiomyomas, and in operative management of a subseptate uterus.

Contraindications to hysteroscopy include pregnancy, acute cervicitis or salpingitis, the presence of STDs, and hemorrhage.

GYNECOLOGIC SURGERY

Dilatation and Curettage (D & C)

Dilatation of the cervix and curettage of the endometrium (D & C) is the most common gynecologic surgical procedure. If D & C is being performed for suspected endometrial or cervical cancer, specimens must be taken first from the endocervix (before sounding and dilatation) and submitted separately from those of the endometrium. This is *fractional curettage*. The indications for D & C are summarized in Table 29-1.

D & C is almost always accomplished in office or outpatient surgical settings. For D & C, the patient is placed in the dorsal lithotomy position. Although local anesthetics (e.g., paracervical blocks) are most commonly used, general anesthetic occasionally will be necessary.

The usual *steps in a D & C* are as follows. Repeat the pelvic examination. Cleanse the vagina and perineum with an antiseptic and place the drapes. Insert a weighted speculum into the posterior vagina. Visualize then grasp the cervix with a tenaculum or Allis clamp. Curette the endocervical canal with a Kevorkian or similar curette. Sound the uterus. Dilate the cervix using progressive dilators (e.g., Hegar) to 8 mm (Figs. 29-8 and 29-9). Introduce a polyp forceps and gently rotate before closing (in an attempt to grasp any polyps present). Introduce a standard sharp curette and begin the curettage by taking strokes across the fundus. Next, start at a given point and proceed around the entire uterus by bringing the curette from the fundus to the endocervix. Remove the curette after each stroke. This facilitates obtaining strips of tissue, all of which are submitted for analysis. Proceed until a gritty sensation (myometrium) is noted.

Table 29-1. Indications for dilatation and curettage

Diagnostic	Therapeutic
Irregular menstrual bleeding	Endometrial hyperplasia
Heavy menstrual bleeding	Endometrial polyps
Postmenopausal bleeding	Pedunculated submucous myomas
	Retained products of conception following abortion
	Missed abortion

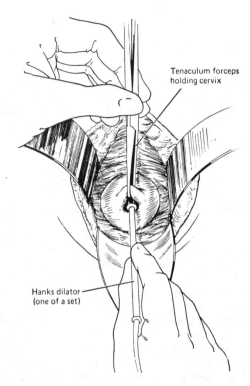

Tenaculum forceps
holding cervix

Hanks dilator
(one of a set)

Figure 29-8. Cervical dilatation.

The most common *complications* of D & C are hemorrhage, infection, uterine perforation, and cervical laceration.

CERVICAL CONIZATION

Cervical conization may be used to diagnose possible cancer or to excise CIN or other abnormal (on colposcopy) tissue extending beyond the field of vision up the cervical canal (10%–15% of cervical cancers develop in the upper cervical canal).

Most cervical conizations are performed as outpatient surgical procedures. Paracervical or general anesthesia may be required. Antiseptic solutions may be used, but care is taken not to touch the external cervical os. Suspicious areas that should be biopsied

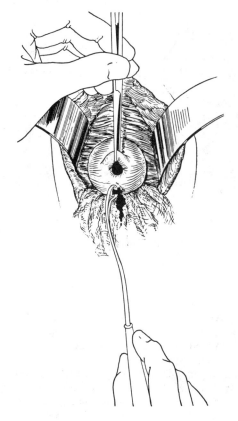

Figure 29-9. Curettage.

have generally previously been mapped by colposcopy. Conization is most commonly accomplished by LEEP scalpel (*cold
conization*) (Fig. 29-10), or laser and involves removing a thin
circular portion of the cervix exterior to the squamocolumnar
junction and extending variably up the endocervical canal. Rarely
should the excision extend to the level of the internal os. Scalpel
cervical conization may be facilitated by introduction of a uterine
sound to or just beyond the internal os so the tip of the blade
approximates the sound. Generally, the tissue removed exceeds
0.3 cm in thickness. A suture usually is inserted at the top of the
cone to aid the pathologist in tissue orientation for histology.

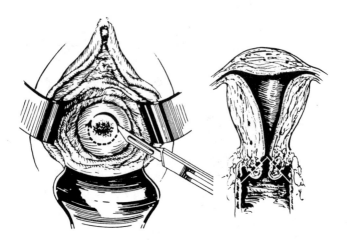

Figure 29-10. Conization of the cervix.

If the cervix is deeply lacerated, *segmental excision* of tissue may be required to constitute a complete sample. Each fragment must be identified, and a diagram to aid the pathologist facilitates accurate analysis.

Bleeding is generally less using the LEEP procedure and is easily controlled using that device, whereas sutures may be necessary with scalpel conization. Hemorrhage necessitates vaginal packing or deeply placed sutures or both. Secondary hemorrhage (related to infection of the surgical site) occurs in 10% of cases and may occur as late as 7–14 days. It is treated with antibiotics and vaginal packing but occasionally requires suturing. Another *late complication* of conization is incompetent cervix (from taking the specimen too far up the endocervical canal).

Conization of the cervix during pregnancy is fraught with hemorrhage and pregnancy wastage. Therefore, it has largely been replaced by colposcopically directed biopsies.

LAPAROSCOPY

Laparoscopy (Fig. 29-11) is a transperitoneal endoscopic technique for visualization of the abdominal and pelvic contents. It is an intraabdominal operation performed through a small subum-

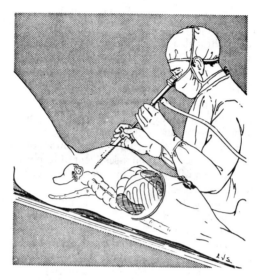

Figure 29-11. Pelvic laparoscopy with patient in Trendelenburg position. (From A.E. Long, *Current Obstetric & Gynecologic Diagnosis & Treatment,* 4th ed. R.C. Benson, ed. Lange, 1982.)

bilical incision, and it provides excellent visualization of the pelvic structures, permitting *diagnosis* of many gynecologic abnormalities and limited surgery without laparotomy. Considerable experience is required to achieve facility with the instrumentation, but in capable hands, laparoscopy is a well-tolerated surgical method that can supplant laparotomy for diagnosis or treatment of intraabdominal problems.

Laparoscopy is almost always a same-day surgery (i.e., the procedure is performed under anesthesia in an operating room, but the patient recovers and goes home the same day) procedure. Fiberoptic illumination and carbon dioxide pneumoperitoneum are used. General anesthesia with endotracheal intubation is employed. With the patient in the supine position, the abdomen is prepared, and sterile drapes are applied. Then, a Veress needle is inserted near the projected site of surgery, and the abdomen is insufflated with CO_2. Once it is certain the pneumoperitoneum is sufficient to displace the bowel, a trochar bearing the laparoscope sleeve is inserted. Next the laparoscope is inserted, and pneumoperitoneum is maintained by continued smaller amounts of CO_2.

In addition to the equipment used for observation, a variety of accessories for biopsy, coagulation, aspiration, and manipulation can be passed through a separate cannula (second puncture technique) or inserted through the same cannula as the laparoscope. There are numerous indications for laparoscopy.

A. *Diagnosis.* Examples are uterine anomaly, endometriosis, biopsy of ovarian tumors, omentum, spleen, or liver, and differentiation between ectopic pregnancy and salpingitis or between psychogenic and organic pelvic pain.

B. *Evaluation.* Examples include investigation of infertility, e.g., tubal patency test, and assessment of response to treatment in women with ovarian or other pelvic cancer.

C. Therapy
   1. Tubal sterilization by fulguration, application of Silastic rings, or metal clips.
   2. Lysis of adhesions.
   3. Elimination of a disorder, e.g., fulguration of endometriosis.
   4. Removal of foreign body, e.g., an extruded intrauterine device.

Absolute *contraindications* to laparoscopy are intestinal obstruction and general peritonitis. Severe cardiac or pulmonary disease is a relative contraindication.

Complications depend on the problem, the status of the patient, and the expertise of the person performing the laparoscopy. Minor problems, e.g., abdominal or shoulder pain, are common but rarely serious. Complications include perforation of a viscus, thermal burn of the bowel, severe bleeding, or cardiac arrest (rare but often critical). If not noted at the time of surgery, thermal bowel injuries do not generally become apparent until several days later, when peritonitis occurs. The incidence of major complications (mostly with bipolar instruments) in the United States is <5%. The overall mortality rate in laparoscopic sterilization is <2/100,000

Other complications of laparoscopy include insufflation of the abdominal wall from improper placement of the Veress needle and hypercarbia from improper anesthetic management of CO_2 insufflation.

STERILIZATION

Sterilization is the permanent prevention of pregnancy. There are as many reasons for sterilization as there are for contraception. Nonetheless, elective sterilization is rapidly becoming the most used method of limiting family size in developed countries. Little controversy surrounds voluntary sterilization in the United States, and it is legal in all states. Sterilization is used as a contraceptive means by about one third of all married couples in the United States. It is most commonly used when no more children are desired, the wife is >30 years of age, or the marriage is of >10 years duration.

Methods

Tubal closure is the most commonly used sterilization procedure. This may be accomplished by ligation, diversion, or excision. Ligation may be done with segmental resection (Pomeroy, Fig. 29-12) or with crushing and ligation (Madlener). Excision may be effected by salpingectomy, removal of the infundibular portion of the tube, resection of the isthmic portion of the tube (cornual resection), burial of the proximal extremity of the tube beneath the visceral or parietal peritoneum (Irving, Fig. 29-13, or Uchida, Fig. 29-14), or cauterization-occlusion of the uterotubal ostia through the uterine cavity.

Most tubal sterilizations in the United States are done by laparoscopy on an outpatient basis. The tubes are either fulgurated in their midportion, occluded by clips of various material or by Silastic rings, or closed by a combination of techniques. The

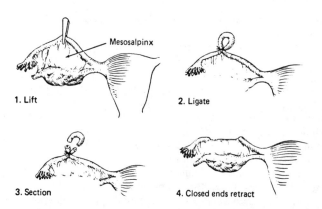

Figure 29-12. Pomeroy method of sterilization.

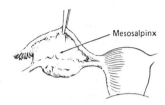

1. Uterine tube lifted and cut.

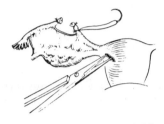

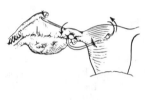

2. Double ligation with gut; one tie left long for traction (special traction suture). Mesosalpinx stripped back.

3. Special traction suture inserted in tunnel in anterior uterine wall.

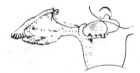

Figure-of-eight fixation suture

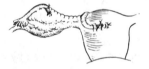

4. Implantation of the proximal tubal limb into a tunnel in the anterior uterine wall.

5. Traction suture tied and proximal tube sutured in tunnel.

Figure 29-13. Irving method of sterilization.

methodology and *complications* of laparoscopy are noted on pages 750–751. Because bipolar coagulation is safer and has a higher reanastomosis success rate, it is the fulguration method of choice. The total *complication rate* of laparoscopic tubal fulguration is 1%–6%, with major problems (hemorrhage or bowel injury) occurring in 0.6% of cases.

Minilaparotomy, a limited celiotomy procedure for tubal sterilization, can be performed on an outpatient basis. This procedure requires a small (usually transverse) skin incision with

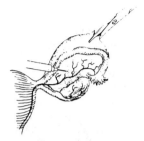

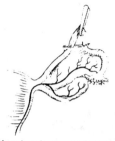

1. Saline with epinephrine injected below serosa, which becomes inflated locally. Muscular tube, and even blood vessels, can be separated from serosa, which is then cut open.

2. Muscular tube emerges through opening or is pulled out to form a U shape.

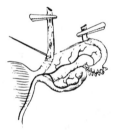

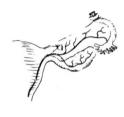

3. Fimbriated end is untouched, while the end leading to the uterus is stripped of serosa. This can usually be done without damaging blood vessels.

4. About 5 cm of muscular tube is cut away; the end is buried automatically in serosa. Fimbriated end and serosa opening are closed and tied together.

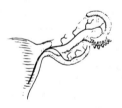

5. Blood supply continues normally between ovary and uterus. Hydrosalpinx or adhesion has not been noted.

Figure 29-14. Uchida method of sterilization.

dissection into the peritoneal cavity. This operation is often performed under analgesia and local anesthesia.

The uterus is elevated (by a uterine sound inserted before surgery or by use of a small intraabdominal retractor), and adequate visualization is afforded by small angular retractors. Both the ovary and the fimbriated end of the tube should be inspected to differentiate the tube from the round ligament. Tubal ligation may be carried out by any of the techniques noted previously.

Minilaparotomy is contraindicated when the patient is obese or has an enlarged or immobile uterus or when adnexal disease or endometriosis is suspected. Nonetheless, in some circumstances, minilaparotomy is simpler, safer, and less costly than laparoscopy for sterilization.

Counseling

All forms of sterilization have reported failures (occasional pregnancies occur). Abdominal and tubal pregnancies have been reported (rarely) even after total hysterectomy. Contemporay failure rates for the various procedures are shown in Table 29-2.

About 1% of sterilized women request reversal. Pregnancy rates following microsurgical tubal reanastomosis are at least 50%, depending on the method used for tubal ligation. The laparoscopic band techniques afford the best reversal rates (75%) and should be considered in the younger patient.

It is useful to have more than one counsellor when sterilization is requested by any woman <25 years of age and in a nulliparous woman <40 years old without children. The health care provider usually explains that with tubal interruption alone, no organ is removed. Tubal sterilization merely prevents conception. The benefits and risks of the operative procedure must be explained. The operation is not desexing and will not reduce libido or alter her appearance. There is usually no adverse change in sexual function following tubal sterilization. On the contrary, many women who feared pregnancy before the operation report increased satisfaction in sexual intercourse and are pleased with the operative result. However, 5%–10% report less frequent orgasm and regret the procedure.

Sterilization in Men

Male sterilization by vas ligation (an office procedure) is far less dangerous than female sterilization. This alternative should be offered to the couple who desire limitation of childbearing,

Table 29-2. Failure rates of minilaparotomy and laparoscopy sterilization procedures

Procedure	Failure rate (%)
Minilaparotomy procedure	
Uchida	<0.1
Fimbriectomy	<0.1
Irving	<0.1
Pomeroy	<0.4
Salpingectomy	<1.9
Madlener	0.3–2
Simple ligation	20
Laparoscopy procedure	
Coagulation and excision	<0.6
Coagulation and division	0.1–2
Coagulation (only)	1–2
Silastic (Falope) rings	0.23
Spring loader (Hulka) clips	0.2–0.6

Data from Department of Medical and Public Affairs, George Washington University Medical Center. *Popul Rep* (May) 1976; Series C, No. 7.

particularly when the woman is not an appropriate candidate for surgery. Impotence does not result. Sterility cannot be assumed until ejaculates are found to be completely free of sperm (1–2 months or 15–20 ejaculations), however. *Disadvantages* of vasectomy include occasional and unlikely spontaneous recanalization (<1%), the occasional development of a spermatocele, and the possible development of antisperm antibodies. Hematoma formation, epididymitis, and psychologic problems are occasional complications. Atrophy of the testes may result if the vasculature is inadvertently ligated.

In the United States, 6%–7% of men who have had vasectomy request reversal. Reanastomosis of vasectomy results in 45%–60% pregnancy rates.

HYSTERECTOMY

Hysterectomy may be the third or fourth most common operation in the United States. Critics have charged that hysterectomy is too often employed for otherwise correctable menstrual problems or for sterilization. In any event, with recent advances, hysterectomy is performed increasingly for conditions refractory to other therapy.

A number of modifiers are used to more accurately describe hysterectomy. Hysterectomy is used interchangeably with *total hysterectomy,* both meaning complete removal of the uterus, including the cervix. *Subtotal hysterectomy* is the removal of the uterine corpus only. *Abdominal hysterectomy* is removal of the uterine corpus and cervix through an abdominal incision. *Vaginal hysterectomy* is removal of the cervix and corpus through the vagina. *Extrafascial hysterectomy* is removal of the uterus and cervix together with the outer fascial layer of the cervix (endopelvic fascia). *Intrafascial hysterectomy* is the removal of the uterus and cervix from within the cervical endopelvic fascia. *Radical hysterectomy* involves dissection and isolation of each ureter as well as the uterine artery and vein, followed by the en bloc removal of the uterine corpus, uterine cervix, a portion of the upper vagina, parametrial tissue, and uterosacral ligaments. Radical hysterectomy is usually combined with adnexectomy and pelvic lymphadenectomy.

Indications

The indications for hysterectomy are summarized in Table 29-3.

Preoperative Evaluation

Cervical cytology (to detect occult cancer) should be performed within 3 months of planned hysterectomy, and any abnormalities should be evaluated. Endometrial assessment (hysteroscopically directed biopsies, D & C) is recommended to detect occult cancer before hysterectomy in any woman >35 years of age who is experiencing abnormal uterine bleeding.

Preoperative workup should include CBC, UA, coagulation profile, chest x-ray and ECG for those ≥45 years, and a stool guaiac determination. Uncomplicated hysterectomy rarely requires transfusion. Hence, type and screen for possible transfusion is often used in many institutions, as opposed to the more costly and time-consuming type and crossmatch procedures. The vagina should be prepared with povidone-iodine douches or a similar antiseptic the night before or the morning of surgery.

Table 29-3. Indications for hysterectomy

Gynecologic malignancy
  Cervical
  Uterine
  Ovarian
  Tubal
Benign gynecologic diseases (refractory to other therapy)
  Uterine leiomyoma
  Symptomatic adenomyosis
  Symptomatic endometriosis
  Symptomatic pelvic relaxation syndromes
  Chronic incapacitating central pelvic pain
  Severe pelvic inflammatory disease or pelvic abscess
  Intractable uterine bleeding
Obstetric complications
  Uncontrollable uterine bleeding
  Molar gestation

Technique

Abdominal Hysterectomy

The patient is placed in the supine position, and a Foley catheter is placed in the bladder. The abdomen is prepared using an antiseptic solution (e.g., povidone-iodine), and sterile drapes are applied. Although the skin incision depends on the nature of the problem, for most benign conditions a low transverse (Pfannenstiel) incision may be used. For malignancy or complicated cases, a lower midline (symphysis pubis to umbilicus) incision affords better exposure and potential for extension.

With a transverse incision, the fascia is incised transversely, laterally curving superiorly to avoid the inguinal area. The pyramidalis muscles are separated together with the rectus muscles. Then, the posterior rectus sheath and peritoneum are entered carefully. The peritoneum is generally incised vertically.

The cecum and appendix are visualized, and the upper abdomen (kidneys, liver, gallbladder, stomach and proximal small bowel, pancreas) is explored. The bowel is packed gently into the upper abdomen. This is facilitated by placing the patient in a slight Trendelenburg position. The round ligaments are suture ligated and cut. By sharp dissection, an incision is carried along the anterior broad ligament, allowing the leaves of the broad ligament to separate and the retroperitoneal space to be opened. This incision passes just superior to the uterovesical fold. By sharp and then blunt dissection, the bladder is separated from the cervix. At this point, with minimal additional blunt dissection, the pelvic vessels and ureters may be identified. The midline dissection is extended toward the vagina until the anterior lip of the cervix is palpated. At that point, blunt dissection is carried out laterally to remove the ureters from the uterine vessels.

If oophorectomy is to be performed, the posterior peritoneum is incised vertically just lateral to the infundibulopelvic ligament for 1 cm. Once it is ascertained that the ureter is clear, the infundibulopelvic ligament is doubly ligated. The posterior broad ligament is incised under direct visualization from the ovary and tube until near the uterus, when the incision is directed toward the uterosacral ligament insertion into the uterus. The ovaries are brought medial. If the adnexa are to remain, each uteroovarian ligament is clamped and ligated at its uterine insertion in a pedicle including the fallopian tube, and the posterior peritoneum is incised toward the uterosacral ligament insertion.

The pelvic vessels are identified and isolated at the level of the internal os. The artery and vein are clamped and doubly ligated. The cardinal ligament is clamped (usually by sliding the clamps off the cervix), incised, and ligated in several segments on each side. When the uterosacral ligaments are encountered, they are clamped, ligated, and incised. At this point, the cervix may be palpated, and the vagina is entered (usually anteriorly) by sharp dissection. A circumferential incision is carried out, and the specimen is removed. Both uterosacral and cardinal ligaments are sutured to the angles of the vagina to ensure vaginal support, and the vagina is closed with sutures. The vaginal closure may be mucosa to mucosa by suturing the vagina closed (anterior to posterior), or the vaginal lumen may be left open (generally for drainage) by simply suturing about the vagina. In both cases, absorbable sutures are used. The pelvic peritoneum is often closed, but recent studies indicate that this may not always be necessary.

Following a correct count of all sponges, needles, and instruments, the parietal peritoneum is closed and the fascia reapproximated with sutures. The subcutaneous tissue is closed, and the skin is closed with sutures or clips. A dry dressing is applied to end the procedure.

Vaginal Hysterectomy

Vaginal hysterectomy should be undertaken with caution if the uterus is >10 weeks gestation or if there are numerous adhesions from pelvic inflammatory disease, endometriosis, or previous surgery (especially cesarean section). The procedure is facilitated if there is uterine prolapse.

The patient is placed in the dorsal lithotomy position, and the vagina and pudendum are prepared with an antiseptic solution. Sterile drapes are applied, and a posterior weighted speculum is placed in the vagina. The cervix is grasped, and mobility is reconfirmed. A circumferential incision is made to the fascia at the cervicovaginal junction, and the cul-de-sac is entered. Once it is ascertained that the cul-de-sac is clear, the uterosacral ligaments are identified, clamped, incised, and ligated. At this point, it is advisable to suture the posterior vaginal mucosa to the peritoneum to arrest bleeding from this area.

If the anatomy allows, modified sharp and blunt dissection is used to free the bladder from the cervix to incise the anterior peritoneum. If this is difficult, one or more segments of the cardinal ligaments may be clamped, incised, and ligated. Once the anterior peritoneum is entered, blunt dissection is carried laterally to retract the ureters from the uterine vessels, whereupon a retractor is placed to elevate and retain the bladder. The uterine vessels are identified, clamped, ligated, and incised bilaterally. Following clamping, ligating, and incising the broad ligaments bilaterally, uteroovarian ligaments, fallopian tubes, and round ligaments are clamped, incised, and ligated in one pedicle. The ovaries are inspected, and hemostasis is secured. The peritoneum is closed using a pursestring suture so that all pedicles are extraperitoneal. The lowermost segment of the cardinal ligament and the uterosacral ligaments are sutured to the superior vaginal angle, and generally the uterosacral ligaments are sutured together in the midline. Finally, the vaginal cuff is closed with absorbable sutures.

Laparoscopic-assisted vaginal hysterectomy recently has begun to be widely applied. In this procedure, the infundibulopelvic ligament (if the ovaries are to be removed) or ovarian ligament and fallopian tube (if the ovaries are not to be removed), round ligament, and often the uterine vessels are hemostatically transacted through the laparoscope. The hysterectomy is completed by vaginally resecting the uterosacral ligaments and lower portion of the cardinal ligaments. Vaginal closure techniques similar to those for vaginal hysterectomy are used.

Complications (see p. 716 for urinary complications)

(see p. 716 for urinary complications)

The most common complications of hysterectomy include bleeding, atelectasis, wound sepsis or disruption, urinary tract injury or infection, thrombophlebitis, and pulmonary embolism.

Bleeding is the most common intraoperative complication of either vaginal or abdominal hysterectomy. This is most commonly from the infundibulopelvic pedicle, the uteroovarian pedicle, the uterine pedicle, or an angle of the vagina. The only site of bleeding accessible for ligation without reoperation is the angle of the vagina. Nonetheless, if bleeding is persistent or sufficient to cause tachycardia, hypotension, or other signs of serious compromise, reoperation may be necessary.

Wound infection may occur about 3–5 days postoperatively and is associated with fever, pain, redness, swelling, and increased warmth about the wound. *Treatment* includes systemic antibiotics, opening the incision, local debridement, and proper wound care. Wound disruption may occur 4–8 days postoperatively as a result of infection but is most often a combination of sutures or suture technique, infection, and altered healing. Wound dehiscence is heralded by an obvious serous discharge from the wound. When evisceration is suspected, the patient should be taken to the operating room, and the incision should be explored. Usually, only retention sutures must be placed in the incision.

Ureteral compromise may occur by sutures, crushing injury, or actual division. *Ureteral injury* may be the most serious complication of hysterectomy. The most common site of ureteral injury is just lateral to the cervix, and the second most common site is at the pelvic brim beneath the infundibulopelvic ligament.

Common symptomatology of ureteral compromise includes fever, flank pain, and a ureterovaginal or ureteroperitoneal fistula. Fistulas occur 5–21 days postoperatively (see p. 720 for a discussion of this and other urinary complications of hysterectomy).

ANTERIOR COLPORRHAPHY

Anterior colporrhaphy is used for repair of cystocele. However, with a large cystocele, care must be taken not to overcorrect, i.e., reduce the cystocele so completely that incontinence results. Anterior colporrhaphy is less useful for treatment of stress incontinence.

Anterior colporrhaphy is performed with the patient in the dorsal lithotomy position. General or spinal, epidural anesthesia is required. After preparation and draping, the vagina mucosa is incised in the midline from the superior extent of the defect to the urethra. Then, the pubocervical fascia is separated from the vaginal mucosa by blunt and sharp dissection. Particular attention must be given to the urethrovesical junction. Often a Foley catheter will identify the area where sutures must be placed.

A plicating suture (e.g., 2-0 polyglycolic) is placed on either side of the junction. This may be followed by an additional suture to reinforce the urethrovesical junction. Bladder plication is performed by placing sutures in the paravaginal tissues. After the vaginal mucosa is sutured, the procedure is terminated.

Complications of the technique include hemorrhage, infection, vesicovaginal or urethrovaginal fistula, incontinence of urine, and failure of repair (recurrence of cystocele).

POSTERIOR COLPORRHAPHY

Rectocele repair is accomplished by posterior colporrhaphy. The preparation for surgery is similar to that for anterior colporrhaphy. The vaginal mucosa is incised at the introitus, and the vaginal mucosa is freed from the endopelvic fascia and perineal muscles to the level of the uterosacral ligaments. If the uterosacral ligaments have not been plicated, they are sutured together.

Starting at the height of the vaginal apex (just below the uterosacral ligaments), the endopelvic fascia and perineal muscles are reapproximated in the midline using slowly absorbed sutures (e.g., polyglycolic). Care should be taken not to perforate the rectum and not to markedly reduce the vaginal diameter. The lower portion of the repair is similar to that of an episiotomy closure. Care must be taken to properly reconstitute the introitus and perineal body.

Complications include bleeding, hematoma, infection, rectovaginal fistula, and excessive narrowing or shortening of the vagina.

REPAIR OF AN ENTEROCELE

Enterocele is *primary* (developmental) or *secondary,* as after inadequate closure of the cul-de-sac or after an abdominal or vaginal hysterectomy. Enterocele correction follows the principles of hernia repair. Repair of enterocele may be accomplished vaginally or abdominally. The sac contents are reduced (adherent contents complicate the repair). The peritoneal pouch must be obliterated and the opening closed. Then, the defect is reinforced by approximating stronger tissues over the defect. In enterocele, the tissues available for closure are the peritoneum, the uterosacral ligaments, and the levator ani fascia and muscles. In both, the uterosacral ligaments are brought together and plicated in the midline. Some surgeons use nonabsorbable suture for this. If the uterosacral ligaments cannot be identified, the cul-de-sac may be obliterated by concentric sutures in the endopelvic fascia. If the procedure is accomplished abdominally, the status of the posterior vagina should be investigated because a posterior colporrhaphy may be necessary for a lasting repair.

In addition to the usual surgical complications, enterocele repair may damage the ureters, rectum, or sigmoid colon.

Chapter 30

Sexual Assault (Rape)

The legal definition of rape varies from state to state, but for medical purposes, rape is *physical assault involving the genitalia of either the victim or the assailant.* Thus, rape is also termed sexual assault. Sexual assault is perpetrated primarily against women or children. Far fewer rape victims are males. Rape is increasing, especially the number of elderly victims, but only 20% of rapes are reported to the police. The relative lifetime risk that a woman will be raped is 10%. About 40% of rapists are known to the victim or have been seen by the victim, and most rapes occur in the victim's home (50%) or neighborhood (80%).

Rape is perpetrated by men <25 years in 45% of cases. Many rapists have serious psychologic or sociologic problems and rape to terrify, humiliate, and degrade rather than to achieve sexual gratification (as evidenced by the high rate of nonejaculation). The average rapist has committed many rapes before being apprehended. Rape can be divided into three categories: power rape (>50%), anger rape (40%), and sadistic rape (5%).

Power rape is usually premeditated. The perpetrator is often a young male (<18 years) who wants to show his dominance over the victim, occasionally resorting to kidnap and multiple assaults. Serious physical injury of the victim is not typical, but multiple assailant rapes fall into this category.

Anger rape is not usually premeditated and is often on impulse, but the victim is more likely to be injured than in power rape. The victim is subject to the assailant's rage and may receive threats of death if the crime is reported.

Sadistic rape frequently results in death or serious injury. The crime is most often premeditated, and torture or mutilation may ensue. Sadistic rape assailants are more likely to be psychotic than other rapists and often have a history of abuse of a wife or child.

The *victim's most common response* during the attack is to survive. Many do not fight for fear of being killed or seriously injured. Lack of resistance may lead to later guilt feelings because they did not try to protect themselves. Disorientation, isolation, anguish, and fear of a later attack are common reactions of victims. During medical evaluation and treatment, the victim may be reluctant to talk and try to establish self-control by appearing detached and calm.

DIAGNOSIS

Since the examining physician is a potential trial witness, the chart should include "findings consistent with the history obtained" or "alleged assault" rather than "rape," which is a legal conclusion. Legally and medically, it is crucial to record the site, type, and extent of the assault, the degree of physical injury, the risk of pregnancy and possible acquisition of STD, and the treatment administered. Emotional aspects of the assault must be addressed because emotional trauma can be devastating, regardless of the degree of physical injury.

Be empathetic. Begin with a statement such as, "This is a terrible thing that has happened to you. I want to help." Medical personnel should carefully avoid further emotional trauma to the rape victim. Show respect, support, and concern. Be aware of the impact of talking to co-workers. If the victim hears herself referred to as "the rape case in treatment room 1," she will feel even more degraded and shamed.

HISTORY AND PHYSICAL EXAMINATION

A brief *gynecologic history,* as well as full details of the assault, should be recorded. Activities between the assault and examination should be noted (e.g., bathing, douching, defecation, voiding, drinking, and eating).

Since a meticulous pelvic examination is required, anesthesia may be required to enable patient cooperation. With witnesses present (and named in the records), inspect the perineum and vulva for abrasions, ecchymoses, and lacerations. Ideally, photographs of all external injuries should be taken, accompanied by a written description and location of each. An ultraviolet or Wood's lamp (fluorescence) should be used to check the patient and her clothing for semen. Positive areas should be blotted with saline-moistened filter paper, labeled, and packaged separately. Pubic hair should be combed, and both the comb and material obtained should be packaged together. Pubic hair cuttings should be obtained, as well as scrapings from under the fingernails. Each specimen should be packaged separately and labeled with source, patient's name, and date. All assembled items should be sealed individually, then sealed in a large container to verify that they were unaltered during transfer to the law enforcement agency. The person who accepts the evidence should sign for the material, and this transfer should become part of the chart.

The vaginal speculum should be moistened with saline only, and careful inspection of the vagina should be performed. Saline-moistened cotton swabs may be used to obtain fluid from the vaginal pool and the endocervix and placed in labeled, corked sterile glass tubes for culture for *Neisseria gonorrhoeae.* The same fluid should be applied to glass slides and air-dried but not fixed. Next, deposit 2 ml of saline in the vaginal vault, and with aspiration, search for motile sperm (often motile even 4–6 h after ejaculation). A cytologic (Pap) smear should be performed to show sperm if present.

If the mouth or anus was invaded, similar cultures should be obtained. Blood should be drawn for VDRL and blood type. HIV testing at this time and later should be offered. A pregnancy test is advisable if the patient may have become pregnant during the assault. Proper labeling of all samples is essential.

TREATMENT

Treatment centers on treatment of physical injuries and prevention of STDs and pregnancy, together with the psychologic problems of the patient.

Treat physical injuries as indicated. For prophylaxis against STD (gonorrhea, syphilis, *Trichomonas, Candida,* and *Gardnerella* infection), follow standard treatment protocols. Tetanus prophylaxis is suggested for possibly contaminated external injury.

Prevention of pregnancy should be discussed if pertinent. Endocrine postcoital pregnancy prophylaxis is effective if administered <72 h after the assault, but before hormonal therapy is initiated, one must determine whether or not the woman is pregnant. Several hormonal regimens are effective, i.e., ethinyl estradiol 50 μg and norgestrel 0.5 μg, 2 tablets at examination and 2 tablets 12 h later, is effective and has few side effects. Ethinyl estradiol 5 mg PO daily for 5 days also is effective, but antiemetics should be given also because 80%–90% will be significantly nauseated.

Initiate follow-up emotional counseling and support of the victim.

PROGNOSIS

Physical recovery almost always precedes emotional recovery. Some women and children never fully recover emotionally.

The acute phase reaction lasting days or weeks includes initial agitation or surprising calmness, followed by somatic complaints of sleep disturbances, nightmares, nausea, headache, or musculoskeletal pain (from tension). Emotional lability is common, fluctuating from fear and guilt to anger and desire for revenge. Inability to concentrate and easy startle and fear reactions are frequent. Since a rape affects the attitude of friends and family as well as the victim, unexpected changes in interpersonal relationships are not unusual.

The long-term reaction may be a permanent behavior modification of the victim. Changing jobs, home, phone number, and city is typical. Some victims will fear isolation, and others will fear men or crowds. Sleep disturbances may persist. Reestablishing normal sexual responses is difficult for 50% of victims. This negative effect is more pronounced in women who have never been sexually active. Victims of sexual assault have an increased likelihood of substance abuse, suicide, neurosis, and psychosis.

CHILD SEXUAL ABUSE

In the case of children who are suspected of being victims of sexual abuse, written informed consent (witnessed) must be obtained from the child's legal guardian, giving permission for examination, collection of evidentiary samples, photographs, release of information to the appropriate authorities, and treatment.

The history should be obtained from the child, if possible, and recorded in the child's own words. Note the type of injury sustained and who is the alleged perpetrator. The child's behavior should be carefully detailed, as well as composure, mental state, and his or her responses.

The examination should follow the techniques outlined in

Chapter 1, with the addition of an ultraviolet (Wood's lamp) examination for semen on the skin and clothing. Collection of foreign materials (e.g., hair, sand, grass) is essential with proper labeling as to site of removal. Fingernail scrapings should be obtained. Semen stains should be sampled in the same manner as with adult victims. Vaginal fluid should be obtained using sterile moistened cotton swabs for culture, wet preparation, cytology, and acid phosphatase determination. Cultures of the pharynx, anus, vagina, and urethra should be taken regardless of history. All specimens must be individually labeled, sealed, and stored in the same meticulous manner as with adult sexual assault to ensure a proper chain of evidence admissible in court.

In suspected child sexual abuse, the local child advocacy or protection agency should be contacted for temporary placement when a parent is suspected of sexual molestation until further investigation can be effected.

Index

Page numbers followed by the letter f *indicate figures; those followed by* t *indicate tables.*